D0267673

172.59
WL 400

UHB TRUST LIBRARY
WITHDRAWN FROM STOCK

UHB TRUST LIBRARY
QUEEN ELIZABETH HOSPITAL
NUFFIELD HOUSE
EDGBASTON
BIRMINGHAM B15 2TH

Spinal Cord Diseases

Diagnosis and Treatment

NEUROLOGICAL DISEASE AND THERAPY

Series Editor

WILLIAM C. KOLLER

Department of Neurology
University of Kansas Medical Center
Kansas City, Kansas

1. Handbook of Parkinson's Disease, *edited by William C. Koller*
2. Medical Therapy of Acute Stroke, *edited by Mark Fisher*
3. Familial Alzheimer's Disease: Molecular Genetics and Clinical Perspectives, *edited by Gary D. Miner, Ralph W. Richter, John P. Blass, Jimmie L. Valentine, and Linda A. Winters-Miner*
4. Alzheimer's Disease: Treatment and Long-Term Management, *edited by Jeffrey L. Cummings and Bruce L. Miller*
5. Therapy of Parkinson's Disease, *edited by William C. Koller and George Paulson*
6. Handbook of Sleep Disorders, *edited by Michael J. Thorpy*
7. Epilepsy and Sudden Death, *edited by Claire M. Lathers and Paul L. Schraeder*
8. Handbook of Multiple Sclerosis, *edited by Stuart D. Cook*
9. Memory Disorders: Research and Clinical Practice, *edited by Takehiko Yanagihara and Ronald C. Petersen*
10. The Medical Treatment of Epilepsy, *edited by Stanley R. Resor, Jr., and Henn Kutt*
11. Cognitive Disorders: Pathophysiology and Treatment, *edited by Leon J. Thal, Walter H. Moos, and Elkan R. Gamzu*
12. Handbook of Amyotrophic Lateral Sclerosis, *edited by Richard Alan Smith*
13. Handbook of Parkinson's Disease: Second Edition, Revised and Expanded, *edited by William C. Koller*
14. Handbook of Pediatric Epilepsy, *edited by Jerome V. Murphy and Fereydoun Dehkharghani*
15. Handbook of Tourette's Syndrome and Related Tic and Behavioral Disorders, *edited by Roger Kurlan*
16. Handbook of Cerebellar Diseases, *edited by Richard Lechtenberg*
17. Handbook of Cerebrovascular Diseases, *edited by Harold P. Adams, Jr.*
18. Parkinsonian Syndromes, *edited by Matthew B. Stern and William C. Koller*
19. Handbook of Head and Spine Trauma, *edited by Jonathan Greenberg*
20. Brain Tumors: A Comprehensive Text, *edited by Robert A. Morantz and John W. Walsh*

21. Monoamine Oxidase Inhibitors in Neurological Diseases, *edited by Abraham Lieberman, C. Warren Olanow, Moussa B. H. Youdim, and Keith Tipton*
22. Handbook of Dementing Illnesses, *edited by John C. Morris*
23. Handbook of Myasthenia Gravis and Myasthenic Syndromes, *edited by Robert P. Lisak*
24. Handbook of Neurorehabilitation, *edited by David C. Good and James R. Couch, Jr.*
25. Therapy with Botulinum Toxin, *edited by Joseph Jankovic and Mark Hallett*
26. Principles of Neurotoxicology, *edited by Louis W. Chang*
27. Handbook of Neurovirology, *edited by Robert R. McKendall and William G. Stroop*
28. Handbook of Neuro-Urology, *edited by David N. Rushton*
29. Handbook of Neuroepidemiology, *edited by Philip B. Gorelick and Milton Alter*
30. Handbook of Tremor Disorders, *edited by Leslie J. Findley and William C. Koller*
31. Neuro-Ophthalmological Disorders: Diagnostic Work-Up and Management, *edited by Ronald J. Tusa and Steven A. Newman*
32. Handbook of Olfaction and Gustation, *edited by Richard L. Doty*
33. Handbook of Neurological Speech and Language Disorders, *edited by Howard S. Kirshner*
34. Therapy of Parkinson's Disease: Second Edition, Revised and Expanded, *edited by William C. Koller and George Paulson*
35. Evaluation and Management of Gait Disorders, *edited by Barney S. Spivack*
36. Handbook of Neurotoxicology, *edited by Louis W. Chang and Robert S. Dyer*
37. Neurological Complications of Cancer, *edited by Ronald G. Wiley*
38. Handbook of Autonomic Nervous System Dysfunction, *edited by Amos D. Korczyn*
39. Handbook of Dystonia, *edited by Joseph King Ching Tsui and Donald B. Calne*
40. Etiology of Parkinson's Disease, *edited by Jonas H. Ellenberg, William C. Koller, and J. William Langston*
41. Practical Neurology of the Elderly, *edited by Jacob I. Sage and Margery H. Mark*
42. Handbook of Muscle Disease, *edited by Russell J. M. Lane*
43. Handbook of Multiple Sclerosis: Second Edition, Revised and Expanded, *edited by Stuart D. Cook*
44. Central Nervous System Infectious Diseases and Therapy, *edited by Karen L. Roos*
45. Subarachnoid Hemorrhage: Clinical Management, *edited by Takehiko Yanagihara, David G. Piepgras, and John L. D. Atkinson*

46. Neurology Practice Guidelines, *edited by Richard Lechtenberg and Henry S. Schutta*

47. Spinal Cord Diseases: Diagnosis and Treatment, *edited by Gordon L. Engler, Jonathan Cole, and W. Louis Merton*

Additional Volumes in Preparation

Spinal
Cord
Diseases

Diagnosis and Treatment

edited by
Gordon L. Engler

Los Angeles County Hospital
University of Southern California Medical Center
Los Angeles, California

Jonathan Cole

University of Southampton
Southampton, Hampshire
and Poole Hospital
Poole, Dorset, England

W. Louis Merton

St. Mary's Hospital
and Portsmouth Hospitals NHS Trust
Portsmouth, England

MARCEL DEKKER, INC.   NEW YORK · BASEL · HONG KONG

Library of Congress Cataloging-in-Publication Data

Spinal cord diseases : diagnosis and treatment / edited by Gordon
    Engler, Jonathan Cole, William L. Merton.
            p. cm. -- (Neurological disease and therapy ; v. 47)
        Includes bibliographical references and index.
        ISBN 0-8247-9489-3 (alk. paper)
        1. Spinal cord--Diseases. 2. Spinal cord--wounds and injuries.
    I. Engler, Gordon. II. Cole, Jonathan. III. Merton,
    William L. IV. Series.
        [DNLM: 1 . Spinal Cord Diseases--diagnosis. 2. Spinal Cord
    Diseases--therapy. WL 400 S756879 1998]
    RC400.S654 1998
    617.4'82--dc21
DNLM/DLC
for Library of Congress   98-4261
                                                                               CIP

This book is printed on acid-free paper.

Headquarters
Marcel Dekker, Inc.
270 Madison Avenue, New York, NY 10016
tel: 212-696-9000; fax: 212-685-4540

Eastern Hemisphere Distribution
Marcel Dekker AG
Hutgasse 4, Postfach 812, CH-4001 Basel, Switzerland
tel: 44-61-261-8482; fax: 44-61-261-8896

World Wide Web
http://www.dekker.com

The publisher offers discounts on this book when ordered in bulk quantities. For more information, write to Special Sales/Professional Marketing at the headquarters address above.

Copyright © 1998 by Marcel Dekker, Inc. All Rights Reserved.

Neither this book nor any part may be reproduced or transmitted in any form or by any
means, electronic or mechanical, including photocopying, microfilming, and recording, or
by any information storage and retrieval system, without permission in writing from the
publisher.

Current printing (last digit):
10 9 8 7 6 5 4 3 2 1

PRINTED IN THE UNITED STATES OF AMERICA

Series Introduction

Diseases of the spinal cord are an important part of neurology. Many of these diseases can have devastating consequences, particularly if treatment is not initiated quickly. *Spinal Cord Disease: Diagnosis and Treatment*, edited by Drs. Engler, Cole, and Merton, covers all aspects of disorders of the spinal cord and their treatment. The book is a practical and thorough discussion of these disorders. Following the introduction, the first two parts of the book cover the developmental and genetic diseases of the spinal cord and the important topic of spinal cord injuries and their management. The third part deals with infections of the spinal cord, and tumors are discussed in the fourth part. Next, other neurological diseases of the spinal cord, including multiple sclerosis, ALS, and vascular and decompression disorders, are reviewed. Part six deals with investigations of the spinal cord, including imaging and neurophysiological studies. The final part addresses additional problems related to spinal cord injury: pain associated with spinal cord disease, sexual dysfunction, and care of the patient with injury to the spinal cord. This text is incredibly thorough, covering all aspects of spinal cord disease, the pathophysiology of these disorders, and their treatment. Health care professionals, physicians, and nonphysicians who deal with patients who have spinal cord dysfunction will find this textbook an invaluable resource and reference.

William C. Koller, M.D., Ph.D.

Preface

The spinal cord is infrequently considered in medicine, yet injury to this area shows us how important it is to a whole range of function. In part, this is because spinal pathology is comparatively rare in mainstream medical and surgical practice. When established spinal cord injury is present, it is then considered appropriate for a specialist. In the United Kingdom, specialized spinal injury centers are located in smaller hospitals and, although a full range of specialist treatments are available, these units are seen in the context of rehabilitation. Few doctors see spinal cord injury during their training. In contrast, in the United States spinal treatment centers are found attached to, and part of, larger hospitals; this may enable earlier intervention, but spinal cord injury is still a specialist's field. This marginalization is not confined to spinal cord injury: in motor neuron disease (amyotropic lateral sclerosis), diagnosis and subsequent care may take place within the field of neurology or at a hospice; with spinal disc disease, surgeons naturally lead the treatment. Medical and surgical conditions of the spinal cord concern many specialties that do not overlap; each specialist hardly knows what the others bring to the care of the same part of the body. To remedy this compartmentalization, the book includes work from a variety of physicians and surgeons who give accounts of their own medical practice related to the spinal cord.

In our work on this book we were faced with an immediate dilemma over definition of the spinal cord. If we had considered the spinal cord to be that and no more, then diseases of its surrounding tissues would have been excluded. We would have had no room for a consideration of the rheumatological conditions of the spinal column, which can have severe effects on spinal cord function. Had we limited ourselves to the cord level, we would not have considered various developmental abnormalities that affect cord function but originate above it. In both cases, we have expanded the definition of "spinal cord" and been inclusive in our approach.

We also had to consider the depth and detail of the contributions. We were torn between the need to be both comprehensive and readable. While maintaining respect for our authors' style and individuality, we asked for their ideas and current practice rather than an encyclopedic response, happy to include both their theories and their interpretation of the current orthodoxy. The book is aimed at medical graduates at any stage of their career; we hope that the text will enable surgeons to learn more about the whole of both surgical and medical spinal cord disease and that physicians will gain some insight into the surgical conditions of the spinal cord. With this in mind, we have included some strictly surgical chapters side by side with medical ones; for instance, we consider terminal care as well as research-oriented techniques such as omental transplantation.

The book is divided into various parts. In Chapter 1, Cole and Weller begin with a short introduction to the anatomy and physiology of the spinal cord. The first part of the book is concerned with developmental abnormalities of the cord. In their chapter, "Myelodysplasia," Coyne and Fehlings give a comprehensive review of the subject from developmental anatomy through diagnosis to surgical treatment. In Chapter 3, Hurlbert and Fehlings consider the Chiari malformations and develop a thesis for their etiology and pathogenesis. Their account goes into great detail on prognosis and morbidity. Set against these anatomical abnormalities, we have placed Chapter 4, on the nosologically difficult spastic paraplegias and spinocerebellar degenerations and late abnormalities of neurological function, to compare with the earlier, grosser problems. Here, Ormerod and Davies stress the importance of accurate diagnosis in allowing a better knowledge of prognosis when alteration in the natural history of the condition is not possible.

The second part is concerned with spinal cord injuries. In Chapter 5, Miz begins by considering the epidemiological frequency and financial costs of these conditions; of course, no one can quantify the human cost. He goes on to detail cervical injuries to the cord in terms of presentation and treatment. In their consideration of thoracolumbar injuries, Main and Engler offer a complementary perspective, giving the presentation, investigation, and treatment, but also discussing long-term management of both the primary condition as well as complications such as syrinx and spasticity. Patrick makes an eloquent and important plea for recognition of spinal injuries at birth in Chapter 7, suggesting that birth injury to the central nervous system does not affect only the brain itself. In Chapter 8, the last in this part, Perin considers posttraumatic syrinx.

Infections and other medical conditions of the spinal cord are discussed in the third part. It is important to consider bacterial infections from a wider perspective than is seen in many of our practices, and so this topic has been covered by Peiris and Gunatilake from Colombo, Sri Lanka. They have great practical experience with bacterial disease of the spinal cord that many of us have only read about. Winer has considerable experience of postinfectious myelopathy and radiculopathy, which he discusses in Chapter 10, while Manji considers the increasingly recognized cord and root complications of HIV infection in Chapter 11.

Tumors are the subject of the fourth part. Their anatomy and pathology is considered first by Weller in Chapter 12. A chapter by Rezai, Lee, and Abbott on benign tumors follows, pointing out that for such benign disease, surgery is the treatment of choice; they document the improvements in prognosis that have arisen from better diagnosis and treatment. Constantini and Epstein cover intramedullary tumors of the cord in Chapter 14. Their aim is high—they suggest that these rare tumors can be treated aggressively by extensive surgical removal with significant improvements in prognosis—and they make their case with enthusiasm and force. In Chapter 15, Paonessa and Halperin consider the wide-ranging topic of metastatic disease of the spine. Their extensive review considers various types of tumors and multiple approaches to treatment and summarizes a great deal of work.

The next part branches out to include topics traditionally regarded as medical and surgical. In Chapter 16, Hawkins gives a comprehensive analysis of spinal features of multiple sclerosis, a specific but complex topic. Lloyd and Leigh give an overview of amyotropic lateral sclerosis and more recent treatments; it is an exciting time for those working in this area. To counterbalance the predominantly surgical approach of the earlier sections, Cooper and Cawley next consider inflammatory diseases of the spinal cord, focusing on long-term nonsurgical care of these important conditions. In Chapter 19, on ischemic disease of the cord, Merton distills much work to give the core areas of controversy in the field. Murrison, Francis, and Sedgwick give a detailed review of decompression sickness, which, although uncommon, is something about which doctors often hear much about but know little. Its pathology and treatment offer an interesting comparison to those of other diseases. Duffill and Iannotti consider the European perspective in treatment of cervical myelopathy in Chapter 21, allowing comparison with earlier work on the acute management of cord injury. In Chapter 22, the last in this part, Martin and Kent consider another more chronic and yet anatomical cord problem—ossification of the posterior longitudinal ligament. This chapter gives a good review of this important subject.

The next part consists of three chapters on the subject of investigation. Although many chapters include discussions of radiology, Barker's chapter gives an up-to-date review of current practice in the United Kingdom. In Chapter 24, on clinical neurophysiology, Merton and Cole combine an explanation of their techniques with information on their clinical utility. Finally, Chandiramani, Thomas, and Fowler consider urological investigations of spinal disease, shedding light on what is often a difficult area for nonurologists and yet is important for all those dealing with spinal cord dysfunction.

The final part contains four chapters. Gerber, Neil-Dwyer, and Lang give an account of omental transposition in spinal injury. This technique has not shown itself worthy of widespread use, and may never do so. It does show, however, one way of trying to maintain or restore cord viability through a method owing something to lateral thinking, and as such alerts us all that we need to keep our minds open. This volume begins with a medical model, or more precisely a strictly surgical one, that treats anatomical abnormalities structurally; the book ends with a more patient-oriented approach. In Chapter 27, Cole describes chronic pain associated with spinal cord disease. In their chapter on the sexual aspects of established spinal cord injury, Tromans and Cole consider the practical problems and the problems of personality, as well as the experience of altered sexual identity after cord injury. In the final chapter, O'Brien writes about terminal care of people with spinal injury. We do not expect that all our readers will be involved in such care, but we think it is important to make such information available to them.

This volume's writers include established senior clinicians and their junior colleagues; approaches vary from the comprehensive to the provocative. It is our hope that most, although perhaps not all, of the subject of spinal cord disease is covered here. It may be that the volume emphasizes surgical conditions, and may therefore be especially useful for such specialists. Our main hope, however, is that the chapters will be read as a series of views on the spinal cord and its disease, so that a surgeon may learn about current practice as well as the wide range of conditions affecting the cord that are outside the field of surgery. If we have contributed to such cross-fertilization in this relatively neglected area, then we will have achieved a measure of success.

Gordon L. Engler
Jonathan Cole
W. Louis Merton

Contents

Series Introduction   *iii*

Preface   *v*

Contributors   *xiii*

1   **Introduction to the Clinical Presentations of Spinal Cord
    Disease from a Pathophysiological Perspective**   **1**
    Jonathan Cole and Roy O. Weller

I.   DEVELOPMENTAL/GENETIC DISEASE

2   **Myelodysplasia**   **15**
    Terry J. Coyne and Michael G. Fehlings

3   **The Chiari Malformations**   **65**
    R. John Hurlbert and Michael G. Fehlings

4   **Spastic Paraplegia, Bulbar Palsy, and Spinocerebellar
    Degeneration**   **101**
    Ian E. C. Ormerod and Paul T. G. Davies

II. INJURIES TO THE SPINAL CORD AND COLUMN

5   **Injuries to the Cervical Spine and Spinal Cord**   **121**
    George S. Miz

6   **Thoracolumbar Spine Trauma**   **155**
    Kenneth Main and Gordon L. Engler

7   **Birth Injuries**   **175**
    Kent Patrick

8   **Posttraumatic Syrinx: Diagnosis and Treatment**   **199**
    Noel I. Perin

III. INFECTIONS

9   **Infections of the Spinal Cord**   **211**
    J. B. Peiris and S. B. Gunatilake

10 **Guillain-Barré Syndrome and Postinfective
    Neuroradiculoneuropathies**   **241**
    John Winer

11 **HIV Disease of the Spinal Cord and Nerve Roots**   **259**
    Hadi Manji

IV. TUMORS

12 **Pathology of Spinal Tumors**   **275**
    Roy O. Weller

13 **Benign Spinal Tumors**   **287**
    Ali R. Rezai, Mark Lee, and Rick Abbott

14 **Primary Intramedullary Spinal Cord Tumors of Children
    and Adults**   **315**
    Shlomi Constantini and Fred Epstein

15 **Metastatic Disease of the Spine**   **335**
    Kenneth J. Paonessa and Michael J. Halperin

V.   NEUROLOGICAL AND SYSTEMIC DISEASE

16 Spinal Features of Multiple Sclerosis   399
Clive Paul Hawkins

17 Motor Neuron Disease (Amyotrophic Lateral Sclerosis)   413
Catherine M. Lloyd and P. Nigel Leigh

18 Rheumatological Aspects of Spinal Disease   443
Cyrus Cooper and Michael I. D. Cawley

19 Spinal Vascular Disease   463
W. Louis Merton

20 Decompression Illness   471
A. W. Murrison, T. James R. Francis, and E. M. Sedgwick

21 Cervical Spondylosis and Myelopathy   495
Jonathan Duffill and Fausto Iannotti

22 Ossification of the Posterior Longitudinal Ligament   517
Robert Jeffrey Martin and Christopher S. Kent

VI.   INVESTIGATION OF SPINAL CORD DISEASE

23 Imaging of Spinal Disease   533
Simon Barker

24 Clinical Neurophysiology of Spinal Cord Disorders   559
W. Louis Merton and Jonathan Cole

25 Urological Aspects of Spinal Cord Disease   579
Vijay Chandiramani, David Thomas, and Clare J. Fowler

VII.   ADDITIONAL PROBLEMS

26 Omental Transposition in Spinal Cord Injury   599
C. J. Gerber, Glenn Neil-Dwyer, and Dorothy A. Lang

27 Pain Associated with Disease of the Spinal Cord   611
Jonathan Cole

28 Sexual Problems Associated with Spinal Cord Disease   **629**
Anthony Matthew Tromans and Jonathan Cole

**29 The Palliative and Terminal Care of Patients with Spinal
Cord Disease**   **645**
Tony O'Brien

Index   *665*

Contributors

Rick Abbott, M.D. Associate Professor, Department of Neurosurgery, Institute for Neurology and Neurosurgery, Beth Israel Medical Center, North Division, New York, New York

Simon Barker, M.B., Ch.B., M.R.C.P., F.R.C.R. Consultant Neuroradiologist, Wessex Neurological Centre, Southampton General Hospital, Southampton, Hampshire, England

Michael I. D. Cawley, M.D., F.R.C.P. Consultant Neuroradiologist, Medical Research Council Environmental Epidemiology Unit, Southampton General Hospital, Southampton, Hampshire, England

Vijay Chandiramani, M.S., F.R.C.S. Senior Registrar in Urology, University Hospital of South Manchester, Manchester, England

Jonathan Cole, M.A., M.Sc., D.M., F.R.C.P. Honorary Senior Lecturer, Clinical Neurological Sciences, University of Southampton, Southampton University Hospital, Southampton, Hampshire, and Consultant in Clinical Neurophysiology, Poole Hospital, Poole, Dorset, England

Shlomi Constantini, M.Sc., M.D.   Director, Division of Pediatric Neurosurgery, Tel-Aviv-Sourasky Medical Center and Dana Children's Hospital, Tel Aviv, Israel

Cyrus Cooper, M.A., D.M., F.R.C.P.   MRC Clinical Scientist and Professor of Rheumatology, Medical Research Council Environmental Epidemiology Unit, Southampton General Hospital, Southampton, Hampshire, England

Terry J. Coyne, M.B., B.S., F.R.A.C.S.   Division of Neurosurgery, The Toronto Hospital and University of Toronto, Toronto, Ontario, Canada

Paul T. G. Davies, M.A., M.D., M.R.C.P.   Consultant Neurologist, Department of Neurology, Northampton General Hospital, Cliftonville, Northampton, England

Jonathan Duffill, M.B., Ch.B., F.R.C.S.   Research Registrar, Department of Clinical Neurological Sciences, University Clinical Neurological Sciences, Southampton General Hospital, Southampton, Hampshire, England

Gordon L. Engler, M.D.   Professor of Clinical Orthopaedics and Neurological Surgery, Director of Scoliosis and Spinal Surgery, Los Angeles County Hospital/University of Southern California Medical Center, Los Angeles, California

Fred Epstein, M.D.   Head, Department of Neurosurgery, Institute of Neurology and Neurosurgery, Beth Israel Medical Center, North Division, New York, New York

Michael G. Fehlings, M.D., Ph.D., F.R.C.S.(C)   Division of Neurosurgery, The Toronto Hospital and University of Toronto, Toronto, Ontario, Canada

Clare J. Fowler, M.B.B.S., M.Sc., F.R.C.P.   Senior Lecturer and Consultant, Department of Uro-Neurology, Institute of Neurology, London, England

T. James R. Francis, Ph.D., M.F.O.M.   Naval Submarine Medical Research Laboratory, Groton, Connecticut

C. J. Gerber, M.D., F.R.C.S.   Research Registrar, Department of Clinical Neurological Sciences, Southampton General Hospital, Southampton, Hampshire, England

S. B. Gunatilake, M.D., F.R.C.P.(Lond), F.R.C.P.(Edin)   Consultant Neurologist and Senior Lecturer, Department of Medicine, University of Kelaniya, Colombo, Sri Lanka

Michael J. Halperin, M.D.   Spinal Surgeon, Department of Orthopedic Surgery, William W. Backus Hospital, Norwich, Connecticut

Clive Paul Hawkins, B.Med.Sci., D.M., F.R.C.P.   Senior Lecturer in Neurology, Keele Postgraduate Medical School and Royal Infirmary, Stoke-on-Trent, England

R. John Hurlbert, M.D., Ph.D, F.R.C.S.C.   Assistant Professor of Spinal Neurosurgery, Department of Clinical Neurosciences, University of Calgary, Calgary, Alberta, Canada

Fausto Iannotti, M.D., F.R.C.S.(S.N.)   Professor of Neurosurgery, Department of Clinical Neurological Sciences, University Clinical Neurological Sciences, Southampton General Hospital, Southampton, Hampshire, England

Christopher S. Kent, M.D., L.C.D.R.   Division of Neurosciences, Navy Regional Medical Center, San Diego, California

Dorothy A. Lang, F.R.C.S.(Glasg), F.R.C.S.(Eng)   Consultant Neurosurgeon, Wessex Neurological Centre, Southampton University Hospitals Trust, Southampton, Hampshire, England

Mark Lee, M.D., Ph.D.   New York University Medical Center, New York, New York

P. Nigel Leigh, Ph.D., F.R.C.P.(Lond)   Professor of Neurology, Department of Clinical Neurosciences, Institute of Psychiatry, London, England

Catherine M. Lloyd, M.D., M.R.C.P.   Research Fellow, Department of Neurology, Institute of Psychiatry, London, England

Kenneth Main, M.D. New York, New York

Hadi Manji, M.A., M.D., M.R.C.P.   Consultant Neurologist, Department of Clinical Neurology, National Hospital for Neurology and Neurosurgery, London, and Ipswich Hospital, Suffolk, England

Robert Jeffrey Martin, M.D.   Department of Neurosciences, Harbin Clinic, Rome, Georgia

W. Louis Merton, B.Sc., F.R.C.P.   Consultant in Clinical Neurophysiology, Department of Clinical Neurophysiology, St. Mary's Hospital, and Director of

Clinical Support Services, Portsmouth Hospitals NHS Trust, Portsmouth, England

George S. Miz, M.D.   Orthopaedic Specialists, Oak Lawn, Illinois

A. W. Murrison, M.D., M.F.O.M.   Undersea Medicine Division, Institute of Naval Medicine, Alverstoke, Hants, England

Glenn Neil-Dwyer, M.S., F.R.C.S., F.R.C.S.E.   Consultant Neurosurgeon, Wessex Neurological Centre, Southampton University Hospital, Southampton, Hampshire, England

Tony O'Brien, M.B., F.R.C.P.I.   Consultant Physician in Palliative Medicine, Marymount Hospice, St. Patrick's Hospital, and Cork University Hospital, Wilton, Cork, Ireland

Ian E. C. Ormerod, M.D.   Department of Neurology, Frenchay Hospital, Bristol, England

Kenneth J. Paonessa, M.D., F.A.A.O.S.   Spinal Surgeon, Norwich Orthopedic Group, Norwich, Connecticut

Kent Patrick, M.D.   Spinal Surgeon, Private Practice, Sacramento, California

J. B. Peiris, M.D., F.R.C.P.(Lond), F.R.C.P.(Edin), F.R.C.P.(Glas), Hon.-F.R.A.C.P.   Senior Consultant Neurologist, National Hospital, and Director, Postgraduate Institute of Medicine, University of Colombo, Colombo, Sri Lanka

Noel I. Perin, M.D., F.R.C.S.(Edin), F.A.C.S.   Assistant Professor, Department of Neurosurgery, Mount Sinai Medical Center, New York, New York

Ali R. Rezai, M.D.   Chief Resident, Department of Neurosurgery, New York University Medical Center, New York, New York

E. M. Sedgwick, B.Sc., M.D., F.R.C.P.   Professor, Department of Clinical Neurological Sciences, University of Southampton, Southampton, Hampshire, England

David Thomas, F.R.C.S., M.R.C.P.   Consultant Urologist, Spinal Unit, Lodge Moor Hospital, Sheffield, England

Anthony Matthew Tromans, M.B., Ch.B., F.R.C.S.   Consultant in Spinal Injuries, Duke of Cornwall Spinal Treatment Centre, Salisbury District Hospital,
Salisbury, Wiltshire, England

Roy O. Weller, B.Sc., Ph.D., M.D., F.R.C.Path.   Professor of Neuropathology, Department of Pathology (Neuropathology), University of Southampton
Medical School, Southampton, Hampshire, England

John Winer, M.Sc., M.D., F.R.C.P.   Senior Lecturer in Neurology, Neuroscience Centre, University Hospital Birmingham NHS Trust, Edgbaston, Birmingham, England

1

Introduction to the Clinical Presentations of Spinal Cord Disease from a Pathophysiological Perspective

Jonathan Cole

Southampton University Hospital, Southampton, Hampshire, and Poole Hospital, Poole, Dorset, England

Roy O. Weller

University of Southampton Medical School, Southampton, Hampshire, England

Interpretation of the signs and symptoms of spinal disease, its effective management and appropriate treatment depends on an understanding of the anatomy and physiology of the spine, spinal cord and its coverings. In this short chapter, these anatomical and physiological features will be considered in relation to their influence on the clinical presentation of spinal disease.

I. THE ANATOMY OF THE SPINE, SPINAL CORD, AND ITS COVERING

A. The Vertebral Column

The spine, although a poorly defined structure, comprises support for not only the spinal cord but for the body as a whole. This supporting vertebral column relies for its stability upon the bony vertebrae, the intravertebral ligaments and spinal musculature.

Within the bony structure, the spinal canal extends from the foramen magnum at the base of the skull to the tip of the sacrum and contains a variety of structures (Fig. 1). Its walls are composed of the vertebral bones, with the

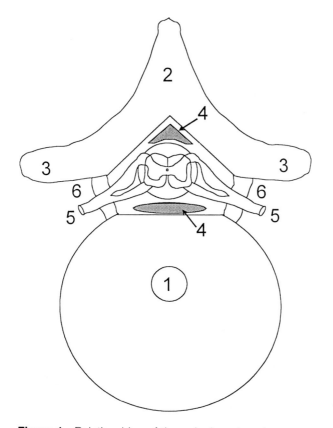

Figure 1 Relationships of the spinal cord and nerve roots to the vertebral column. A diagram showing a transverse section of a vertebral body (1), vertebral spine (2), and transverse processes (3). The spinal cord in the center of the spinal canal is surrounded by the dura, and epidural fat (4) fills the spinal canal, both posteriorly and anteriorly. Anterior and posterior nerve roots join to form spinal nerves (5) as they pass through the intervertebral foramina between the pedicles (6).

bodies of the vertebrae anteriorly and the laminae behind. Ligaments, in particular the elastic yellow-colored ligamentum flavum, run in a longitudinal direction along the posterior aspect of the spinal canal and provide inelastic stability to the structure. The column, however, manages to combine this necessary rigidity with a degree of flexibility. This allows for much subtle movement which is only noticed when the consequences of stiffening of the spine are seen, for example, in ankylosing spondylitis. Much of this flexibility, as well as part of the structural integrity of the whole, is given by the action of the surrounding muscles (1,2). Just how significantly muscular action contributes to this may be seen in such diseases as idiopathic scoliosis, or some myopathies that are strictly outside the scope of this book.

B. The Dura and Extradural Space

The spinal cord is encased in the dura mater, a tough sheet of compacted fibrous tissue that forms a tube extending from the foramen magnum to the lower end of the sacrum. The extradural space between the dural tube and the bony lining of the spinal canal is filled by adipose tissue that is more abundant posteriorly than anteriorly. As nerve roots pass from the spinal cord or cauda equina through the intervertebral foramina, they are ensheathed by an extension of the dura mater. The dura forms an important barrier that largely prevents the invasion of metastatic tumor from bone or the extradural space into the spinal cord. The spread of infection from the extradural compartment into the subarachnoid space is probably also delayed by the dura.

C. The Leptomeninges

As the dura mater is opened, either at surgery or post mortem, the diaphanous translucent arachnoid mater is revealed and, through it, the spinal nerve roots and spinal cord are visible. The complexity of the arachnoid mater as it covers the spinal cord is shown in Figure 2 (3,4). The outer layer of arachnoid comprises multiple layers of closely packed cuboidal cells that confine the cerebrospinal fluid (CSF) to the subarachnoid space. In addition to the outer layer of arachnoid mater, there are several layers of intermediate arachnoid, the middle of which forms a web-like coating over the nerve roots and vessels, which may dampen movements of CSF. They also form the dorsolateral and anterior ligaments of the spinal cord.

The pia mater is a thin layer of cells coating the surface of the spinal cord. A subpial layer forms a sheath around the cord itself and is extended into the dentate ligaments, along the lateral aspect of the spinal cord, which are anchored into the dura at their lateral extremities.

D. The Subarachnoid Space

The spinal cord is surrounded by CSF confined between the outer impervious layer of arachnoid mater and the pia mater coating the spinal cord and nerve roots. As the spinal cord only normally extends down to the first lumbar vertebra (L1), the subarachnoid space below L1 is filled by the nerve roots of the cauda equina. The CSF supports the spinal cord, which is further stabilized by the presence of the dentate ligaments and the dorsal and dorsolateral ligaments

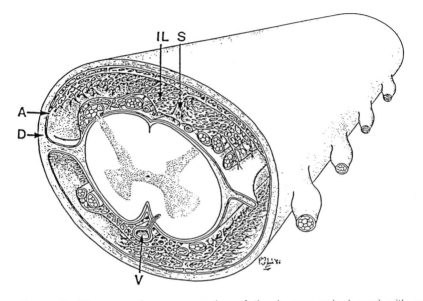

Figure 2 Diagrammatic representation of the human spinal cord with surrounding meninges. The arachnoid mater (A) is closely applied to the thick outer dura (D). An intermediate leptomeningeal layer (IL) lies between the arachnoid mater and the pia mater. This layer is fenestrated and is attached to the inner aspect of the arachnoid mater. It is reflected to form the dorsal septum (S). The intermediate layer spreads over the surface of the cord and is connected to blood vessels, nerve roots, and pia mater by fine trabeculae. Dentate ligaments are present on either side of the cord and are covered by a layer of pia arachnoid. The collagenous core of the dentate ligaments fuses with subpial collagen medially and at intervals laterally with dural collagen, as shown on the left side of the diagram. Blood vessels (V) within the subarachnoid space are coated by a leptomeningeal sheath continuous with the pia mater. (Reproduced with permission from Ref. 1.)

of arachnoid. In normal individuals, there is free passage of CSF between the cranial and subarachnoid space; interference with this free passage may result in disorders of the spinal cord such as syringomyelia.

Inflammatory changes within the subarachnoid space may cause subsequent fibrosis of the intermediate arachnoid sheets, not only interfering with CSF flow within the space, but also by the tethering of nerve roots, resulting in the pain of arachnoiditis (5). Dorsal and ventral nerve roots arising from the spinal cord occupy much of the subarachnoid space (Figs. 2 and 3). Blood vessels on the surface of the cord are also exposed to the CSF in the subarachnoid space. Thus toxic, infectious, or therapeutic agents introduced into the

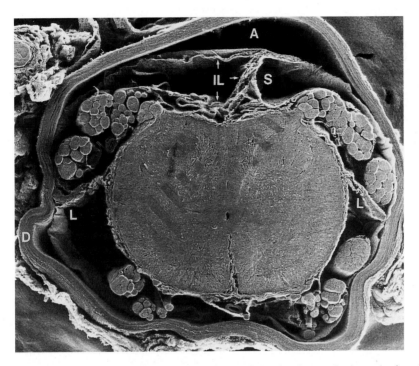

Figure 3 Scanning electron micrograph of the lumbar spinal cord of a 15-month-old child. An intermediate leptomeningeal layer (IL) is closely applied to the inner aspect of the arachnoid (A). It reflects to form the dorsal septum (S) and arborizes over the dorsal surface of the cord. The dentate ligaments (L) are seen on each side of the cord; that on the left merges with the dura (D). On the right, the free margin of the dentate ligament abuts the arachnoid mater. (Reproduced with permission from Ref. 1.)

subarachnoid space are in contact with both spinal nerve roots and the vessels supplying the spinal cord.

E. The Nerve Roots

The nerve roots themselves are coated by a thin layer of arachnoid cells enclosing the endoneurial compartment of the nerve and comprising myelinated and nonmyelinated nerve fibers, together with their accompanying Schwann cells and endoneurial blood vessels. In the upper cervical region, the nerve roots pass out of the spinal canal through the intervertebral foramina, almost at the level at which they leave the spinal cord. However, as the spinal cord only extends to L1, the segmental level of the cord is above the intervertebral foramina at most levels. Roots, therefore, pass obliquely down from the cord to intervertebral foramina. Thus, the lower sacral roots leave the cord at L1 and extend several centimeters down to the sacral region before leaving the spinal canal.

Such a dissociation of level needs to be considered when determining the level at which spinal nerve roots are affected, particularly by diffuse processes such as carcinomatous meningitis, which may not necessarily be detected by computerized tomography or magnetic resonance imaging. The size of nerve roots depends on the level of the cord at which they enter or leave. For example, the largest roots of the cord are found in the cervical and first thoracic segments, carrying nerve fibers to and from the upper limbs.

F. The Spinal Cord

The spinal cord is approximately 30-cm long and has a soft paste-like consistency that is easily distorted by compression. Centrally, the gray matter forms the dorsal sensory and ventral motor horns of nerve cells; the white matter, containing the long motor and sensory tracts, is distributed around the periphery. The blood supply of the spinal cord is from the one anterior and two posterior longitudinal spinal arteries (Figs. 2 and 3). Arising from the vertebral artery at the foramen magnum, the anterior spinal artery receives supplementary branches from radicular arteries entering the spinal canal along nerve roots, as does the posterior artery. There are several large radicular arteries, particularly in the midthoracic region. Branches of the anterior and posterior spinal arteries form an encircling network around the spinal cord and penetrate the cord from the outside. They are, therefore, fully exposed to the CSF in the subarachnoid space and can be damaged by tumor, infection, or toxins in that space.

Within the cord itself, the anterior spinal artery supplies mainly the anterior two-thirds, whereas the posterior spinal arteries perfuse the posterior one-third, something which allows differentiation of the anatomical origin of spinal stroke and which is considered in greater detail in Chapter 19.

II. THE CLINICAL NEUROPHYSIOLOGY OF THE SPINAL CORD

Although it is anatomy that preoccupies much of clinical practice, what patients are concerned about is not structure but function, so that some knowledge of underlying physiology is necessary (Fig. 4). The cord may be divided into the spinal gray, which contains the cell bodies and dendritic processes of segmental and local cells, and the white matter, which is made up of the ascending and descending spinal and supraspinal pathways. The spinal gray is largest in the cervical and lumbosacral enlargements where many of the efferent and afferent relays and cells in connection with the limbs are contained. Much of the detailed physiology of the cord is abstruse, but some of it has clinical relevance.

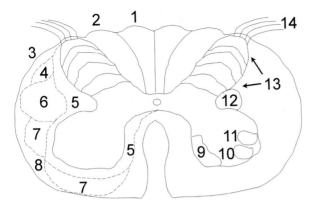

Figure 4 Cross-sectional diagram of the spinal cord.

White matter tracts:
1 and 2, Dorsal Columns—Low threshold mechanoreceptors, cutaneous, joint, and muscle afferents.
  1. Gracile tract containing fibers from ~ S5 to T7.
  2. Cuneate tract containing fibers from ~ T6 to C4.
  3. Dorsal spinocerebellar tract.
  4. Raphespinal tract—motor.
  5. Propriospinal tracts (spinal–spinal tracts).
  6. Lateral corticospinal (pyramidal) tract—motor.
  7. Reticulospinal tracts—motor.
  8. Spinothalamic tracts (temperature, nocioception, etc.); also spinoreticular and spinocerebellar tracts.

Gray matter areas:
  9. Ventral horn—medial motor nuclei.
 10. Ventral horn—axial motor nuclei.
 11. Ventral horn—lateral motor nuclei.
 12. Intermediolateral cell column—autonomic.
 13. Dorsal horn laminae (including substantia gelatinosa)—segmental synapsing of afferents, including nocioception.

Nerve roots:
14. Dorsal root afferents.

A. The Sensory Pathways

Sensory afferent neurones have their cell bodies in the dorsal root ganglia outside the intervertebral space. This has important consequences: radiculopathies may affect motor neurons and the proximal portion of the sensory axon but leave the sensory cell body and distal axon intact, allowing, for instance, for normal peripheral sensory nerve conduction on clinical neurophysiology tests, even in a complete root avulsion injury.

The proximal parts of the sensory axons enter the cord through the dorsal roots (almost without exception). Their subsequent paths depend on the modalities of sensory information they convey and their paths within the cord. Large myelinated sensory fibers, conveying low threshold cutaneous mechanoreceptor and muscle and joint information, pass through the dorsal horn and ascend in the ipsilateral dorsal column nuclei to synapse in the dorsal column nuclei at the rostral end of the cord. These cells do give off some segmental synapses *en passage,* and a percentage of dorsal column cells actually have segmental synapses and ascend as second order cells.

Small myelinated and unmyelinated fibers, conveying information about temperature, pain, and muscle fatigue, synapse in the laminae of the dorsal horn, in an exquisitely arranged array, before ascending in the contralateral spinothalamic pathways. It is, of course, this crossing at, or close to, the segmental level in the anterior part of the cord, close to the central canal, that renders such fibers vulnerable to the pressure effects associated with syrinx and leads to the classical dissociated sensory loss.

Intramedullary damage to, or extramedullary pressure on, these various pathways gives classical clinical findings such as posterior syndromes of loss of cutaneous sensation and loss of position and movement sensibility, and lateral and central cord damage that can be associated with loss of pain and temperature sensation.

The physiological properties of the cells also have clinical consequences that reflect altered response properties of cells. Chronic and even some acute pain is known to involve altered receptive field sensitivities, both peripherally, in their cutaneous receptive fields, and in the dorsal horn within the cells of the nociceptive pathway. Spasticity involves segmental alterations in responsiveness as a result of altered descending control. The phenomenon of allodynia, in which even light touch leads to pain, suggests synaptive reorganization between low threshold/dorsal column afferents and nociceptive neurons, probably at a dorsal horn level. In fact, inflammatory peripherally originating pain has recently been shown to amplify transmission through large low threshold myelinated inputs too, so that these fibers can switch to resemble nociceptors fibers (6).

B. Segmental Reflexes

As well as sending ascending fibers, many sensory afferents synapse at their segmental level with other sensory neurons or with motor neurons. Such synapses can be disclosed clinically, via the tendon jerks and other reflexes that have cutaneous afferent limbs, and may involve single synapses or a number of interneurons (7). [Some cortical reflexes can also be observed with special physiological techniques (8).] Testing of segmental reflexes is an important part of each clinical examination via stretch reflexes. Reduced tendon reflexes point to either a sensory problem or to reduced motor output at a segmental level. Enhanced reflexes indicate reduced descending inhibition and so are associated with upper motor neuron problems. Altered or more widely elicited reflexes are also seen with upper motor neuron lesions and sometimes with the segmental disorganization seen, for instance in cervical myelopathy.

C. Motor Pathways

The main descending motor pathways from the brain occupy the lateral part of the cord and enter the ventral horn from there to synapse in segmental motor nuclei. From there, the lower motor neurons, both alpha and gamma, leave the cord via the ventral roots to innervate their target muscle fibers, both extrafusal and intrafusal. Classically clinical examination of motor function in the cord has concerned itself mainly with tests of the pyramidal tract. The other motor tracts from extrapyramidal areas are considered to be involved with more proximal automatic movements. The relation between descending tracts and motor function is an extraordinarily complex matter that is not of great clinical or physiological significance in spinal cord pathology.

The hallmarks of spinal cord motor damage—weakness, with a spinal level with reduced increased reflexes—allow reasonable localization in most cases of the area of damage. The specific type of descending pathway damaged is less important clinically, possibly because the cord, being so small, usually suffers damage to more than one pathway. Classically, upper motor neuron weakness has been said to affect particularly the forearm extensors and lower limb flexors, although the true situation may not be quite so clear.

D. Autonomic Pathways

The great outflows of the sympathetic and parasympathetic systems via the sympathetic chain from T1 to L2 and the craniosacral chain are well known. The system controls circulation, gut functions, the urogenital system, thermoregulation, and sweating. Often, these functions are best observed and understood by looking at their dysfunction (9,10).

In acute cervical spinal cord injury (SCI), for instance, although the catastrophic losses of movement sensation dominate, there is also loss of thermoregulation, something noticed on the battlefields of the First World War by Gordon Holmes (11). At a similar time, Head and Riddoch (12) noted the characteristics of the autonomic dysreflexiae, which may begin a few weeks after injuries to the cord at and above the midthoracic level, with sweating above the lesion, paroxysmal hypertension, headache after bowel evacuation, and bladder problems, all of which show the effect of disorganization in the autonomic system.

The authors became interested in bladder control after SCI and found that not only was there disorganization of the normal voiding and storage functions of the bladder, but that voiding led to far more widespread effects than normal, involving flexor spasm and excessive sweating. Disruption of normal autonomic control led to loss of the "local sign" of reflexes and the emergence of a "mass reflex." After the Second World War, Guttman and Whitteridge (13) described autonomic dysreflexiae in more detail (facial flushing, nasal passage edema, pupillary distension, rise in temperature above the lesion) and realized the role of the rise in blood pressure in the symptom complex.

1. Blood Pressure Effects

During acute spinal shock, blood pressure is lower than usual (14), then during rehabilitation tetraplegics, with a level above T5, have profound postural hypotension if raised from the horizontal, such that syncope may occur (15). This is in part due to the lack of co-ordinated sympathetic vasoconstriction (16,17). With time however this postural problem is reduced, though how is not completely clear but may include reduced orthostatic hypotension, changes in hormonal body fluid regulation and alterations in vasomotor reflexes.

Individuals with tetraplegia are more at risk of hypertensive strokes as a consequence of their loss of autonomic control of systemic and, possibly, cerebral blood pressure. They tend to have lower ambient blood pressures, but occasionally they also have to face paroxysmally large pressures due to autonomic dysreflexiae, or "sympathetic storms." In addition, there is some evidence that the sympathetic nerves contribute to the upper limits of cerebral autoregulation of blood pressure, and that those with tetraplegia normally shift their limits for that autoregulation downwards with time, compounding their risk from short periods of hypertension (18,19).

2. Gastrointestinal, Renal, and Metabolic Effects

There is an increased risk of acute gastrointestinal bleeding immediately after SCI, probably due to a complex of factors, including increased vagal activity. Paralytic ileus and acute gastric dilatation may also occur. Later loss of sacral parasympathetic regulation leads to atony of the bowel and retention of feces. Some lower bowel reflexes may recover, possibly because of the development of a low spinal cord "centre" (20). Complex alterations in the metabolic effects of hypoglycemia have been found in tetraplegics, often without the normal clinical signs of this condition (21).

In acute spinal shock there is bladder atony. Retention is then followed by distension with voiding by overflow. As the tetraplegic person rehabilitates, the bladder may develop some local reflex activity so that emptying may be possible by tapping the abdominal wall. A subsequent problem in some persons, however, is dyssynergia between the bladder neck and detrusor bladder muscles leading to abnormal or interrupted flow. Similarly, in the male initially there is an absence of penile erection or ejaculation. Later, due to the return of some local sympathetic and parasympathetic reflexes, erection can occur, although ejaculation usually requires assistance (see Chapter 28). Menstrual cycle alteration also may occur soon after injury but usually recovers.

Such alterations in function, as described above, are not simply a consequence of the loss of coordinated autonomic control due to the interruption of transmission up and down the cord via the lateral parts of the cord. Many of the abnormalities also reflect alterations in synaptic activity, input/output relations within the cord and in the autonomic ganglia.

Lastly, the autonomic system is often defined in purely efferent motor function. This, of course, ignores the sensory afferents from blood vessels, muscles, and bladder, which provide feedback to the system. Their pathway to the cord may be via blood vessels and with somatic nerves. Disorganization of the autonomic system may represent losses of both afferents and efferents.

The pathophysiology and consequences of the autonomic lesion associated with SCI have become much better understood for they, as much as the loss of sensation and movement, have profound consequences for rehabilitation after injury. Although largely outside the scope of this book (but see Chapters 5, 6, and 25), it is the autonomic problems, especially with the bladder, that can greatly affect the daily lives of those with SCI.

III. CLINICAL SIGNS AND SYMPTOMS OF SPINAL CORD DISEASE

Given the physiology of the spinal cord and a simplified account of its function, the nature of the signs and symptoms of dysfunction of the cord are not difficult to work out. Varieties of motor weakness, sensory disturbance, autonomic problems, and pain encompass nearly the whole gamut of clinical problems associated with cord disease. The only problem, then, is to try to determine the site and cause of the various combinations of such symptoms and findings. Many clues are provided by the speed of onset of a problem and the relative components of motor, sensory, and autonomic symptoms and signs. In addition, in some cases, systemic symptoms are also present and associated with spinal problems, e.g., a pyrexia in infections, or preceding infection in some cases of postinfective radiculopathy.

Perhaps the most common and devastating symptom is weakness. The acute onset and severe weakness associated with a spinal stroke, bleed, or injury, have very different signs, with spinal shock and hyporeflexia, to the gradual onset of weakness due to a slow myelopathy, usually with an upper motor neuron weakness with hyperreflexia. Although the distribution of weakness tends to be different between upper and lower motor neurones weakness, often a firm distinction requires examination when the differences in distribution of weakness and reflexes can be brought out. Reflex changes in the legs but not the arms, or hyperreflexia in the legs and reduced reflexes in the legs, may suggest a thoracic or cervical problem. Whereas weakness either as a symptom or sign is always enquired after, more subtle motor deficits may also occur. Patients may sometimes complain of having to think about their movements, for instance. The type of cord problem may also have some relevance to the rapidity with which weakness occurs. Pyramidal tract function is usually considered to be more sensitive to intramedullary tumors than to extramedullary ones.

Sensory change is also common with spinal cord problems, affecting both long tracts and segmental function. The distribution of parasthesiae and sensory loss can help determine the nature of the problem. Thus, altered sensation in a dermatomal distribution makes one consider a radiculopathy, whereas a more generalized sensory disturbance with a sensory level points to a cord myelopathy. Often, mixed sensory and motor syndromes are seen, of which the most famous is the Brown-Séquard syndrome, which includes both motor weakness and sensory disturbance of the segment involved and of the long tracts below. This leads to bilateral segmental spinothalamic loss (classically pain and temperature), and below-level contralateral spinothalamic and ipsilateral dorsal column loss. Motor weakness is lower motor neuron in type at the level of the lesion and upper motor neuron below that. Although rare, this syndrome is famous for revealing functional anatomy. On rare occasions only is there such a clear relation between the two.

Pain is a frequent and distressing accompaniment of spinal cord disease. Its character and distribution again can give important clues to both the cause and location of the problem. Pain in the back, sometimes with a root distribution, may suggest vertebral body problems, whereas pure root pain is in favor of a radiculopathy. Diffuse pain in contrast may be seen in intramedullary spinal disease. The character of pain also differs; root pain is severe and lancinating, whereas spinal cord pain is often more unpleasant and difficult to describe.

In addition to clues from the distribution of signs and symptoms and their combination, there are also clues from the evolution and the age of the patient. Thus a paroxysmal onset suggests a spinal stroke, whereas a slow, progressive deterioration is more in favor of a neoplasm. Some pathologies show differences according to age; in younger people, root problems often are associated with more severe pain and sensory motor deficits for a comparatively mild problem on MRI than in older people, in whom lumbosacral degenerative change is almost the norm regardless of symptoms.

Thus far, symptoms and signs of spinal cord disease have been discussed in almost anatomical terms. Some cord problems, however, do not follow such strict anatomical distributions and this itself suggests particular pathologies. Motor neurone disease may involve the whole of the cord progressively, or it may begin with a localized distribution. Spinal demyelination may present with a localized deficit or with several of them having no clear anatomical localization. Subacute combined degeneration may suggest both peripheral nerve disease and more central cord problems. In this case, the lack of a clear anatomical locus may aid diagnosis.

In a book concerned with acute medicine and surgery, it is natural that acute signs and symptoms will be stressed. There are, however, more chronic findings associated with spinal disease, including chronic pain (see Chapter 27) and autonomic problems of great importance for the patient, even though they are not usually useful in diagnosis. In one case however, autonomic dysfunction may be used in diagnosis: i.e., electromyography of the pelvic floor musculature may be useful in considering function in the neurons of the nucleus of Onuf to distinguish between Parkinson's disease and Steele-Richardson-Olszewski syndrome (pan autonomic failure) (22).

REFERENCES

1. Bogduk N. Anatomy of the spine. In: Klippard JH, and Dieppe PA. Rheumatology. St Louis: Mosby, 1994; pp. 5.2.1–14.
2. Cole J. Pride and a Daily Marathon. Boston: MIT Press, 1995.
3. Nicholas DS., Weller RO. The fine anatomy of the human spinal meninges. J Neurosurg 1988; 69:276–282.
4. Weller RO. Fluid compartments and fluid balance in the central nervous system. In: Williams PI, et al. ed. Gray's Anatomy. 38th ed. Edinburgh: Churchill Livingstone, 1995.
5. Dolan RA. Spinal adhesive arachnoiditis. Surg Neurol 1993; 39:479–484.
6. Neumann S, Doubell TP, Leslie T, and Woolf CJ. Inflammatory pain hypersensitivity mediated by phenotypic switch in myelinated primary sensory neurons. Nature 1996; 386:360–364.
7. Katz R, Mmeunier S, and Pierot-Deseilligny. Changes in presynaptic inhibition of 1a fibres in man while standing. Brain 1988; 111:417–437.
8. Marsden CD, Merton PA, Morton PA, and Adam J. The effect of lesions of the sensorimotor cortex and capsular pathways on servo responses from the human long thumb flexor. Brain 1977; 100:503–526.
9. Bannister, Sir Roger, ed. Autonomic Failure: A Textbook of Clinical Disorders of the Autonomic Nervous System. London: Oxford University Press, 1983.

10. Cole JD. The pathophysiology of the autonomic nervous system in spinal cord injury. In: Illis LS ed. Spinal Cord Dysfunction: Assessment. Oxford: Oxford University Press, 1988; pp 201–235.
11. Holmes G. Spinal injuries of warfare. Brit Med J 1916; 2:769–774, 815–821, 855–861.
12. Head H, and Riddoch G. The autonomic bladder, excessive sweating and some reflex conditions in gross injuries of the spinal cord. Brain 1917; 40:188–263.
13. Guttman L, and Whitteridge D. Effects of bladder distension on autonomic mechanisms after spinal cord injuries. Brain 1947; 361–404.
14. Walsh JJ. Cardiovascular complications in paraplegia. Proceedings of Scientific Meeting, International Stoke Mandeville Games, Rome, 1960, pp 37–45.
15. Corbett JL, Frankel HL, and Harris PJ. Cardiovascular responses to tilting in tetraplegic man. J Physiol 1971; 215:411–432.
16. Wallin BG, and Nerhed C. Relationship between spontaneous variations of muscle sympathetic activity and succeeding changes of blood pressure in man. J Autonomic Nervous System 1984; 6:293–302.
17. Matthias CJ, and Frankel HL. Autonomic failure in tetraplegic man. In: Bannister, R, ed. Autonomic Failure. London: Oxford University Press, 1983.
18. Bill A, and Linder J. Sympathetic control of cerebral blood flow in acute arterial hypertension. Acta Physiol Scand 1976; 96:114–121.
19. Bevan AT, Honour AH, and Stott FH. Direct arterial recording in unrestricted man. Clin Sci 1969; 36:329–344.
20. Guttman L. Spinal Cord Injuries. 2nd ed. Oxford: Blackwell Scientific Publications, 1976.
21. Matthias CJ, Frankel HL, Turner RC, and Christiansen NJ. Physiological responses to insulin hypoglycaemia in spinal man. Paraplegia 1979; 17:319–326.
22. Pramstaller PP, Wenning GK, Smith SJM, Beck RO, Quinn NP, and Fowler CJ. Nerve conduction studies, skeletal muscle EMG, and sphincter EMG in multiple system atrophy. J Neurol Neurosurg and Psych 1995; 58:618–621.

2

Myelodysplasia

Terry J. Coyne and Michael G. Fehlings
The Toronto Hospital and University of Toronto, Toronto, Ontario, Canada

Congenital anomalies of the spinal cord (myelodysplasia) and associated mal-developed midline structures are the most common congenital abnormalities of the central nervous system, and thus occupy a significant role in pediatric neurological and orthopedic surgery. These anomalies may be classified as open or closed, depending on whether an intact layer of skin is present over the malformation. A number of terms describing these malformations are used interchangeably in the literature. Spinal dysraphism literally refers to a defective fusion process, but is used to describe these malformations regardless of whether a fusion abnormality has occurred. The terms spina bifida aperta (open) and occulta (closed) have also been used to describe abnormalities of midline development. Spina bifida occulta, or occult dysraphism, takes the form of minor vertebral anomalies, such as an absent spinous process, without any neural malformation. This chapter will focus on abnormalities of neural development along with accompanying major vertebral anomalies.

To understand the spectrum of abnormalities encountered in myelodysplasia, along with the principles of appropriate management, it is necessary to have a fundamental understanding of the normal development of the spinal cord. This chapter will, therefore, briefly review the embryology of the spinal cord before discussing the theories of embryogenesis, clinical features, and principles of management of open and closed forms of myelodysplasia.

I. EMBRYOLOGY

A. Normal Development

The embryonic period has been divided into 23 morphological stages or "horizons" of 2–3 days each (67,93). The end of this time corresponds to approximately 60 days after fertilization and a crown-rump length of 30 mm. During this period, the primitive central nervous system is formed, and the primary malformations responsible for the open and closed forms of myelodysplasia occur. Subsequent events before and after birth may further modify the malformation and influence its clinical presentation. Although the morphological changes of embryonic development are well described, the inability to study human embryos dynamically has meant that the regulatory mechanisms involved in cell migration and differentiation are poorly understood, with most information coming from animal studies.

Embryonic stages 1–5, occurring during the first 2 weeks after fertilization, result in a bilaminar embryonic disc contained within an amniotic cavity. The outer layer, lying adjacent to the amniotic cavity, is termed the epiblast, and the inner layer, adjacent to the primary yolk sac, is the hypoblast. During days 13–15 (stage 6), hypoblastic cells form a thickening, the prochordal plate, which marks the future rostral end of the embryo.

1. Gastrulation

During the latter part of stage 6, the process of transformation into a trilaminar embryo (gastrulation) commences. The primitive streak, a midline caudal thickening in the epiblast, appears (Fig. 1). The primitive streak enlarges and lengthens and develops a thickening at its rostral aspect, the primitive or Hensen's node. At the same time, a central depression, the primitive groove, develops along the primitive streak, forming the primitive pit at the level of Hensen's node. Proliferating cells from the epiblast migrate into the primitive streak and groove, and then move rostrally between the epiblast and hypoblast to form the third embryonic layer, the mesoblast.

2. Notochord Development

During days 16–17 (stage 7), mesoblastic cells migrate in the midline rostral to Hensen's node to form the notochordal process (Fig. 2). Mesoderm originating from the primitive streak then condenses along each side of this process. Subsequently, the primitive pit at Hensen's node extends into the notochordal process, creating a central notochordal canal (Fig. 3a,b,c). The canalized notochordal process then fuses with the adjacent ventral entoderm (hypoblast). These two cell layers degenerate where they have fused, thus creating a longitudinally

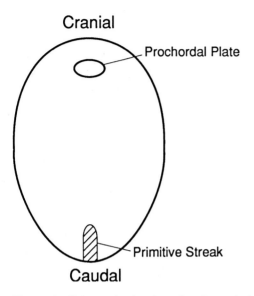

Cranial

Prochordal Plate

Primitive Streak

Caudal

Figure 1 Schematic drawing of embryo during stage 6 (gastrulation).

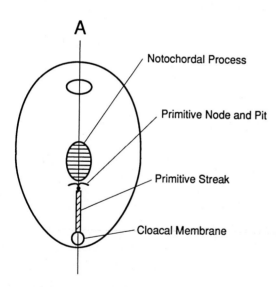

A

Notochordal Process

Primitive Node and Pit

Primitive Streak

Cloacal Membrane

Figure 2 Embryo at early stage 7, at the time of formation of the notochordal process.

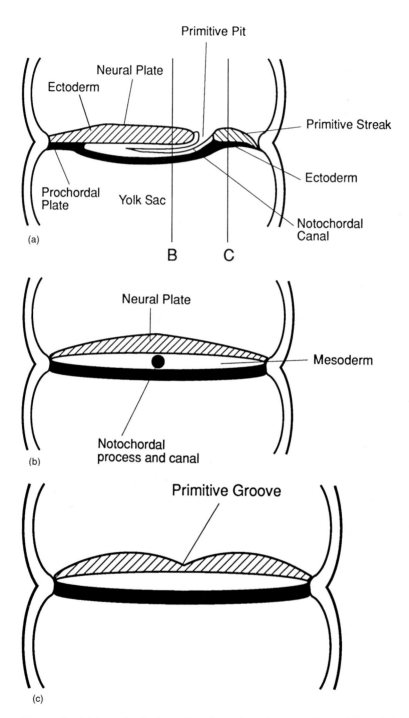

Figure 3 (a) Longitudinal section through embryo, at level of line A in Fig. 2, during stage 7, at the time of development of notochordal canal. (b), (c) Transverse sections of embryo through lines B and C, respectively, of Fig. 3(a).

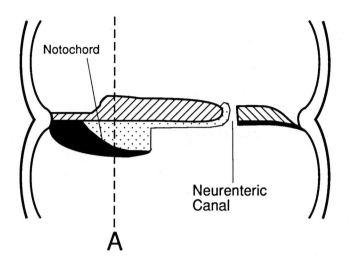

Figure 4 Longitudinal section through embryo at late stage 7, at time of neurenteric canal.

grooved notochordal plate in the roof of the yolk sac and allowing the notochordal canal to communicate with the yolk sac. At the caudal end of the notochordal plate, where the primitive pit initially began extending into and canalizing the plate, a communication called the neurenteric canal now extends from the dorsal to ventral surface of the embryo, linking the amniotic cavity and yolk sac (Fig. 4). Beginning at the cranial end, the notochordal plate then infolds to form the solid notochord. This process allows the entoderm to again become a continuous layer ventrally, and obliterates the neurenteric canal. The notochord is believed to play a key role in inducing the overlying ectoderm to form the neural tube and acts as the structure around which mesoderm will form the vertebral column. It later regresses and is represented in the adult only as the nucleus pulposus. Disorders of notochord and neurenteric canal development are the likely mechanisms responsible for diastematomyelia, neurenteric cyst, and combined anterior and posterior spina bifida.

3. Neurulation

Neurulation, the process of neural tube formation, occurs during days 18–27 (stages 8–12). Rostral to Hensen's node, ectoderm overlying the notochordal process initially thickens, forming the neural plate. The edges of the neural plate become heaped, creating the neural folds and a midline neural groove (Fig. 5). Changes occur first in the middorsal region of the embryo, the site of

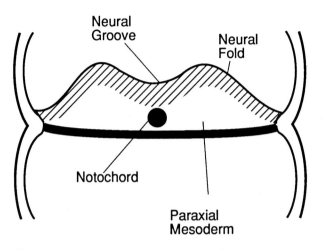

Figure 5   Transverse section at level of line A of Fig. 4, during stage 8, at the beginning of neurulation.

the future cervical cord, and proceed caudally. Stage 10 (days 22–23) marks a deepening of the neural groove and convergence of the neural folds in the dorsal midline to create the neural tube (Fig. 6a,b,c). Closure first occurs at the region of the third or fourth somite, the future cervicomedullary junction, and continues both rostrally and caudally simultaneously. At days 24–25 (stage 11), the neural tube completes its rostral closure at the anterior neuropore, which will become the site of the lamina terminalis. During days 26–27 (stage 12), caudal closure of the neural tube occurs at the posterior neuropore, corresponding to the L1/L2 segment of the spinal cord. The more caudal cord segments do not develop by neurulation, but subsequently by the process of canalization. Neurulation abnormalities are implicated in the majority of open spinal cord malformations.

   Other tissues develop simultaneously with the primitive nervous system. While the neural plate is developing, the mesoderm on each side of the notochord condenses to create the paired somites. Beginning about day 20 (stage 9), these first form rostrally at the region of the future occipital bone and progress caudally, eventually to comprise up to 44 pairs extending to the coccygeal level. Eventually the first occipital pair and the caudal 5–7 coccygeal ones will regress. The segmental arrangement also alters, such that the caudal half of one somite condenses with the cephalic half of the adjacent caudal sclerotome. These masses will fuse around the notochord and neural tube to form the vertebrae, so that each vertebra contains components of 4 somites. The ectoderm

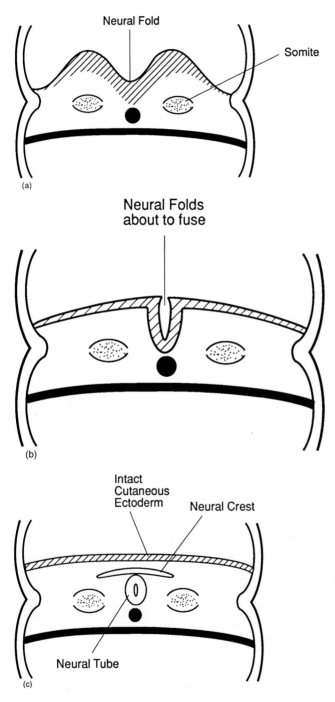

Figure 6 Closure of the neural folds to form the neural tube (stages 10–12).

UHB TRUST LIBRARY
QEH

continuous with the lateral edges of the neural folds, which will become the epidermis, moves medially with the folds and fuses along the midline. It then separates from the neural tube, with mesoderm moving in to form muscular and skeletal structures. Incomplete separation of this ectoderm may be involved in the pathogenesis of congenital dermal sinuses and intraspinal epidermoid and dermoid tumors.

4. Canalization

Formation of the most caudal part of the neural tube occurs during days 28–48 (stages 13–20). Prior to this, the cell mass of the primitive streak caudal to the posterior neuropore has remained undifferentiated. This cell mass develops vacuoles that coalesce to create a neural tube, which in turn fuses with the rostral neural tube (Fig. 7a,b,c).

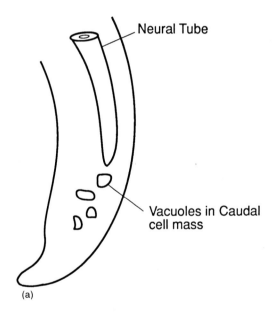

Neural Tube

Vacuoles in Caudal cell mass

(a)

Figure 7   Formation of caudal part of neural tube by the process of canalization (stages 13–20).

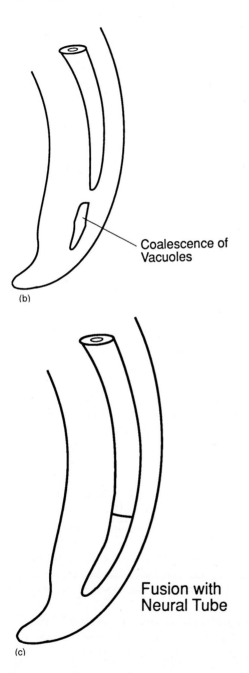

Coalescence of
Vacuoles

(b)

Fusion with
Neural Tube

(c)

Table 1   Stages of Spinal Cord Development and Associated Anomalies

Stage	Gestational age, in days	Process	Potential anomaly
1–5	1–14	Bilaminar embryonic disc forms	
6	13–15	Gastrulation (trilaminar embryo forms)	
7	16–17	Notochord and neur-enteric canal development	Diastematomyelia, neur-enteric cyst, combined anterior and posterior spina bifida
8–12	18–27	Neurulation formation of somites	Open spinal cord malformations, congenital dermal sinus, epidermoid and dermoid tumors
13–17	28–42	Canalization	Lipomyelomeningocele
18–20	43–48	Regression	Thick filum terminale

5. Regression

Regression describes the process of formation of the filum terminale and cauda equina and the migration of the conus medullaris to its level in the adult opposite the L1/L2 vertebral body. During days 43–48 (stages 18–20), the future site of the conus medullaris, known as the ventriculus terminalis, develops. Initially, it lies at the level of the second coccygeal vertebra. The caudal neural tube then regresses, allowing the ventriculus terminalis to rise within the spinal canal. This at first is relatively rapid, so that by 18 weeks it lies at the level of the L4 vertebral body. Ascent then slows, the tip of the spinal cord lying at the level of the L2-3 interspace at birth and reaching the adult level of the L1-2 interspace by the first three postnatal months. As the neural tube ascends, a fibrous band remains between the ventricularis medullaris and the tip of the coccygeal vertebrae, which becomes the filum terminale. In the course of this ascent, the nerve roots, originally exiting the spinal canal opposite their spinal cord segmental origin, are forced to elongate, and become the cauda equina.

Closed malformations, such as lumbosacral lipoma and lipomyelomeningocele, and tethering of the spinal cord by thickened filum terminale are attributed to defects of canalization and regression. Table 1 summarizes the stages of development of the spinal cord and times at which anomalies occur.

II. OPEN SPINAL CORD MALFORMATIONS

Open spinal cord malformation anomalies have been written about for a long time, having attracted the attention of both Hippocrates and Aristotle. Unfortunately, even today the genesis of these problems is poorly understood, and they continue to present a formidable medical and social challenge.

A. Classification

These malformations are generally classified morphologically, although their form is very much dependent on the stage of embryological development at which the malformation occurred.

1. Myeloschisis

In myeloschisis, the neural tube at the site of the defect is completely open, taking the form of a filletted placode without any surrounding meninges. Either the neural folds have not fused or a newly formed neural tube has reopened. The malformation, therefore, occurs on or prior to day 28. It most commonly occurs at the thoracolumbar junction, where the parts of the spinal cord formed by neurulation and canalization meet, and there is associated spina bifida of the entire lumbar and sacral spine. The central canal of the more cranial neurulated cord is continuous with a central groove in the exposed flat neural plaque, and escape of cerebrospinal fluid (CSF) is often visible. The exposed neural tissue has degenerated, and there is usually a complete neurological deficit below the level of the lesion (4,49).

2. Meningocele

This is a skin- or membrane-covered cystic lesion consisting of meninges only, and although continuous with the neural canal, contains only CSF and no neural tissue. The dorsal half of one or more vertebrae is absent, with the spinal cord running through the ventral part of the dysraphic spinal canal. Meningoceles make up approximately 10% of open spinal cord anomalies and are uncommonly associated with hydrocephalus or other central nervous system anomalies (37,80). Although the prognosis for normal development is generally good, meningocele may mask other more occult myelodysplasias (98).

3. Myelomeningocele

The most common form of open neural tube defect, myelomeningocele, describes a posterior midline cystic mass, apparent at birth, that contains CSF,

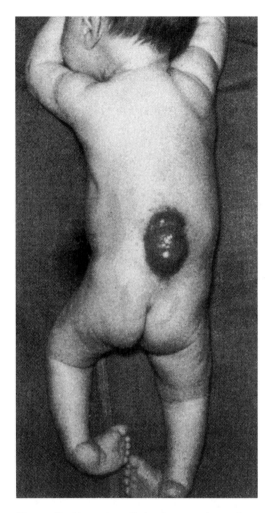

Figure 8   Neonate with lumbar myelomeningocele.

meninges, malformed spinal cord, and nerve roots (Fig. 8). The roots may head toward their normal dural exits or end blindly in the lateral or dorsal dural encasement or overlying tissue. The neural malformation is covered by a gliotic membrane, which has commonly ruptured. In meningocele and myelomeningocele, the malformation occurs during or after neurulation (and therefore more than 28 days after fertilization).

B. Theories of Embryogenesis

Open neural tube defects are believed to be the result of a disorder of neurulation, and theories of embryogenesis essentially fall into two groups—those of defects of closure of the neural folds and those of reopening of the neural tube after normal closure. The former group of theories includes those of developmental arrest and overgrowth, and the latter group includes those of hydrodynamic forces and neuroschisis. However, none of these theories are sufficient in themselves to account for the spectrum of abnormalities seen with open neural tube defects.

1. Developmental Arrest

First proposed by von Recklinghausen in 1886, this theory holds that the neural plate fails to close because of arrest of development with subsequent changes in secondary tissues (101,105). Although this may account for myeloschisis, it does not adequately explain neurulated malformations or those formed by disorders of canalization.

2. Overgrowth Theory

This theory proposes that an overgrowth of neural plate tissue everts the neural folds before neurulation, thus preventing their fusion. Also having its origin in the 1880s, after studies of chick embryos (16), Patten subsequently related this theory to observations in human embryos (75,76). There has been debate as to whether the overgrowth is a primary event, or whether it is secondary to some other phenomenon. As with the theory of arrested development, this theory cannot explain open lesions with a central canal (indicating neurulation has occurred), or open lesions of levels of the cord formed by canalization beneath an intact epidermal layer.

3. Hydrodynamic Theory

First suggested by Morgagni (64) and Virchow (11), this theory proposes that increased fluid pressure within the central canal of the developing spinal cord leads to its cystic dilatation, with eventual rupture through the posterior bony and soft tissues. This theory was developed in detail by Gardner, who maintained that a build-up of fluid within the neural tube leads to overdistension and rupture (25). The principle criticism of this theory is that extensive open lesions are difficult to attribute to overdistension, because the initial rupture would presumably decompress the neural tube and limit the extent of the lesion (24). Nonetheless, hydrodynamic abnormalities are believed to play a role in some of the malformations associated with open forms of myelodysplasia, such as Chiari anomalies and aqueduct stenosis.

4. Neuroschisis Theory

Elaborated by Padget, this theory holds that after closure of the neural tube, a dorsal midline cleft develops and the tube reopens (69,70). This allows protein-rich fluid from the central canal to escape and cause first an elevation (the "neuroschistic bleb"), then a breakdown of the overlying mesodermal and epidermal tissue. However no etiology for this reopening is suggested.

5. Other Theories

Other theories of embryogenesis include: (1) The traction theory of Penfield and Coburn (77), now discounted, which held that the spinal cord became fixed to the skin at a low level and was thus unable to migrate cranially in its usual fashion; (2) A caudal displacement of the site where fusion of the neural folds begins, causing a dyssynchrony between normal neuroectodermal and mesodermal tissue at this caudal level (43); and, (3) A primary disturbance of the gastrulation process, causing secondary abnormalities of neural tube closure (19).

C. Epidemiology

The overall incidence of open spinal cord malformations in North America is approximately 1–2 per 1000 live births. There is considerable geographic variability, however, with the incidence increasing from the west to the east coast (48,54). The incidence is as high as 8 per 1000 live births in northern and western regions of Great Britain, whereas it is 2–3 per 1000 live births in the eastern and southern regions of that country (10). Women are afflicted more than men by a factor of 2:1, and incidence increases with lower socioeconomic level (95). However, these observations have not led to the discovery of an etiological agent.

D. Genetics

The genetic basis of most myelodysplasias does not fit a Mendelian inheritance pattern. Although some forms may be a feature of a purely genetic disorder (chromosome or single gene defects), the great majority are multifactorial in origin, with a combination of genetic susceptibility and environmental factors acting to produce the malformation (91,95). There is an established familial tendency—when one sibling is afflicted with an open neural tube lesion, the risk for other siblings increases to 5%, and if there are two affected siblings, this risk is 12–15% (23).

E. Etiology

Although it is suggested that environmental factors likely play a role in the etiology of these malformations, it has been difficult to establish definite responsibility for any particular agent. Numerous dietary substances have been examined (e.g., blighted potatoes), as have other potential teratogens such as alcohol and anticonvulsant agents, without any firm conclusions being reached (13). Various nutritional deficiency states, particularly that of folic acid deficiency, have also been studied. A recent well-designed, prospective trial from the United Kingdom found that folic acid supplementation around the time of conception significantly reduced the incidence of neural tube defects (65), but there are no similar studies of other potential environmental factors.

F. Prenatal Diagnosis

The prenatal diagnosis of open neural tube defects is possible using alpha-fetoprotein (AFP) measurements and ultrasonography. Amniocentesis in this setting was first described in 1972 by Brock and Sutcliffe (9), who noted that amniotic fluid AFP levels were markedly elevated in pregnancies that had resulted in children with open neural tube defects. AFP passes from CSF to amniotic fluid in the presence of an open defect and reaches peak levels at around the sixteenth week of pregnancy. AFP also crosses the placenta, and so may be assayed in maternal serum (95). It has been recommended that screening be offered to women with high-risk pregnancies (those with a child, sibling, or parent with an open neural tube defect). Maternal serum AFP levels have been found to be reliable for screening purposes, and mothers with positive screening results should be considered for amniocentesis and serial ultrasound examinations (26,63,102). With early intrauterine diagnosis, there is the opportunity for parents to prepare for the delivery of the child, the ability to plan early postnatal intervention, and the option of termination of the pregnancy. For further discussion of the risks of spina bifida with elevations of AFP, see Chapter 3.

G.   Clinical Features and Evaluation

1. Initial Assessment

In addition to neurological and lesion evaluation, the initial evaluation of the neonate with an open neural tube defect includes an assessment of general well-being and a search for other system anomalies. Hydrocephalus is present at birth or develops in the neonatal period in 80% of patients (57), and head circumference should be monitored. Upper limb function and the nature of the infant's cry should be noted, as these may change if an Arnold-Chiari anomaly later becomes symptomatic.

2. The Lesion

The site and size of the lesion are determined. The rostral margin of the lesion provides an approximation of the neurological level. In addition to location and size of the lesion, the size and shape of the skin defect and integrity of the sac are noted to help in surgical planning. Overall, 45% of lesions are at the level of the thoracolumbar junction, 20% are lumbar, 20% are at the level of the lumbosacral junction, and 10% lie over the sacrum, with the remainder located at more rostral spinal levels (37). The degree of cord malformation, and thus the neurological deficit, is variable.

3. Neurological Deficit

The neurological examination of the neonate may be difficult. Reflex spinal movements may be mistaken for voluntary movement, and hypothermia or maternal sedation administered during labor may worsen the neurological deficit. The infant should be examined at rest and spontaneous movements noted. The effects of a painful stimulus applied to the upper and lower limbs and the perineum are then noted. Lower limb movements in response to pain that are associated with crying and continue beyond the application of the stimulus are likely to be voluntary, whereas stereotyped movements that cease when the stimulus ceases and are not accompanied by crying are likely to be reflex responses.

Motor loss may be of upper or lower motor neuron type. Most commonly, it is a combination of both, creating a mixture of flaccid paralysis and involuntary reflexes (24,37). Generally, the voluntary motor deficit is complete below the upper segmental level of the lesion and is usually symmetrical within one or two segments. Innervation of the lower limb muscle groups is shown in Table 2.

Sensory loss usually correlates with the motor deficit to within one or two segmental levels, usually being slightly higher (24,37). Sensory examination relies on the sleeping or resting infant's response to a painful stimulus. The lowest sensory dermatomes in the perineal region are tested first, and the examination continues proximally until the sensory level is established.

Bladder dysfunction occurs in more than 90% of patients with myelomeningocele, with normal urinary sphincter function requiring the S2-S4 spinal cord segments to be intact. Of these patients, two-thirds have an upper motor disturbance, with reflexive, often uncoordinated, detrusor and external sphincter activity. The remaining one-third have lower motor dysfunction, with a flaccid external sphincter and lax detrusor (82,90). Examination includes observation of any spontaneous voiding (indicating detrusor activity) and nature of the urinary stream. It is difficult to predict accurately future bladder function in the

Table 2 Innervation of Lower Limb
Muscle Groups

Hip	
flexion	L1-L3
adduction	L2-L4
abduction	L5-S1
extension	L5-S2
Knee	
extension	L2-L4
flexion	L5-S2
Ankle	
inversion	L4
dorsiflexion	L4-L5
eversion	L5-S1
plantar flexion	S1-S2
Toe	
extension	L5-S1
flexion	S2-S3
Intrinsic foot muscles	S2-S3
Perineal muscles	S2-S3

Source: Ref. 86.

neonate. The bladder may initially appear flaccid, with upper motor neuron reflexes appearing later, and early surgery may affect final function.

Bowel continence, controlled by pelvic floor innervation by spinal cord segments S3-S4, generally parallels bladder continence. Upper motor neuron lesions result in constipation but may allow control of defecation and satisfactory continence, whereas lower motor lesions produce anal laxity and rectal prolapse.

4. Vertebral Abnormalities

A wide range of vertebral maldevelopment has been described in association with open cord lesions (4). The failure of normal neural tube development prevents formation of the posterior vertebral elements, so that the spinous processes and laminae are absent, and the pedicles are displaced laterally, creating a widened spinal canal. If T12 and L1 have normal posterior elements, the posterior spina bifida is in the region of the open cord lesion, and may only span two or three levels. Should T12 and L1 be abnormal, the entire lumbar and sacral spine will be bifid (24). Other anomalies, not necessarily confined to the level of the cord lesion, include aplasia, incomplete vertebral development (hemivertebrae and wedged vertebrae), and failure of segmentation leading to bony bars (Fig. 9).

Scoliosis is a frequent accompaniment of open cord lesions and may be classified as congenital or developmental (81). Congenital scoliosis, apparent at birth and the result of structural vertebral anomalies, is present in 30% and is almost invariably progressive. The group with developmental scoliosis usually have straight spines at birth and vertebral abnormalities limited to posterior spina bifida at the level of the lesion. One-half of patients with these findings will develop a scoliosis between the ages of 5 and 10 years. Thoracic and

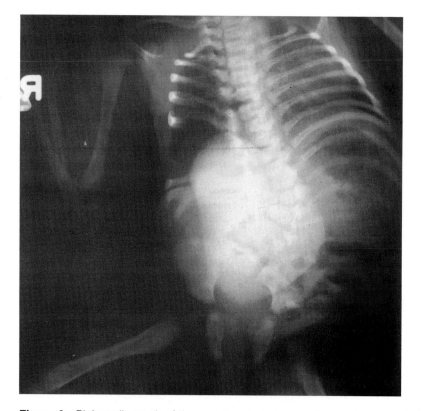

Figure 9 Plain radiograph of the chest and abdomen of a newborn myelodysplastic girl, demonstrating hemivertebrae, segmentation abnormalities, and scoliosis. The myelomeningocele is apparent as a superimposed soft tissue mass. Also noted are fused and absent ribs.

thoracolumbar scolioses usually have a concomitant kyphosis, whereas lumbosacral scolioses are usually associated with lordosis. Kyphosis may occur independently of scoliosis, as a consequence of deficient laminae, separated and everted pedicles, or maldevelopment of vertebral bodies, and most commonly occurs in the lumbar region.

Lumbar lordosis is commonly seen developing during childhood in patients with L1/2 motor levels as a compensatory mechanism to maintain upright trunk posture in the presence of hip flexion contractures (87).

5. Other Associated Abnormalities

Neurological

The majority of anomalies occurring with open neural tube defects also involve the nervous system or its associated mesoderm. An Arnold-Chiari hindbrain malformation is virtually always present and contributes to a 90% incidence of hydrocephalus at or soon after birth. Other abnormalities of brain development include cerebral aqueduct stenosis, cerebellar dysgenesis, agenesis of the corpus callosum, midline lipoma, and microgyria (24,37) (Fig. 10).

Other intraspinal lesions may exist in addition to the open neural tube defect. Syringomyelia, split cord malformations, intraspinal lipomas, epidermoid and dermoid cysts, and various tethering bands and adhesions may all be encountered, alone or in combination (20).

Other

Cranial anomalies that may be present include a small posterior fossa and low-lying tentorial attachment and torcular (37). Lower limb deformities may occur and usually reflect muscle imbalance secondary to the neurological deficit (87). Associated anomalies of other organ systems are uncommon, although craniofacial anomalies and involvement of the cardiovascular, pulmonary, and gastrointestinal systems have all been described. The most frequently seen abnormalities are in the genitourinary system, where problems such as hydronephrosis and hydroureter occur as a consequence of sphincter dysfunction (37).

H. Investigation

Imaging studies of the spine contribute little to the early management of the neonate with an open neural tube defect, although they obviously become important in the follow-up of late neurological deterioration or the development of spinal curvature, as will be discussed later.

Hydrocephalus is readily monitored with serial ultrasound examinations. Cranial computed tomography (CT) has been recommended as a baseline investigation and in follow-up, if progressive clinical hydrocephalus is suspected (59,92).

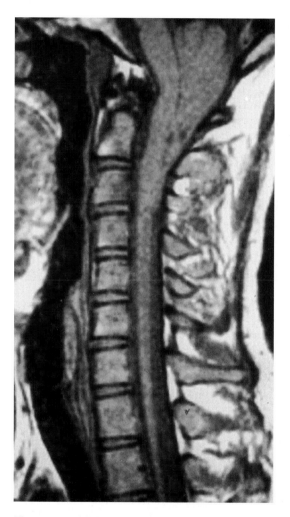

Figure 10 MRI scan of an Arnold-Chiari type II malformation, demonstrating herniation of the cerebellum, hindbrain, and fourth ventricle, along with kinking of the cervicomedullary junction.

I. Management

The treatment of open neural tube defects has undergone considerable evolution since the time of Aristotle, who recommended infanticide for infants with these lesions. Untreated, the natural history of infants with myelomeningocele is bleak, with a mortality of 80–90% in the first year of life, primarily from central nervous system (CNS) infection or hydrocephalus. A significant proportion of the remainder die during the next few years, from problems such as renal failure and respiratory failure secondary to spinal deformity (84). Operative closure of the back lesion was recommended in the early 18th century, although the outcome was almost invariably fatal (97). The 1950s saw the advent of effective hydrocephalus treatment and antibiotics, which led to improved outcomes. There have been two subsequent areas of controversy continuing to the present time: whether to selectively offer treatment only to less severely affected children, and whether to close the back lesion early (within 48 hours of birth) or late.

The Sheffield group in the early 1960s proposed aggressive therapy with immediate closure of the back defect in all infants (85), and this policy was widely followed for a period of time. However, dismay at an increased number of severely disabled survivors led to the proposal of not treating those infants with high lesions (paralysis at L3 or above), severe hydrocephalus, kyphosis, other major congenital anomalies, or birth trauma (52,53). Nonetheless, most major centers currently advocate treatment of all viable infants, citing objections to the reliability of selection criteria in predicting future function and the fact that some nontreated infants do survive but are significantly more impaired than if they had been treated (24,37,79).

The optimal time for closure of the back lesion has also been debated. Current consensus favors closure within 36–48 hours, as the placode is colonized by bacteria after this time and surgery carries a significant risk of CNS infection (24,37,62,85). Should a child be referred after 36–48 hours, the lesion should be managed by frequent dressings, with topical and systemic antibiotic therapy as necessary, and surgery should be postponed until after three consecutive negative 24-hour cultures. Progressive hydrocephalus may require treatment during this time, although a shunt should not be internalized until a CSF culture (ventricular puncture) is negative.

The 36–48 hour time frame implies that closure is not a surgical emergency and allows some time for parental counseling, along with early involvement of the multidisciplinary team (including neurosurgeon, pediatrician, orthopedic surgeon, urologist, nurses, therapists, and social workers) who will be involved in the care of the child.

1. Closure of the Back Defect

The goals of early surgery are to prevent infection and preserve existing neurological function. Prior to surgery, correct fluid balance and normothermia are maintained. The general principles of the procedure are preservation of the exposed neural tissue, restoration of the spinal cord into the spinal canal, and anatomical reconstitution of tissue layers. The use of magnification is advisable.

The child is positioned prone on bolsters, with temperature controlled by heating blankets and appropriate operating room temperature. The skin surrounding the lesion is prepared with an iodine-based solution, but such potentially neurotoxic agents are not applied to the lesion itself. If the sac is intact, it is aspirated, and the fluid is sent for culture. A circumferential incision is made around the placode, along the white line marking the boundary between skin and meninges. Any adhesions between the arachnoid and the ventral and lateral dura are divided, and the entire placode is dissected out. Anomalous roots are identified, and any ending blindly in the dome of the sac are divided. Arachnoid and dural remnants are trimmed away flush with the edges of the placode. Some surgeons advocate approximating the lateral arachnoid edges with fine sutures and so reconstituting a neural tube (28,55).

The dura is then identified. This is best done by identifying normal dura rostrally (beneath the most caudal intact lamina) and caudally, then dissecting laterally until enough has been mobilized to allow the edges to meet in the midline and reconstitute the dural sac around the placode (Fig. 11). The dural closure should be watertight, with a capacious subdural space. If insufficient dura is available to achieve this, fascia lata or a sheet of Silastic may be used.

The next step is to dissect out and approximate flaps of lumbodorsal fascia, which can be identified at its attachment to the posterior iliac crest and sacrum. This may not always be possible, as the caudal fascia may be deficient or the reapproximation may leave the dural sac constricted. Finally, the subcutaneous tissue and skin are closed in separate layers without tension.

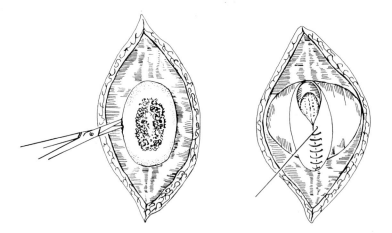

Figure 11   Dissection and mobilization of the dura around the placode (left), to allow a capacious watertight closure (right).

Occasionally, more extensive procedures are required. A minority of patients will require construction of myocutaneous flaps to achieve skin coverage. Prominent laminae should be removed to avoid areas of pressure on the skin closure. Spinal osteotomy (kyphectomy) for marked kyphosis is sometimes necessary to reduce the deformity and obtain adequate skin coverage.

Meningocele repair follows similar principles. The sac can usually dissected out easily, and occasionally a herniated nerve root or minor herniation of the spinal cord needs to be replaced inside the dural tube and spinal canal. The dura is closed over the neck of the sac, and the remainder of the closure is as for meningomyelocele.

2. Postoperative Care

If there is some concern about the viability of the wound closure, the infant should be nursed face down until it is known the wound is healthy. Feeding can commence when bowel sounds are present, usually within 24 hours after the surgery. A CSF leak from the wound will usually resolve spontaneously if associated hydrocephalus has been treated. If a fistula does not close, treatment options are ventricular drainage if a shunt is not yet in place, or secondary wound closure.

3. Management of Hydrocephalus

Hydrocephalus may be present at birth but more often becomes clinically apparent in the first 1–2 weeks after the surgical repair (37). After ultrasound or CT confirmation, and providing the wound appears clean and intact, a ventriculoperitoneal shunt should be inserted. If hydrocephalus is present at the time of, or before, the myelomeningocele closure, a shunt may be performed before or simultaneously with the back repair. If CSF or wound cultures suggest colonization or infection, hydrocephalus is best managed by external ventricular drainage and antibiotic therapy until cultures are negative.

4. Management of Arnold-Chiari Malformation

The Arnold-Chiari malformation associated with myelomeningocele may become symptomatic in 10–20% of infants in the first months of life (73). Symptoms include feeding difficulties and regurgitation, a change in the nature of the infant's cry, and apneic periods. Surgical decompression is required.

J. Long-Term Outcome

After back closure and treatment of hydrocephalus, 80% of all infants with myelomeningocele can be expected to survive the first 2 years of life, after which the mortality rate levels off (24,59). The most common cause of death in this time is hindbrain dysfunction. The intellectual development of these children is variable; 30–40% will show some degree of mental retardation, which is more common with high lesions and active hydrocephalus. Episodes of shunt infection and obstruction further decrease intellectual function (18).

The potential for ambulation depends on the segmental motor level. Theoretically, L3 level is compatible with orthotic-assisted ambulation, but factors such as intelligence, spinal and lower limb deformities, and coordination may influence this ability. The ease of ambulation also decreases with age, as body weight increases more than muscle strength (37). Practically, L5 is the highest level likely to be associated with long-term ambulation.

K. Late Neurological Deterioration

Delayed neurological deterioration is not part of the natural history of meningocele or myelomeningocele, and the development of new neurological symptoms or signs requires investigation and appropriate intervention.

1. "Retethering" of the Spinal Cord

Approximately 3% of patients will develop late symptoms related to a low-lying spinal cord held by scar tissue to the site of the initial back repair (24) [Fig. 12]. Other causes of a tethered cord include lesions such as thickened filum terminale, diastematomyelia, dermoid and epidermoid tumors, and arachnoid cysts. Clinical features include back pain radiating into the legs, increasing spasticity, changing motor and sensory levels, a change in bladder or bowel function, and the development of scoliosis or neuromuscular lower limb deformities. A second untethering procedure generally brings an arrest of the neurological deterioration (80,99).

2. Arnold-Chiari Malformation

Occasionally the Arnold-Chiari malformation associated with myelomeningocele continues to be symptomatic or occurs beyond infancy. Occipital and neck pain, lower cranial nerve dysfunction, nystagmus, spasticity, and upper limb weakness may occur.

3. Syringohydromyelia

Fifty to eighty percent of patients with myelomeningocele have syringo- or hydromyelia, the most common features being progressive scoliosis, spasticity, and upper limb weakness (21) [Fig. 13].

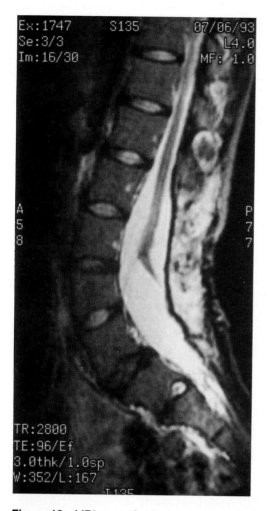

Figure 12 MRI scan of spinal cord tethered at the site of a previous myelomeningocele repair at the L3-L4 level.

The initial step in the investigation of these entities is to exclude shunt dysfunction. After this, magnetic resonance imaging (MRI) is appropriate to demonstrate the state of the hindbrain, the spinal cord, and any tethering lesion. In the presence of spinal deformity, coronal plane MRI is helpful. Occasionally, CT myelography is required when severe spinal curvature creates difficulty in obtaining a good quality MRI study.

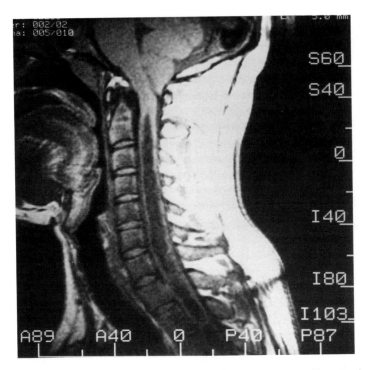

Figure 13 MRI scan demonstrating Arnold-Chiari type II anomaly, with associated syringomyelia.

III. CLOSED SPINAL CORD MALFORMATIONS

These congenital spinal anomalies have in common an intact epidermal covering, and most commonly presents with neurological deterioration in childhood or, less commonly, in later life. Occasionally, they may present with a fixed neurological deficit at birth due to the primary effect of the malformation. The classical delayed clinical presentation has become known as "tethered cord syndrome." The term originally referred primarily to deterioration from traction on a low lying conus by a thickened filum terminale but has come to encompass a number of abnormalities (Table 3). It is also now acknowledged that these malformations and the accompanying clinical syndrome may occur with the conus lying at a normal level (31,104).

These closed anomalies have many pathophysiological and clinical features in common, and these along with general investigation and management principles will be considered prior to discussion of specific lesions.

Table 3 Lesions Presenting as Occult Malformations

Split-cord malformations (diastematomyelia, diplomyelia)
Thickened filum terminale
Lumbosacral lipomyelomeningocele
Dermoid and epidermoid tumor
Congenital dermal sinus
Neurenteric cyst
Previous myelomeningocele repair
Anterior sacral meningocele
Sacrococcygeal teratoma
Caudal regression syndrome

A. Pathophysiology

Neurological deficits occurring with a tethered cord may result from one or a combination of traction effects, compression, inflammation, or the effects of the primary neurological malformation (24). When there has been a failure of normal ascent and the cord is low lying, it has a stretched appearance, with the surface vessels appearing taut. Neurological dysfunction is thought to result from repetitive stretching and distortion with activity and growth, resulting in eventual microvascular injury and chronic ischemia (44,79). Lesions such as intraspinal lipomas, dermoid tumors, and neurenteric cysts may cause mechanical compression of the spinal cord. Meningitis may occur with a dermal sinus and may cause or worsen a neurological deficit. Lastly, a fixed neurological deficit may be present at birth as a result of the neural malformation itself, such as may occur with lipomyelomeningocele. This deficit remains susceptible to worsening from the effects of traction or compression.

B. Clinical Features

1. Cutaneous

Hair tufts, subcutaneous lipomas, hemangiomatous nevi, skin tags, and skin dimples may all occur on the back in conjunction with an occult spinal malformation. The lesions occur on or adjacent to the midline, usually in the lumbosacral region. Hair tufts are more common in diastematomyelia than in other forms of malformation (28) (Fig. 14). Atretic meningoceles (areas of thin, pearly skin with a red-pink halo) are occasionally seen. These represent open lesions that have healed spontaneously (94).

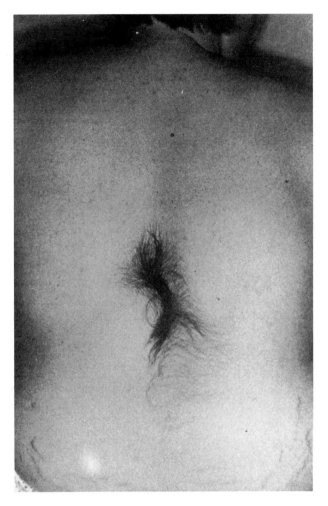

Figure 14   Hair tuft overlying diastematomyelia.

2. Neuromusculoskeletal

Clinical presentation frequently features a mixture of related orthopedic and neurological symptoms and signs, which are appropriately considered together. Some combination of lower limb deformity, weakness, sensory loss, gait disturbance, and reflex abnormality occurs in two-thirds of patients with closed spinal cord malformations (24). A combination of upper and lower motor neurone signs may exist. Involvement of a nerve root or anterior horn cells at the conus by tethering lesion can cause lower motor deficits, and traction more proximally causes upper motor neuron dysfunction. This may result in spasticity and extensor plantar responses in addition to weakness. Sensory loss is usually patchy and nondermatomal in distribution, and this type of deficit may be manifest in a younger child by trophic changes. Orthopedic abnormalities are found in 75% of patients, the most common being valgus, varus, and cavus foot deformities (60). The affected limb may be smaller or shorter than the other, with atrophic musculature. Neuromuscular symptoms may first appear during phases of increased activity or rapid growth, such as when the child is learning to walk and in early adolescence, at which time the tethered cord is liable to undergo increased stretching (44).

3. Spinal Curvature

In 12% of patients a scoliosis or other progressive curvature develops, which may or may not be at the site of the primary spinal cord abnormality (34). The tethering effect of the lesion is apparently a factor in the etiology of at least some curves, as untethering of the cord can improve or arrest the scoliosis in more than 50% of patients (47,60). In some patients, the scoliosis is secondary to hemivertebrae or other segmentation anomalies and would not be expected to improve with untethering of the cord.

4. Sphincter Disturbance

Up to 30% of patients will have some form of sphincter dysfunction, usually in association with neuromuscular symptoms (24). Abnormalities in early childhood may be manifest by an absence of dry periods between diaper changes, continuous dribbling, nocturnal enuresis, or recurrent urinary tract infections. After early childhood, urinary frequency, urgency, incomplete voiding, and stress or overflow incontinence may occur (72).

5. Back or Leg Pain

Pain commonly accompanies tethering of the cord, usually in association with other neurological or musculoskeletal symptoms (10). It often radiates into the anterior thigh and/or perineum and genitals and can frequently be aggravated by toe-touching or flexing of the neck on the trunk.

C. Investigation

1. Radiological

Plain x-ray and myelography with CT have been the procedures of choice for the investigation of suspected occult spinal cord malformations (41,42). Plain x-rays show abnormalities in 95% of patients, the most common findings being posterior spina bifida, widening of the spinal canal, and vertebral body abnormalities such as failure of segmentation and hemivertebrae (2,12). Myelography can demonstrate the position of the conus, the diameter of the filum terminale, the presence of a midline septum or two dural tubes, and the presence of any space occupying lesions. CT scanning post-myelography further defines any intraspinal abnormality, the bony spinal elements, and the relationship between these entities.

More recently MRI has replaced these as the primary imaging modality, having the advantages of excellent imaging of soft tissue in multiple planes, noninvasiveness, and absence of ionizing radiation (72,94). A low-lying conus and lesions such as thickened filum and lumbosacral lipoma are well visualized. However, MRI in some complex lesions can be difficult to interpret, such as with complex lipomyelomeningoceles or postmyelomeningocele repair. It has been suggested that MRI is an appropriate screening test for occult spinal cord malformations, with no further radiological investigations required if this is entirely normal or shows an uncomplicated lesion. However, should MRI be able to definitively exclude a lesion, or should it show a complicated lesion requiring more precise anatomical detail for surgical planning, a CT myelogram should also be performed (72).

2. Electrophysiological

Any symptoms of urinary dysfunction require clarification with urodynamic studies. This will establish a baseline for assessment of any future neurological deterioration, help predict future function, and help guide therapy (5).

When somatosensory evoked potentials (SSEPs) after peroneal nerve stimulation have been monitored serially in patients with tethered cord syndrome, a reduction in amplitude and an increase in latency of responses have been found during the 6–12 months prior to surgery, with a decrease in latency after surgery (79).

D. Management

Surgical treatment is clearly indicated for the development or progression of any neurological deficit in a patient with an occult malformation, with the goals of undoing any cord tethering and relieving any compression that may be present. There has been considerable controversy regarding the role of surgery for a tethering anomaly without neurological deficit. Prophylactic surgery in asymptomatic and neurologically stable children within 2 years after birth has been strongly advocated in the past (27,61), whereas others have advised that, as neurological progression is not invariable and surgery carries some potential risks, conservative management is preferable unless deterioration occurs (39,107). However, with increasing knowledge of the natural history of these lesions, it is recognized that the incidence of neurological deterioration is ultimately very high, and that once established, a new deficit may not be reversible (35). It is also known that these patients are susceptible to precipitous deterioration after minor trauma (72), and for these reasons prophylactic repair is now considered the appropriate standard of care (10,24,72).

Specific surgical aspects for each lesion will be discussed below. These procedures have in common the principles of the use of magnification, a plan of working from normal tissue to abnormal, and the use of electrophysiological monitoring. Common peroneal nerve SSEPs monitor the spinal cord from the S1 dorsal root entry zone upward. Although directly assessing the dorsal columns, in practice they are sensitive to anterior and lateral column traction or pressure (72). The S2-S4 ventral roots should be monitored by cystometry or by external anal sphincter myography/manometry. Pudendal SSEPs have been used to monitor S2-S4 dorsal roots (30).

Although the prevention of further neurological deterioration has been regarded as the primary reason for surgery (62,96), a number of series report pain relief in almost all symptomatic patients and an improvement in motor and bladder function in 30–50% (24,60).

IV. SPECIFIC LESIONS

A. Split-Cord Malformations

Diastematomyelia refers to congenital splitting of the spinal cord into two hemicords, usually but not invariably of approximately equal size. Although usually occurring as an occult malformation, it may occur in association with an open lesion. A bony, cartilaginous, or thick fibrous septum may be present between the two hemicords, with each hemicord having its own dural sheath (type I diastematomyelia). Less commonly, the septum is an incomplete fibrous band, and the dural tube around the two hemicords is single, with the medial surface of each hemicord tethered to the midline band (type II). Diplopmyelia is occasionally incorrectly used as a synonym for diastematomyelia. This term implies a true duplication, with two fully formed spinal cords and sets of nerve roots.

Theories of the embryogenesis of split-cord malformation (SCM) are of two types—primary maldevelopment of the neural ectoderm, and primary maldevelopment of extraneural tissue resulting secondarily in a split cord. In the first group of theories, Herren and Edwards suggested that the neural folds may turn inwards and fuse with the neural plate before fusing with each other, thus creating two neural tubes (32). The surrounding mesoderm would then migrate around the neural tubes, with the possibility of the mesenchyme between the tubes forming pia only (and therefore a single dural/arachnoid tube), or the mesenchyme forming arachnoid, dura, cartilage, and bone to create two dural tubes and a midline osteocartilaginous septum. Kapsenberg and Van Lookeren Campagne suggested that an overgrowth of neural ectoderm may make it impossible for the neural folds to reach each other, resulting in each fold turning in on itself to form separate neural tubes (46). The overlying mesenchyme is then induced to form two bony canals that fuse in the midline to form a septum. Gardner has postulated a hydrodynamic theory, in which an overdistended neural tube ruptures without breach of the overlying cutaneous ectoderm. The edges of the neural tube then reunite to form two tubes (25). Another theory of primary neural tissue abnormality invokes an abortive form of twinning (60).

The most plausible theory of the second group is that of Bremer, who suggested that, at the time of formation of the neurenteric canal, an accessory canal may develop and persist (7). This would cause the neural plate and notochord to be divided, accounting for the hemicords and the mesenchymal abnormalities often associated with diastematomyelia, such as hemivertebrae and butterfly vertebrae. Other theories propose a primary mesodermal midline septum

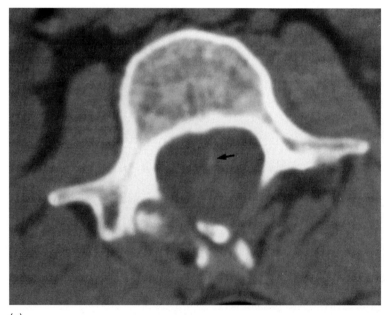

(a)

Figure 15   Diastematomyelia. (a) Plain CT scan showing a midline bony spicule (arrow); (b) CT scan after the administration of intrathecal contrast; and (c) coronal MRI scan, demonstrating split dural sacs.

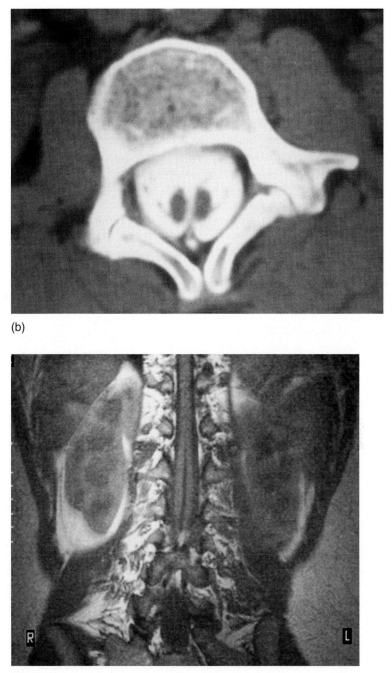

(b)

(c)

that splits the neural plate (51), and a primary split of the notochord inducing a split in the neural plate (6).

SCM occurs more often in women than men by a ratio of 4:1 or more (29,60) and is usually accompanied by hair tufts or nevi on the skin overlying the lesion. The septum is located at the lumbar spine level in 70% (usually from L1–L3), and in the thoracic spine in 28%. Approximately 60% of patients present before the age of 5, and 25% between the ages of 5 and 10 (24,33,47). Plain radiographs demonstrate spina bifida in almost all patients, and a wide range of other vertebral anomalies may be seen, including block vertebrae, hemivertebrae, and a widened interpedicular distance. An ossified septum is seen in two-thirds of patients (24,29). MRI has supplanted CT myelography as the investigation of choice for SCM, noninvasively demonstrating the split cord and septum. CT myelography also demonstrates these lesions well and may be required on occasion, such as in the presence of significant scoliosis (Fig. 15).

The goal of surgery for diastematomyelia is to free the spinal cord by removing the tethering median septum. For type I lesions, the dura over each hemicord is opened to allow full visualization of the split cord during removal of the septum. The bony or cartilaginous septum is removed from its attachment to the ventral vertebral body with rongeurs or a high-speed diamond drill. Any bands between the spinal cord and dura are divided. The anterior dural defect may be left open, but the posterior dura is reconstructed to form a single dural tube. With type II lesions, the dura is opened, and the incomplete fibrous septum, (which may even be ventral to the hemicords), is located and divided.

B. Thickened Filum Terminale

Any form of occult spinal cord malformation may be associated with fibrous bands, adhesions, or both attaching the cord, conus, filum terminale, or spinal roots to the dura. In some cases, these represent an aborted or regressed meningeal sac, termed *meningocele manqué* (40). Occasionally the clinical syndrome of tethered cord is due to thickened (i.e., more than 2 mm diameter) filum terminale alone (71,94).

The neural tube normally atrophies beyond the 42nd somite, accompanied by lengthening of the filum and nerve roots. The syndrome of thickened filum is postulated to result from a failure of this process of neural tube involution and/or root lengthening (44).

Plain radiographs in these patients usually demonstrate posterior lumbosacral spina bifida, but definitive diagnosis requires the visualization of a tethered cord and a thickened filum in the absence of another lesion. MRI again is the investigation of choice, although CT myelography images the filum well and should be considered if the clinical picture is suggestive of a tethered cord and the MRI study is equivocal (94) (Fig. 16). Surgery requires dural opening and sectioning of the filum as low as possible.

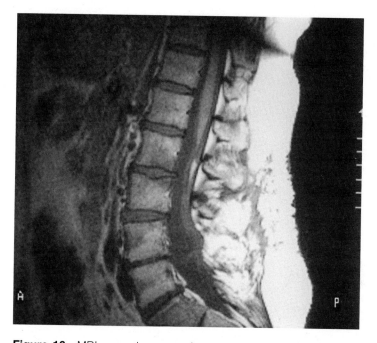

Figure 16 MRI scan demonstrating a thickened filum terminale, tethering the thecal sac at the L2-L4 levels. The conus is in a normal position. The area of bright signal in the filum terminale represents a small lipoma. An L4-L5 laminectomy, through which the dural sac is bulging, had been performed before referral (symptoms had been presumed to be the result of lumbar canal stenosis).

C. Lumbosacral Lipomyelomeningocele

Lipomatous tissue within the intradural space may take the form of spinal cord lipoma, lipomyelomeningocele, or filum terminale fibrolipoma, which is commonly found in association with a thickened filmum terminale. Spinal cord lipomas are usually located in the thoracic region, appear in adulthood, and are not uniformly regarded as myelodysplastic lesions.

Lipomyelomeningocele describes a lipoma of a caudally tethered spinal cord that extends out of an overlying dural and vertebral defect into the subcutaneous tissues and accounts for one-third of closed myelodysplastic lesions (24,60). It is suggested that lipomyelomeningocele results if the neural ectoderm prematurely separates from the cutaneous ectoderm, allowing the paraxial mesenchyme access to the as yet unclosed neural tissue. Closure of the neural tube is impeded, and the adjacent mesenchyme can only be induced to form fat, leading to lipoma formation between the splayed dorsal columns (56). Other theories of embryogenesis suggest that lipomas may result from the over-

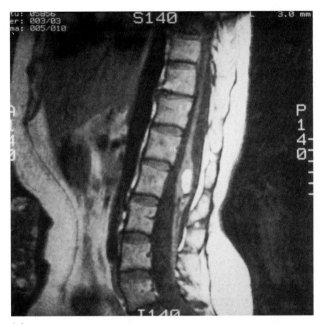

(a)

Figure 17   (a) Sagittal and (b) axial MRI images of an intradural lipoma and associated tethered spinal cord.

growth of mesenchymal cells included in the neural tube during the process of canalization, or from perivascular mesenchyme that invades the spinal cord during vascularization. Tethering occurs during subsequent development of this abnormal tissue, restricting the ascent of the conus (60).

Lipomyelomeningoceles are located in the lumbosacral region in 90% of instances and are usually apparent at birth as a soft subcutaneous mass. Over one-half of patients have associated cutaneous lesions, such as a hair tuft, hemangioma, or dermal sinus tract. Most infants do not have any neurological deficits at birth, although the natural history during the next few months to years is of progressive neurological dysfunction and musculoskeletal deformity resulting from a combination of tethering of the cord and compression by the lipoma. However, the clinical course is variable—some patients show early rapid progression in the weeks after birth, whereas others may not have any symptoms until adulthood (24,60,66).

Plain radiographs are virtually always abnormal, demonstrating posterior spina bifida in most patients, with vertebral segmentation and sacral anomalies

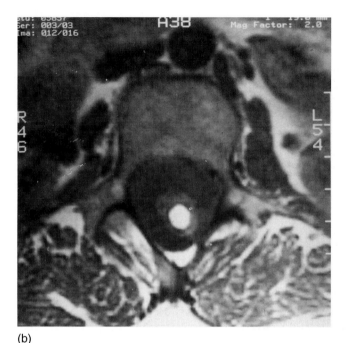

(b)

present in 50% (100). MRI again accurately demonstrates the anatomy of the malformation and has replaced CT myelography as the investigation of first choice (Fig. 17).

As with other tethering lesions, surgery is the recommended treatment for both symptomatic and asymptomatic lipomyelomeningoceles. Although it has not been absolutely proven that prophylactic surgery for neurologically intact infants is the correct course of therapy, the evidence that most patients progressively lose function that may not be recoverable, and that the risk of neurological injury with surgery is low (less than 5% have permanent worsening), has led to a strong endorsement of prophylactic surgery (24,60,66,71,94).

The goals of surgery are to relieve traction on the spinal cord and to alleviate compression by the lipoma. The procedure may be technically challenging, and it is important for the surgeon to appreciate the pathological anatomy. The dura is deficient deep to the lipoma in the dorsal midline, with the edges of the dural defect seeming to attach to the edges of the neural plate dorsal to the dorsal root entry zone. The lipoma inserts into the exposed dorsal surface of the neural plate and may extend to the central canal of the cord (60). The junction between lipoma and spinal cord may lie either within or be external to the spinal canal. The latter implies that there is some spinal cord herniation.

Surgery begins with a midline excision above and below the subcutaneous lesion and the establishment of a circumferential plane around the lipoma. The "stalk" where the lipoma has herniated through the lumbar fascia is identified. A laminectomy cephalad to the lesion is performed, and normal dura is identified. Epidural fat is removed and the caudal aspect of the dural defect found. The dura is opened cephalad to the defect and neural tissue and the intradural extension of the lipoma identified. Working laterally, the dura is carefully dissected from the lateral spinal cord and nerve roots on each side. The lipoma may then be freed from the dura caudally. The whole lipoma may be lifted to identify the junction of caudal neural tissue and lipoma and to allow assessment of whether the roots of the cauda equina can be separated from the undersurface of the lipoma. The lipoma can now be removed from the dorsal surface of the spinal cord. The use of the CO_2 laser is helpful in facilitating this. Chapman and Beyerl have described two basic forms of lipoma that may be appreciated at this stage (14). The dorsal variant attaches directly onto the dorsal aspect of the conus, with all nerve roots emerging from the ventral or lateral cord and lying in the subarachnoid space. These lipomas can be removed from the dorsal aspect of the cord in a plane superficial to the lateral margin of fusion of the lipoma, conus, and dura. With the caudal variant, seen at the sacral level, the lipoma emerges from the terminal conus or filum terminale, so that the cord becomes progressively larger caudally, and nerve roots do traverse the lipoma. Sectioning of the lipoma must be distal to any functional roots, which may be identified with stimulation. It is not necessary to remove the entire lipoma; good clinical results are achieved if decompression and untethering are accomplished, and neurological function should not be risked in the pursuit of total lipoma excision.

After decompression and untethering, the neural tube is approximated with pia-to-pia sutures if possible (in an effort to prevent retethering), and a watertight but capacious dural repair is carried out. There may be insufficient dura to achieve this, and the use of Silastic sheeting or fascia may be required.

D. Neurenteric Cyst

Also known as enterogenous cysts, neurenteric cysts are rare intraspinal cysts of entodermal derivation. They are held to arise as a result of abnormalities relating to development of the entoderm-lined neurenteric canal, which transiently connects the yolk sac (destined to become the gut) and the dorsal surface of the embryo. Failure of regression of this canal could conceivably give rise to a variety of potential sinuses, cysts, or fistulae along its course. Thus, an intraspinal neurenteric cyst may result if the intraspinal portion of the canal persists (6,7). Persistence of the entire canal in association with maldevelopment of the midline dorsal ectoderm causes a combined anterior and posterior spina bifida. Histologically, neurenteric cysts are lined with simple or pseudo-stratified columnar epithelium and may contain gastric parietal and chief cells, or mucin-producing goblet cells (50).

Neurenteric cysts are usually located in the cervical and thoracic regions and may be intramedullary or intradural and extramedullary. Fifty percent of patients will have an associated posterior mediastinal cyst, with the two lesions usually connected through a defect in the adjacent anterior vertebral bodies. The most common presentation is in early childhood, with a cervical or thoracic mass, or with symptoms of spinal cord compression (24). However, neurenteric cysts may present with spinal cord compression in older children or adults, or rarely with meningitis caused by bowel organisms (38).

Plain radiographs may show a widened interpedicular distance and vertebral segmentation anomalies. MRI demonstrates the anatomy of the cyst and its relationship with the spinal cord and dura, but in the presence of an associated posterior mediastinal mass, CT myelography may be required to determine if the two lesions are in communication (24,94).

Treatment of a neurenteric cyst varies according to its location and the presence of a prevertebral lesion. Wide laminectomy with cyst drainage and conservative removal of the cyst wall has been found to be successful treatment. An anterior dural defect may be plugged with muscle and fascia at the time of the laminectomy or repaired via a thoracotomy, if this is being performed for treatment of a prevertebral lesion (24,94).

E. Congenital Dermal Sinus and Dermoid and Epidermoid Cyst

A congenital dermal sinus is an epithelium-lined tract extending inward from the skin overlying the spine. These tracts may occur anywhere from the cervical to the sacral regions and vary in depth from ending in the subcutaneous tissues to ending in neural tissue. With the deeper lesions, there is a potential communication between the skin and the intradural space. These lesions are postulated to arise as a result of defective separation of the cutaneous and neural ectoderm. Incomplete separation of these layers creates a sinus, and with closure of the neural groove, cutaneous elements that may subsequently develop into an intraspinal dermoid or epidermoid are incorporated into the neural tube (103).

Sinus tracts occur most frequently in the lumbar (40%), lumbosacral (10%), and sacral (25%) regions. Fifty percent of patients have an associated intraspinal inclusion tumor, of which 85% are dermoids. Epidermoids make up 15% of these tumors, and teratomas 5% (36,78). The appearance of the sinus may range from an obvious opening to an almost invisible pinhole, and associated cutaneous nevi or hair tufts may be present. In addition to having an obvious lesion, patients may present with purulent discharge from the sinus, meningitis, or the symptoms of an intraspinal mass lesion (inclusion tumor or abscess). Recurrent bouts of meningitis in an infant, or meningitis with unusual or multiple organisms requires a search for a sinus tract.

As with other forms of occult lesions, plain radiographs will frequently show abnormalities of the posterior vertebral elements. MRI will not always demonstrate the intraspinal extent of the sinus if it should extend that far, but is indicated in the presence of a sinus to determine whether an inclusion tumor exists (Figs. 18 and 19). Lumbar puncture in the investigation of meningitis may not return CSF if an intraspinal tumor is present. Probing or injection of contrast material into the sinus is potentially dangerous and should be avoided.

The treatment of a congenital sinus is excision of the entire tract once it has been diagnosed. The skin around the sinus opening is excised, and the tract is followed down to its termination. If it continues to the dura, a laminectomy

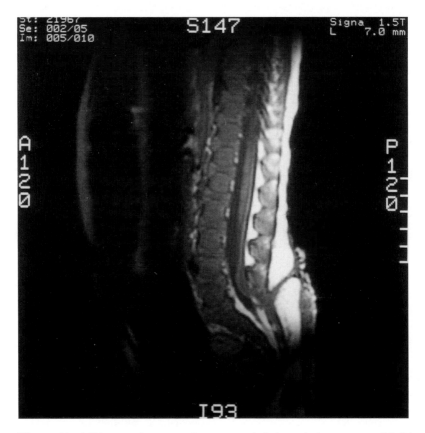

Figure 18 MRI scan demonstrating congenital dermal sinus tract at L5-S1, associated with thickened filum terminale tethering the cord at this level.

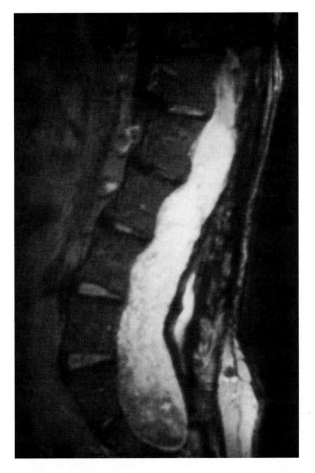

Figure 19 Large spinal dermoid tumor, filling the lumbosacral canal and causing scalloping of the posterior margins of the lumbar vertebral bodies. No nerve roots of the cauda equina are visible.

is performed, the dura opened, and the intradural contents explored. If possible, intradural cysts are removed with their capsule intact, although dense adhesions of the tumor capsule to neural tissue may make total removal impossible.

Congenital dermal sinuses are to be distinguished from the sacrococcygeal dimples that occur in 4% of children. Dimples are thought to arise as a result of the sacrococcygeal ligament attaching to the skin and placing traction on it as the spine elongates. There is no connection with the spinal canal, and no treatment is required other than maintaining local cleanliness (15,36).

F. Caudal Regression Syndrome

Also termed sacral agenesis, the caudal regression syndrome refers to a failure of formation of the coccygeal, sacral, and occasionally lumbar vertebrae, along with the corresponding segments of the spinal cord. This anomaly may be associated with malformations of the lower limbs, genitourinary system, and anorectal area. The areas of the child affected principally develop in conjunction with the final stages of neurulation. Theories of embryogenesis include nondevelopment of the notochord and neural ectoderm (45) and constriction of the embryo (e.g., by a too small amniotic sac), impairing distal neurulation (58). The cause of this syndrome is unknown, although there is a strong association with maternal diabetes mellitus (74).

The most common presentation is that of a 3-year-old to 5-year-old child with failure of development of sphincter control, recurrent urinary tract infections, or chronic constipation. Unless upper sacral or lumbar segments are involved, neurological deficit and orthopedic abnormalities are absent. Unless obvious abnormalities of other systems are present, external findings are limited to flattening of the buttocks and a shallow gluteal cleft. The absent vertebral segments may be apparent on palpation, and the anal sphincter is usually lax. Perianal sensation may be normal and is not a reliable indicator of bladder function (89,106).

Plain radiographs show missing sacral segments, although the difficulty of identifying segments precisely makes it hard to correlate the radiographs with neurological impairment. Investigation of urinary tract function is essential. Although other forms of myelodysplasia in association with this abnormality are uncommon, MRI is indicated if the clinical picture or plain radiograph suggests this possibility.

In the absence of an associated tethering lesion, treatment is primarily aimed at establishing urinary continence and preventing the sequelae of urinary obstruction.

G. Sacrococcygeal Teratoma

Teratomas of the sacrococcygeal region develop from totipotential cells originating in the region of Hensen's node and comprise elements of all three germ layers. They occur with an once in every 40,000 births, with a female-to-male preponderance of 3:1 (24).

These tumors usually present at birth as obvious masses extending out from the sacrum and coccyx. Up to 45% have a significant pelvic or presacral component, and 10% are located entirely within the pelvis. Entirely intrapelvic lesions may only be diagnosed clinically by rectal examination. The majority are asymptomatic, although birth trauma may cause significant hemorrhage.

Symptoms, when present, are generally caused by the presacral component, which may obstruct the urinary and gastrointestinal tracts (22). The differential diagnosis of a presacral mass presenting with obstructive uropathy or constipation is varied, and anterior meningocele, retrorectal abscess, rectal duplication, and other tumors such as neuroblastoma, dermoid, chordoma, and chondroma need to be considered.

Sacrococcygeal teratomas may be benign, cystic, or mixed. The majority (70–90%) are benign, although the incidence of malignancy increases with age after early infancy. After 3 months of age, 30% are malignant, whereas more than 50% are malignant after 1 year (22,83).

Plain radiographs are usually normal. MRI has replaced ultrasound and CT as the investigation of choice to demonstrate the anatomy and relationships of the tumor. Angiography may be useful in planning surgery by demonstrating the tumor's blood supply, particularly in the case of malignant tumors.

The appropriate treatment for sacrococcygeal teratomas is complete resection. This can usually be done via a posterior approach, with careful dissection of the tumor and excision of the coccyx required. Occasionally, a transabdominal approach will be necessary if a large intrapelvic extension is present. There is some evidence that patients with malignant tumors benefit from adjuvant radiotherapy and chemotherapy (3). Tumors excised in the neonatal period, which are usually benign, rarely recur. Malignant, incompletely excised tumors have a poor outcome, with few long-term survivors.

H. Anterior Sacral Meningocele

Anterior sacral meningocele is a herniation of the sacral meninges through a defect in the anterior sacrum. The lesion results from a failure of fusion of sclerotomes on one side, producing a hemisacrum of variable extent, through which the meninges bulge (1,8) (Fig. 20). Frequently there are pelvic organ anomalies, but the spinal cord and cauda equina develop normally. The meningocele lies in the presacral, retroperitoneal space, and contains CSF. Neural elements are only rarely contained in the sac.

Symptoms generally result from mass effect of the sac on pelvic organs such as the rectum, bladder, uterus and sacral nerve roots. Although symptoms may occur in young children, these lesions most commonly present in the second and third decades with chronic constipation and urinary difficulties, or as obstetrical complications in women. Occasionally, headache while straining at stool (the result of CSF shift into the sac), or back pain and sciatica from nerve root irritation occurs. True neurological dysfunction of the lower limbs or bladder is rare (17,88). Meningitis is a well-recognized complication and may follow spontaneous microperforation of the rectum, rupture during labor, or attempted aspiration of the sac (94). Rectal or vaginal palpation will reveal a

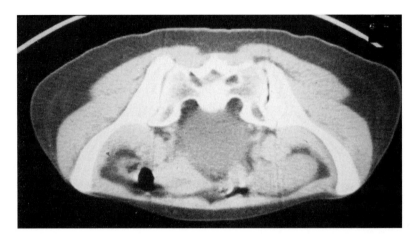

Figure 20   Plain CT scan demonstrating an anterior sacral meningocele.

smooth, cystic mass. Only if the mass is very large will it be palpable on abdominal examination.

Plain radiographs usually reveal some abnormality of the sacrum, classically the sickle-shaped "scimitar" deformity. Intravenous pyelography and cystography are necessary to delineate any accompanying urinary tract anomalies and will show displacement of the bladder and ureters by the mass. MRI demonstrates pelvic and spinal anatomy and may show the communication between the sac and the spinal canal. CT myelography is necessary if the presence or site of the communication remains doubtful after MRI.

Surgery is recommended for symptomatic lesions, as symptoms do not resolve spontaneously, and in women, where there is a risk of obstructed labor in pregnancy. Asymptomatic lesions may be followed of nonsurgically, provided pregnancy is not anticipated and the meningocele is not enlarging (1,68). In most cases, the lesion may be successfully managed by a sacral laminectomy, which allows inspection of nerve roots, division of any adhesions, and, after division of the filum terminale, identification of the opening of the meningocele. Removal of the entire pelvic cyst is unnecessary, and the goals of surgery are to decompress the sac, obliterate the fistula, and undo any tethering that may be present. An anterior transabdominal approach may be required if the dura is friable, or if the defect is too large to repair securely via a posterior approach.

REFERENCES

1. Amacher AL, Drake CG, McLaughlin AD. Anterior sacral meningocele. Surg Gynecol Obstet 1968; 126:986–994.
2. Anderson FM. Occult spinal dysraphism: A series of 73 cases. Pediatrics 1975; 55:826–835.
3. Applebaum H, Exelby PR, Wollner N. Malignant presacral teratoma in children. J Pediatr Surg 1979; 14:352–355.
4. Barson AJ. Spina bifida: The significance of the level and extent of the defect to the morphogenesis. Dev Med Child Neurol 1970; 12:129–144.
5. Bauer SB, Hallett M, Khoshbin S, Lebowitz RL, Winston KR, Gibson S, Colodny AH, Retik AB. Predictive value of urodynamic evaluation in newborns with myelodysplasia. JAMA 1984; 252:650–652.
6. Bentley JFR, Smith JR. Developmental posterior enteric remnants and spinal malformations: The split notochord syndrome. Arch Dis Child 1960; 35:76–86.
7. Bremer JL. Dorsal intestinal fistula; accessory neurenteric canal; diastematomyelia. Arch Pathol 1952; 54:132–138.
8. Brihaye J, Gerard A, Kiekens R, Retif J. Recto-meningeal fistulae in dysraphic states. Surg Neurol 1978; 10:93–95.
9. Brock DGH, Sutcliffe R.G. Alphafetoprotein in the antenatal diagnosis of anencephaly and spina bifida. Lancet 1972; 2:197–199.
10. Brock DGH. Alpha-fetoprotein and the prenatal diagnosis of neural tube defects. J R Coll Surg Edin 1978; 23:184–192.
11. Brocklehurst G. Spina Bifida for the Clinician. London: William Heinemann Medical Books, 1976.
12. Carr TL. The orthopedic aspects of 100 cases of spina bifida. Postgrad Med J 1956; 32:201–210.
13. Carter CO. Clues to the etiology of neural tube malformations. Dev Med Child Neurol (Suppl), 1974; 32:3–15.
14. Chapman PH, Beyerl B. The tethered spinal cord, with particular reference to spinal lipoma and diastematomyelia. In: Hoffman H. J., Epstein F, eds. Disorders of the Developing Nervous System: Diagnosis and Treatment. Boston: Blackwell Scientific Publishers, 1986; pp 109–131.
15. Cheek WR, Laurent JP. Dermal sinus tracts. Concepts Pediatr Neurosurg 1985; 6:63–75.
16. Cleland J. Contribution to the study of spina bifida, encephalocele and anencephalus. J Anat Physiol 1883; 17:257–292.
17. Cohn J, Bay-Nielson E. Hereditary defect of the sacrum and coccyx with anterior sacral meningocele. Acta Paediatr Scand 1969; 58:268–274.
18. Dennis M, Fitz CR, Netley CT, Sugar MA, Harwood-Nash DCF, Hendrick EB, Hoffman HJ, Humphreys RP. The intelligence of hydrocephalic children. Arch Neurol 1981; 38:607–615.
19. Dias MS, Walker ML. The embryogenesis of complex dysraphic malformations: A disorder of gastrulation? Pediatr Neurosurg 1992; 18:229–253.
20. Emery JL, Lenden RG. Clinical implications of cord lesions in neurospinal dysraphism. Dev Med Child Neurol (Suppl) 1972; 27:45–51.

21. Emery JL. The cervical cord of children with myelomeningocele. Spine 1986; 11:318–322.
22. Filston HC. Sacrococcygeal teratomas. In: Wilkins RH, Rengachary SS, eds. Neurosurgery. New York: McGraw-Hill, 1985; pp 2077–2080.
23. Fraser F. Genetic counselling in some common pediatric diseases. Am J Human Genet 1974; 26:636–661.
24. French BN. Midline fusion defects and defects of formation. In: Youmans JR, ed. Neurological Surgery. Philadelphia: WB Saunders, 1990; pp 1081–1235.
25. Gardner WJ. The Dysraphic States from Syringomyelia to Anencephaly. Amsterdam: Excerpta Medica, 1973.
26. Globus MS, Loughman WD, Epstein CJ, Halbasch G, Stephens JD, Hall BD. Prenatal genetic diagnosis in 3000 amniocenteses. N Engl J Med 1979; 300:157–163.
27. Guthkelch AN. Diastematomyelia with median septum. Brain 1974; 97:729–742.
28. Guthkelch AN, Pang D, Vries JK. Influence of closure technique on results in myelomeningocele. Child's Brain 1981; 8:350–355.
29. Guthkelch AN. Diastematomyelia. In: Wilkins RH, Rengachary SS, eds. Neurosurgery. New York: McGraw-Hill, 1985; pp 2058–2061.
30. Haldeman S, Bradley WE, Bhatia NN. Pudendal evoked responses. Arch Neurol 1982; 39:280–283.
31. Hendrick EB, Hoffman H, Humphreys RP. The tethered spinal cord. Clin Neurosurg 1983; 30:457–463.
32. Herren RY, Edwards JE. Diplomyelia (duplication of the spinal cord). Arch Pathol 1940; 30:1203–1214.
33. Hilal SK, Marton D, Pollack E. Diastematomyelia in children. Radiology 1974; 112:609–621.
34. Hoffman HJ, Hendrick EB, Humphreys RP. The tethered spinal cord: Its protean manifestations, diagnosis and surgical correction. Child's Brain 1976; 2:145–155.
35. Hoffman HJ. The tethered spinal cord. In: Holtzman RNN, Stein BM, eds. The Tethered Spinal Cord. New York: Thieme-Stratton, 1985, pp 91–115.
36. Howarth JC, Zachary RB. Congenital dermal sinuses in children—their relation to pilonidal sinuses. Lancet 1955; 2:10–14.
37. Humphreys RP. Spinal dysraphism. In: Wilkins RH, Rengachary SS, eds. Neurosurgery. New York: McGraw-Hill, 1985; pp 2041–2058.
38. Jackson FE. Neurenteric cysts. Report of two cases of neurenteric cyst with associated meningitis and hydrocephalus. J Neurosurg 1961; 18:678–682.
39. James CCM, Lassman LP. Diastematomyelia. A critical survey of 24 cases submitted to laminectomy. Arch Dis Child 1964; 39:125–130.
40. James CCM, Lassman LP. Spinal Dysraphism–Spina Bifida Occulta. New York: Appleton-Century-Crofts, 1972.
41. James HE, Oliff M. Computed tomography in spinal dysraphism. J Comput Assist Tomogr 1977; 1:391–397.
42. James HE, Walsh JW. Spinal dysraphism. Curr Probl Pediatr 1981; 11:1–25.
43. Jennings MT, Clarren SK, Kokich VG, Alvord EC Jr. Neuroanatomic examination of spina bifida aperta and the Arnold-Chiari malformation in a 130-day human fetus. J Neurol Sci 1982; 54:325–338.

44. Jones PH, Love JG. Tight filum terminale. Arch Surg 1956; 73:556–566.
45. Källén B. Early embryogenesis of the central nervous system with special reference to closure defects. Dev Med Child Neurol (Suppl) 1968; 16:44–53.
46. Kapsenberg JG, Van Lookeren Campagne JA. A case of spina bifida combined with distematomyely, the anomaly of Chiari and hydrocephaly. Acta Anat (Basel) 1949; 7:366–388.
47. Keim HA, Greene AF. Diastematomyelia and scoliosis. J Bone Joint Surg 1973; 55A:1425–1435.
48. Khoury MJ, Erickson JD, James LM. Etiologic heterogeneity of neural tube defects: Clues from epidemiology. Am J Epidemiol 1982; 115:538–548.
49. Lemire RJ. Embryology of the central nervous system. In: Davis JA, Dobins JA, eds. Scientific Foundations of Paediatrics. London: William Heinemann Medical Books, 1974; pp 547–564.
50. Levin P, Anton SP. Intraspinal neurenteric cyst in the cervical area. Neurology 1964; 14:727–730.
51. Lichtenstein BW. Spinal dysraphism, spina bifida and myelodysplasia. Arch Neurol Psychiatry 1940; 44:792–810.
52. Lorber J. Results of treatment of myelomeningocele. An analysis of 524 unselected cases, with special reference to possible selection for treatment. Dev Med Child Neurol 1971; 13:279–303.
53. Lorber J. Spina bifida cystica. Results of treatment of 270 cases with criteria for selection for the future. Arch Dis Child 1972; 47:854–873.
54. McLaughlin JF, Shurtleff DB. Management of the newborn with myelodysplasia. Clin Pediatr 1979; 18:463–476.
55. McLone DG. Techniques for closure of myelomeningocele. Child's Brain 1980; 6:65–73.
56. McLone DG, Mutluer S, Naidich TP. Lipomeningoceles of the conus medullaris. Concepts Pediatr Neurosurg 1983; 3:170–177.
57. McClone DG, Dias L, Kaplan WE, Sommers MW. Concepts in the management of spina bifida. Concepts Pediatr Neurosurg 1985; 5:97–106.
58. McLone DG. Embryonic deformation and caudal suppression. In: Marlin AE, ed. Concepts in Pediatric Neurosurgery. Basel: S Karger, 1987; pp 169–171.
59. McLone DG, Naidich TP. Myelomeningocele: Outcome and late complications. In: McLaurin RL, Schut L, Venes JL, Epstein F, eds. Pediatric Neurosurgery. Philadelphia: WB Saunders, 1989; pp 53–70.
60. McLone DG, Naidich TP. The tethered spinal cord. In: McLaurin RL, Schut L, Venes JL, Epstein F, eds. Pediatric Neurosurgery. Philadelphia: WB Saunders, 1989; pp 71–96.
61. Matson DD, Woods RP, Campbell JR, Ingraham FD. Diastematomyelia (congenital clefts of the spinal cord): Diagnosis and surgical treatment. Pediatrics 1950; 6:98–112.
62. Matson DD. Neurosurgery of Infancy and Childhood. 2nd ed. Springfield, Ill: Charles C Thomas, 1969.
63. Milunsky A, Alpert E, Neff RK, Frigoletto FD Jr. Prenatal diagnosis of neural tube defects. IV. Maternal serum alpha-fetoprotein screening. Obstet Gynecol 1980; 55:60–66.

64. Morgagni JB. The Seats and Causes of Disease Investigated by Anatomy. London: A Millar and T Cadell, 1769.

65. MRC Vitamin Study Research Group. Prevention of neural tube defects: Results of the Medical Research Council vitamin study. Lancet 1991; 2:131–137.

66. Oakes WJ. Management of spinal cord lipomas and lipomyelomeningoceles. In: Wilkins RH, Rengachary SS, eds. Neurosurgery Update II. Vascular, Spinal, Pediatric, and Functional Neurosurgery. New York: McGraw-Hill, 1991; pp 345–352.

67. O'Rahilly R. Developmental Stages in Human Embryos, Part A: Embryos of the First Three Weeks (Stages 1 to 9). Washington, DC: Carnegie Institute of Washington, 1973.

68. Oren M, Lorber B, Lee SH, Truex RC Jr, Gennaro AR. Anterior sacral meningocele. Report of 5 cases and review of the literature. Dis Colon Rectum 1977; 20:492–505.

69. Padget DH. Spina bifida and embryonic neuroschisis—a causal relationship: Definition of postnatal confirmations involving a bifid spine. Johns Hopkins Med J 1968; 128:233–252.

70. Padget DH. Neuroschisis and human embryonic maldevelopment: New evidence on anencephaly, spina bifida and diverse mammalian defects. J Neuropathol Exp Neurol 1970; 29:192–216.

71. Page LK. Occult spinal dysraphism and related disorders. In: Wilkins RH, Rengachary SS, eds. Neurosurgery. New York: McGraw-Hill, 1985; pp 2053–2058.

72. Pang D. Tethered cord syndrome: Newer concepts. In: Wilkins RH, Rengachary SS, eds. Neurosurgery Update II. Vascular, Spinal, Pediatric, and Functional Neurosurgery. New York: McGraw-Hill, 1991; pp 336–344.

73. Park TS, Hoffman HJ, Hendrick EB, Humphreys RP. Experience with surgical experience of the Arnold-Chiari malformation in young infants with myelomeningocele. Neurosurgery 13 1983; 147–152.

74. Passarge E, Lenz W. Syndrome of caudal regression in infants of diabetic mothers. Pediatrics 1966; 37:672–675.

75. Patten BM. Embryological stages in the development of spina bifida and myeloschisis. Anat Rec 1946; 94:487.

76. Patten BM. Overgrowth of the neural plate in young human embryos. Anat Rec 1952; 113:381–393.

77. Penfield W, Coburn DF. Arnold-Chiari malformation and its operative treatment. Arch Neurol Psychiatry 1938; 40:328–336.

78. Powell KR, Cherry JD, Hougen TJ, Blinderman EE, Dunn MC. A prospective search for congenital dermal abnormalities of the craniospinal axis. J Pediatr 1975; 87:744–750.

79. Reigel DH. Tethered spinal cord. In: Humphreys RP, ed. Concepts in Pediatric Neurosurgery. Vol. 4. Basel: S Karger, 1983; pp 142–164.

80. Reigel DH. Spina bifida. In: McLaurin RL, Schut L, Venes JL, Epstein F, eds. Pediatric Neurosurgery. Philadelphia: WB Saunders, 1989; pp 35–52.

81. Rosen MJ. Pathophysiology and spinal deformity in myelomeningocele. In: McLauren RL, ed. Myelomeningocele. New York: Grune and Stratton, 1977; pp 565–579.

82. Rudy DC, Woodside JR. The incontinent myelodysplastic patient. Urol Clin North Am 1991; 18:295–308.

83. Schey WL, Shkolnik A, White H. Clinical and radiographic considerations of sacroccygeal teratomas: An analysis of 26 new cases and review of the literature. Radiology 1977; 125:189–195.

84. Sharpe N. Spina bifida. An experimental and clinical study. Ann Surg 1915; 61:151–165.

85. Sharrard WJW, Zachary RB, Lorber J, Bruce AM. A controlled trial of immediate and delayed closure of spina bifida cystica. Arch Dis Child 1963; 38:18–22.

86. Sharrard WJW. The segmental innervation of the lower limb muscles in man. Ann R Coll Surg Engl 1964; 35:106–122.

87. Sharrard WJW. Lordosis and lordo-scoliosis in myelomeningocele. In: McLauren RL, ed. Myelomeningocele. New York: Grune and Straton, 1977; pp 591–607.

88. Silvis RS, Riddle LR, Clark GC. Anterior sacral meningocele. Am Surg 1956; 22:554–566.

89. Smith ED. Congenital sacral anomalies in children. Aust N Z J Surg 1959; 29:165–176.

90. Stark G. The pathophysiology of the bladder in myelomeningocele and its correlation with the neurological picture. Dev Med Child Neurol (Suppl) 1968; 16:76–86.

91. Steegers-Theunissen, Smithells RW, Eskes TKAB. Update of new risk factors and prevention of neural tube defects. Obstet Gynecol Surv 1993; 48:287–293.

92. Stein SC, Schut L. Hydrocephalus in meningomyelocele. Child's Brain 1979; 5:413–419.

93. Streeter GL. Developmental Horizons in Human Embryos. Age Groups XI–XXIII. Embryology Reprint. Vol 11. Washington, DC: Carnegie Institute Of Washington, 1951.

94. Sutton L. Congenital anomalies of the spinal cord. In: Rothman RH, Simeone FA, eds. The Spine Philadelphia: WB Saunders, 1992; pp 315–348.

95. Thompson MW, Rudd NL. The genetics of spinal dysraphism. In: Morley TP, eds. Current Controversies in Neurosurgery. Philadelphia: WB Saunders, 1976; pp 126–146.

96. Till K. Spinal dysraphism. A study of congenital malformations of the lower back. J Bone Joint Surg 1969; 51B:415–422.

97. Trowbridge A. Three cases of spina bifida, successfully treated. Boston Med Surg J 1828; 1:753.

98. Tryfonas G. Three spina bifida defects in one child. J Pediatr Surg 1973; 8:75–76.

99. Venes JL, Stevens EA. Surgical pathology in tethered cord secondary to myelomeningocele repair: Implications for initial closure technique. Concepts Ped Neurosurg 1983; 4:165–185.

100. Villarejo FJ, Blazquez MG, Gutierrez-Diaz JA. Intraspinal lipomas in children. Child's Brain 1976; 2:361–370.

101. Von Recklinghausen F. Untersuchungen über die Spina bifida. Virchows Arch [Pathol Anat] 1886; 105:243–373.

102. Wald NJ, Cuckle H, Brock JH, Peto R, Polani PE, Woodford FP. Maternal serum-

alpha-fetoprotein measurement in antenatal screening for anencephaly and spinal bifida in early pregnancy. (Report of United Kingdom collaborative study on alpha-fetoprotein in relation to neural tube defects.) Lancet 1977; 1:1323–1332.

103. Walker AE, Bucy PC. Congenital dermal sinuses; a source of spinal meningeal infection and subdural abscesses. Brain 1934; 57:401–421.

104. Warder DE, Oakes WJ. Tethered cord syndrome and the conus in a normal position. Neurosurgery 1993; 33:374–378.

105. Warkany J. Morphogenesis of spina bifida. In: McLaurin RL, ed. Myelomeningocele. New York: Grune and Stratton, 1977; pp 31–39.

106. Williams DI, Nixon HH. Agenesis of the sacrum. Surg Gynecol Obstet 1957; 105:84–88.

107. Winter RB, Haven JJ, Moe JH, Lagaard SM. Diastematomyelia and congenital spinal deformities. J Bone Joint Surg 1974; 56A:27–39.

3

The Chiari Malformations

R. John Hurlbert
University of Calgary, Calgary, Alberta, Canada

Michael G. Fehlings
The Toronto Hospital and University of Toronto, Toronto, Ontario, Canada

I. HISTORICAL PERSPECTIVE

Although named Chiari malformations, the first description of such hindbrain abnormalities was provided in a series of nine fetal and infant autopsies and two chick embryo dissections by Cleland in 1883 (23). In a full-term infant with meningomyelocele, Cleland described an elongated brainstem with fourth ventricular herniation into the cervical spinal canal.

Hydrocephalus, tectal beaking, and cervical hydromyelia (without fourth ventricular communication) were also detailed. Another autopsy in the series described herniation of the cerebellum and cerebrum into an occipital encephalocele. Although in his discussion Cleland explored the pathophysiology in the development of these anomalies, attributing them to fetal hydrocephalus, he did not choose to subclassify them, but instead preferred to consider all as arising from a common etiology.

A decade later, Chiari presented four types of congenital hindbrain anomalies associated with hydrocephalus, pioneering the classification system still in use today (18–20). A few years after this, Arnold published a report of meningomyelocele, noting the associated caudal displacement of the cerebellum and brainstem (8). His students would later point out this similarity to the type II anomaly described by Chiari, unfortunately originating the term "Arnold-Chiari" malformation (82). Predictably, the use of this term has lead to widespread confusion, primarily because of loose application to both the type I and II conditions. Hence, it has come to have historical significance only. The original and unambiguous "Chiari II malformation" is much preferred.

The first description of an abnormal, fluid-filled space within the spinal cord was published in 1546 by Estienne (35). Cavitation within the spinal cord in continuity with the fourth ventricle was noted by Ollivier d'Angers in 1824 and subsequently termed syringomyelia (69,70). The Greek origin of this word translates literally to tubular cavitation of the spinal cord. As a disorder of the central nervous system (CNS), syringomyelia has many causes. However, it is most commonly associated with developmental hindbrain abnormalities and, therefore, its treatment is an important facet in the management of the Chiari malformations. In 1892, Abbe and Coley performed the first successful operation directed at decompressing a syringomyelic cavity (1). It was not until well into the 1950s that Gardner put forth his hydrodynamic theory and described craniocervical decompression as being of benefit in the treatment of patients with syringomyelia when associated with abnormalities at the foramen magnum (39). This remains the cornerstone of treatment today. The terminal ventriculostomy was proposed in 1977 as a means to drain syrinx fluid in the setting of failed craniocervical decompression (40). The procedure involved excision of the filum terminale along with the tip of the conus (terminal ventricle) in an effort to drain a communicating syrinx through a patent central canal. However, subsequent reports were unable to reproduce the success of the initial claims and the operation has become one of historical note only (99).

Cerebellar tonsillar herniation arising from iatrogenic causes was first described by Hoffman and Tucker in 1976 in 8 children undergoing ventriculoperitoneal or lumboperitoneal shunting (45). Since then, several other reports have been added to the literature, including some with radiographic documentation of normalcy at the craniocervical junction prior to the shunting procedure (21,74,88,94). The incidence of acquired Chiari may be as high as 70% after lumboperitoneal shunting, with two-thirds or more of the symptomatic patients requiring surgical intervention for progressive or disabling symptomatology (21,74). Although the proportion of patients with acquired Chiari who are symptomatic is variable (4–60%), sudden death due to respiratory arrest has been reported, underscoring the potential severity of the disorder (21,74). The time to onset of symptoms from shunt placement ranges from a few months to several years. The postoperative outcome in this group of patients is generally good to excellent (80–100% resolution of symptoms not related to myelopathy), with removal of the lumbar shunt followed by insertion of a ventriculoperitoneal catheter or craniocervical decompression as indicated (21,45,74,88,94). Follow-up magnetic resonance (MR) sequences have demonstrated return of the tonsils to a normal position above the foramen magnum in a number of these patients (74,88).

II. DEFINITIONS

Chiari classified congenital hindbrain herniations based on their location and the degree of herniation (Table 1) (18–20). The type I Chiari malformation is represented by caudal descent of the cerebellar tonsils through the foramen magnum (Figs. 1 and 2). It is associated with arachnoidal adhesions between the cerebellar tonsils and hydromyelia or syringomyelia (Figs. 3 and 4). The aqueduct is frequently elongated and narrowed, and the fourth ventricle may be stretched and thinned. Kinking of the lower medulla is common, but herniation of the medulla itself through the foramen magnum is rare (85). Except in severe cases, the upper cervical nerve roots project inferiorly as they exit the spinal cord. The posterior fossa is more shallow than usual, with flattening of the squamous occipital bone. In addition, the diameter of the foramen magnum is enlarged. With the advent of MR imaging, strict criteria have been adopted to assist in making the diagnosis of a Chiari I malformation (see below).

The type II Chiari malformation is associated with much more extensive pathology throughout the craniospinal axis. It typically occurs in the setting of meningomyelocele and hydrocephalus (see Chapter 2). In addition to herniation of the cerebellar tonsils, the cerebellar vermis, fourth ventricle, and medulla also protrude through the foramen magnum. Because the cervical cord is supported by the dentate ligament, the downward migration of the medulla produces a kink just caudal to the cuneate and gracile nuclei. In more severe cases, the medulla, cerebellar vermis, and pons are all displaced below the level of the foramen magnum. The upper cervical roots project superiorly as they leave the spinal cord. The pons is thin and elongated, and the fourth ventricle

Table 1   Classification of Chiari Malformations

	Herniation	Associated anomalies
Type I	Foramen magnum tonsils only	Shallow post fossa Syringomyelia
Type II (Arnold-Chiari)	Foramen magnum tonsils, vermis fourth ventricle medulla, pons	Shallow post fossa Meningomyelocele Syringomyelia Hydrocephalus
Type III	Meningocele high cervical suboccipital	—
Type IV	None	Cerebellar hypoplasia
Acquired Chiari	Same as Type I	Usually none

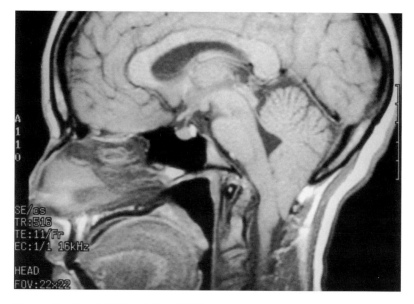

Figure 1 Sagittal T1-weighted MRI of type I Chiari malformation illustrating the downward herniation of tonsils with compression of the cervicomedullary junction.

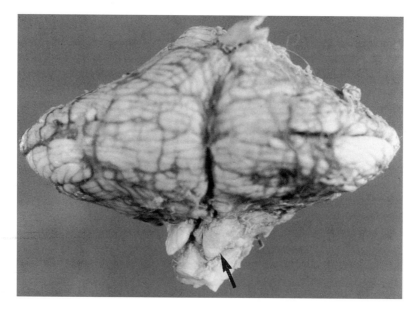

Figure 2 Postmortem case of type I Chiari malformation. Note the compressed, gliotic tonsils (arrow) and the effect of the shallow posterior fossa on the appearance of the cerebellum.

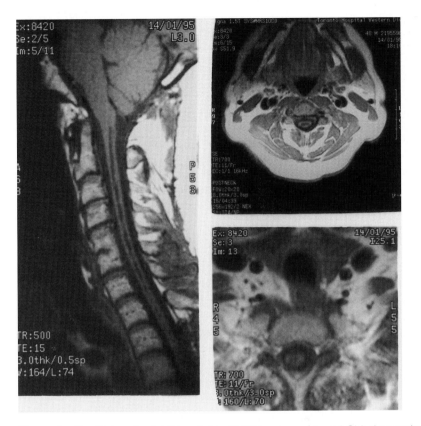

Figure 3   Sagittal and axial T1-weighted MRI images of type I Chiari associated with syringomyelia.

is typically slit-like in its course through the foramen magnum. The tentorium cerebelli are low lying, often with the superior cerebellum displaced upwards through the incisura. Several other CNS abnormalities occur with variable frequency (Table 2).

Abnormalities in the skull and dural partitions are commonly associated with Chiari II malformations. Lacunae of the skull, also referred to as lückenschädel, can be identified in utero and are present in 85% or more of patients at birth (66). The lacunae disappear in most cases by 6 months of age. Erosion of the posteromedial aspect of the petrous pyramids (petrous scalloping) and enlargement of the foramen magnum are frequently noted. Partial absence, hypoplasia, or fenestrations in the falx cerebri are also common, leading to tight apposition between the left and right cerebral hemispheres with interdigitation or even pial fusion appreciated on MRI or computed tomography (CT). In asso-

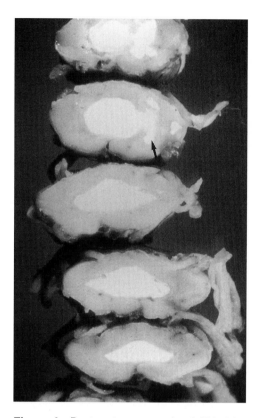

Figure 4 Postmortem example of Chiari I associated syringomyelia. The syringomyelic cavity has been filled with barium. Note the eccentric cavity (arrow) in communication with the expanded central canal in the cervical cord. Cross-sections are through the cervical and upper thoracic cord.

ciation with the small posterior fossa, the tentorium is hypoplastic, creating a wide incisura, and attaches to the caudal aspect of the occiput near the foramen magnum.

In certain instances, there may be some confusion in the distinction between Chiari I and II malformations. Kinking of the cervicomedullary junction and caudal dislocation of the medulla have been used to diagnose Chiari II malformations presenting in adults in the absence of a neural tube defect (32). However, brainstem descent has been described as a feature in the Chiari I malformation even as far back as Chiari's original accounting (20,49,73,84). Similarly, varying degrees of hindbrain herniation have been observed in patients with known myelomeningocele, sometimes with only the tonsils protrud-

Table 2 Associated Features of Chiari II

Supratentorial
  Lückenschädel of the skull
  Polygyria
  Cortical heterotopia
  Dysgenesis or agenesis of the corpus callosum
  Hypertrophy of the massa intermedia
  Arachnoid cysts
  Tectal beaking

Infratentorial
  Small shallow posterior fossa
  Scalloping of the petrous bone
  Low-lying tentorium cerebelli
  Enlarged incisura
  Loss of the pontine flexure
  Aqueductal forking or stenosis
  Caudal displacement of the basilar artery

Source: Modified from Ref. 58.

ing through the foramen magnum, more in keeping with the "idiopathic" adult-onset variety (17,91). The clinical relevance of attempting to differentiate hindbrain malformations into Chiari I and II based on poorly defined anatomical criteria has not been established. Furthermore, the pathogenesis of the two conditions has not been shown to be absolutely distinct; rather, current theories have much in common. Consequently, we agree with others in defining the Chiari II malformation as cerebellar ectasia in the presence of a neural tube defect, regardless of associated abnormalities or age of onset (75).

Caudal displacement of the cerebellum and brainstem into a high cervical or suboccipital meningocele constitutes the Chiari III anomaly. The incidence is rare. A Chiari IV malformation is represented by cerebellar hypoplasia without cerebellar herniation. These last two categories are mentioned for the sake of completeness only and will not be further discussed, as their neurosurgical relevance is very restricted.

The final subgroup of the Chiari classification has become more prevalent in the last few decades as a result of neurosurgical practices. The iatrogenic or "acquired Chiari" malformation is not a congenital herniation nor was it a clinically recognized entity at the time of Chiari's original classification. This condition presents in adulthood with all the signs and symptoms attributable to the Chiari I malformation. Cerebellar herniation through the foramen magnum (which is usually normal in size) arises from alterations in normal cerebrospinal fluid (CSF) dynamics either as a result of posterior fossa/upper cervical spinal cord surgery or from the introduction of a lumboperitoneal shunt.

Hydromyelia refers to a cavity within the spinal cord that is lined with ependyma and therefore involves the central canal. A cyst outside of the central canal, and thus without an ependymal lining, is referred to as a syrinx (resulting in the diagnosis of syringomyelia). Differentiation between the two conditions is made purely on a histological basis and has little, if any, role in treatment planning. Therefore, the distinction between the two entities as they pertain to Chiari malformations is not relevant and for the purposes of this chapter, they will both be considered under the heading syringomyelia.

III. EPIDEMIOLOGY

A. Chiari I

The incidence of asymptomatic Chiari I malformations is not known. With the advent of noninvasive screening, a large segment of the population has been exposed to MRI and a relatively high prevalence of the condition has become apparent (2,12). In a review of sequential MR studies at one institution, the incidence of Chiari I malformation has been estimated to be as high as 0.6%, or 1 in every 200 people (33).

Up to 31% of all Chiari I malformations may become symptomatic (33). When tonsillar ectasia does become problematic, presentation is typically well into adulthood. Most patients note the onset of symptoms in the third to fifth decades (32,33,62,73,75); 75% then seek medical attention in the fourth to sixth decades, whereas only 5% present later. Thus, as is apparent, the symptoms may have experienced for a few months to many years. Women may have a higher preponderance toward this condition than men, on the order of 3:2 (33,49,80). Although most cases are sporadic, familial tendencies have been described, suggesting transmission through an autosomal dominant pattern in rare instances (24,86).

B. Chiari II

Neural tube defects occur in approximately 1 of every 1000 live births in North America, with a higher incidence reported in the United Kingdom and Hungary (61). Approximately 10–20% of children with meningomyelocele develop symptoms referrable to cranial nerve, cerebellar, or brainstem dysfunction (13,44). However, 90% of children with meningomyelocele have various degrees of hindbrain herniation at autopsy, arguing for a large asymptomatic group in this population as well (91). There is a higher incidence when the neural tube defect is at or above L3 (17).

Despite aggressive medical and surgical intervention, hindbrain abnormalities constitute the principle cause of death in patients born with neural tube defects (58). Symptoms of the Chiari II malformation present in infancy, typically before 3 months of age (13). As a direct result of the association now established between neural tube defects and folic acid, a reduction in the incidence of Chiari II malformations by 50% or more may be expected through food fortification (61,64).

C. Acquired Chiari

Acquired Chiari malformations occur in patients after some type of neurosurgical intervention. The most common procedure associated with this abnormality is insertion of a lumboperitoneal shunt either for the treatment of communicating hydrocephalus or benign intracranial hypertension. Although the true incidence is not known, tonsillar herniation may occur in up to 70% of these patients (74).

D. Syringomyelia

Syringomyelia occurs in about 30–40% of Chiari I malformations (2,6,33,72,73,87), although incidences of 60% or more have been reported (28,75,81). The frequency may be less in Chiari II malformations (15,87).

IV. ETIOLOGY AND PATHOGENESIS

A. Chiari I

The pathogenesis of Chiari I malformations is unknown. There remains some debate as to the actual nature of the syndrome presenting in adulthood. In his original descriptions, Chiari described hindbrain anomalies in infants and preterms; hence the congenital association. Subsequent descriptions of tonsillar herniation in adults assumed the condition to have been present since birth. However, this assumption has been challenged. Trauma at birth has also been postulated as a factor in the development of Chiari I in certain cases (96,98). Excessive molding of the skull plates during a difficult delivery was thought to press the brain down into the foramen magnum with resulting anoxia, hemorrhage, and hydrocephalus setting the stage for chronic ectopia. Alternatively, tonsillar ectopia may not be a secondary event but may represent a primary developmental defect in which genetic factors are important (84,86). However, the role of a craniospinal CSF pressure gradient in the pathogenesis of this condition is at least suggested by similarity of the presenting features, radiographic evidence of tonsillar herniation sometimes with syringomyelia, and favorable outcome with surgical intervention in those cases arising from iatrogenic causes. Welch has proposed that spontaneous Chiari I malformations arise as a result of impaired cranial CSF absorption in the presence of maintained spinal CSF absorption, leading to a relative craniospinal pressure gradient (94).

The reasons why patients with Chiari I malformation may remain asymptomatic or present well into adulthood are not known. Clinical symptoms may be related to arachnoidal scarring and adhesions near the foramen magnum, perhaps caused by the movement of tonsils against bone over many years. The resulting interference with CSF dynamics is certainly related to the development of syringomyelia. That syringomyelia is a secondary event arising as a consequence of tonsillar herniation is supported by observations of discordance in monozygotic twins (87). Arachnoidal adhesions are also likely to be a secondary phenomenon as a distinct lack of adhesions has been observed in children undergoing surgery for Chiari I malformation (25).

B. Chiari II

Although we clinically distinguish between Chiari I and II malformations based on the presence or absence of a neural tube defect, abnormal CSF flow patterns may simply provide a "common final pathway" for different degrees of tonsillar herniation. The larger extent of tonsillar herniation generally seen in the type II anomalies compared with those encountered in type I may be linked to a greater disruption of normal CSF flow at a time when the nervous system is still developing. The importance of CSF shunting in spina bifida aperta is underscored by the high incidence of hydrocephalus after repair of an open meningomyelocele. Recently, the midbrain distortion and beaking of the tectal plate seen in Chiari II malformations has been likened to changes seen in the midbrain of patients with *acquired* Chiari malformation, lending further support to the importance of CSF venting from meningomyelocele in the pathogenesis of tonsillar herniation in Chiari II (21). The rarity of Chiari malformations in closed forms of meningomyelocele also argues for altered CSF flow as a causative factor. The brainstem dysfunction associated with Chiari II malformations appears to be acquired rather than congenital (76). Thus, the cerebellar displacement of Chiari I and Chiari II malformations may represent a common spectrum of a single clinical disease state.

The dysraphic condition occurring in the setting of a Chiari II malformation has been proposed to arise from many causes including: (1) an arrest of normal closure of the neural tube; 2) overgrowth during neurulation; 3) reopening of a closed neural tube; or 4) as an event secondary to altered CSF dynamics (see Chapter 2). Recent evidence has linked the condition to maternal vitamin B_6 (thiamine) levels. Preconceptual vitamin supplementation can significantly reduce the incidence of meningomyelocele and the associated Chiari II malformation.

After an extensive study of animal and human material, McLone has proposed a unified theory to explain the development of Chiari II malformations (57,58). He suggests that a series of interrelated, time-dependent defects occurs in the developing ventricular system, resulting in not only the Chiari II malformation of the hindbrain but also in the other associated CNS anomalies. As a result of failed neurulation, a dorsal myeloschisis is created that leads to excessive drainage of ventricular CSF through the defect. Subsequently, the ventricular system is unable to distend as it normally would, altering the inductive effect of pressure and volume on the surrounding mesenchyme and on endochondral bone formation. A small posterior fossa results, within which the developing cerebellum and brainstem expand and herniate through the incisura and foramen magnum. Close approximation of the thalami because of ventricular collapse leads to hypertrophy of the massa intermedia. Nondistention of the telencephalic vesicles leads to migrational defects (dysgenesis of the corpus callosum, cortical heterotopias, polygyria) and disorganized ossification of the skull (lückenschädel).

As opposed to Gardner's unifying theory in which hydrocephalus is proposed to *initiate* tonsillar and brainstem herniation, McLone suggests that hydrocephalus arises as a *result* of the hindbrain herniation. Specifically, outflow may be impaired by "collapse-induced" developmental abnormalities (blockage) at the cerebral aqueduct, obstruction of the outlets of the fourth ventricle, or obstruction at the level of the incisura. It is equally possible that the abnormally low CSF pressure, as a result of overdrainage, may have an adverse effect on developing arachnoid granulations, eventually leading to hydrocephalus, especially after closure of the neural tube defect.

C. Acquired Chiari

Two theories have been put forward to explain the development of the acquired Chiari malformation. In the pediatric population, shunting procedures can be associated with the arrest of skull growth. The cephalocranial disproportion theory suggests that after insertion of a lumboperitoneal shunt, the cranial contents grow faster than the surrounding cranial vault, resulting in downward displacement of the cerebellar tonsils (45,74). Skull growth is again eventually stimulated as the brain continues to expand, but not before a transient increase in intracranial pressure produces herniation of the cerebellar tonsils through the foramen magnum. However, this theory does not explain why acquired Chiari malformations are so rare after routine ventriculoperitoneal shunting procedures. In addition, this theory does not account for the syndrome arising in patients whose shunting procedures were performed after normal cessation of brain and skull growth. Finally it does not allow for resolution of cerebellar displacement after removal of a shunt.

The cranialspinal pressure gradient theory invokes a relatively low pressure in the spinal CSF compartment as the cause of the acquired Chiari malformation (36). The resulting cranial-to-caudal directed pressure gradient eventually drives the tonsils down into the foramen magnum. Progression through worsening degrees of herniation could take months or years to become symptomatic. This theory is similar to the cranialspinal pressure dissociation theory proposed by Cameron and modified by Williams to explain the development of syringomyelia in patients with hindbrain herniation (17,95,98).

D. Syringomyelia

Altered CSF flow arising from tonsillar herniation has long been thought to contribute to the formation of syringomyelia. O'Connel was among the first to link movement of the brain to movement of CSF in 1943 (48). Although CSF pulsations were later proposed to arise from the choroid plexus, subsequent studies linked CSF flow to the cardiac cycle and elasticity of the cerebral arteries and veins (14,27,28). The normal pattern of CSF flow is closely related to the cardiac cycle (7,22,27). The pulsations in the basal cisterns arise from expansion of the cerebral hemispheres and are an order of magnitude greater in volume than the concordant pulsations within the ventricular system (28). Caudal CSF pulsations in the cisterns are greatest in systole, whereas cranial pulsations are greatest in diastole. The direction of flow at the foramen magnum and at C2 during the very early phase of systole (within the first 100 msec) is in a cranial direction. This represents isovolumetric contraction of the left ventricle before blood leaves the aortic valve. Then, as the stroke volume is pumped into the cerebral arterial tree, caudally oriented CSF flow is produced and lasts through middle systole to late systole. The end of systole (corresponding to the dichrotic notch) sees a second but smaller caudal efflux of CSF, which reverses to cranially directed flow once again in early diastole, as blood leaves the brain and hemispheric volume diminishes. In general, caudally directed CSF flow patterns predominate over cranially directed flow and are of higher velocity. Pediatric flow rates tend to be higher than adult rates.

In normal subjects, the brainstem and cerebellum remain motionless within the posterior fossa despite this pulsatile movement of the cerebral hemispheres and CSF. However, in patients with Chiari malformations, pulsatile movements of the cerebellar tonsils are noted in a downward direction into the upper cervical canal during systole followed by retraction during diastole (28). As a result, obstruction of CSF flow occurs at the craniocervical junction. In type I Chiari malformations, both the velocity and the duration of caudal CSF flow are reduced at the foramen of Magendie and foramen magnum. Indeed, flow direction across the foramen magnum during middle-to-late systole actually tends to be cranially directed, in direct contrast to the caudal flow seen in normal individuals. Cranial CSF flow velocities are also reduced (7). Farther down the spinal column, CSF surrounding the cervical spinal cord and within an associated syrinx cavity moves caudally during systole and cranially during diastole (68). The cord and syrinx both constrict during systole and expand during diastole.

During craniospinal decompression, pulsatile systolic constrictions of the spinal cord and syrinx cavity cease immediately after opening of the dura (with preservation of the arachnoid), as do the downward movements of the cerebellar tonsils. Postoperatively (after lysis of adhesions and duraplasty), CSF flow patterns through the foramen magnum are markedly changed. Up to a threefold increase in the peak velocity of CSF flow results, with a dramatic prolongation of caudal flow through middle-to-late systole. The restoration of a more normal pattern of CSF flow is associated with improvement or resolution of clinical symptomatology and radiographic collapse of associated syringomyelia (7,68).

Thus, in summary, expansion of the cerebral hemispheres during systole causes downward flow of CSF through the tentorial incisura (and to a lesser degree through the aqueduct of Sylvius). It appears that in Chiari malformations, as a result of a small posterior fossa and reduced cisterna magna, systolic CSF outflow through the foramen magnum is restricted, and a "ball-valve" mechanism further impacts the herniated cerebellar tonsils against the foramen. Hence, the normal caudal flow of CSF throughout most of systole is severely restricted. A craniospinal pressure gradient is created and then relieved during diastole with relaxation of the brain. More normal CSF flow patterns are restored through surgical decompression by providing a route for CSF to travel past the cervicomedullary junction and are associated with clinical improvement. However, the mechanism by which these altered CSF dynamics contribute to syrinx formation and expansion is purely speculative and the subject of much debate. Nonetheless, a better understanding of this mechanism is critical to the development of improved treatment strategies. Several hypotheses have been proposed.

1. The Hydrodynamic Theory

Gardner's hydrodynamic theory was put forth in the late 1950s and early 1960s to replace the long-held belief that syringomyelia arose from areas of cystic degeneration in nests of glial proliferation scattered throughout the spinal cord. Gardner suggested that syringomyelia arose from dilatation of the central canal of the spinal cord (39). The cavitations were created by exaggerated ventricular pulsations, produced by the choroid plexus, in the face of obstruction of normal fourth ventricular outflow (foramina of Luschka and Magendie). A failure to develop permeability to CSF flow in the roof of the fourth ventricle between weeks 6 and 8 of embryonal development prevented CSF from escaping through its normal pathways. The subsequent hydrocephalus caused posterior displacement of the primitive transverse sinus and herniation of the posterior hindbrain and cerebellum through the foramen magnum. Because of obstruction at the foramina of Luschka and Magendie, the water-hammer effect of the choroid plexus-driven CSF not only maintained patency of the central canal through the obex but caused dilatation and hydromyelia and syringomyelia. Increased intracranial venous pressure from a Valsalva maneuver or jugular venous pressure was felt to distend the intracranial venous compartment, causing further caudal displacement of CSF from the fourth ventricle into the central canal, contributing to syrinx expansion. In the most severe cases, occurring early in utero, expanding syringomyelia resulted in decompression of the neural tube through the ectoderm or myelomeningocele. Subsequently, Gardner proposed relieving outflow obstruction through lysis of arachnoidal adhesions and treatment of the syrinx by plugging the obex. This procedure is still in use today.

2. The Cranial-Spinal Pressure Dissociation Theory

The cranial-spinal pressure dissociation theory was initially proposed by Cameron and later modified by Williams (17,95,96,98). Obstruction of cranial CSF flow downward into the spinal subarachnoid space was felt to occur at the foramen magnum as a result of tonsillar herniation. A cranial-spinal pressure gradient was thus created that caused CSF to flow from the fourth ventricle into the central canal, ultimately resulting in syrinx formation. In contrast to Gardner's theory, syrinx expansion was believed to be due to increases in intrathoracic pressure, not intracranial pressure. Sneezing or coughing expanded the epidural spinal veins and moved CSF into the cranial subarachnoid spaces through the foramen magnum. In doing so, the syrinx cavity was compressed, propelling fluid up and down the central canal and expanding the cavity ("slosh" effect). At the end of the Valsalva maneuvre, the return of CSF into the spinal subarachnoid space from the cranial cisterns was restricted by tonsillar herniation, maintaining an increased intracranial CSF pressure in the face of a much lower spinal CSF pressure. The pressure gradient forced CSF through the obex into the central canal, leading to further syrinx expansion ("suck" effect). Syrinx initiation was held to be primarily due to the suck mechanism in the face of hindbrain herniation. Measurements in patients with Chiari malformations in vivo have documented gradients in excess of 100 mm Hg after coughing episodes, lending support to these arguments (96,98).

Both Gardner's hydrodynamic and Williams' cranial-spinal pressure dissociation theories invoke flow of CSF through a patent communication between the fourth ventricle and the syrinx. However, Gardner believed obstruction to CSF flow arose from scarring of the fourth ventricular outlets, whereas Williams perceived CSF flow obstruction to be at the foramen magnum as a result of tonsillar herniation. In further contrast, the hydrodynamic theory proposes an arterial pulse pressure (from the choroid plexus) to act from within the neural axis in generating a syrinx, whereas the cranial-spinal pressure dissociation theory suggests a relatively prolonged intrathoracic venous pulsation to act initially on the syrinx cavity from outside (slosh) and then from inside (suck).

In a series of animal and human experiments, DuBoulay established that the periodic movements of CSF in the basal cisterns were due to expansion of the cerebral hemispheres in response to arterial inflow during systole (27,28). He proposed that in patients with tonsillar herniation, these movements produced a ball-valve plugging of the foramen magnum with the cerebellar tonsils. As a result of this impaction during systole, CSF was rerouted from the basal cisterns back into the fourth ventricle and into the central canal. Retraction of the tonsils and brainstem during diastole was proposed to create a "milking" action at the level of the foramen magnum, further propelling CSF along the central canal. Over time this resulted in the formation and expansion of a cervical syrinx. An increase in spinal venous pressure was felt to be more important than intracranial venous pressure in contributing to syrinx expansion after the Valsalva maneuver, as a large upward displacement of CSF throughout the spinal axis associated with up to 50% narrowing of the anteroposterolateral diameter of the thecal sac was noted with coughing.

3. Syringomyelia Without a Patent Central Canal

Ball and Dayan proposed that syringomyelia arose from the migration of CSF into the cord from dilated perivascular spaces (9). They observed prominent small arteries and veins in the walls of syrinxes studied at necropsy and noted that the dilated perivascular spaces were likely to represent enlarged Virchow-Robin spaces. India ink injected into the lumen of the syrinx spread centrifugally from the lumen by tracking around the blood vessels and could be found in the dorsal subarachnoid space. With obstruction at the foramen magnum, the authors proposed that CSF might dissect into the cord along the Virchow-Robin spaces. More recently, using cardiac-gated phase-contrast cine MRI imaging, Oldfield et al. have expanded on this theory after observing that abrupt caudal movement of syrinx fluid during systole was rendered stationary after craniocervical decompression (68). They suggest that cerebellar ectopia results in a continuous but partial block of CSF flow through the foramen magnum during both systole and diastole (caudal and cranial flow respectively). An accentuated systolic pressure wave in the upper cervical spinal canal is produced by the "piston-like" movement of the cerebellar tonsils into the foramen magnum during contraction of the left ventricle. The authors feel that the syrinx cavity is likely to originate from ceaseless systolic pressure waves driving CSF into the intramedullary compartment, through the surface of the spinal cord, through enlarged perivascular spaces, or perhaps through the dorsal root entry zones as originally suggested by Aboulker (3). Syrinx expansion, however, occurs as the pressure wave is transmitted to the walls of the syrinx causing compression of the cavity and propulsion of syrinx fluid caudally, much in the way of Williams' "slosh" phenomenon (but independent of venous pressure). This theory does not rely on communication between the fourth ventricle and central canal for formation or expansion of the syrinx.

4. A Perspective

There are many arguments either against or in favor of each of these hypotheses, alone or in various combinations. A few points are noteworthy however. The foramina of Luschka and Magendie have been shown to be patent in a large proportion of patients with Chiari malformations (28). Additionally, hydrocephalus is rare in patients with Chiari I malformations. Thus the foraminal obstruction and hydrocephalus of Gardner's hypothesis do not account for many instances of Chiari malformation with or without syringomyelia. Syringomyelia occurs predominately in the upper cervical region and is rare in the thoracic cord, suggesting the pathogenesis to be in the vicinity of the foramen magnum or herniated tonsils rather than widely dispersed throughout the spinal axis. Many of the theories discussed above have been heavily criticized because the human central canal has been thought to be vestigial, with obliteration occurring during childhood. However, although a progressive degree of stenosis does develop with age, a recent large autopsy series has demonstrated that most adults maintain a patent central canal in the upper cervical region throughout life (60). Therefore, it remains appropriate to consider a patent central canal in the pathogenesis of Chiari-associated syringomyelia. A combination of hydrodynamic and progressive degenerative mechanisms has been proposed to account for those patients who fail to benefit from craniocervical decompression (49).

The presence or absence of syringomyelia does not seem to be directly linked to the degree of tonsillar herniation (33).

V. PATHOLOGY

A.   Chiari Malformations

The hallmark of the Chiari I and II malformations is flattening of the cerebellar tonsils. This can easily be appreciated intraoperatively where indentation from the foramen magnum provides clear demarcation between the intracranial and extracranial tonsillar segments (Fig. 5). Associated abnormalities of the mid-brain and pons have recently been described in association with the Chiari I malformation (47). The midbrain can be enlarged, low in position, with an exaggerated cleft between it and the pons anteriorly. The pons can also be situated in a more inferior location than normal. Abnormal dilatations, aberrant course, and anomalous branches of the posterior inferior cerebellar artery can be present (73). Commonly, the cranial loop of the posterior inferior cerebellar

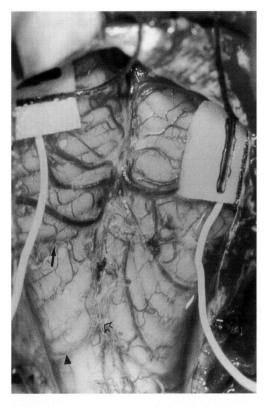

Figure 5 Intraoperative photograph of Chiari I malformation after posterior fossa decompression and opening of the dura for expansile duroplasty. The compressive effect of the foramen magnum is seen by the "kink" at the superior end of the tonsil (large arrow). Note the inferior extent of the tonsil (arrowhead) and intra-arachnoidal adhesions (open arrow). Incidental note is made of sub-dural recording electrodes (covered by cottonoids) used for cerebellar evoked potential recording.

artery is below the foramen magnum. Caudal displacement of the brainstem can sometimes be appreciated. The upper cervical cord and cervicomedullary junction may appear to be of normal diameter despite the presence of an underlying syrinx. A thick transverse cervicomedullary dural band, arachnoid adhesions with occlusion of the foramen of Magendie, and upward nerve root deviation may or may not be identified both intraoperatively or in postmortem specimens.

Paraffin-embedded specimens of the herniated tonsils demonstrate disorganization of all three cellular layers of the cerebellum (6). In the more severe Chiari II malformations, cerebellar cortical heterotopia is often manifested as displaced, discrete islands of Purkinje, granular, and basket cells deep within the cerebellar white matter (17). The pia-arachnoid is markedly thickened in the region of the herniation and contains prominent collections of thin-walled vessels and arteriovenous shunts. These vascular anomalies have been postulated to contribute to ischemia or anoxia of the brainstem with resulting symptomatology (6). Herniation of the tonsils and vermis produces atrophy in the form of neuronal dropout in all three cortical layers supplanted by a reactive astrocytic proliferation.

Postmortem examination of the brainstem region in children dying of meningomyelocele and Chiari II malformation shows vascular engorgement, hemorrhage, and focal areas of neuronal and axonal loss with hemosiderin deposition and gliosis (17). These changes are confined to that part of the hindbrain below the level of the foramen magnum. Partial obliteration of the subarachnoid space is due to thickening and adhesions between the pia and arachnoid. Cleft-like spaces are seen in the inferior vermis communicating with the fourth ventricle. Associated abnormalities consisting of thickening of the interthalamic ramus, hypoplasia of the falx cerebri, and partial obliteration of the interhemispheric fissure are commonly encountered. Cortical heterotopia (in the form of ependyma-lined nodules projecting into the walls of the lateral ventricles), cerebral microgyria, stenosis (disorganized ependyma and gliosis), and forking of the aqueduct are also frequently observed.

B. Syringomyelia

The dimensions of the syrinx cavity, both transverse and rostrocaudal, can vary widely. The cervical spinal cord is most usually affected, typically in the upper cervical region (33,41,75,87). When thoracic involvement is present, it extends from a cervical origin, except in very rare instances.

The cavities are incompletely lined by ependyma, the remaining being lined by subependymal astrocytic glial cells. Strands or septations of glial tissue partially divide the cavity into compartments to variable degrees. At least one pathological study has demonstrated communication between the cavity of eccentrically located syringomyelia and the central canal in 100% of cases (34) (Fig. 4). Furthermore, patency of the central canal has been shown to be a function of age and proximity to the cervicomedullary junction (60). Thus, communication between a syrinx and the fourth ventricle, although difficult to detect radiologically, is likely to occur in most instances.

VI. CLINICAL PRESENTATION

A. Chiari I

The clinical presentation of Chiari I malformations is usually delayed until the third to fifth decades, although pediatric presentations have been described (10,25,30–33,62,75,81). The mean duration from onset of symptoms to diagnosis varies depending on the series but has been reported from 1 month to 30 years, with an average duration of 3–7 years (49,80). Headache and neck pain are the most common presenting complaints (10,32,33,49,72,75,81). The common clinical findings can generally be considered to arise from cerebellar, bulbar, or spinal cord dysfunction. Nystagmus is the most frequent abnormality encountered on physical examination. Nystagmus is classically downbeat on neutral or horizontal gaze and rotatory on lateral gaze, but other forms can be observed. Lower cranial nerve palsies in the form of impaired swallowing (IX/X), shoulder or neck weakness (XI), and dysarthria or difficulty with food manipulation (XII) are also relatively frequent. Impaired function of cranial nerves V, VI, VII, and VIII has also been reported but is considerably more uncommon (32,83). Extremity weakness or numbness is usually related to the presence of a syrinx but can also be related to brainstem compression. The more common clinical findings are summarized in Table 3 (32,33,49,72,73,75,80,84). Although up to 40% of patients complain of gait disturbance, ataxia tends to be detected somewhat less frequently. The remaining patients are accounted for with extremity weakness or numbness. Trauma may aggravate existing symptoms or even precipitate the onset of new symptoms in a previously asymptomatic patient (84).

   The classic Chiari headache is described as a dull or throbbing occipital or suboccipital discomfort, originating days to years before the diagnosis is made. The headache is worsened by sudden changes of intracranial pressure either through an increase in intrathoracic pressure (cough, sneeze, straining) or postural changes of the head. Oral analgesics may or may not provide relief. Migraine prophylactic medications are typically ineffectual. This classic presentation is relatively rare, occurring in about 28% of patients with Chiari I, being more common in patients with more severe tonsillar herniation (72). It is un-

Table 3 Presenting Signs and Symptoms in Chiari I Malformations

Clinical findings	Frequency (%)
Headache/neck pain	50–70
Nystagmus	30–50
Extremity weakness/numbness (may be syrinx related)	10–55
Hyperreflexia/spasticity	10–50
Cranial nerve palsies (IX–XII)	10–20
Gait disturbance	5–40
Ataxia	5–20
Dysphagia	5–15
Dysarthria	5–10
Sleep apnea	0–10

clear whether the headache originates from dural irritation or stretching of the upper cervical nerve roots. Migraine and tension-type headaches are seen in the remaining Chiari I patients presenting with headache.

Dysphagia from IX and X dysfunction is manifest clinically as choking, gagging, pharyngonasal regurgitation, and recurrent pneumonia due to aspiration. The pathophysiology of dysphagia in Chiari malformations is not known but is likely due to a variety of causes, including developmental brainstem anomalies, brainstem compression, disruption of medullary gray matter from syringomyelia, and traction on peripheral nerves. The reversible nature of symptoms after craniocervical decompression argues for a non-destructive cause. The end result is a sensory, motor, or combined deficit contributing to the clinical presentation. The signs and symptoms result from either incomplete upper esophageal sphincter relaxation or pharyngoesophageal incoordination, evaluated by manometric or esophagographic testing. Although thought to be due to separate and distinct neuropathological substrates, the distinction between failed relaxation and incoordination in both Chiari I and II malformations has not been found to be clinically relevant (77). Manometry appears to be the most sensitive test currently available with which to monitor these patients. The presence of dysphagia is an ominous symptom that heralds an unremitting and relentless progression of swallowing difficulties, usually accompanied by the onset of other signs of brainstem compromise (76).

As previously mentioned, less common findings include trigeminal distribution pain, diplopia, facial weakness, and sensory neural deafness. Sudden cardiorespiratory arrest, sometimes resulting in death, has been associated with Chiari I malformations (37,53,90). Children with Chiari malformations may be more prone to spinal cord injury (16,93).

B. Chiari II

Signs and symptoms of the Chiari II malformation are similar to those described for Chiari I above, localizable to the cerebellum, brainstem, or spinal cord. However, there is considerable overlap with the presenting features of hydrocephalus, which must always be kept in mind. Symptoms tend to develop most frequently during the first 3 months of infancy and include stridor, apnea, and feeding difficulties (13). Irritability and neck stiffness can also be observed. Dysphagia is detected in the neonatal setting as poor feeding, prolonged feeding time, pooling of secretions in the oropharynx, and coughing or choking episodes during feeding (76). Apneic episodes, vocal cord paralysis, and a weak cry occur more frequently than with Chiari I malformations, probably as a result of the more extensive brainstem abnormalities associated with the Chiari II condition. When symptoms arise during childhood or adolescence, presenting abnormalities include hemiparesis, quadraparesis, oscillopsia, nystagmus, and opisthotonus. Long-tract findings suggestive of brainstem or spinal cord pathology may be obscured by the neurological changes accompanying the dysraphic state.

C. Acquired Chiari

The presentation of the acquired Chiari malformation is essentially the same as for Chiari I disorders.

D. Syringomyelia

Syringomyelia can present with almost any combination of spinal cord symptoms and signs. Pain is the most common presenting complaint, usually described as aching or burning in nature and typically lateralized to the face, trunk, or extremities. Neurological examination classically demonstrates a dissociated sensory loss in a cape-like distribution, involving deficits in pain and temperature appreciation with relative sparing of vibration and proprioception. Disruption of the decussating fibers of the spinothalamic pathways with sparing of the uncrossed primary afferents in the dorsal columns accounts for this presentation. With extension into the brainstem, medullary white matter can become involved leading to lower cranial nerve palsies, ataxia, and nystagmus. Often associated with these findings are back pain, muscular wasting, and spasticity. Occasionally trophic changes in the skin of the upper extremities can be detected. Weakness in the upper extremities is generally associated with atrophy and hyporeflexia, indicative of a lower motor neuron disorder, whereas in the

Table 4 Presenting Signs and Symptoms in Chiari I
Associated Syrinx

Clinical finding	Frequency (%)
Extremity numbness	45–65
Extremity weakness	40
Extremity pain	30 (40)[a]
Gait disturbance	10–70
Spasticity/hyperreflexia	10–50 (100)[a]
Headache/neck pain	10–40 (55)[a]
Nystagmus	10 (55)[a]
Bowel/bladder dysfunction	10 (10)[a]
Decreased facial sensation	10
Neuropathic joint	0–10
Scoliosis	Up to 100% in children (35)[a]

[a]( ) indicates pre-MRI.

lower extremities there is hyperreflexia and spasticity indicating an upper motor
neuron disorder. A major motor deficit is usually contralateral to the most prominent sensory disturbance. The clinical presentation and course are extremely
variable, but stepwise progression over months or years is the rule (15,52,56).
The symptoms at presentation of Chiari-associated syringomyelia, in order of
decreasing incidence, are summarized in Table 4 (33,41,50,87). Other studies on syringomyelia from any cause confirm that the most common presenting features are numbness, weakness, or pain in the upper extremities
(11,15,41,43,51,56,63). Patients often complain that pain or parasthesias are
aggravated by sneezing, coughing, or other Valsalva-like maneuvers. The mechanism underlying this transient or sometimes permanent worsening is unknown
but may involve more complete obstruction of the foramen magnum with neck
flexion (89).

The presence of a syrinx does not appear to be directly related to the
severity of tonsillar herniation but, in fact, may be most commonly associated
with an intermediate degree of herniation (75,87). However, when syringomyelia is present in a patient with Chiari I malformation, it (rather than the hindbrain anomaly) almost always accounts for the presenting signs and symptoms
(33,75). In children, syringomyelia from Chiari malformation is often associated with scoliosis (25).

The relatively low incidence of long-tract signs in more recent studies
compared to the pre-MRI era may reflect a trend toward earlier diagnosis.

VII. DIAGNOSIS

A. Chiari Malformations

The sagittal and parasagittal images of MR sequences have brought the precision of intraoperative and postmortem diagnosis into the preoperative clinical mainstream, especially with respect to the diagnosis of Chiari I malformations and syringomyelia. Radiographic evidence of a Chiari malformation has previously included failure of subarachnoid contrast (or air) to pass above the foramen magnum on myelography (pneumoencephalography) or inferior descent of the posterior inferior cerebellar artery or its tonsillar branches on vertebral angiography. With the advent of computerized tomography (CT), the diagnosis of tonsillar herniation was more readily made, especially with intrathecal metrizamide contrast. The midbrain enlargement sometimes seen in association with Chiari I anomalies has been difficult to distinguish from a brainstem glioma on the basis of CT findings alone (47). Magnetic resonance imaging has quickly become the gold standard for making the radiological diagnosis of Chiari malformation.

The foramen magnum can be precisely localized by MR techniques (Fig. 1). High signal intensity characteristics of CSF on T2-weighted images serve to obscure definition of the cerebellar tonsils; thus measurements of tonsillar position are made on T1 or proton-density images. Fat within the marrow of the clivus and basi-occiput gives off a high signal intensity on T1 images that can help to establish the level of the foramen magnum. However, it is the lack of signal (indicating the presence of cortical bone) at the lowest end of the clivus (basion) and the posterior lip of the foramen magnum (opisthion) that defines the line separating posterior fossa from spinal compartments (2,12,67). Magnetic resonance radiographic criteria used for diagnosis of Chiari I malformations have been developed based on patients with symptomatic tonsillar ectopia compared to normal controls. These include (1) Herniation of one or both cerebellar tonsils 5 mm or more below the plane of the foramen magnum; (2) Herniation of both cerebellar tonsils 3 mm below the foramen magnum if accompanied by other features consistent with a Chiari I malformation (e.g., syrinx, cervicomedullary kinking); and (3) The absence of clinical or radiographic evidence of a Chiari II malformation, prior cranial or cervical spinal surgery, previous shunting procedure, or intracranial mass lesion (2,12). These criteria have been widely adopted (33,75,87). The usual position of the cerebellar tonsils is 1–3 mm above the foramen magnum, but 14% of normal patients have tonsils that extend below the foramen by up to 3 mm (2,12). Ectopia of less than 2 mm is unlikely to be of clinical significance.

Asymmetry in the degree of tonsillar herniation by 5 mm or more is not uncommon, yet it is not associated with asymmetric neurological signs (33).

However, more extensive tonsillar herniation (mean = 12.3 mm) is associated with the presence of objective cranial nerve deficits. Conversely, less extensive tonsillar descent is found in incidental Chiari I anomalies (mean = 7.3 mm).

One-quarter to one-half of patients with symptomatic Chiari I malformation have associated skeletal, cerebral, or craniofacial anomalies (10,32,33,49, 50). These include:

- Atlanto-occipital assimilation
- Platybasia
- Basilar invagination
- Abnormal odontoid segmentation
- Fused cervical vertebrae
- Cervical ribs
- Fused thoracic ribs
- Lipoma of the corpus callosum
- Septo-optic dysplasia
- Choanal atresia
- Aqueductal stenosis
- Kyphoscoliosis (syrinx associated)

Chiari II malformations are usually defined in the presence of a known meningomyelocele. Magnetic resonance imaging is the diagnostic procedure of choice in this group of hindbrain anomalies as well. The degree of tonsillar herniation is generally more severe than that seen in Chiari I malformations (87). The various other brain abnormalities previously discussed are also evident.

B. Syringomyelia

One of the most significant advances in medicine this century has been the markedly improved means available to diagnose syringomyelia. Magnetic resonance imaging (Fig. 3) has become the first noninvasive procedure, not only to determine the exact location and dimensions of an intramedullary spinal cord lesion, but also the first to accurately distinguish between solid and cystic components. Magnetic resonance imaging has quickly established itself as the gold standard for the evaluation of syringomyelia because of its unprecedented degree of sensitivity and specificity. This imaging technique has proven far superior to the myelographic and delayed contrast CT imaging techniques of the past, where syrinxes were poorly defined as a routine, and completely missed in 1–5 out of every 10 patients (4,11,32,100).

On MR images, syrinx cavities are visualized as areas of low signal intensity on T1-weighted images and high signal intensity on T2 images, similar to the signal characteristics of CSF. Septations can often be visualized, especially on sagittal cuts, giving the syrinx a loculated type of appearance. Although sagittal views provide an excellent overall appreciation of the extent of a syrinx (and the craniocervical junction), axial images are more sensitive in detecting medium or small syrinxes (100).

It is important to note that the radiological extent of the syrinx does not correlate well with either the degree of neurological deficit or the duration of the symptoms (41,54). Therefore it is likely that current imaging techniques do not adequately visualize the true extent of the disease, arguing for even better techniques than MRI to evaluate these lesions in the future. The sensitivity for detecting clinically significant syringomyelia is not yet 100%, as patients with findings localized to the spinal cord without MRI evidence of syringomyelia have been reported (33).

In patients with or suspected of having dysphagia, swallowing studies in the form of a cine-esophagogram and (in less severe cases) pharyngoesophageal manometry are indicated. These studies are not only helpful in determining whether supplemental nutrition is required, but they also aid in determining which alternate feeding technique is best suited to the individual patient's needs. These quantitative assessments provide an objective means by which to follow patients' progress postoperatively and also bear directly on overall prognosis (76).

VIII. TREATMENT

A. Chiari I and II

As described earlier, the natural history of Chiari malformations is not known. In addition, there have been no randomized prospective trials evaluating the short-term or long-term efficacy of surgical intervention of Chiari malformations. Subsequently, guidelines for management as we enter the 21st century can only be based on "common-sense" principles and the historical experience of others. The treatment of Chiari malformations must be tailored to the clinical condition of the patient and not the radiographic findings alone. In the increasing number of patients with tonsillar herniation detected coincidently, observation in the form of routine follow-up is indicated. Similarly, the dimensions of a syrinx alone provide no indication for surgical intervention (41,54). When operative intervention is indicated, either by progressive or disabling symptomatology, the "top-down" approach suggested by Williams 12 years ago still applies today (shunt for hydro, postfossa decompression, then syringopleural shunt) [42,99].

Surgical decompression for Chiari I and II malformations consists of an occipital craniectomy or craniotomy with wide decompression of the foramen magnum. At our institutions, the bone of the foramen magnum is removed until the dura is receding away from the operative field at 90 degrees to the horizontal plane on either side of midline. Laminectomies are performed at C1 and C2, extending lower to accommodate more severe degrees of cerebellar or brainstem herniation. A generous duraplasty with tensor fascia lata is used to close a "Y"-shaped dural incision made over the cerebellar hemispheres extending the full length of the laminectomy. Brisk hemorrhage can be expected from relatively large intradural venous channels in the infant population undergoing decompression and should be aggressively controlled with metal clips (13). A running, nonabsorbable, multistranded synthetic suture is used to fasten the fascia graft to native dura and the edges are sealed with fibrin glue in an effort to decrease the incidence of CSF leak. The paraspinal musculature is closed snugly but not tightly. Closely spaced interrupted sutures are placed through the subcutaneous fascia/ligamentum nuchae and tightened securely.

It is not our practice to lyse arachnoidal adhesions or to shunt an associated syrinx at the time of primary surgery. Similarly, we have abandoned plugging of the obex as an initial form of treatment as it adds unnecessary morbidity to the procedure, has not been shown to improve outcome, and is not necessary to achieve postoperative collapse of a syrinx (7,32,50,68,81,89,97). Nevertheless, some surgeons still prefer to use a piece of muscle or fat to plug the obex after microsurgical lysis of arachnoidal adhesions (42,59,75) Follow-up clinical evaluation and MR studies are obtained at routine intervals. In those patients who remain symptomatic or deteriorate with evidence of a persistent syrinx on MR imaging, a shunting procedure is considered.

First-line surgical intervention for those few patients presenting with hydrocephalus is a ventriculoperitoneal shunt

B. Acquired Chiari

The treatment of an acquired Chiari malformation is to remove the lumboperitoneal shunt, replacing it if necessary with a ventriculoperitoneal shunt or some other cranial diversionary technique. Stereotactic placement of ventricular catheters can be used in cases in which ventricles are normal or small. Removal of the lumbar shunt will usually result in resolution of the symptoms coinciding with radiographic evidence of improvement (74). In those cases of symptomatic acquired Chiari due to bony removal at the posterior fossa, a duraplasty may be indicated, depending on the severity of the presenting complaints.

C. Syringomyelia

The first-line surgical treatment for a symptomatic syrinx in the presence of a Chiari malformation remains craniocervical decompression. Only after this surgery has failed should a direct approach to the syrinx be considered. Shunting of a cervical or thoracic syrinx is a complicated procedure with a relatively high potential for serious morbidity and even mortality. If possible, the shunt should be placed in the thoracic extension of the syrinx at T3 or lower. Alternatively, the lowest cervical level where the syrinx is accessible should be chosen. This serves to decrease or eliminate the potential for upper limb dysfunction as a result of the procedure and also decreases the length of shunt tubing required. A two- or three-level laminectomy is performed. Using microsurgical techniques, the dura is opened and the syrinx entered through a small myelotomy where the syrinx most closely approaches the posterior surface of the spinal cord. Intraoperative ultrasound has proven to be a valuable tool in confirming correct localization, especially in cases where the syrinx does not obviously extend near the posterior surface of the spinal cord. If the cyst is not immediately apparent near the dorsal surface of the cord, we prefer to make a small myelotomy in one of the dorsal root entry zones, thus traumatizing only one dorsal column. A midline myelotomy may also be considered, splitting the dorsal columns and sacrificing the dorsal spinal vein if necessary. However this procedure significantly increases the risk of a bilateral dorsal column deficit. A variety of shunting devices are available. We prefer to use a single piece of Silastic tubing with a blunted fenestrated proximal tip and an open distal end. We do not use a pressure- or flow-regulated valve. A 4-0 nonabsorbable, multistranded synthetic suture is used to snugly affix the shunt tubing to the arachnoid. The dura is closed by placing interrupted sutures on either side of the shunt tubing, running them rostrally and caudally and sealing with fibrin glue. We routinely use evoked potential monitoring as a measure of dorsal column integrity during this procedure, although low amplitude or absent responses are not uncommon in the setting of tonsillar herniation (63).

We have enjoyed most success with shunting into the pleural space. The pleural cavity is more readily available and also has a relatively negative pressure compared to the abdominal cavity. A syringoperitoneal shunt is an alternative procedure. We do not recommend syringosubarachnoid shunting, because our experience has shown that scarring in the subarachnoid space eventually blocks the shunt. Other institutions have also had poor experience with this technique (5,11,52). Intraoperative syringography and neuroendoscopy may come to play a role in the direct surgical decompression of syringomyelia (46,79).

Lumboperitoneal shunting, both with and without myelotomy, has been described as a surgical intervention for the treatment of syringomyelia (71,92).

However, in view of the small number of patients reported, the questionable benefits of surgery, and the absence of long-term follow-up, the hypothetical yet potentially disastrous risk of aggravating a pre-existing Chiari malformation weighs against recommending this procedure at this time.

D. Morbidity and Mortality

The postoperative complications vary, depending on the series, from 3–23% (32,49,73,80). Respiratory depression tends to occur most frequently at night and has led to a number of postoperative deaths (49,73). It is not related to intraoperative dissection of tonsillar arachnoidal adhesions. In surviving patients, the condition is transient, usually resolving within the first week of surgery. The more common complications are presented in Table 5 (32,49,73,80). The incidence of aseptic meningitis has been dramatically reduced since closure of the dura has become widespread practice.

Complications from syrinx-related operations include meningitis, shunt infections, neurogenic bladder (associated with urinary tract infections and sepsis), neurogenic pain syndrome, overdrainage (headache), underdrainage (obstruction), and sometimes worsening neurological defect. The overall complication rate tends to be high with these procedures, approaching 26% in some series (11).

Operative mortality has been historically quoted to be as high as 15% due to nonspecific causes such as air embolism, as well as related complications such as postoperative hemorrhage or respiratory compromise (26,38,49,97). However, this high mortality rate has not been borne out in other retrospective

Table 5 Complications from Craniocervical
Decompression

Complication	Incidence
Overall	3–23
Respiratory depression	0–14
CSF leak (including pseudomenigocele)	1–3
Meningitis (aseptic)	0–10
Meningitis (bacterial)	< 1
Wound hematoma	1–3
Weakness (temporary or permanent)	0–3
Sensory loss (temporary or permanent)	0–3
Cranial nerve palsy	0–1
Death (temporary or permanent)	0–1

reviews of relatively large surgical populations, including more recent ones, where postoperative deaths are in the order of 0–1% (32,50,73,75,80).

IX. PROGNOSIS

The natural history for patients with Chiari I malformations remains largely a mystery. Comparable proportions of nonsurgical patients have been found to deteriorate or remain stable when observed for a number of years for symptomatic Chiari I (62). When observed for long enough periods most patients, including those having undergone a previous surgical procedure, demonstrate long periods of stability interrupted by step-wise neurological deterioration (49). It is important to note however, that in unoperated patients, spontaneous remission of symptoms has not been recorded. This is in distinct contrast to patients undergoing surgical intervention in whom objective evidence of improvement is routinely reported. Nonetheless, there are no long-term studies to demonstrate that surgery significantly alters the overall natural course of the Chiari disorders.

The prognosis for relief from headache and neck pain in those patients undergoing posterior fossa decompression for Chiari I malformation is very good, with 85% claiming significant improvement or complete resolution (72). Cerebellar dysfunction also responds well to surgery (80). Up to 100% of patients with parasthesias and sensory deficits have been reported to experience improvement or resolution postoperatively (7), but most other series offer much more conservative figures on the order of 40% (80). Scoliosis has been reported to remain stable or improve in 70–100% of patients after craniocervical decompression with or without a secondary syrinx drainage procedure (25,65).

The long-term outcome for treated patients with Chiari II malformations is variable, depending to a large degree on the severity of their associated anomalies. Progressive neurological, orthopedic, or urological deterioration has been well documented in the face of early myelomeningocele repair associated with retethering of the spinal cord. However, relatively good success (80% improved) after second surgical intervention has been reported (78). Although the natural history is not fully understood, patients can enjoy freedom from neurological deterioration over prolonged periods (even through "growth spurts"), in spite of significant associated craniospinal anomalies (55).

Resolution of dysphagia after craniocervical decompression has been reported. In patients with both Chiari I and II malformations treated with manometry, esophagography, and pH testing for gastroesophageal reflux, alleviation of symptoms is reported as high as 100% (77). A more modest success rate of 30–70% has been observed in a larger series of patients (13,76). Not surprisingly, postoperative outcome is highly correlated with preoperative function. Chronic ventilatory dependence and death can ensue in cases presenting with advanced progression of brainstem dysfunction, underscoring the need for aggressive early surgical intervention in this particular group of patients (76).

In large operative series, overall outcome for craniocervical decompression with or without syrinx shunting ranges from a conservative estimate for improvement of 50% based on objective findings alone, to an estimate of 85% based on both objective and subjective criteria (32,49,59,73,75,80). Six to twenty-five percent have been reported to be worse over long-term follow-up, with the better outcomes being reported more recently. No particular difference has been observed between success rates for Chiari I vs. Chiari II decompression (32,44); however, patients with syringomyelia have a less favorable prognosis for improvement, where roughly one-third improve, one-third remain stable, and one-third get worse (10,50,75,80). Delayed deterioration back to preoperative morbidity has been reported in 20% of improved patients within 2–3 years of surgery, emphasizing the need for long-term postoperative follow-up (73). However, other long-term studies have failed to verify this high rate of recurrence (50,62,75,80). Infants with symptomatic Chiari II malformations have a high incidence of mortality (50% or higher in both surgical and nonsurgical groups), but good outcomes are reported in survivors (13). The prognosis for children and adolescents with symptomatic type II ectopia appears to be at least as good as that of adults with type I malformations.

Progressive neurological deficit in a postoperative setting can arise from a number of causes. Attention should be paid to the possibilities of recurrent syringomyelia, occipital-C1-C2 instability, pseudomeningocele, meningitis (bacterial or fungal), and extradural abscess. "Sagging" or "slumping" of the cerebellum has been attributed to excessive decompression of the posterior fossa (29,59). Further impaction at the newly formed foramen magnum has been thought to re-create the craniospinal pressure dissociation, leading to recurrence or progression of neurologic deficits. However, more recent evidence has challenged this concept. Sahuquillo et al. have found that the creation of an artificial cisterna magna through a generous posterior fossa decompression and duraplasty using "tent-up" sutures is associated with significant *upward* migration of the cerebellum and brainstem documented on preoperative and postoperative MR studies (81). Care is taken to keep the arachnoid mater intact. Although long-term follow-up results are not yet available, they provide convincing evidence that the extra CSF under the inferior surface of the cerebellum (and associated lack of dural adhesions) lends buoyancy or support to the posterior fossa structures, hopefully reducing or eliminating recurrence of symptomatology.

In those cases that present late in the progression of these disorders, or those that continue to progress despite surgical intervention, recurrent pneumonia represents the most common cause of death (76).

X. SUMMARY

The Chiari malformations represent a spectrum of clinical conditions sharing various degrees of cerebellar ectasia or herniation. The Chiari I malformation generally presents in adulthood, whereas the Chiari II malformation typically presents in the pediatric population. Although midbrain and hindbrain abnormalities are more common in the Chiari II syndrome, they can also be seen in type I malformations. The distinction between the two conditions should be based on the presence or absence of a neural tube defect. The acquired Chiari malformation can result in serious neurological deficit or death. For this reason, lumboperitoneal shunting procedures should be avoided unless all other surgical options have been exhausted. Patients presenting with dysphagia should be treated aggressively with early surgical intervention. The imaging modality of choice for diagnosis of a Chiari malformation is a T1-weighted sagittal MRI. Because of the high incidence of associated syringomyelia, the cervical spinal cord should also be routinely visualized. Craniocervical decompression followed by duraplasty is the surgical procedure of choice for symptomatic tonsillar herniation with or without associated syringomyelia, in the absence of hydrocephalus. Good to excellent results can be expected in the majority of patients over long periods of postoperative follow-up.

REFERENCES

1. Abbe R, Coley WB. Syringo-myelia, operation—exploration of cord—withdrawal of fluid—exhibition of patient. J Nerv Ment Dis 1892; 19:512–520.
2. Aboulezz AO, Sartor K, Geyer CA, Gado MH. Position of the cerebellar tonsils in the normal population and in patients with Chiari malformation: A quantitative approach with MR imaging. J Comput Assist Tomogr 1985; 9(6):1033–1036.
3. Aboulker J. La syringomyelia et les liquides intra-rachidiens. Neurochirurgie 1979; 25(suppl 1):1–144.
4. Aichner F, Poewe W, Rogalsky W, Wallnofer K, Willeit J, Gerstenbrand F. Magnetic resonance imaging in the diagnosis of spinal cord diseases. J Neurol Neurosurg Psychiatry 1985; 48:1220–1229.
5. Anderson NE, Willoughby EW, Wrightson P. The natural history and the influence of surgical treatment in syringomyelia. Acta Neurol Scand 1985; 71:472–479.
6. Archer CR, Horenstein S, Sundaram M. The Arnold-Chiari malformation presenting in adult life: A report of thirteen cases and a review of the literature. J Chronic Dis 1977; 30:369–382.
7. Armonda RA, Citrin CM, Foley KT, Ellenbogen RG. Quantitative cine-mode magnetic resonance imaging of Chiari I malformations: An analysis of cerebrospinal fluid dynamics. Neurosurgery 1994; 35(2):214–224

8. Arnold J. Myelocyste, Transposition von Gewebskeimen and Sumpodie. Beitr Path Anat 1894; 16:1–28.
9. Ball MJ, Dayan AD. Pathogenesis of syringomyelia. Lancet 1972; 2:799–801.
10. Banerji NK, Millar JHD. Chiari malformations presenting in adult life: Its relationship to syringomyelia. Brain 1974; 97:157–168.
11. Barbaro NM, Wilson CB, Gutin PH, Edwards MSB. Surgical treatment of syringomyelia: Favorable results with syringoperitoneal shunting. J Neurosurg 1984; 61:531–538.
12. Barkovich AJ, Wippold FJ, Sherman JL, Citrin CM. Significance of cerebellar tonsillar position on MR. AJNR 1986; 7:795–799.
13. Bell WO, Charney EB, Bruce DA, Sutton LN, Schut L. Symptomatic Arnold-Chiari malformation: Review of experience with 22 cases. J Neurosurg 1987; 66:812–816.
14. Bering HA. Choroid plexus and arterial pulsations of cerebrospinal fluid: Demonstration of the choroid plexus as a cerebrospinal fluid pump. Arch Neurol Psychiatry 1955; 73:165–173.
15. Boman K, II, Iivanainen M. Prognosis of syringomyelia. Acta Neurol Scandinav 1967; 43:61–68 1967.
16. Bondurant CP, Oro JJ. Spinal cord injury without radiographic abnormality and Chiari malformation. J Neurosurg 1993; 79:833–838.
17. Cameron AH. The Arnold-Chiari and other neuro-anatomical malformations associated with spina bifida. J Path Bact 1957; 73:195–211.
18. Chiari H. Ueber Veraderungen des Kleinhirns infolge von Hydrocephalie des Grosshirns. Deutsch Med Wschr 1891; 17:1172–1175.
19. Chiari H. Ueber Veranderungen des Kleinhirms, des Pons und der Medulla oblongata in Folge von congenitaler Hydrocephalie des Grossshirns. Denschr Akad Wiss Wien 1896; 63:71–116
20. Chiari H. Concerning alterations in the cerebellum resulting from cerebral hydrocephalus. Pediatr Neurosci 1987; 13:3–8.
21. Chumas PD, Armstrong DC, Drake J, Kulkarni AV, Hoffman HJ, Humphreys RP, Rutka JT, Hendrick EB. Tonsillar herniation: The rule rather than the exception after lumboperitoneal shunting in the pediatric population. J Neurosurg 1993; 78:568–573.
22. Citrin CM, Sherman JL, Gangarosa RE, Scalon D. Physiology of the CSF flow void sign: Modification by cardiac gating. AJNR 1986; 7:1021–1024.
23. Cleland J. Contribution to the study of spina bifida, encephalocele and anencephalus. J Anat Physiol 1883; 17:257–291
24. Coria F, Quintana F, Rebollo M, Combarros O, Berciano J. Occipital dysplasia and Chiari Type I deformity in a family: Clinical and radiological study of three generations. J Neurol Sci 1983; 62:147–158.
25. Dauser RC, DiPietro MA, Venes JL. Symptomatic Chiari I malformation in childhood: A report of 7 cases. Pediatr Neurosci 1988; 14:184–190.
26. Donauer E, Rascher K. Syringomyelia: A brief review of ontogenic, experimental and clinical aspects. Neurosurg Rev 1993; 16:7–13.
27. DuBoulay G, O'Connell J, Currie J, Bostick T, Verity P. Further investigations on pulsatile movements in the cerebrospinal fluid pathways. Acta Radiol Diagnosis 1972; 13:496–523.

28. DuBoulay GH, Shah SH, Currie JC, Logue V. The mechanism of hydromyelia in Chiari type I malformations. Br J Radiol 1974; 47:579–587.
29. Duddy JM, Williams B. Hindbrain migration after decompression for hindbrain hernia: A quantitative assessment using MRI. Br J Neurosurg 1991; 5:141–152.
30. Dure LS, Percy AK, Cheek WR, Laurent JP. Chiari I type malformation in children. J Pediatr 1989; 115:573–576.
31. Dyste GN, Menezes AH. Presentation and management of pediatric Chiari malformations without myelodysplasia. Neurosurgery 1988; 23:589–597.
32. Eisenstat DDR, Bernstein M, Fleming JFR, Vanderlinden RG, Schutz H. Chiari malformation in adults: A review of 40 cases. Can J Neurol Sci 1986; 13:221–228.
33. Elster AD, Chen MYM. Chiari I malformations: Clinical and radiologic reappraisal. Neuroradiology 1992; 183:347–353.
34. Emery JL, MacKenzie N. Medullo-cervical dislocation deformity (Chiari II deformity) related to neurospinal dysraphism (meningomyelocele). Brain 1973; 96:155–162.
35. Estienne C. La Dissection du Corps Humain. Paris: Simone de Colines, 1546; pp 3–42.
36. Fischer EG, Welch K, Shillito J Jr. Syringomyelia following lumboureteral shunting for communicating hydrocephalus. Report of three cases. J Neurosurg 1977; 47:96–100.
37. Fish DR, Howards RS, Wiles CM, Simon L. Respiratory arrest: A complication of cerebellar ectopia in adults. J Neurol Neurosurg Psychiat 1988; 51:714–716.
38. Gardner WJ. Hydrodynamic mechanism of syringomyelia: Its relationship to myelocele. J Neurol Neurosurg Psychiat 1965; 28:247–259.
39. Gardner WJ, Angel J. The mechanism of syringomyelia and its surgical correction. Clinical Neurosurgery 1958; 14:591–607.
40. Gardner WJ, Bell HS, Poolos PN, Dohn DF, Steinberg M. Terminal ventriculostomy for syringomyelia. J Neurosurg 1977; 46:609–617.
41. Grant R, Hadley DM, MacPherson P, Condon B, Patterson J, Bone I, Teasdale GN. Syringomyelia: Cyst measurement by magnetic resonance imaging and comparison with symptoms, signs and disability. J Neurol Neurosurg Psychiat 1987; 50:1008–1014.
42. Haines SJ, Berger M. Current treatment of Chiari malformations types I and II: A survey of the pediatric section of the American Association of Neurological Surgeons. Neurosurgery 1991; 28(3):353–357.
43. Hida K, Iwasaki Y, Imamura H, Abe H. Posttraumatic syringomyelia: Its characteristic magnetic resonance imaging findings and surgical management. Neurosurgery 1994; 35(5):886–891.
44. Hoffman HJ, Neill J, Crone KR, Hendrick EB, Humphreys RP. Hydrosyringomyelia and its management in childhood. Neurosurgery 1987; 21(3):347–351
45. Hoffman HJ, Tucker WT. Cephalocranial disproportion. Child's Brain 1976; 2:167–176.
46. Huewel N, Perneczky A, Urban V, Fries G. Neuroendoscopic technique for the operative treatment of septated syringomyelia. Acta Neurochir 1992; 54(suppl): 59–62.
47. Hunter JV, Youl BD, Moseley IF. MRI demonstration of midbrain deformity in association with Chiari malformation. Neuroradiology 1992; 34:399–401.

48. O'Connel JEA. Vascular factor in intracranial pressure and maintenance of cerebrospinal fluid circulation. Brain 1943; 66:204–228.

49. Levy WJ, Mason L, Hahn JF. Chiari malformation presenting in adults: A surgical experience in 127 cases. Neurosurgery 1983; 12:377–390.

50. Logue V, Edwards MR. Syringomyelia and its surgical treatment—an analysis of 75 patients. J Neurol Neurosurg Psychiatry 1981; 44:273–284.

51. Love JG, Olafson RA. Syringomyelia: A look at surgical therapy. J Neurosurg 1966; 24:714–718.

52. Mariani C, Cislaghi MG, Barbieri S, Filizzolo F, DiPalma F, Farina E, Aliberti GD, Scarlato G. The natural history and results of surgery in 50 cases of syringomyelia. J Neurol 1991; 238:433–438.

53. Martinot A, Hue V, Leclerc F, Vallee L, Closset M, Pruvo JP. Sudden death revealing Chiari type 1 malformation in two children. Intensive Care Med 1993; 19: 73–74.

54. Masur H, Oberwittler C, Fahrendorf G, Heyen P, Reuther G, Nedjat S, Ludolph AC, Brune GG. The relation between functional deficits, motor and sensory conduction times and MRI findings in syringomyelia. Electroencephalogr Clin Neurophysiol 1992; 85:321–330.

55. McEnery G, Borzyskowski M, Cox TCS, Neville BGR. The spinal cord in neurologically stable spina bifida: A clinical and MRI study. Dev Med Child Neurol 1992; 34:342–347.

56. McIlroy WJ, Richardson JC. Syringomyelia: A clinical review of 75 cases. Can Med Assoc J 1965; 93(14):731–734.

57. McLone DG, Knepper PA. The cause of Chiari II malformation: A unified theory. Pediatr Neurosci 1989; 15:1–12.

58. McLone DG, Naidich TP. Developmental morphology of the subarachnoid space, brain vasculature, and contiguous structures, and the cause of the Chiari II malformation. AJNR 1992; 13:463–482.

59. Menezes AH. Chiari I malformations and hydromyelia—complications. Pediatr Neurosurg 1991; 17:146–154.

60. Milhorat TH, Kotzen RM, Anzil AP. Stenosis of the central canal of spinal cord in man: Incidence and pathological findings in 232 autopsy cases. J Neurosurg 1994; 80:716–722.

61. Mills JL, Simpson JL. Prospects for prevention of neural tube defects by vitamin supplementation. Cur Opion Neurol Neurosurg 1993; 6:554–558.

62. Mohr PD, Strang FA, Sambrook MA. The clinical and surgical features in 40 patients with primary cerebellar ectopia (adult Chiari malformation). QJ Med 1977; 46:82–96.

63. Morioka T, Kurita-Tashima S, Fujii K, Nakagaki H, Kato M, Fukui M. Somatosensory and spinal evoked potentials in patients with cervical syringomyelia. Neurosurgery 1992; 30(2):218–222.

64. MRC Vitamin Study Research Group: Prevention of neural tube defects: Results of the Medical Research Council vitamin study. Lancet 1991; 338:131–137.

65. Muhonen MG, Menezes AH, Sawin PD, Weinstein SL. Scoliosis in pediatric Chiari malformations without myelodysplasia. J Neurosurg 1992; 77:69–77.

66. Naidich TP, Pudlowski RM, Naidich JB, Gornish M, Rodriguez FJ. Computed

tomographic signs of the Chiari II malformation part I: Skull and dural partitions. Radiology 1980; 134:65–71.

67. O'Connor S, DuBoulay G, Logue V. The normal position of the cerebellar tonsils as demonstrated by myelography. J Neurosurg 1973; 39:387–389

68. Oldfield EH, Muraszko K, Shawker TH, Patronas NJ. Pathophysiology of syringo-myelia associated with Chiari I malformation of the cerebellar tonsils. Implications for diagnosis and treatment. J Neurosurg 1994; 80:3–15.

69. Ollivier d'Angers CP. De la Moelle Epiniere et des Ses Maladies. Paris: Chez Crivot 1161824.

70. Ollivier d'Angers CP. Vol. 1, Paris and Brussels: Crevot, 1827; p 178.

71. Park TS, Cail WS, CBW, Walker MG. Lumboperitoneal shunt combined with mye-lotomy for treatment of syringomyelia. J Neurosurg 1989; 70:721–727.

72. Pascual J, Oterino A, Berciano J. Headache in type I Chiari malformation. Neurol-ogy 1992; 42:1519–1521.

73. Paul KS, Lye RH, Strang FA, Dutton J. Arnold-Chiari malformation. Review of 71 cases. J Neurosurg 1983; 58:183–187.

74. Payner TD, Prenger E, Berger TS, Crone KR. Acquired Chiari malformations: Incidence, diagnosis, and management. Neurosurgery 1994; 34(3):429–434.

75. Pillay PK, Awad IA, Little JR, Hahn JF. Symptomatic Chiari malformation in adults: A new classification based on magnetic resonance imaging with clinical and prognostic significance. Neurosurgery 1991; 28(5):639–645.

76. Pollack MD, Pang D, Kocoshis S, Putnam P. Neurogenic dysphagia resulting from Chiari malformations. Neurosurgery 1992; 30(5):709–719.

77. Putnam PE, Orenstein SR, Pang D, Pollack IF, Proujansky R, Kocoshis SA. Crico-pharyngeal dysfunction associated with Chiari malformations. Pediatrics 1992; 89(5):871–876.

78. Reigel DH. Tethered spinal cord. Concepts Pediatr Neurosurg 1983; 4:142–164.

79. Robertson DP, Narayan RK. Intraoperative endomyelography during syrinx drain-age: Technical note. Neurosurgery 1992; 30(2):246–249.

80. Saez RJ, Onofrio BM, Yanagihara T. Experience with Arnold-Chiari malformation, 1960 to 1970. J Neurosurg 1976; 45:416–422.

81. Sahuquillo J, Rubio E, Poca MA, Rovira A, Rodriguez-Baeza A, Cervera C. Pos-terior fossa reconstruction: A surgical technique for the treatment of Chiari I mal-formation and Chiar I / syringomyelia complex. Neurosurgery 1994; 35(5):874–885.

82. Schwalbe E, Gredig M. Ueber Entwicklungsstorungen des Kleinhirns, Hirnstamms und Halsmarks bei Spina bifida (Arnold'sche und Chiari'sche Misbildung). Bietr Pathol Ana U Allg Pathol 1907; 40:132–194.

83. Sclafani AP, DeDio RM, Hendrix RA. The Chiari-I malformation. Ear Nose Throat J 1991; 70:208–212.

84. Spillane JD, Pallis C, Jones AM. Developmental abnormalities in the region of the foramen magnum. Brain 1957; 80:11–48.

85. Spinos E, Laster DW, Moody DM, Ball MR, Witcofski RL, Kelly DL Jr. MR evaluation of Chiari I malformations at 0.15 T. AJNR 1985; 6:203–208.

86. Stovner LJ, Cappelen J, Nilsen G, Sjaastad O. The Chiari type I malformation in two monozygotic twins and first-degree relatives. Ann Neurol 1992; 31:220–222.

87.	Stovner LJ, Rinck P. Syringomyelia in Chiari malformation: Relation to extent of cerebellar tissue herniation. Neurosurgery 1992; 31(5):913–917.
88.	Sullivan LP, Stears JC, Ringel SP. Resolution of syringomyelia and Chiari I malformation by ventriculoatrial shunting in a patient with pseudotumor cerebri and a lumboperitoneal shunt. Neurosurgery 1988; 22:744–747.
89.	Tachibana S, II, Iida H, Yada K. Significance of positive Queckenstedt test in patients with syringomyelia associated with Arnold-Chiari malformations. J Neurosurg 1992; 76:67–71.
90.	Tomaszek DE, Tyson GW, Bouldint T, Hansen AR. Sudden death in a child with an occult hindbrain malformation. Ann Emerg Med 1984; 13:136–138.
91.	Variend S, Emery JL. Cervical dislocation of the cerebellum in children with meningomyelocele. Teratology 1976; 13:281–290.
92.	Vengsarkar US, Panchal VG, Tripathi PD. Percutaneous thecoperitoneal shunt for syringomyelia. Report of three cases. J Neurosurg 1991; 74:827–831.
93.	Vicek BW, Ito B. Acute paraparesis secondary to Arnold-Chiari Type I malformation and neck hyperflexion. Ann Neurol 1987; 21:100–101.
94.	Welch K, Shillito J, Strand R, Fischer EG, Winston KR. Chiari I "malformation"—an acquired disorder? J Neurosurg 1981; 55:604–609.
95.	Williams B. The distending force in the production of "communicating syringomyelia." Lancet 1969; 2:189–193.
96.	William B. On the pathogenesis of the Chairi malformation. Zeitschrift fur Kinderchirurgie und Grenzegebiete 1977; 22:533–553.
97.	Williams B. A critical appraisal of posterior fossa surgery for communicating syringomyelia. Brain 1978; 101:223–250.
98.	Williams B. On the pathogenesis of syringomyelia: A review. J Royal Soc Med 1980; 73:798–806.
99.	Williams B, Fahy G. A critical appraisal of "terminal ventriculostomy" for the treatment of syringomyelia. J Neurosurg 1983; 58:188–197.
100.	Yeates A, Brant-Zawadzki M, Norman D, Kaufman L, Crooks LE, Newton TH. Nuclear magnetic resonance imaging of syringomyelia. AJNR 1983; 4:234–237.

4

Spastic Paraplegia, Bulbar Palsy, and Spinocerebellar Degeneration

Ian E. C. Ormerod
Frenchay Hospital, Bristol, England

Paul T. G. Davies
Northampton General Hospital, Cliftonville, Northampton, England

Weakness of the legs and lower trunk, if complete, is termed paraplegia or diplegia; if incomplete, it is called paraparesis (although the terms are often used interchangeably). In clinical practice, the term paraparesis implies an upper motor neurone (UMN) lesion. The first part of this chapter concerns the clinical assessment and investigation of spastic paraplegia, which is usually, but not always, a sign of spinal cord dysfunction (i.e., a similar clinical picture can be seen with pathology occurring in the parasagittal region of the motor cortex or in the brain stem). Recognizing signs of cerebral disease, particularly bulbar palsy, may be crucial to the assessment of spastic paraplegia; therefore, some aspects of bulbar palsy will also be covered in this chapter. In the final section, rarer causes of walking difficulties, the spinocerebellar degenerations, will be considered.

Spastic paraplegia/paraparesis is, of course, merely a descriptive term for a common clinical picture produced by a wide spectrum of diseases. Other features of spinal cord disease such as sensory or urinary symptoms may be present, and more prominent, with patients seeking treatment from many different medical and surgical specialities.

I. SPASTIC PARAPLEGIA

A. Acquired Spastic Paraplegia

Whereas some diseases causing spastic paraplegia are confined to the nervous system, e.g., multiple sclerosis (MS), motor neuron disease (MND)/amyotrophic lateral sclerosis (ALS), many are multisystem disorders, such as carcinomatosis and vitamin B_{12} deficiency. A full history and examination are of paramount importance and will give the diagnosis in many cases. Although the elucidation of the neurological signs will allow correct anatomical localization of pathology, clues as to its nature come largely from the history. Presentation in early life may represent cerebral palsy, whereas in older patients, cord compression due to cervical spondylosis or tumor are more common. General examination of the patient may point to the cause of spastic paraplegia; a short neck may suggest an Arnold-Chiari malformation or Klippel-Feil syndrome, whereas systemic signs of rheumatoid arthritis or neurofibromatosis may point to associated and related cord disease. Figure 1 is a transverse section of the spinal cord showing the main ascending and descending pathways.

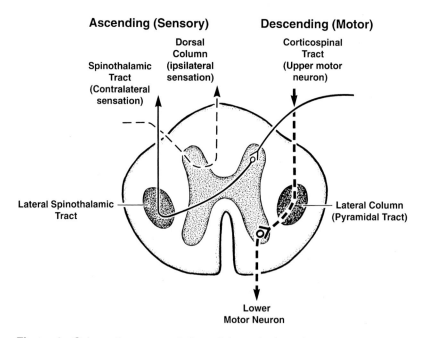

Figure 1 Schematic representation of the spinal cord in transverse section illustrating the main ascending (sensory) and descending (motor) pathways. Spinothalamic sensory modalities = pain and temperature; dorsal column sensory modalities = light touch, joint position, and vibration.

1. Symptoms

Motor

An evolving paraplegia may cause clumsiness of leg movement, an unsteady or stiff gait, a tendency to drag one leg or to trip on uneven ground, an inability to run, or uneven shoe wear. Undue limb fatigue after customary exercise may be a complaint. Spasticity, which generally takes weeks to develop after an UMN lesion, may produce muscle cramps and "jumping" in the legs, which may be painful. These spasms may be evoked by a sensory stimulus. Exacerbation of symptoms by heat is characteristic of demyelination.

Sensory

These symptoms may be absent, e.g., MND/ALS, or wide ranging if the long sensory tracts of the spinal cord are affected. Tingling, numbness, or pins and needles may be felt in different parts of the legs and trunk, although these sensations may also occur in disease of the peripheral sensory system. Deep, poorly localized pain suggests spinothalamic involvement. In contrast, peripheral involvement of pain fibers tends to produce burning pain, dysesthesiae, and hypersensitivity. Feelings of constricting tight bands around a limb, tightness of the skin, "running-water" sensations, and the sensation of "electric" paresthesiae that radiate downward on neck flexion (L'Hermitte's phenomenon) suggest dorsal column disease. The latter is a common symptom in multiple sclerosis. The so-called "reverse L'Hermitte's phenomenon," produced by extension of the neck, can be seen in cervical spondylosis.

Bladder

The bladder is bilaterally innervated and the tracts lie medially in the lateral columns. In cord compression, micturition is often affected late, whereas in intrinsic cord lesions it is affected early, often with only mild signs of cord disease. The symptoms produced by a UMN lesion to the bladder are urinary frequency, urgency, and dribbling. This contrasts with a lower motor neurone (LMN) lesion, e.g., in cauda equina disease, in which there is likely to be a large and poorly contracting bladder producing urinary retention with overflow.

2. Signs

Whereas limb weakness may be due to muscle, neuromuscular junction, or LMN disease, in cord disease the weakness may be associated with the hallmarks of spasticity (hypertonicity, clonus, hyperreflexia, and extensor plantar responses). If the leg weakness is particularly noticeable in hip and knee flexion and ankle dorsiflexion, then the term "pyramidal" distribution is given. The presence of these signs denotes spinal cord and/or brain pathology. It is important to realize that the degrees of spasticity, weakness, and hyperreflexia are often unrelated to each other; spastic legs may be quite strong, whereas weak legs may show little spasticity. In general, the degree of hyperreflexia correlates with the degree of increased tone felt when attempting to move the limb quickly. The more significant the pyramidal tract dysfunction, the greater the sensory area from which the Babinski response can be elicited.

3. Causes

In considering the etiology of spastic paraplegia, it is useful to determine whether symptoms have a subacute or chronic onset. Trauma to the cord, hemorrhage into the cord (hematomyelia), and infarction (e.g., anterior spinal artery thrombosis), produce a rapid-onset paraplegia that is often initially flaccid due to spinal shock. The longer the limbs remain flaccid, the worse the prognosis. Flexor spasticity gradually emerges, but later extensor spasticity predominates (see "Rehabilitation and Treatment of Spasticity").

Onset of paraplegia over 2 to 3 days is usually due to an inflammatory cause (transverse myelitis) but may be due to cord compression associated with an infection (e.g., extradural abscess) or secondary carcinoma of the spine, both being an acute neurosurgical emergency. An insidious onset, over months, is often due to cervical cord compression from cervical spondylosis, although in this case there are usually neurological signs in the arms as well. Other diseases presenting with a spastic paraplegia include multiple sclerosis, other causes of cord compression, vitamin B_{12} deficiency (subacute combined degeneration of the cord), and MND/ALS (Table 1). The most common cause of spastic paraplegia is trauma with fracture dislocation followed by thoracic cord compression.

B. Inherited Spastic Paraplegia

1. Clinical Features

Hereditary spastic paraplegia (HSP), also known as familial spastic paraparesis and Strümpell-Lorrain syndrome, is not a single disease but a group of unusual disorders that most often demonstrate autosomal dominant (AD) inheritance (Table 2). They can present in infancy or old age but in most, the onset of symptoms occurs during the second to fourth decades with a gait disorder that progresses insidiously. Both within and between HSP kindreds, the age of symptom onset, rate of symptom progression, and extent of disability are variable. In contrast, within HSP kindreds, the range of neurological deficits is invariant. Although type I is of early onset, its prognosis appears to be better than the more rapidly progressive but later-onset type II. As these conditions proceed, involvement of the arms and sphincters is also seen, but there is no corticobulbar tract disease. Occasionally sensory disturbance, distal muscle thinning, and deformities of the spine and limbs may occur (uncomplicated

Table 1   Causes of Spastic Paraplegia

1. Demyelinating
   Multiple sclerosis
   Acute disseminated encephalomyelitis (postinfectious)
   Inflammatory transverse myelitis
   Central pontine myelinolysis
2. Trauma
3. Compression syndromes including tumors
4. Infections
   Bacterial, e.g., pyogenic, tuberculous
   Viral, e.g., HTLV-1, HIV
   Parasitic, e.g., hydatid, schistosomiasis
   Other infections, e.g., syphilis, Lyme, mycoplasma
5. Granuloma, e.g., sarcoid, Wegener's
6. Vascular
   Vasculitis
   Spinal artery occlusion
   Decompression sickness
   Arteriovenous malformation
   Postradiation
7. Metabolic
   B_{12} and folate deficiency
   Hyperthyroidism
   Diabetes
   Mitochondrial disease
   Leucodystrophy
8. Motor neurone disease
   Sporadic/familial
9. Paraneoplastic
10. Inherited disorders, e.g., spinocerebellar disorders
11. Syringomyelia/Chiari malformation
12. Hydrocephalus
13. Drugs and toxins
    Methotrexate
    Cytosine arabinoside
    Alkylating agents
    Intravenous heroin abuse
    Lathyrism
14. Perinatal/cerebral palsy

Source: Ref. 8.

Table 2   Classification of Inherited Spastic Paraplegias

A. Isolated paraplegia
      Type I (dominant; onset before age 35)
      Type II (dominant; onset after age 35)
      Recessive inheritance
B. Paraplegia "plus"
      LMN features
      Cerebellar features
      Kjellin syndrome (macular degeneration and mental retardation)
      Chorea/dystonia
      Others

Source: Ref. 8.

HSP). The clinical picture in the autosomal recessive (AR) kindreds appears to be similar to the more common AD families. Sporadic cases may represent recessively inherited conditions. The diagnosis of HSP, given a family history of progressive spastic paraparesis as an isolated symptom, is straightforward, but it must be distinguished from other inherited conditions that may affect gait, e.g., DOPA-responsive dystonia and familial ALS.

Of the inherited spastic paraplegias associated with other neurological deficits (complicated HSP), amyotrophy is the most usual feature. This may be with a peripheral neuropathy (hereditary motor and sensory neuropathy [HMSN] type V) and a clinical appearance of Charcot-Marie-Tooth disease (1). In others there is a marked wasting of the small hand muscles (2). There remains a heterogeneous and rare group of inherited conditions with spastic paraplegia and a variety of other neurological abnormalities. Some display dominant inheritance (optic atrophy, chorea, or dystonia). Others are recessive (with cerebellar features or optic atrophy and mental retardation).

2. Genetics

The genetic basis for HSP has been revealed in part in recent years. Loci for autosomal dominant HSP have been identified on chromosomes 2p, 14q, and 15q. One locus (in one family Xq22) has been found for uncomplicated X-linked HSP and shown to be due to a proteolipoprotein gene mutation in one family. It has been postulated that the gene products from different HSP loci participate in some common biochemical pathway which, once disturbed, results in axonal degeneration in the longest motor neurones (3).

Investigation of Spastic Paraplegia

Identifying treatable disease is a priority, and imaging to exclude cord compression is usually essential (Fig. 2). Cervical and dorsal spine x-rays may also be helpful. Lumbar spine x-rays may suggest root and cauda equina pathologies but do not help the investigation of spastic paraplegia. The possibility of cere-

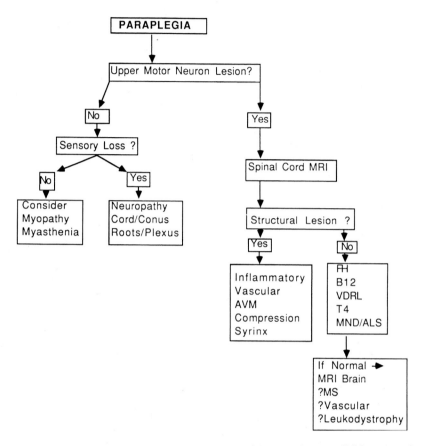

Figure 2 An outline for the investigation of leg weakness. AVM = arteriovenous malformation, FH = family history, B12 = vitamin B12, VDRL = venereal disease reference laboratory, T4 = thyroxine, MND/ALS = motor neuron disease/amyotrophic lateral sclerosis, MS = multiple sclerosis.

bral disease (e.g., a parasagittal tumor affecting the leg area of the motor strip) must not be forgotten and a brain computed tomography (CT) scan may be required. Magnetic resonance imaging (MRI) is the imaging method of choice for most spinal cord lesions. It may show pathology within the spinal cord not previously imaged e.g., demyelination, sarcoid granuloma, toxoplasmosis, tuberculous myelitis, and HTLV-1. Computed tomographic scanning, only able to generate images in the axial plane, is still useful if directed at a particular spinal level and often better than MR at identifying bony abnormalities. Brain MR scanning is now widely used to assist in the diagnosis of MS.

If a diagnosis has not been made after MR scanning, cerebral spinal fluid (CSF) examination should be carried out but, provided MS has been excluded, it provides little specific diagnostic data in chronic states. Neurophysiological tests (electromyogram [EMG], visual evoked response [VER], somatosensory evoked potentials [SSEP]) and blood tests (e.g., vitamin B_{12}, VDRL, HTLV-1) may be helpful.

Prevention of Spasticity
After spinal shock, nociceptive stimuli from bladder, bowel, and skin seem to affect neuronal connections within the damaged cord. They promote the generation of unhelpful flexor spasticity, leading to paraplegia in flexion. Skilled nursing is needed to avoid these nociceptive stimuli. Physiotherapy, to maintain joint mobility, may reduce the final severity of spasticity and generate the more helpful extensor tone.

Rehabilitation and Treatment of Spasticity
There is considerable variability in the disability produced by spasticity. In severe spinal spasticity, flexor or extensor spasms may be painful, making self care and nursing difficult. Adductor spasms in women may produce problems with bladder and bowel care. In less severe spasticity, scissoring of the thighs and forced plantar flexion and inversion of the feet may hinder walking. On the other hand, extensor spasms in the legs may aid walking and transfer in some cases. The prevention and treatment of spasticity may alleviate disability in some patients but in others, excessive antispasticity treatment may worsen disability. Treatment must be suited to the individual's needs. Established spasticity may be reduced in various ways.

(1) Drug Treatment. Baclofen (Lioresal) is generally regarded as the first-line drug in the treatment of spasticity. It is a gamma-aminobutyric acid (GABA) analogue that binds GABA-B receptors and thereby suppresses the release of excitatory neurotransmitters. It diminishes spasticity of cerebral and spinal origin. The dose should be increased slowly over days and weeks. Drowsiness is a common side effect that may limit its use.

Dantrolene (Dantrium) depresses the release of sarcoplasmic reticulum calcium to reduce all forms of spasticity. It may be used together with baclofen.

Diazepam (Valium) in small doses can be useful but it frequently produces drowsiness and dependancy.

Botulinum toxin injected directly into muscle reduces spasticity, but its benefit lasts only 2–3 months. The cost of injecting large volumes of muscle is often prohibitory, and there are risks of more generalized weakness.

Baclofen Pumps for Intrathecal Delivery. In about 30% of patients with spinal spasticity, oral doses of baclofen produce unacceptable side effects or fail to alleviate symptoms adequately. (Baclofen, being poorly lipid soluble, does not easily cross the blood-brain barrier.) Intrathecal administration allows good control of spasticity when oral doses have failed. Administration can be by a mechanical device operated by external pressure, which produces bolus delivery of baclofen solution, or via programmable infusion devices (4). In this way, the quality of life is improved in a high proportion of patients although, in general, motor function is not greatly improved. In many cases, an improvement in bladder function is also seen.

(2) Operative Procedures. There is a wide variety of orthopaedic and neurosurgical operations for the management of spasticity. They are generally carried out in specialized centers and are beyond the scope of this chapter.

II. BULBAR PALSY

A. Bulbar Dysfunction

The muscles of the tongue, palate, larynx, and pharynx, collectively termed the bulbar muscles, are supplied mainly by the tenth and twelfth cranial nerves, whose nuclei lie in the bulb-like structure, the medulla oblongata, on the ventral surface of the lower brain stem. Bulbar dysfunction usually presents with dysarthria, dysphonia, dysphagia, choking, or aspiration. A full clinical history and examination, including examination of bulbar function, can often identify the etiology of the problem. Examination of the mouth, tongue and palate, speech, swallowing, and cough are all relatively easy at the bedside. Lower motor neuron signs produce a bulbar palsy whereas, due to bilateral cortical representation, UMN disorders must be bilateral to produce bulbar symptoms (pseudobulbar palsy). Although the symptoms may be similar, the signs of bulbar and pseudobulbar palsy are quite different, as are their causes (Table 3). Both bulbar and pseudobulbar palsy may occur together in conditions that affect UMN and LMN, e.g., MND/ALS.

B. Causes of Bulbar Palsy and Their Investigation

A wide variety of neurological diseases may produce bulbar dysfunction so that when considering the possibilities, it may be helpful to think in anatomical terms. Some produce only bulbar palsy (malignant meningitis, poliomyelitis), others pseudobulbar palsy (cerebrovascular disease affecting both hemispheres); some conditions (MND/ALS) may produce signs of both. It is important to remember that symptoms of bulbar dysfunction, such as dysarthria, may have some other neurological basis, for example cerebellar or extrapyramidal disease. Further clues as to the etiology of bulbar dysfunction come from the rate of progression of symptoms. An acute onset is seen in vascular disease and in some infections (diphtheria, herpes zoster), although slow progression might

Table 3   Causes of Bulbar and Pseudobulbar Palsy

Bulbar Palsy
  Acquired
  Common
      Brain stem vascular disease
      Lower brain stem tumors (extrinsic/intrinsic)
      Motor neuron disease
      polyneuropathy
      Myasthenia
      Malignant meningitis
  Uncommon
      Trauma
      Syringobulbia
      Chiari malformation
      Myopathy
      Bulbar poliomyelitis
Pseudobulbar Palsy
  Common
      Cerebrovascular disease
      MS
      ALS/MND
      Tumors (upper brain stem)
  Uncommon
      Trauma
      Spinocerebellar degenerations
      Leukodystrophies
      Steele-Richardson syndrome (progressive supranuclear palsy)
Hereditary (uncommon)
  Childhood onset
      Fazio-Londe disease (progressive bulbar and cranial nerve palsies)
      Vialetto-van Laere syndrome (characteristically, progressive lower
        cranial motor nerve palsies)
      Spinal muscular atrophy (SMA) types I and II (AR)
  Adult onset
      Autosomal dominant
      X-linked bulbospinal neuronopathy (Kennedy syndrome)
      Familial motor neurone disease
      SMA type III (AR and AD)

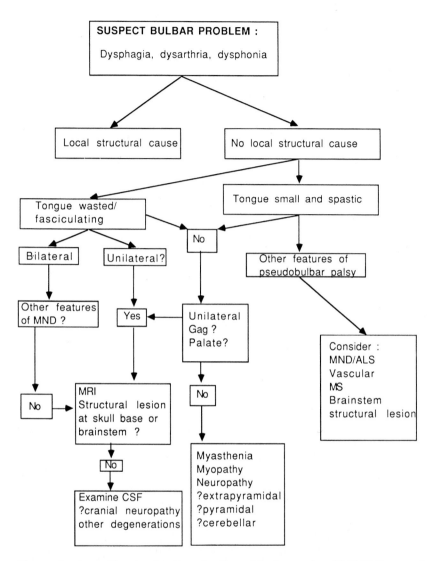

Figure 3   An outline for the investigation of bulbar palsy. MND/ALS = motor neuron disease/amyotrophic lateral sclerosis. MS = multiple sclerosis.

suggest tumor, granulomatous disease, or neurodegenerative disorders. A flow chart for the investigation of bulbar palsy is shown (Fig. 3).

1. Muscle Disease

Muscle disease affecting the tongue, pharyngeal, and laryngeal muscles is uncommon and seldom a presenting feature, but it may occur in dystrophia myotonia, polymyositis, and oculopharyngeal myopathy. Investigations may include creatinine kinase (CK), EMG, and muscle biopsy.

2. Neuromuscular Disorders

Myasthenia gravis, a purely motor disorder, commonly causes bulbar palsy. The hallmark is fluctuating weakness, worsened by continued muscular activity and improved by rest. Onset is usually insidious with variable and sometimes intermittent ptosis, diplopia, and bulbar dysfunction being common presentations. Bulbar involvement in the Lambert-Eaton myasthenic syndrome is unusual. Investigation includes the edrophonium (Camilon) test, antiacetylcholine receptor antibody titers in the blood, and EMG.

3. LMN (Bulbar Palsy)

Extra-Axial Lesions

Neuronal involvement may be outside the brain stem. Here, adjacent cranial nerves are affected, often in succession, with late and relatively mild affliction of long tract and other brain stem structures. Skull-base fractures, Paget's disease, tumurs, and granulomata may all produce bulbar palsy. Tumors of the jugular foramen may produce a particular pattern with ipsilateral ninth, tenth and eleventh cranial nerve involvement. Investigation will involve imaging of the posterior fossa. Magnetic resonance scanning, with and without gadolinium enhancement, is often the most informative imaging method. For extra-axial lesions, CSF examination may be diagnostic, for instance, in malignant meningitis.

Intrinsic Brain Stem Lesions

Intramedullary lesions usually produce crossed sensory or motor signs in the limbs. There are a number of distinctive syndromes produced by brain stem vascular disease, such as lateral medullary syndrome.

4. UMN (Pseudobulbar Palsy)

This is usually due to bihemispheric vascular disease, advanced MS, or brain stem tumors. In a series of 91 consecutive patients presenting with acute unihemispheric stroke, some with a background of diffuse cerebral ischemia, 37 were dysphagic. These patients had more severe limb paresis and higher mortality when compared with those without dysphagia. In those who survived, dysphagia lasted, on average, 8.5 days (5).

Assessment and Treatment of Bulbar Dysfunction

Even if the underlying cause of bulbar dysfunction has no specific treatment, much can be done to help patients' symptoms, which are usually dysphagia, dysarthria, dysphonia, salivary dribbling, and choking (for review see 6).

Dysphagia can be assessed at the bedside by watching the patient swallow a little water. Nasal regurgitation implies palatal dysfunction, whereas choking and coughing mean that water has entered the larynx. The time taken to swallow should also be assessed. The presence of a palatal or pharyngeal gag does not necessarily mean a safe swallow. In some cases, further assessment using videofluoroscopy may be informative. Often, the severity of dysphagia is underestimated and may result in major morbidity, particularly from recurrent aspiration. Drowsy patients and those with poor respiratory function, hence cough, are especially vulnerable.

The problems produced by dysphagia may be tackled in several ways. Difficulties maintaining adequate nutrition may be helped by diétary advice concerning the type and consistency of food. Altering head position while swallowing may be very helpful for some patients. Baclofen may be tried when swallowing is hindered by spasticity; physostigmine (Mestinon) may be useful when there is denervation. If swallowing is considered unsafe a fine-bore nasogastric tube may be inserted. If hold-up of contrast is seen at the cricopharyngeus on videofluoroscopy, then cricopharyngeal myotomy can be considered, although this is a controversial area.

A feeding gastrostomy, inserted by endoscopic control, is simple and effective and can easily be reversed. It is frequently used in patients with the form of MND/ALS called progressive bulbar palsy.

The management of dysarthria often requires a skilled speech therapist. There are now many communication aids ranging from the simple alphabet board to portable electronic communicators. Dysphonia may be helped through sound amplification. Coating the vocal cord with teflon can be used when inadequate cord adduction occurs in lower motor neurone lesions.

Salivary dribbling may be difficult to manage, but may be helped by altering head posture. Atropine or hyoscine also may be helpful.

III. SPINOCEREBELLAR DEGENERATION

A. Cerebellar Dysfunction

The term ataxia is often used interchangeably with cerebellar deficit in the mind of the clinician. This is rather misleading. What the clinician may call ataxia, the patient will broadly refer to as clumsiness of the limbs or gait. This clearly covers a wider spectrum of conditions than cerebellar dysfunction. Diseases of the cerebellum and its connections are associated with some characteristic features, which include dysarthria and nystagmus as well as dysmetria, poor rapid alternating movements (dysdiadochokinesia), and abnormal displacement reactions in the limbs. Some of the clinical features seen in the limbs in cerebellar ataxia may be seen in other conditions. Patients with pyramidal and extrapyramidal dysfunction may have slow movement and clumsiness. Patients with marked proprioceptive loss may have clumsiness and unsteady gait. In some conditions, there will be a combination of systems involved, and the deficits and physical signs may be complex and difficult to unravel. An outline for the investigation of unsteadiness of gait is shown in Figure 4.

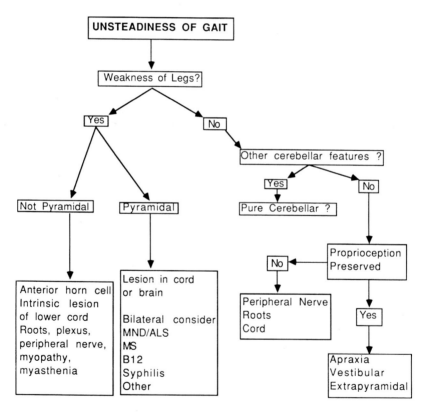

Figure 4   An outline for the investigation of unsteadiness of gait. MND/ALS = motor neuron disease/amyotrophic lateral sclerosis, MS = multiple sclerosis, B12 = vitamin B12.

Table 4 Metabolic Disorders Associated With Ataxia

Leukodystrophies (metachromatic, adrenoleukodystrophy)
Hexosaminidase deficiency
Sphingomyelin storage disease (Niemann-Pick)
Mitochondrial cytopathy
Vitamin E deficiency (betalipoprotein deficiency or malabsorption)
Wilson's disease
Sialidosis
Ceroid lipofuscinosis (Kufs' disease)

Source: Ref. 8.

B. Spinocerebellar Degenerations

This is a group of degenerative ataxic disorders with diverse clinical features. Some clearly have an inherited basis, others are sporadic without a known cause, and a further group is associated with metabolic multiple system problems in which the neurological deficit may not be the most prominent feature. The neurological involvement may consist of a pure syndrome of ataxia caused by damage to the cerebellum and its connections, but other groups have a combination of neurological deficits involving the central and peripheral nervous system.

The classification is confusing despite detailed studies; Harding (7,8) has produced the most widely accepted method of categorizing these disorders. One of the problems in classifying the ataxic disorders has been whether to differentiate by inheritance pattern, clinical features, pathological and radiological findings, or combinations of these. Ultimately, many will be classified by the genetic defect underlying the disorder. Recent developments in the understanding of the genetics of these disorders have already lead to new insights into the phenotypic variation and classification. The term idiopathic or sporadic will hopefully become redundant as the genetic changes underlying these conditions become clarified in due course. The division of the inherited ataxias into those thought to be recessively inherited, dominantly inherited, and those thought to be sex-linked may be reasonable at this state of knowledge and follows on from the classification proposed by Harding (9).

1. Ataxic Disorders with Metabolic Defects

Some metabolic deficits produce ataxia only intermittently. This is usually not the only clinical feature. These conditions are associated with disorders of amino acid metabolism (e.g., Hartnup disease), hyperammonemia (e.g., ornithine transcarbamylase deficiency), and disorders of pyruvate and lactate metabolism. Others are associated with a constant and progressive neurological deficit, although ataxia is rarely the sole or even most prominent feature (Table 4).

2. Autosomal Recessive Ataxic Disorders with Defects in DNA Repair

Ataxia telangectasia (AT) is the most common of these unusual conditions. It usually has an onset in childhood associated with oculocutaneous telangiectasia, immune defects, and an increased incidence of childhood malignancy (particularly lymphoma and leukemia). The serum alpha-fetoprotein is usually elevated. Other motor abnormalities (chorea and dystonia) and neuropathy may occur.

Xeroderma pigmentosa and Cockayne's syndrome are also associated with a failure of repair of damaged DNA. Ataxia, other neurological defects, and skin damage and premature aging are seen in these patients.

3. Other Recessively Inherited Ataxias

The two main groups are Friedreich's ataxia (FA) and the other early-onset ataxias with retained reflexes. Friedreich's ataxia is the most common and best known of these disorders with a prevalence of 1–2/100,000. It is recessively inherited (chromosome 9). The neurological presentation is of a progressive ataxic disorder with pyramidal signs, lost tendon reflexes, and impaired proprioception. Pathologically, there is degeneration of the dorsal root ganglia, dorsal columns, and the corticospinal and spinocerebellar tracts of the spinal cord. The cerebellum itself is little affected. Spinal deformities, diabetes and cardiac abnormalities develop. Abnormalities of the electrocardiogram (ECG) are frequent. It has become clear that FA is caused by a guanine-adenosine-adenosine (GAA) trinucleotide repeat sequence on chromosome 9. Whereas normal chromosomes contain some repeats, the vast majority of FA chromosomes have been found to contain several hundred repeats. The gene product has been called Frataxin, which is a protein of unknown function at present. The application of the new genetic tests has already shown that the previous phenotypic descriptions (10) are probably too restrictive to be an absolute diagnostic guide.

Other early-onset ataxias are rare and are a collection of various disorders of largely unknown etiology and inheritance. Early-onset ataxia with retained reflexes is the most common of this group and may be associated with spasticity. Other conditions may involve optic atrophy, deafness, cataract, mental retardation, myoclonus, hypogonadism, and other deficits. Vitamin E deficiency is a rare cause of ataxia and is associated with peripheral neuropathy and pigmentary retinopathy. Although this is usually an acquired abnormality or related to an abnormality of the lipoproteins, there are reports of rare familial cases of isolated vitamin E deficiency (11).

4. Dominantly Inherited Ataxias

This group of ataxic disorders has given rise to difficulty and controversy in classification for the reasons already mentioned. Harding classified these into four groups (I–IV) on clinical features. Type IV is probably not a useful sub-group, and these patients now may well be considered to have manifestations of mitochondrial disease (9).

Autosomal-dominant cerebellar ataxia (ADCA) type 1 is not associated with pigmentary retinopathy. The onset is from the midteens to 60s, and the usual presentation is with ataxia of gait. Other features develop as the condition progresses to produce ataxia in all limbs. These include pseudobulbar palsy, supranuclear ophthalmoplegia, optic atrophy, dementia, lower motor neuron signs, and sensory loss. Clinical features and abnormalities on cerebral imaging (cerebellar, bráin stem, and cerebral atrophy) both tend to evolve with the pro-gression of the condition. Failure to appreciate this, and to consider disease duration when interpreting imaging studies, has hindered classification in the past (12,13). The genetic analysis for ADCA 1 initially showed evidence of linkage to chromosome 6. Subsequently, this abnormality was identified as an expanded trinucleotide repeat sequence known as the SCAR 1 variant. It seems likely that this genetic abnormality is associated with a fairly specific neuro-pathological change in the brain stem and cerebellum. A SCAR 3 locus has also been identified on chromosome 14 and is associated with the phenotypic variant of Machado-Joseph Disease (MJD), which may have certain specific clinical features including eye staring, dystonic movements and orofacial move-ments (14). It may be difficult to distinguish SCAR 1 and SCAR 3 patients on clinical grounds alone. Other loci exist for patients with ADCA, and these are incompletely analyzed at present.

ADCA type II is associated with pigmentary retinopathy and visual failure. Other neurological features may develop, including pyramidal signs. ADCA type III is a relatively pure late-onset cerebellar syndrome without retinopathy. Some dominantly inherited ataxic disorders may be associated with deposition of cerebral amyloid and prion diseases such as Gerstmann-Straussler-Scheinker disease (15).

Other late-onset ataxias occur without family history but may, in part, be recessively inherited. Their clinical features are variable.

5. Periodic Ataxias

Rare familial (dominantly inherited) periodic ataxic disorders occur and may be associated with abnormalities of ion channels in membranes. They may be treated with acetazolamide successfully in some cases. Chromosomes 12 and 9 have been suggested as sites of the abnormal genes.

Table 5   Drugs and Toxins That May Cause Ataxia

Alcohol
Anticonvulsants
Piperazine
5-fluorouracil
Cytosine arabinoside
Lithium
Organic solvents (toluene, carbon tetrachloride)
Organic mercury

---

6. Cerebellar Ataxic Syndromes with Drugs and Toxins

A number of drugs and toxins can cause ataxic syndromes that may or may not be reversible (Table 5).

7. Differential Diagnosis

In degenerative disorders without a clear family history, the diagnosis may be uncertain without further specific investigations. Additional neurological features or evidence of a metabolic defect may help. Understandably, some of these patients are labelled as having MS without any clear evidence for that diagnosis. Although the label of MS may provide a useful handle for the doctor and patient, it does tend to lead to a lack of clarity of thought and may not help in counseling patients about prognosis and genetic implications. Some patients with inherited ataxic disorders demonstrate cerebral MRI abnormalities, although the characteristics of these changes do not usually lead to misdiagnosis (12) and other investigations may help (evoked potentials, CSF analysis). Specific genetic studies may also help to classify these patients; some tests are now available and more will be developed in the coming years.

REFERENCES

1. Harding AE, Thomas PK. Peroneal muscular atrophy with pyramidal features. J Neurol Neurosurg Psychiatry 1986; 29:135–139.
2. Silver JR. Familial spastic paraplegia with amyotrophy of the hands. J Neurol Neurosurg Psychiatry 1966; 29:135–139.
3. Fink JK, Heiman-Patterson T, et al. Hereditary spastic paraplegia: Advances in genetic research. Neurology 1996; 46:1507–1514.
4. McLean BN. Intrathecal baclofen in severe spasticity. Br J Hosp Med 1993; 49:262–267.
5. Gordon C, Langton Hewer R, Wade DT. Dysphagia in stroke. BMJ 1987; 295:411–414.

6. Wiles CM. Neurogenic dysphagia. J Neurol Neurosurg Psychiatry 1991; 54:1037–1039.
7. Harding AE. Classification of the hereditary ataxias and paraplegias. Lancet 1983; 1:1151–1155.
8. Harding AE. The hereditary ataxias and related disorders. Edinburgh: Churchill Livingstone, 1984.
9. Hammans SR. The inherited ataxias. J Neurol Neurosurg Psychiatr, 1996; 61:327–332.
10. Harding AE. Friedreich's ataxia. A clinical and genetic study of 90 families with an analysis of early diagnostic criteria and intrafamilial clustering of clinical features. Brain 1981; 104:589–620.
11. Belal S, Hentati F, BenHamida C, et al. Friedreich's Ataxia—Vitamin E responsive type. Clin Neuroscience 1995; 3:39–42.
12. Ormerod IEC, Harding AE, Miller DH, Johnson G, Macmanus P, duBoulay EPGH, Kendall BE, Moseley IF, McDonald WI. Magnetic resonance imaging in degenerative ataxic disorders. J Neurol Neurosurg Psychiatry 1994; 57:51–57.
13. Klockgether T, Wullier U, Dichgans J, Grodd W, Nagele T, Pekersen D, Schroth G, Schmidt O, Voigt K. Clinical and cord imaging correlations in inherited ataxias. In: Harding A E, Dentel T, eds. Advances in neurology. Vol 61. New York: Raven Press, 1993; pp. 77–96.
14. Junck L, Fink JK. Machado-Joseph disease and SCA3: The genotype meets the phenotypes. Neurology 1996; 46:4–8.
15. Hudson AJ, Farell MA, Kalmins R, Kaufman JCE. Gerstmann-Straussler-Scheinker disease with coincidental familial onset. Ann Neurol 1983; 14:670–676.

5

Injuries to the Cervical Spine and Spinal Cord

George S. Miz
Orthopaedic Specialists, Oak Lawn, Illinois

I. EPIDEMIOLOGY

Nowhere is the spinal cord so vulnerable than in the neck where the spinal column has to support the head yet allow its mobility, as well as protecting the cord itself. In traumatic injury to this area, spinal cord injury often, but not always, follows injury to the spinal column. This chapter will discuss cervical spine injuries and their treatment in relation to injuries of the underlying spinal cord.

Traumatic spinal cord injury is a catastrophic event. Spinal cord injury incidence rates are reported to be in the range of 28 to 50 per million annually with approximately 30 per million spinal cord injury survivors (1,2). Cervical spine injuries can be caused by a variety of traumatic events. Most common among these are vehicular accidents, falls (including those from recreational sporting activities), and penetrating trauma, such as gunshot wounds (3). Injuries to the cervical spine range from simple neck sprains to complete quadriplegia and death.

Patients sustaining injuries to the cervical spinal cord can experience varying degrees of motor and sensory impairment as well as dysfunction of the genitourinary system. A 1992 survey indicated that spinal cord-injured persons spent an average of 171 days in the hospital at a cost of more than $95,000. After recovery and rehabilitation, costs of care exceeded $7,000 per year (4).

The mean life expectancy of those surviving the initial injury is nearly 40 years, with older age at injury a stronger predictor of poor long-term survival (5).

The goals of initial management of these serious injuries are accurate diagnostic evaluation of bony, ligamentous, and neurologic injury as well as prompt immobilization of the spine. Long-term goals include restoring spinal stability and providing the neural elements with an anatomical environment allowing the maximum potential for recovery of neural function.

II. PATHOPHYSIOLOGY

The biomechanics of the spinal cord have been described by Breig (6). He showed that the spinal cord with its investing and vascular elements exhibits good elasticity in the axial direction. Spinal extension causes the cord to shorten posteriorly and stretch anteriorly, whereas lateral bending stretches the cord on the convex side and shortens it in the concavity. He also noted that the cord does not slide in the cephalad and caudad direction within the spinal canal. The cord does not accommodate well to translatory forces, which makes them much more potentially injurious to the neural tissues (7). Other than in cases of penetrating trauma, it is this translatory force and the resultant direct pressure on the spinal cord and root that result in the neural dysfunction.

Trauma to the spinal cord causes mechanical destruction of neural tissue as well as hemorrhage within the cord. This axonal loss from direct physical deformation is known as the primary injury (8). This primary injury initiates a cascade of pathochemical events that results in significant further axonal loss, which is the secondary injury.

The histological picture of events immediately after the traumatic insult has been elucidated by animal studies. Hemorrhages appear almost immediately within the gray matter and spread within minutes to the white matter, affecting the microcirculation (9,10). Within approximately 4 hours, this hemorrhage spreads to the periphery of the white matter, resulting in irreversible cystic degeneration.

Underlying this histological picture of the evolution of the secondary injury is a host of chemical events that occur at the cellular level (8). A paradigm of this sequence based on current research is seen in Figure 1. The result of this cascade is cell death with neuronophagia by polymorphonuclear leukocytes. A great deal of emphasis has been placed on posttraumatic axonal membrane lipid derangements because of the potential for pharmacological interruption of this cascade, possibly limiting secondary injury. The events concerned are the activation of membrane phospholipases and lipases leading to the release of fatty acids (lipid hydrolysis) and free radical-induced lipid peroxidation (8). Lipid

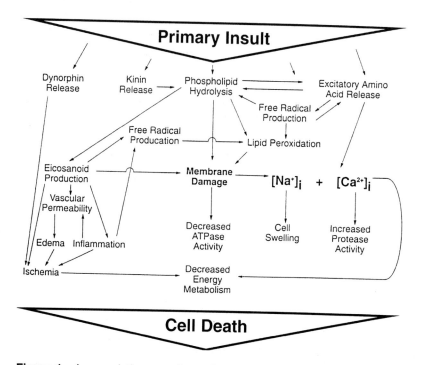

Figure 1 A speculative paradigm of secondary pathophysiologic events after primary traumatic injury to the spinal cord. See text for explanation. (From Ref. 8.)

hydrolysis is evidenced by a marked increase in gray matter total free fatty acid levels in experimental cord compression (11). Nonenzymatic lipid peroxidation is also a very early posttraumatic event. This is evidenced by the rapid loss of tissue vitamin E and membrane cholesterol, as well as an increase in the levels of 25-hydroxycholesterol, an oxidation product of cholesterol (12).

The presence of these phenomena in and of themselves does not mean that they are responsible, however, for perpetuation of secondary injury. This concept is supported by evidence that agents that can block portions of this cascade can limit certain secondary injury events and enhance neurological recovery. Synthetic glucocorticoids with antioxidant capabilities, such as methylprednisolone, have been shown to reduce posttraumatic tissue destruction via the above pathways. Bracken, in the NASCIS II study, has shown that methylprednisolone, when given in high doses within 8 hours of injury, significantly improved posttraumatic neurological recovery (13).

III. PATIENT EVALUATION

A. History

The patient's or an observer's description of the injury often gives a clue as to the mechanism of injury as well as the degree of force involved. Did the patient fall from a height of 5 feet or 20 feet? Did he strike his head? Was there loss of consciousness? Were any symptoms of neurological deficit present immediately postinjury? Symptoms of cervical pain as well as symptoms of paresthesia, hypesthesia, and/or weakness of the upper or lower extremities mandate a thorough evaluation of the cervical spine. The absence of these symptoms, however, should not lower the clinician's index of suspicion (14).

B. Physical Examination

1. General (Associated Injuries)

The first priority in the patient's initial care is evaluation and treatment, as indicated, of impairment of the airway, of ventilation, and circulatory embarrassment. Nearly half of spinal injury patients have significant associated injuries, many of them life threatening (14). Most commonly, these include injuries to the head, chest, and long bones; 10% have three or more such injuries. Unfortunately, missed injuries associated with spinal trauma are not rare, such as pneumothorax, hemopneumothorax, and renal or intra-abdominal injury (16). Hypotension on initial presentation may be the result of neurogenic shock; however, its classic presentation in association with bradycardia is relatively rare, occurring in fewer than 10% of patients with complete cord transection from penetrating injury (17). The presentation of shock, therefore, mandates evaluation for significant blood loss. Clinical signs and symptoms of cerebral trauma may also have another source. Vertebral injuries may also cause vertebral artery occlusion, giving rise to similar symptoms (18,19). Injuries to the head, face, and clavicle raise the index of suspicion for spinal injury but are not reliable predictors. In one study, a Glasgow Coma Score of less than fourteen was associated with a higher incidence of cervical cord injury (15). A high index of suspicion and adherence to accepted trauma protocols should reduce the morbidity and potential mortality of the associated injuries.

2. Neurologic

A thorough neurological examination is then performed and recorded. This should be repeated at appropriate intervals to detect any change in neurological status. The level of injury is, by definition, the lowest cord segment with intact function. The motor level is more functionally important, however, and in most cases corresponds well to the sensory level, especially in complete injuries. The presence and absence of muscle strength, reflexes, and pain, touch, and position sensation need to be accurately documented (20). Figure 2 outlines the muscle groups and dermatomes affected by different levels of injury. Incomplete injuries are those that exhibit preservation of function at some level below that of injury. This function may be preserved motor or sensory function or only the preservation of rectal tone or perineal sensation (21). A complete cord injury may be present if the patient has no distal sparing on initial evaluation. The postconcussive period known as spinal shock is usually over within 48 hours of injury, as evidenced by return of the bulbocavernous reflex. At this point, if there is no function distal to the level of injury, the lesion is considered complete and there is no potential for neural recovery (22).

Most recently, evoked potentials, especially somato-sensory evoked potentials, have shown some promise, both diagnostically and prognostically, in spinal cord injury. When performed early (within 48 hours) postinjury, they can be a more sensitive indicator of sparing of neural function, although they can not predict the degree of recovery potential. They are typically absent in complete injuries (23).

Incomplete injuries to the spinal cord typically result in patterns of damage depending on which portion of the cord is impaired (Fig. 3). Injury to the ventral portion of the cord or anterior spinal artery results in an anterior cord syndrome. This involves mainly loss of function of the corticospinal and spinothalamic tracts with resultant motor paralysis and loss of pain and temperature sensation. There is a varying degree of functional posterior column preservation, that is, preservation of proprioception, deep touch, and vibratory sensation (24). This is the most common incomplete cord syndrome often associated with direct compression from bone fragments of a burst fracture, retropulsed disc material, or tenting of the anterior cord over the lower vertebral body in a fracture-dislocation.

Central cord syndromes occur, usually as the result of a hyperextension injury. In younger patients, they can occur during water sports injury or football (25–27,110). In older patients, they are often the result of a fall. With the resultant hyperextension of the narrowed spinal canal, the cord is thought to be trapped by a "pincer-like" effect between osteophytic ridges and infolding of the hypertrophic ligamentum flavum (21,28,29,111). Anatomically, the greatest impairment is of the pyramidal tracts caused by an expanding hematoma of the central cord (28–30). Clinically, the central cord syndrome presents with marked motor impairment of the upper extremities with lesser impairment of the lower extremities due to the more lateral position of the lower extremity motor pathways. Fine motor function of the hands is usually the most affected and recovers poorly. Sacral level function (bowel and bladder), along with the lower extremities, has a reasonably good prognosis for recovery to ambulatory status (21).

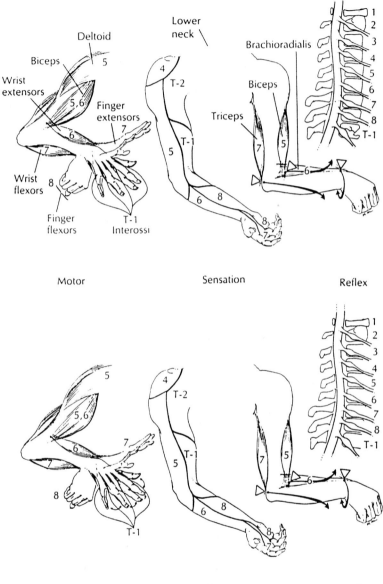

Motor   Sensation   Reflex

Motor   Sensation   Reflex

Figure 2 Segmental motor and sensory examination C-3 to T-1. The diaphragm is innervated from C-3 to C-5, and injuries in this region will weaken it to varying degrees. C-2 supplies sensation to the upper neck, while C-3 supplies the lower neck. The area under the clavicle is supplied by C-4. C-5 supplies sensation to the shoulder area, and a C-5 injury will weaken elbow flexion and paralyze the deltoid. Injury at C-6 will affect the biceps and weaken elbow flexion, causing numbness in the radial digits and palm. C-7 supplies sensation to the middle finger and midpalm, and motor function to the triceps, and injury at this level limits active elbow extension. Injury at C-8 will result in paralysis of the interossei

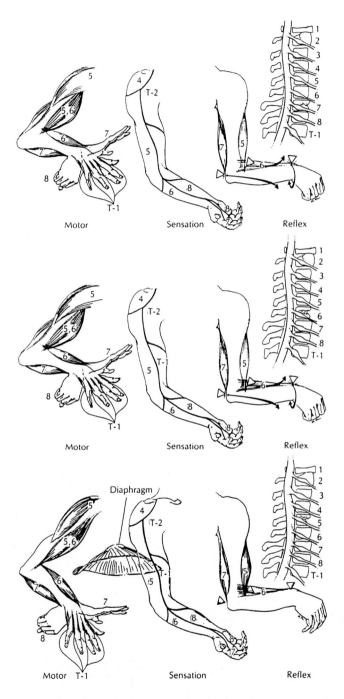

Motor	Sensation	Reflex

Motor	Sensation	Reflex

Motor T-1	Sensation	Reflex

and lumbricals, reducing sensation in the ulnar palm and the last two digits. Spinal injury at the T-1 level will result in incomplete loss of function of the intrinsic hand muscles with compromise of sensation on the undersurface of the proximal arm. (From Ref. 109.)   (*Fig. continues*)

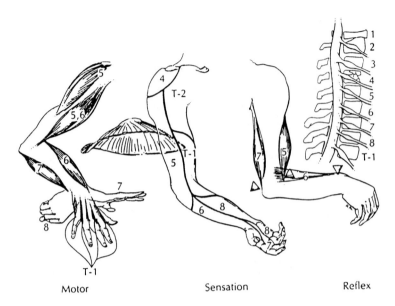

Motor   Sensation   Reflex

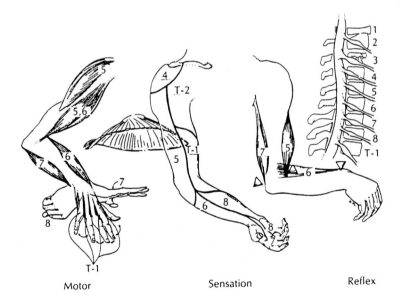

Motor   Sensation   Reflex

Figure 2 Continued

The Brown-Séquard syndrome results more commonly from penetrating injuries with hemisection of the cord. When seen in closed injuries, it is usually due to unilateral facet dislocations or other rotational deformity. The clinical syndrome consists of motor dysfunction of variable degree, ipsilateral to the side of the lesion, with loss of pain and temperature sensation on the opposite side one to two levels below that of the injury (30).

Rarely seen, the posterior cord syndrome can result from posterior impingement of the cord, such as from depressed laminar fractures or a posterior epidural hematoma. This syndrome presents with posterior column dysfunction, such as loss of deep touch, position, and vibratory sensation (31).

C. Radiographic Evaluation

1. Plain Film Evaluation

A high quality lateral film that includes the C7-T1 level will detect 70–90% of cervical fractures or dislocations (32). This should be the initial film obtained and should be examined in an orderly and methodical fashion. The occipitoatlantal articulation is examined first. Secondly, the atlantoaxial articulation is evaluated by using the atlantodental interval. This should not exceed 3 mm in adults or 5 mm in children. Prevertebral soft tissue shadows greater than 7 mm at C2 or 22 mm at C6 may indicate swelling and may be a clue to spinal trauma (32). Lines drawn along the anterior vertebral bodies, the posterior vertebral bodies, and the spinolaminar line are next assessed for deviation or interruption. Deviation of any of these lines may represent a subluxation or dislocation. Lastly, the integrity of each individual segment is assessed.

The next film obtained is the anteroposterior (AP) view. On this view, interspinous distances should be symmetrical and spinous processes must be carefully checked for any rotational malalignment.

The third film to be obtained is the open-mouth odontoid view to examine the C1-C2 region. In this view, the lateral masses of C1 should align over the lateral masses of C2. Lateral displacement may indicate a burst fracture of C1. Most fractures of the dens will be revealed by this view. The sensitivity of this series of films has been estimated to be 93%, with an accuracy of 84% (33,34). Any single view, however, has lower sensitivity and accuracy.

The sensitivity of the plain film evaluation can be increased with the addition of supine oblique views. These films can be obtained without moving the patient's head and are taken by angling the tube 30 degrees from the horizontal (35). When visualization of C7-T1 is difficult, a "swimmer's" view may be helpful (36). It can be somewhat difficult to interpret but may be necessary in the short-necked or uncooperative patient. The examiner must also be aware of normal variants as well as maintain a high index of suspicion in patients with

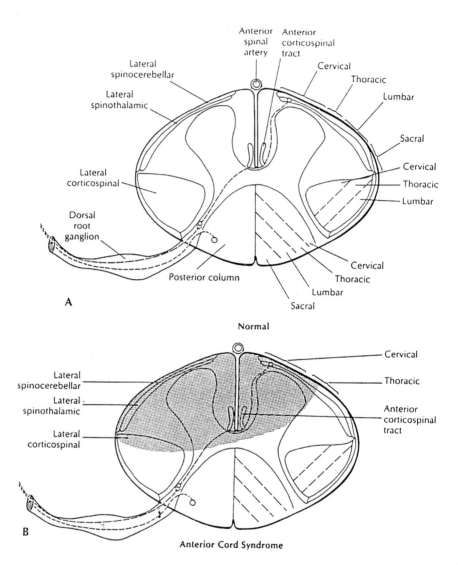

Figure 3 With incomplete motor or sensory injury, neurologic examination may reveal a "cord syndrome," due to injury to specific fiber tracts. The damage can be predicted by knowledge of the cross-sectional anatomy of the cord. (A) The major motor pathways descend in the anterior half of the spinal cord, while the sensory tracts are located in the posterior and lateral aspects of the spinal cord. (B) Anterior cord syndromes are caused by damage to the ventral aspect of the spinal cord; they involve mainly the spinothalamic (pain and temperature) and corticospinal (motor function) tracts. Such damage results in immediate partial or complete paralysis with loss of pain and temperature sensation but with preservation of proprioception, sense of vibration, and deep pressure sensation. (From Ref. 109.) (C) Central cord syndromes cause greater motor impairent of the upper than the lower extremities, with bladder dysfunction and varying degrees of sensory loss below the level of the lesion. (D) Brown-Séquard syndrome

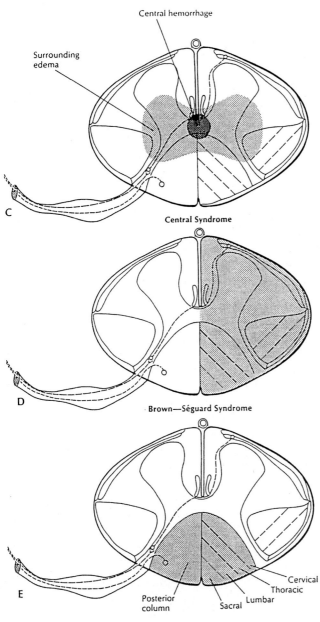

Central Syndrome

Brown—Séguard Syndrome

Posterior Spinal Syndrome

causes a motor weakness on the side of the lesion and decreased pain and temperature sensation on the side contralateral to the injury, beginning one or two segments below the level of injury. (E) The posterior cord syndrome is marked by loss of position and sense of vibration distal to the lesion. It is caused by involvement of the posterior columns.

other risk factors, such as previous spinal fusion or degenerative changes (37–39).

2. Provocative Studies

Flexion-extension films can be useful in detecting occult ligamentous instability that is hidden by initial muscle spasm. When indicated, these films must be performed with the patient positioning himself with the supervision but not assistance of the clinician. They are not indicated if an unstable lesion has been diagnosed on plain films (40).

Provocative testing in the longitudinal direction is probably neurologically safer, as the cord accommodates more readily to longitudinal distraction. White and Panjabi have described the "stretch test" described in Figure 4 (41). Any abnormal separation of anterior or posterior elements or change in neurology is considered a positive test. Using this test and other criteria, they have developed a diagnostic checklist for spinal stability (Table 1).

3. Tomography

Plain or computed tomography is useful both in detected occult injuries as well as more accurately depicting a known injury. Computed tomography accurately displays the cross-sectional anatomy of a given level, particularly the extent of any impingement on the spinal canal. It also gives a limited view of the soft

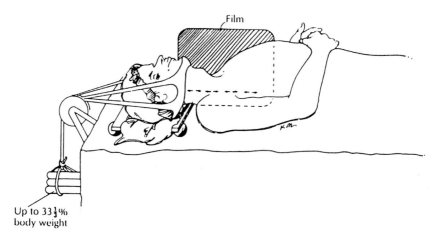

Figure 4 Stretch test—this should be performed only in the presence of a physician who performs periodic neurologic examinations as the loads increase to 33% of body weight or 65 pounds. (From Ref. 7; modified from Ref. 112.)

Table 1 Diagnostic Checklist for Spinal Stability

Elements	Point value	Individual clinical value
Anterior elements destroyed or unable to function	2	—
Posterior elements destroyed or unable to function	2	—
Relative sagittal plane translation >3.5 mm	2	—
Relative sagittal plane rotation >11 degrees	2	—
Positive stretch test	2	—
Cord damage	2	—
Root damage	1	—
Abnormal disk narrowing	1	—
Dangerous loading anticipated	1	—
Congenitally narrow spinal canal	1	—

Instability is defined as a total of 5 points or more, *or* a translation 20% of the anteroposterior diameter of the involved vertebra.
Source: Ref. 112, based on data from Ref. 113.

tissue structures. Sagittal reconstruction can give further information regarding the spinal canal; however, it can completely miss fractures that are in the plane of the scan. Planar tomography is probably a superior diagnostic modality in fractures of dens, subluxation of vertebral bodies, atlanto-occipital dislocation, and possibly in fractures of the lateral masses and articulate processes (42).

4. Myelography

In evaluation of spinal trauma, myelography is performed via C1-C2 puncture using a non-ionic water soluble contrast medium in conjunction with CT. This combination is more accurate than either CT or myelography alone (43). Computed tomography-myelography most commonly is indicated in evaluating injuries of nonosseous origin or when the clinical picture is incongruous with the obvious bony injury. It can detect dural tears or anatomic disruption of the cord; however, in these situations, it probably does not change the course of treatment.

5. Magnetic Resonance Imaging

Magnetic resonance imaging (MRI) is now used routinely when available on patients with neurologic deficit after vertebral injury (44,45). It is useful in the evaluation of cord compression by prolapsed disc or bony fragments. Its greatest utility appears to be in evaluation of the cord itself. An MRI can demonstrate a variety of pathologies, from transection of the cord, hematomyelia, contusion, ischemia, and edema. Ten percent of patients with neurologic injury, however, will have a normal-appearing cord on MRI. Contusion or ischemia are seen as areas of hyperintense signal within the cord. These are most commonly found in incomplete injuries, with the extent of signal changes correlating reasonably well with the extent of neurologic impairment. Cord edema occurs in both complete and incomplete injuries. Its significance from a neurologic recovery standpoint is unclear. Hematomyelia is primarily found in complete injuries and portends a poor prognosis for recovery of neurologic function (46).

IV. INITIAL MANAGEMENT

A. Initial Stabilization of the Spine

Initial stabilization of the potentially injured spine must begin at the accident site. Approximately 10 to 20% of patients with neurological deficit are worsened during extrication from the accident scene and subsequent transport to emergency facilities (47). When intubation is necessary, orotracheal intubation with manual inline stabilization by trained and experienced personnel appears to be safe, although blind or bronchoscopic nasotracheal intubation or tracheostomy may be preferable (48).

Soft collars provide little immobilization and should not be relied upon to provide initial stabilization (49). The least rigid device that affords some protection is the Philadelphia collar (Table 2). Once the diagnosis of an unstable cervical spine injury is made, the spine can be stabilized by Gardner-Wells tongs. These are applied quickly and easily in the Emergency Department. Crutchfield tongs are more difficult to apply and may loosen. A good alternative is the early application of a halo ring (50). The application of a halo-vest often facilitates the performance of further diagnostic and treatment procedures in the patient with multiple injuries. It is particularly appropriate in those patients when the halo-vest may be the definitive treatment of the spine injury.

B. Medical Management

Restoration of normovolemia, correction of hypotension, and maintenance of adequate oxygenation can reduce the risk of further ischemic cord damage. A number of pharmacological agents have been used to attempt to limit the degree of neural injury and to enhance recovery. Mannitol, an osmotic diuretic, has not been shown to be helpful and has the risk of creating hypokalemia (9). Naloxone has shown some promise in animal experiments; however, it has not shown the same clinical benefits in humans (9,13). The well-publicized NASCIS II study (13) published in 1990 compared the use of high-dose meth-

Table 2 Normal Cervical Motion Allowed From the Occiput to the First
Thoracic Vertebra

			Mean % of normal motion		
	Number of subjects	Mean age (yrs)	Flexion-extension	Lateral bending	Rotation
Normal	44	25.8	100	100	100
Soft collar	20	26.2	74.2	92.3	82.6
Philadelphia collar	17	25.8	28.9	66.4	43.7
SOMI brace	22	25.0	27.7	65.6	33.6
Four-poster brace	27	25.9	20.6	45.9	27.1
Rigid cervicothoracic brace	27	25.9	12.8	50.5	18.2
Halo vest	7	40.0	4	4	1

Source: Ref. 114, based on data from Ref. 115.

ylprednisolone, Naloxone and placebo in spinal-injured patients. A dose of
methylprednisolone of 30 mg/kg was given intravenously as soon as possible
after the injury and 5.4 mg/kg more per hour was given for the next 23 hours.
The methylprednisolone treatment was associated with improved motor function, pin-prick and touch sensation 6 months after the injury. The use of high-
dose steroids is a two-edged sword, however, as these patients have longer and
more complicated hospital courses primarily due to pulmonary complications
such as pneumonia (51).

V. SPECIFIC INJURIES

A. Occiput-C1

This injury is rarely encountered clinically and is usually fatal because of injury
to the medulla oblongata or spinomedullary junction. It is the most common
upper cervical injury in victims of fatal motor vehicle accidents (52,53) Survival of this injury has been reported with varying degrees of neurological
deficit (54). Displacement can occur anteriorly, posteriorly, or rotationally and
may be associated with rotary subluxation or dislocation of C1 and C2 in the
opposite direction (55). The diagnosis is made on plain lateral radiographs of
the cervical spine. Treatment of survivors of this injury consists of mechanical
ventilation, closed reduction with halo stabilization and subsequent occipitocervical fusion (54,56)

B.   C1-C2 Complex Injuries

1.   C1 Fractures

The most common fracture of C1 is fracture of the posterior arch. The fracture occurs just posterior to the lateral masses in the thinnest part of the bone. This part of the C1 ring has the lowest sectional inertia against a vertical compression force (57). This injury is usually diagnosed on a high-quality lateral radiograph of C1. This fracture is stable and is treated with orthotic immobilization until the fracture heals.

Jefferson (burst) fractures of C1 result from injuring forces of relatively high magnitude directed caudally. The lateral masses of C1 are driven apart by the occipital condyles (40,58). The classic fracture pattern consists of two fractures of the ring anteriorly and two posteriorly. Most commonly, however, there is one anterior fracture and one posterior fracture (59). The primary radiographic feature of this injury is the spread of the lateral masses of C1 on the open-mouth view. Spence has shown experimentally that if this spread (the combined overhang of the C1 lateral masses) is more than 7 mm then the transverse ligament is most likely ruptured with resultant C1-C2 instability (60). Fracture anatomy is particularly well demonstrated by CT. Comminuted fractures also can present a problem with nonunion, which is unusual in the more common two-and four-part fractures. This can result in functional impairment due to pain and stiffness (58).

Treatment of burst fractures of C1 depends on the degree of displacement. Minimumly displaced (less than 5 mm) fractures can be treated with orthotic protection until healed (61). In fractures with significant displacement, reduction with halo traction is indicated. This traction is continued until early healing occurs, up to 6 to 8 weeks. Premature conversion to a halo-vest risks secondary fracture displacement, as it cannot adequately unload the fracture until late in the healing process (62). If there is evidence of associated transverse ligament disruption with C1-C2 instability, it is preferable to allow healing of the C1 ring and then perform a C1-C2 fusion rather than an occiput-C2 fusion that would be required to obtain stability before fracture healing. This allows significantly better preservation of motion after injury (63). Neurologic injury in C1 fractures is rare.

2.   Atlantoaxial Dislocation and Subluxation

Traumatic displacement of C1 on C2 may be anterior or posterior, or there may be a rotary subluxation. The primary restraint to anterior displacement is the transverse ligament that runs between tubercles on the lateral masses of the atlas. The alar ligaments function as secondary restraints. Experimentally, Fielding was able to produce anterior subluxation of C1 on C2 with about 84 kg of force rupturing the transverse ligament (64).

Diagnosis of this lesion is made on lateral films of the upper cervical spine. If not apparent on static studies, it can usually be detected on flexion-extension films, although initial cervical muscle spasm can result in a false-negative examination. Mild displacement of less than 5 mm indicates a stretch injury of the transverse ligament. Rupture of the transverse ligament is complete at 5 to 10 mm of displacement. More than 10 mm of displacement means that the entire ligament complex is disrupted (62). This degree of displacement endangers the spinal cord.

Treatment of this lesion usually requires surgical stabilization and fusion. Orthotic immobilization will not result in stabilization of the C1-C2 complex. Stabilization is usually performed from a posterior approach using a Brooks or modified Gallie-type construct (62,65). Neurological injury can occur when displacement exceeds 1 cm. More commonly in the elderly, this injury may go unrecognized after a seemingly minor injury until it presents because of chronic myelopathy.

Posterior dislocation of C1 on C2 is a rare injury. It can result from a hyperextension injury that involves a significant distracting force. Rotary subluxation of C1 on C2 is an unusual lesion. When caused traumatically, the injuring force is rotation with disruption of the joint capsules with subluxation or dislocation of one or both joints, potentially compromising the spinal canal (57). Treatment consists of attempted closed reduction with halo traction and subsequent surgical stabilization and fusion (66).

3. Odontoid Fracture

Fractures of the odontoid process of C2 typically occur in two patient populations. They occur in the young as a result of high energy trauma, often caused by a motor-vehicle accident. Less commonly, they are the result of falls in the elderly, which may cause posteriorly displaced fractures (67). Determining the mechanism of injury is somewhat speculative, as odontoid fractures have been difficult to reproduce in cadavers.

Odontoid fractures typically present with muscle spasm and suboccipital pain and occasionally pain in the distribution of the greater occipital nerve. The majority of these patients are neurologically intact; however, up to 20% will exhibit a variety of motor and/or sensory deficits, including high quadriplegia (67).

The open-mouth view will demonstrate most odontoid fractures. If the diagnosis is unclear, AP and lateral plain tomograms will demonstrate the fracture and allow anatomic classification. Computed tomographic scanning may be helpful, particularly in a displaced fracture; however, if the CT cuts are immediately above or below the fracture, it may be missed even with sagittal reconstruction of the images (40,68).

Anderson and D'Alonzo have classified odontoid fractures into three groups (69) (Fig. 5). Type I is an oblique avulsion of the upper portion of the dens. Stability of the motion segment is undisturbed, as the transverse ligament and alar ligaments remain intact. These fractures heal routinely with orthotic immobilization (70).

The type II fracture occurs at the junction of the dens with the vertebral body of the axis. This is the most common odontoid fracture, yet the most difficult to treat. Anterior displacement is clinically more common. Because the fracture interrupts the blood supply to the dens, there is a significant risk of nonunion that increases with age (69,71). Treatment with halo immobilization is considered for minimumly displaced fractures in the young, healthy patient. In patients older than age forty, with more than 4 mm of displacement, stabilization is recommended either with anterior screw fixation (70,72) or with posterior stabilization and C1-C2 fusion (62,72).

Type III fractures occur through the body of the axis at the base of the dens. These fractures are most often mildly displaced and stable once reduced. Definitive treatment consists of halo or cervicothoracic orthosis immobilization, with the expectation of solid union as the end result (70,73).

C. Traumatic Spondylolisthesis of the Axis

This lesion is commonly called the "hangman's fracture." The injury produced by judicial hanging is a fracture of the axis through the pars interarticularis separating the anterior and posterior elements. The use of the submental knot causes an extension-distraction type injury with disruption of the C2-C3 disc and transection of the cord (74).

The modern counterpart of this injury is most commonly the result of a motor vehicle accident. The major injury vector is usually extension without significant distraction. The injury force creates an extension moment on the dens and body with a balancing joint reaction force at the C2-C3 articulation and failure occurs at the pars interarticularis because of its relatively low area moment of inertia to bending in the sagittal plane. If the force is more severe, the anterior longitudinal ligament and finally the disc at C2-C3 may be disrupted, resulting in instability between the cervicocranium and the lower cervical spine (57). Because the spinal canal actually widens in this injury, neurologic injury is rare.

The diagnosis is usually apparent on lateral or oblique plain films. The degree of fracture displacement and disc space deformity determines treatment. Type I fractures—those with no angulation of less than 3 mm of displacement—are treated with a halo-vest and will typically unite in about 12 weeks (75,76).

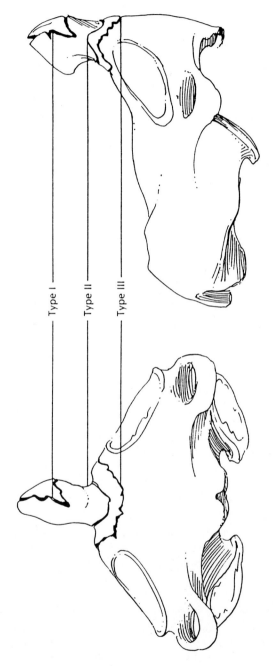

Figure 5 Classification of odontoid fractures is based upon level of fracture, because the level is predictive of the likelihood of nonunion. Type I fractures are avulsion fractures of the tip. Type II fractures occur at the junction of the odontoid process and the body of C-2 in the area of the attachment of the accessory ligaments, and are prone to nonunion. Type III fractions occur through the body of the axis between the junction of the dens and the axis. (From Ref. 109.)

Type II fractures are those with significant translation and angulation. These fractures are treated with closed reduction by halo traction, which is converted to a halo-vest at 5 to 7 days. If there is significant redisplacement, the patient may need to be kept in halo traction for 4 to 6 weeks until early union occurs (62,76). A subset of these fractures involves a distraction component with flexion angulation of the C2-C3 disc (type IIa). Traction may increase their angulation. These injuries are treated in a halo-vest with fracture reduction in extension (76).

Type III fractures additionally consist of unilateral or bilateral C2-C3 facet dislocation. Closed reduction should be attempted by halo traction, but not infrequently, this fails. If necessary, open reduction with stabilization and fusion via a posterior approach is used. Postoperative immobilization with a halo-vest may be necessary in these very unstable injuries (76).

D. Fractures of the Lower Cervical Spine

The subsequent discussion applies similarly to all levels of the lower cervical spine. Torg (77), however, has outlined some specific differences in behavior of the injured spine at the C3-C4 level. In his analysis of twenty-five cases of compressive flexion and vertical compressive injuries, he noted that at this level bony injury is uncommon, with most injuries resulting in unilateral or bilateral facet dislocations. Closed reduction of these injuries was particularly difficult and, if achieved, it was difficult to maintain. He also noted several cases of traumatic disc herniation at this level that resulted in transient quadriplegia.

The cervical spine functionally can be divided into anterior and posterior columns (Fig. 6) (78). The anterior column consists of the anterior longitudinal ligament, the vertebral body or intervertebral disc and the posterior longitudinal ligament. The posterior column consists of the structures dorsal to the posterior longitudinal ligament; the facet joints, the vertebral arch, and the spinous processes with the intraspinous ligament. This concept is useful in describing patterns and mechanisms of injury in the lower cervical spine. Based on this, a comprehensive classification system was developed by Allen and associates in 1982 (79). The usefulness of such a system is that certain patterns of injury will behave in a biologically predictable fashion allowing a more accurate treatment plan.

The first determination to be made is whether the lesion is stable. If not, can it be adequately stabilized by an orthosis or a halo? If surgical stabilization is required, an accurate understanding of the mechanism of injury and of which stabilizing structures are lost will allow prudent decision-making regarding surgical approach and the use of internal or external fixation.

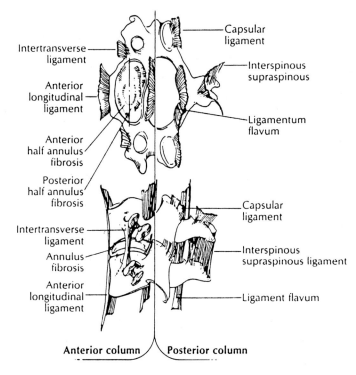

Figure 6 Diagrammatic representation detailing the anatomy and separation of anterior and posterior elements. (From Ref. 7.)

1. Compressive Flexion

This group of injuries is the result of a major injury vector directed caudally and anteriorly (Fig. 7). The injuring force is propagated through the anterior column. This phylogeny is graded in five recognizable stages according to severity. CFS1 injuries consist of blunting of the anterosuperior vertebral margin without injury to the posterior column. In CFS2, there is loss of anterior height of the vertebral body with "beaking" of the anteroinferior body. Again, the posterior column remains intact. In CFS3, there is an oblique shear fracture of the vertebral body centrum. In the next stage (CFS4), there is mild posterior displacement of the posterior inferior body into the spinal canal. In this and CFS5 injuries, there is a component of tension posteriorly that results in failure of the posterior column as well with gross instability in CFS5 injuries.

The simple compression fractures are usually stable; however, if there is

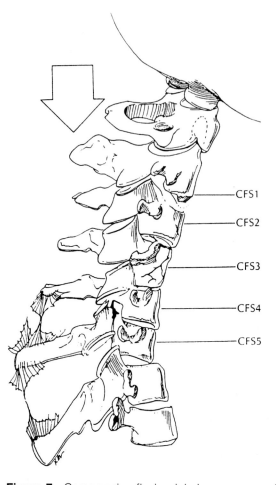

Figure 7 Compressive flexion injuries are caused by a force vector directed inferiorly and anteriorly. CFS1 consists of blunting at the anterior margin of the vertebral body. CFS2 adds obliquity to the anterior vertebral body and loss of some of the anterior height of the vertebral body. In CFS3 the fracture line passes obliquely from the anterior surface through the subchondral plate without displacement. In CFS4 there is less than 3 mm displacement of the inferoposterior margin of the vertebral body into the neural canal. Severe displacement of the body fragment into the canal, with separation of the articular facets and increased distance between spinous processes occurs in CFS5. (From Ref. 109.)

any doubt, a stretch test or flexion-extension film should be performed (80). Treatment of more unstable injuries depends on the neurological status of the patient. Those with incomplete cord injuries and demonstrable anterior compression will require anterior decompression and fusion. Even complete injuries may recover an additional root level with this approach (81). The anterior approach, even with internal fixation, usually needs to be supplemented by posterior stabilization, as the stabilizing anterior longitudinal ligament is sacrificed in the anterior approach leading to two-column instability and potentially recurrent deformity (82–86).

Neurologically intact injuries can be treated with halo traction followed by conversion to a halo vest; however, stability must be assessed during the healing process, and if the lesion is unstable at 3 months, fusion should be considered (87). CFS4 and CFS5 injuries often exhibit bony ankylosis after management with the halo (88).

2. Vertical Compression

In this phylogeny, the major injury vector is directed caudally, resulting primarily in anterior column disruption (Fig. 8). In VCS1 injuries, there is deformity of either the superior or inferior vertebral endplate. Greater body comminution but with minimal displacement is classified as VCS2. In VCS3 injuries, there is compressive failure of the entire vertebral body resulting in the typical "burst" fracture. Body fragments are often displaced posteriorly into the spinal canal. If there is a component of extension, there may be an associated vertebral arch fracture. This group of fractures is often associated with severe incomplete or complete cord injuries (89,90).

Treatment, once again, depends on the neurological status of the patient. Patients with incomplete injuries and selected patients with complete injuries are candidates for anterior decompression to facilitate neurological recovery. As in CF injuries, however, posterior ligamentous injury may be present and posterior stabilization may be necessary (84,85). In the neurologically intact patient, traction is used to restore alignment. A halo-vest is then used to maintain alignment throughout the course of healing with close follow-up to detect the development of posttraumatic kyphosis (91). This can be the result of so-called paradoxical motion, possible in a halo-vest, where one motion segment flexes as the one above or below extends (91,92). Flexion-extension films should be performed after 3 months in the halo-vest and if instability persists, posterior fusion may be indicated.

3. Distractive Flexion

The common characteristic of this group is tension-shear failure of the posterior column, usually the ligamentous complex (Fig. 9). The major injury vector is

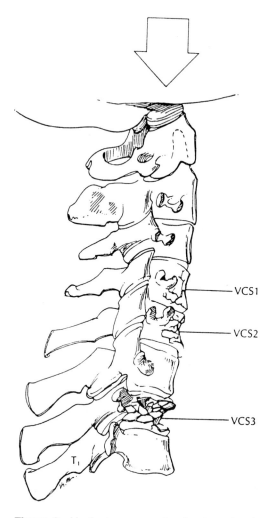

Figure 8   Vertical compression fractures begin with a fracture through the center of either the inferior or superior end-plate of the vertebral body (VCS1). VCS2 consists of fractures through both end-plates but minimal displacement. More force fragments the body (VCS3) and causes it to displace peripherally, abutting on or protruding into the neural canal. (From Ref. 109.)

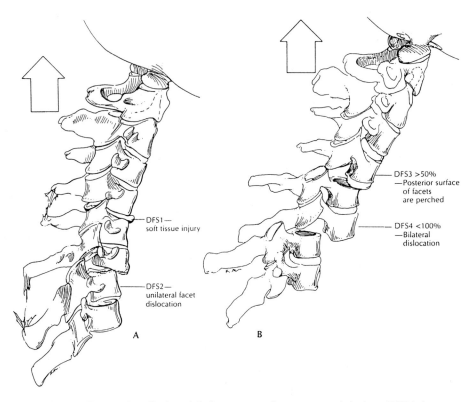

DFS3 >50%
—Posterior surface
of facets
are perched

DFS1—
soft tissue injury

DFS4 <100%
—Bilateral
dislocation

DFS2—
unilateral facet
dislocation

A   B

Figure 9 Distractive flexion injuries cause ligamentous injuries. DFS1 is a "flexion sprain" with failure of the posterior ligamentous complex. DFS2 is a unilateral facet dislocation and DFS3 and DFS4 are bilateral facet dislocations with increasing translation. (From Ref. 109.)

distraction with a minor injury vector of flexion. The DFS1 lesion consists of posterior ligamentous injury with facet subluxation, anterior displacement of the superior vertebral body, and kyphotic angulation of the vertebral bodies with divergence of the spinous processes, the so-called "hyperflexion sprain" (93–97). There may be an associated mild compression fracture of the inferior vertebral body. This injury may be difficult to detect on initial evaluation, especially in the presence of muscle spasm, and accounts for a significant proportion of "occult" injuries to the cervical spine (95). Instability may become apparent on flexion-extension films once the initial spasm subsides (98,99). Herkowitz (100) has described a syndrome of subacute instability wherein after initial elastic deformation of the ligaments, over a period of weeks, plastic deformation occurs with subsequent vertebral displacement. It is apparent that close follow-up of these injuries is indicated.

The unilateral facet dislocation is DFS2. Rather than being caused by a rotational force, it is felt that the rotation necessary to produce this injury is an exaggeration of the normal coupled motion when lateral bending is produced by off-center distraction (101). The vertebral body displacement is less than 50% in this injury, which may involve pure facet dislocation or fracture of the articular processes or pedicle. This lesion may be overlooked at C6-C7 if initial radiographs do not clearly show C7 (101–103). Cord injury is not likely; however, root lesions are common from compression by the inferior articular process of the superior vertebrae. Treatment consists of attempted closed reduction with traction (101,104). If this is unsuccessful, open reduction is required. Reduction may be impossible after 6 weeks, in which case root impingement can be treated with foraminotomy (101).

DFS3 and DFS4 are bilateral facet dislocations with 50% to 100% body displacement in DFS3 and more than 100% displacement in DFS4. These injuries usually result in significant, often complete cord lesions (105). Bilateral facet dislocations can often be reduced with cervical traction with resultant varying degrees of neurological improvement (101,105). These injuries may fuse spontaneously by ossification along the anterior longitudinal ligament after reduction; however, more often they will remain unstable and require posterior stabilization (103). Prior to attempting reduction of unilateral or bilateral facet dislocations, the clinician must rule out an associated disc herniation at that level by myelography or MRI. If reduction is achieved in the face of a disc herniation, it may result in neurological compromise. In these cases, a two-staged approach with anterior discectomy, with or without reduction, is followed by posterior reduction and stabilization (106–108).

4. Compressive Extension

This group of injuries has a major injury vector of axial compression with the spine held in extension (Fig. 10). The CES1 lesion consists of a unilateral vertebral arch fracture with or without displacement. Bilaminar fractures, often at multiple contiguous levels, constitute the CES2 injury. CES3 and CES4 injuries have not been described clinically; however, hypothetically they would consist of greater posterior column comminution with some body displacement in CES4. The CES5 lesion consists of bilateral arch fractures with full vertebral body with displacement anteriorly, essentially a traumatic spondylolisthesis type of injury. Interestingly, serious neurological injury is more common in the CES2 injury (79). Treatment of these injuries consists of immobilization after traction realignment with decompression and stabilization as indicated by the neurological status of the patient.

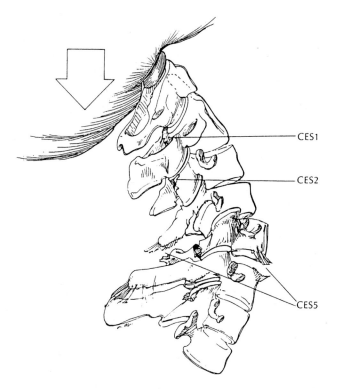

Figure 10 CES1 consists of a unilateral vertebral arch fracture. CES2 consists of bilateral laminar fractures. CES5 consists of bilateral vertebral arch fractures with full vertebral body width displacement anteriorly. (From Ref. 109.)

5. Distractive Extension

This injury phylogeny has a major injury vector of axial distraction with the spine postured in extension. In DES1, failure occurs only in the anterior column (anterior longitudinal ligament, vertebral body, or disc). DES2 injuries also involve disruption of the posterior ligamentous complex, sometimes displacing the upper vertebral body into the spinal canal. There is often minimal residual displacement, and these injuries may go unrecognized (107).

The most common associated neurological injury is a central cord syndrome (108). The bony-ligamentous injury is usually stable and will heal with immobilization. There is usually a significant degree of spontaneous neurological recovery; however, if a compressive lesion (such as a disc herniation) is found on diagnostic studies, decompression is indicated.

6. Lateral Flexion

This group of injuries has a major injury vector of axial compression but offset laterally to the side of lateral bending. In LFS1, the vertebral arch and body both fail on the side of compression without displacement. LFS2 injuries are those with displacement or ligamentous failure and tension on the opposite side. These injuries are uncommon and are treated individually using the previously mentioned determinants of stability.

VI. SUMMARY

In this chapter, we have given an overview of the evaluation and treatment of cervical spine injuries. Accurate evaluation of specific injuries while maintaining a high index of suspicion for lesions that are not readily apparent is extremely important. Once an accurate diagnosis is made, the knowledge of the natural history of an injury will allow the treating clinician to provide the care that will result in the best outcome possible in these potentially devastating injuries.

REFERENCES

1. Gerhart KA. Spinal cord injury outcomes in a population-based sample. Journal of Trauma 1991; 31:1529–1535.
2. Fine PR, Kuhlemeier KV, DeVivo MJ, Stover SL. Spinal cord injury: An epidemiologic perspective. Paraplegia 1979; 17:237–241.
3. Burney RE, Maio RF, Maynard F, Karunas R. Incidence, characteristics and outcome of spinal cord injury at trauma centers in North America. Arch Surg 1993; 128:596–599.
4. Harvey C, Wilson SE, Greene CG, Berkowitz M, Stripling TE. New estimates of the direct costs of traumatic spinal cord injuries: Results of a nationwide survey. Paraplegia 1992; 30:834–850.
5. Samsa, GP, Patrick CH, Feussner JR. Long-term survival of veterans with traumatic spinal cord injury. Arch Neurol 1993; 50:909–914.
6. Breig, A. Biomechanics of the nervous system: Some Basic Normal and Pathologic Phenomena. Stockholm: Almquist & Wiksell, 1960.
7. Miz G. Cervical spine instability and biomechanics of treatment. In: Errico TE, and ed. Spinal Trauma. Philadelphia: J.B. Lippincott, 1991:128.
8. Anderson DK, Hall ED. Pathophysiology of spinal cord trauma. Ann Emerg Med 1993; 22:987–992.
9. de la Torre JC. Spinal cord injury: A review of basic and applied research. Spine 1981; 6:315–335.

10. Albin MS, White RJ. Epidemiology, physiopathology, and experimental therapeutics of acute spinal cord injury. Crit Care Clin 1987; 3:441–452.
11. Demediuk P, Saunders RD, Anderson DK, Means ED, Horrocks LA. Membrane Lipid Changes in Laminectomized and Traumatized Cat Spinal Cord. Proc Nat Acad Sci USA 1985; 82:7071–7075.
12. Anderson DK, Demediuk P, Saunders RD, Dugan LL, Means ED, Horrocks LA. Spinal cord injury and protection. Ann Emerg Med 1985; 14:816–821.
13. Bracken MP, Shepard MJ, Collins WF Jr, et al. A randomized controlled trial of methylprednisolone or naloxone in the treatment of acute spinal cord injury. New Engl J Med 1990; 322:1405–1411.
14. Saboe LA, Reid DL, Davis LA, Warren SA, Grace MG. Spinal trauma and associated injuries. J Trauma 1991; 31:43–48.
15. Williams J, Jehle D, Cottington E, Shufflebarger C. Head, facial, and clavicular trauma as a predictor of cervical spine injury. Ann Emerg Med 1992; 21:719–722.
16. Ryan M, Klein S, Bongard F. Missed injuries associated with spinal cord trauma. Amer Surg 1993; 59:371–374.
17. Zipnick RI, Scalea TM, Trooskin SZ, Sclafani SJ, Emad B, Shah A, Talbert S, Haher T. Hemodynamic responses to penetrating spinal cord injuries. J Trauma 1993; 35:578–583.
18. Schwarz N, Buchinger W, Gaudernak T, Russe F, Zechner W. Injuries to the cervical spine causing vertebral artery trauma: Case reports. J Trauma 1991; 31:127–133.
19. Song W, Chiang Y, Chen C, Lin S, Liu M. A simple method for diagnosing traumatic occlusion of the vertebral artery at the craniovertebral junction. Spine 1994; 19:837–839.
20. Wagner FC, Cheharz B. Neurologic evaluation of cervical spine injuries. Spine 1989; 9:507–511.
21. Cooper PR. Initial evaluation and management. In: Berczeller PH, Bezkor MH, eds. Medical Complications of Quadriplegia. Chicago: Yearbook Medical Publishers, 1986.
22. Stauffer ES. Fractures and dislocations of the spine. Part I—The cervical spine. In: Rockwood CA, Green DP eds. Fractures in Adults. 2d ed. Philadelphia: J. B. Lippincott, 1989:987–1035.
23. Young W. Correlation of somatosensory evoked potentials and neurologic findings in spinal cord injury. In: Tator CH, ed. Early Management of Acute Spinal Injuries. New York: Raven Press, 1982; 153–165.
24. Fielding JW, Hawkins RJ. Roentgenographic diagnosis of the injured neck. In: American Academy of Orthopaedic Surgeons, ed.: Instructional Course Lectures. St. Louis: C. V. Mosby, 1976.
25. Cheng CLY, Wolf AL, Mirvis S, Robinson WL. Bodysurfing accidents resulting in cervical spinal injuries. Spine 1992; 17:257–260.
26. Bailes JE, Hadley MN, Quigley MR, Sonntag VKH, Cerullo LJ. Management of athletic injuries of the cervical spine and spinal cord. Neurosurgery 1991; 29:491–497.
27. Maroon JC. "Burning Hands" in football spinal cord injuries. JAMA 1977; 238:2049–2051.

28. Morse SD. Acute central cervical spinal cord syndrome. Ann Emerg Med 1982; 11:436–439.

29. Schneider RC, Thompson JM, Bebin J. The syndrome of acute central cervical spinal cord injury. J Neurosurg Psychiatry 1958; 21:216–227.

30. Julow J, Szarvas I, Sarvary A. Clinical study of injuries of the lower cervical cord. Injury 1984; 11:38–42.

31. Weir DC. Roentgenographic signs of cervical injury. Clin Orthop 1975; 109:11–17.

32. Berguist TH, Cabanela ME. The spine. In: Imaging of Orthopedic Trauma and Surgery Berquist TH, ed. Philadephia: W. B. Saunders; 1986:91–180.

33. Streitwieser DR, Knopp R, Wales LR, Williams JL, Tonnemacher K. Accuracy of standard radiographic views in detecting cervical spine fractures. Ann Emerg Med 1983; 12:538–542.

34. Holliman CJ, Mayer JS, Cook RT, Smith JS. Is the anteroposterior cervical spine radiograph necessary in initial trauma screening? Am J Emerg Med 1991; 9:421–425.

35. Turetsky DB, Vines FS, Clayman DA, Northup HM. Technique and use of supine obligue views in acute cervical spine trauma. Ann Emerg Med 1993; 22:685–689.

36. Bachulis BL, Long WB, Hynes GD, Johnson MC. Clinical indications for cervical spine radiographs in the traumatized patient. Am J Surg 1987; 153:473–478.

37. Woodring JH, Lee C. Limitation of cervical radiograph in the evaluation of acute cervical trauma. J Trauma 1993; 34:32–39.

38. Gerrelts BD, Petersen EV, Mabry J, Petersen SR. Delayed diagnosis of cervical spine injuries. J Trauma 1991; 31:1622–1626.

39. Macmillan M, Stauffer ES. Traumatic instability in the previously fused cervical spine. J Spinal Disord 1991; 4:449–454.

40. Alker GJ. Radiographic evaluation of patients with cervical spine injury. In: Griffin P, ed. Intructional Course Lectures Vol. 36. Chicago. 1987. American Academy of Orthopaedic Surgeons, 1987.

41. White AA III, Panjabi MM. Update on the evaluation of instability of the lower cervical spine. In: Griffin PP, ed. Instruction Course Lectures—vol. 36. Chicago; American Academy of Orthopaedic Surgeons, 1987.

42. Woodring JH, Lee C. The role and limitations of computed tomographic scanning in the evaluation of cervical trauma. J Trauma 1992; 33:698–708.

43. Nussbaum ES, Sebring LA, Wolf AL, Mirvis SE, Gottlieb R. Myelographic and enhanced computed tomographic appearance of acute traumatic spinal cord avulsion. Neurosurgery 1991; 30:43–48.

44. Daffner RH. Evaluation of cervical vertebral injuries. Sem Roentgenology 1992; 27:239–253.

45. Wilberger JE. Diagnosis and management of spinal cord trauma. J Neurotrauma 1991; 8:521–530.

46. Shaffer DM, Flander A, Bruce NE. Magnetic resonance imaging of acute cervical spine trauma. Spine 1989; 14:1090–1095.

47. Mattox KL. The Injured Patient's Neck. Emerg Med Clin North Am 1984; 16:24–48.

48. Scanell G, Waxman K, Tominaga G, Barker S, Annas C. Orotracheal intubation in trauma patients with cervical fractures. Arch Surg 1993; 128:903–906.
49. Johnson RM, Hart DL, Simmons EF, Ramsby GR, Southwick WO. Cervical orthoses. A study comparing their effectiveness in restricting cervical motion in normal subjects. J Bone Joint Surg 1977; 59-A:332–339.
50. Heary RF, Hunt CD, Krieger AJ, Antonio C, Livingston DH. Acute stabilization of the cervical spine by halo/vest application facilitates evaluation and treatment of multiple trauma patients. J Trauma 1992; 33:445–451.
51. Galandiuk S, Raque G, Appel S, Polk HC. The two-edged sword of large-dose steroids for spinal cord trauma. Ann Surg 1993; 218:419–427.
52. Bucholz RW, Burhead WZ. The pathologic anatomy of fatal atlanto-occipital dislocations. J Bone Joint Surg 1979; 61-A:248–250.
53. Alker GJ, Oh YS, Leslie EV. Postmortem radiology of head and neck injuries in fatal traffic accidents. Radiology 1975; 114:611–617.
54. Zigler JE, Waters RL, Nelson RW. Occipito-cervical-thoracic spine fusion in a patient with occipito-cervical dislocation and survival. Spine 1986; 11:645–646.
55. Pierce DS, Barr JS. Fractures and dislocations. In: Cervical Spine Research Society, eds. The Cervical Spine. Philadelphia: J.B. Lippincott, 1983.
56. Evarts C. Traumatic occipito-atlantal dislocation: Report of a case with survival. J Bone Joint Surg 1970; 52-A:1653–1660.
57. Miz G. Cervical spine instability and biomechanics of treatment. In: Errico TE, ed. Spinal Trauma. Philadelphia: J. B. Lippincott, 1991; 123–143.
58. Segal D, Grimm JO, Stauffer ES. Nonunions of fractures of the atlas. J Bone Joint Surg 1987; 69-A:1423–1434.
59. Hays MB, Alker GJ. Fractures of the atlas vertebra: The two part burst fracture of jefferson. Spine 1988; 13:600–603.
60. Spence KF Jr, Decker J, Sell KW. Bursting atlantal fracture associated with rupture of the transverse ligament. J Bone Joint Surg 1970; 52-A:543–548.
61. Landells CD, van Peteghem PK. Fractures of the atlas: Classification, treatment, and morbidity. Spine 1988; 13:450–452.
62. Fielding JW, Hawkins RJ, Sanford RA. Spine fusion for atlanto-axial instability. J Bone Joint Surg 1976; 58-A:400–406.
63. King AG. Spinal column trauma. In: Anderson, C.D., ed. Instructional Course Lectures, Vol. 35 St. Louis: C.V. Mosby, 1986.
64. Fielding JW, Cochran GVB, Lansing JF III. Tears of the transverse ligament of the atlas: A clinical and biomechanical study. J Bone Joint Surg 1974; 56-A:1683–1687.
65. Levine AM, Edwards CC. Treatment of injuries of the C1-C2 complex. Orthopedic Clin North Am 1986; 17:31–42.
66. Fielding JW. Injuries to the upper cervical spine. In: Griffen, PP., ed. Intructional Course Lectures, Volume 36 Chicago, American Academy of Orthopaedic Surgeons 1987.
67. Pepin JW, Bourne RB, Hawkins RJ. Odontoid fractures with special reference to the elderly patient. Clin Orthopaedics 1985; 193:175–183.

68. Cooper PR, Cohen W. Evaluation of cervical spinal cord injuries with metrizamide myelography CT scanning. J Neurosurg 1984; 61:281–289.

69. Anderson LD, D'Alonzo RT. Fractures of the odontoid process of the axis. J Bone Joint Surg 1974; 56-A:60–64.

70. Fuji E, Kobayashi K, Hirabayashi K. Treatment in fractures of the odontoid process. Spine 1988; 13:604–609.

71. Scheiss RJ, deSaussure RL, Robertson JT. Choice of treatment of odontoid fractures. J Neurosurg 1982; 51:496–499.

72. Karlstrom G, Olerud S. Internal fixation of fractures and dislocations in the cervical spine. Orthopedics 1987; 10:1549–1558.

73. Hanssen A, Cabaneal ME. Fracture of the dens in adult patients. J Trauma 1987; 27:928–934.

74. Francis WR, Fielding JW. Traumatic spondylolisthesis of the axis. Orthopaedic Clin North Am 1978; 9:1011–1027.

75. Effendi D, Roy D, Cornish B. Fractures of the ring of the axis: A classification based upon the analysis of 131 cases. J Bone Joint Surg 1981; 63-B:319–327.

76. Pepin JW, Hawkins RJ. Traumatic spondylolisthesis of the axis: Hangman's fracture. Clin Orthop 1981; 157:138–148.

77. Torg JS, Sennett B, Vegso JT, Pavlov H. Axial loading injuries to the middle cervical spine segment. Am J Sports Med 1991; 19:6–20.

78. Panjabi MM, White AA III, Johnson RM. Cervical spine mechanics as a function of ligament transection. J Bone Joint Surg 1975; 57-A:582–585.

79. Allen BL, Ferguson RL, Lehmann TR, O'Brien RP. A mechanistic classification of closed, indirect fractures and dislocations of the lower cervical spine. Spine 1982; 7:1–27.

80. Mazur JM, Stauffer ES. Unrecognized spinal instability associated with seemingly simple cervical compression fractures. Spine 1983; 8:687–692.

81. Yablon IG, Palumbo M, Spatz E, Mortara R, Reed J, Ordia J. Nerve root recovery in complete injuries of the cervical spine. Spine 1991; 55:18–21.

82. Cybulski GR, Douglas RA, Meyer PR, Rovin RA. Complications in three-column cervical spine injuries requiring anterior-posterior stabilization. Spine 1992; 17:253–256.

83. Capen DA, Nelson RW, Zigler J. Surgical stabilization of the cervical spine: A comparative analysis of anterior and posterior spinal fusions. Paraplegia 1987; 25:111–119.

84. van Peteghem PK, Schweiger JF. The fractured cervical spine rendered unstable by anterior cervical fusion. J Trauma 1979; 19:110–114.

85. Stauffer ES, Kelly EG. Fracture-dislocations of the cervical spine: Instability and recurrent deformity following treatment by anterior interbody fusion. J Bone Joint Surg 1977; 59-A:45–48.

86. Evans DK. Dislocations of the cervicothoracic junction. J Bone Joint Surg 1983; 65-B:124–127.

87. Stauffer ES. Management of spine fractures C3-C7. Orthopaedic Clin North Am 1986; 17:45–53.

88. Garfin SR, Botte MJ, Waters RL, Nickel VL. Complications in the use of halo fixation. J Bone Joint Surg 1986; 68-A:320–325.

89. Levi L, Wolf A, Rigamonti D, Ragheb J, Mirvis S, Robinson WL. Anterior decompression in cervical spine trauma: Does timing affect outcome? Neurosurgery 1991; 29:216–222.

90. Ducker TB, Bellegarrigue R, Salzman M, Walleck C. Timing of operative care in cervical spinal cord injury. Spine 1984; 9:525–531.

91. Whitehall R, Richman JA, Glaser JA. Failure of immobilization of the cervical spine by the halo-vest. J Bone Joint Surg 1986; 68-A:326–332.

92. Koch PR, Nickel VL. The halo-vest and evaluation of motion and forces across the neck. Spine 1978; 3:103–107.

93. Green JD, Harle TS, Harris JH. Anterior subluxation of the cervical spine: Hyperflexion sprain. AJNR 1981; 2:243–250.

94. Paley D, Gillespie R. Chronic repetitive unrecognized flexion injury of the cervical spine (high jumper's neck). Am J Sports Med 1986; 14:92–95.

95. Scher AT. Anterior cervical subluxation: An unstable position. AJR 1979; 133:275–280.

96. Scher AT. Ligamentous injury of the cervical spine: Two radiological signs. South African Medical Journal 1978; 53:802–804.

97. Scher AT. Radiographic indicators of traumatic cervical spine instability. South African Medical Journal 1982; 62:562–565.

98. Plunkett PK, Redmond AD, Billsborough SJ. Cervical subluxation: A deceptive soft tissue injury. J Royal Soc Med 1987; 80:46–47.

99. Rifkinson-Mann S, Mormino J, Sachdev VP. Sub-acute cervical spine instability. Surg Neurol 1986; 26:413–416.

100. Herkowitz HN, Rothman RH. Sub-acute instability of the cervical spine. Spine 1984; 9:348–357.

101. Rorabeck CH, Rock MG, Hawkins RJ. Unilateral facet dislocation of the cervical spine. Spine 1987; 12:23–27.

102. Braakman R, Vinken PJ. Unilateral facet interlocking in the lower cervical spine. J Bone Joint Surg 1967; 49-B:249–257.

103. Savini R, Parsini P, Cervellati S. The surgical treatment of late instability of flexion-rotation injuries in the lower cervical spine. Spine 1987; 12:178–182.

104. Miller LS, Cotler HB, Delucia RA. Biomechanical analysis of cervical distraction. Spine 1987; 12:831–837.

105. Maiman DJ, Barolat G, Larson SJ. Management of bilateral locked facets of the cervical spine. Neurosurgery 1986; 18:542–547.

106. Eismont FJ, Arena MJ, Green BA. Extrusion of an intervertebral disc associated with traumatic subluxation of dislocation of cervical facets. J Bone Joint Surg 1991; 73-A:1555–1560.

107. Zeidman S. Traumatic quadriplegia with Dislocation and Central Disc Herniation. J Spinal Disord 1991; 4:490–497.

108. Berrington NR, van Staden JF, Willers JG, van der Westhuizen J. Cervical intervertebral disc prolapse associated with traumatic facet dislocations. Surg Neurol 1993; 40:395–399.

109. Errico TE, Bauer RD. Cervical spine injuries. In: Errico TE ed. Spinal Trauma. Philadelphia: J.B. Lippincott, 1991.

110. Carter DR, Frankel VH. Biomechanics of hyperextension injuries to the cervical spine in football. Am J Sports Med 1980; 8:302–309.
111. Marar BC. Hyperextension injuries of the cervical spine: The pathogenesis of damage to the spinal cord. J Bone Joint Surg 1974; 56-A:1655–1662.
112. White AA III, Panjabi MM. Clinical Biomechanics of the Spine. Philadelphia, JB Lippincott, 1978.
113. Hartman JT, Palumbo F, Hill BJ. Cineradiography of the braced normal cervical spine. Clin Orthop 1975; 109:97.
114. Sherk HH, Dunn EJ, Eismont FJ et al. The Cervical Spine, Philadelphia, JB Lippincott, 1987.
115. Johnson RM, Hart DL, Simmons EF et al. Cervical orthoses: A study comparing their effectiveness in restricting cervical motion in normal subjects. J Bone Joint Surg (Am) 1977; 59:332.

6

Thoracolumbar Spine Trauma

Kenneth Main
New York, New York

Gordon L. Engler
*Los Angeles County Hospital/University of Southern California Medical Center,
Los Angeles, California*

I. INTRODUCTION

The comprehensive management of trauma to the thoracolumbar spine requires a thorough understanding of both the skeletal and neurological injuries that may result. In the acute setting, the clinical assessment of neurological status and osseous injuries may carry lifelong implications for the patient. Established injuries, with associated disability or deformity, introduce management issues that are often more complex and frequently involve multidisciplinary decision-making. Although not uniformly rewarding, such clinical problems always pose a challenge to the physicians involved in the care of these patients.

The following is a diagnostic and therapeutic overview of thoracolumbar spine injuries that the authors hope will serve as a guide to management in both the acute and chronic phases.

II. BACKGROUND

Ancient Egyptian physicians, who could be put to death if patients died under their care, are said to have regarded spinal cord injury (SCI) as "an ailment not to be treated" (2). As recently as 1927, military surgeon Harvey Cushing reported that 80% of all spinal cord-injured patients died within 2 weeks of in-

155

jury. He noted that only those cases survived in which the lesion was "partial." Although complete spinal cord lesions continue to be among the most devastating life-altering injuries, such therapeutic nihilism is no longer justified. The past half-century has witnessed dramatic improvements in the outlook for victims of spinal trauma.

During World War II, the British Medical Research Council proposed a more aggressive approach to the management of SCI. At that time, SCI was almost universally fatal, due to either collateral injuries or the breakdown of dermal, renal, or pulmonary systems with debilitation from the system's failure and/or secondary infection (13). A specialized SCI unit, Stoke Mandeville Hospital, was opened in 1944 in Aylesbury, England under the direction of Sir Ludwig Guttmann (14). Guttmann, Frankel, and their contemporaries pioneered a comprehensive approach to the acute management and long-term rehabilitation of SCI (25). Holdsworth, Denis, and others have advanced our understanding of spinal anatomy and biomechanics, and their work has served as a foundation for subsequent advances in stabilization and instrumentation (15–17,32,33). Surgical stabilization procedures are now performed routinely throughout the world on a daily basis, permitting a more aggressive approach to rehabilitation. Pharmacological developments continue to be a source of optimism for those involved in the care of these patients.

III. EPIDEMIOLOGY

The incidence of SCI in the United States is between 30 and 50 per million per year, or approximately 10,000–12,000 new injuries annually. Spinal cord injuries primarily affect young adults between the ages of 16 and 30, of which 82% are men, and 60% are single and employed. An estimated 225,000 individuals in the United States live with an SCI (55).

Motor vehicle accidents are the single largest cause of SCI (40%), followed by falls (21%), acts of violence (15%), and sports-related injuries (14%). Of the last group, two-thirds are diving injuries and are most likely to occur in the summer and on weekends (55,61).

The mortality from SCI peaks during the initial hospitalization and period of treatment. Thereafter, survival is similar to that of the general population. Pneumonia (approximately 80%), heart disease, accidents, poisoning, and septicemia are the most frequent causes of death in these patients (55). Renal failure was once the primary cause of death, but its incidence has been reduced by improvements in urological management. Genitourinary complications continue to be among the greatest sources of morbidity, along with pulmonary complications, pressure sores, deep venous thrombosis, and musculoskeletal complications such as heterotopic ossification and contractures (2).

The financial implications of SCI are enormous. The aggregate cost to society, according to the 1989 National Consensus Conference on Catastrophic Illness and Injury, is estimated at $6.2 billion per year. Direct costs of acute care and rehabilitation and lifelong chronic care amount to approximately $2.5 billion each year. Indirect costs, predominantly those that result from loss of lifetime wages and productivity, are placed at $3.7 billion annually (2).

IV. INITIAL MANAGEMENT

As a result of dramatic improvements in emergency medical services, the care of the trauma victim is usually initiated by ancillary personnel at the site of injury. Basic Cardiac Life Support (BCLS) and frequently Advanced Cardiac Life Support (ACLS) are instituted long before the patient arrives at a health care facility. Airway management, resuscitative measures, hemodynamic support, along with a preliminary neurologic assessment, are carried out. Most trauma victims arrive on a spinal board, often with a cervical collar in place, and spinal immobilization is continued until the presence of spinal injury is excluded.

A. Systemic Effects of SCI

Injury to the spinal cord at or above T6 can result in neurogenic shock. The interruption of sympathetic outflow to the heart and peripheral vasculature causes bradycardia and hypotension, which can worsen neurological injury. Pressor agents such as dopamine may be needed and atropine is given for profound bradycardia. In the trauma victim, neurogenic shock must be differentiated from hemorrhagic shock and managed accordingly. Lower extremity paralysis predisposes to deep vein thrombosis with the potential for pulmonary embolism. Gastric hyperacidity, paralytic ileus, and dysfunction of the pancreatic sphincter lead to stress ulceration, vomiting, aspiration, fecal impaction, and pancreatitis. Bladder dysfunction results in urinary stasis, which in turn predisposes to cystitis, pyelonephritis, hydronephrosis, stone formation, and renal failure.

Autonomic dysreflexia characterized by hypertension, headaches, flushing, palpitations, an increase in spasticity, and profuse sweating can be triggered by noxious stimuli in sympathectomized patients. When autonomic dysreflexia presents, a search for its cause (bladder distention, fecal impaction, decubitus ulcer, occult infection) should be initiated (58).

Immobilization leads to demineralization of the long bones of the lower extremities with risk of pathological fracture. Pressure sores occur over bony prominences such as the sacrum, buttocks, trochanters, and heels, and may become infected. Plastic surgical consultation is often required for established ulcers that require skin grafting or flap coverage. Chronic osteomyelitis developing under poorly managed ulcers can lead to amputation, hip disarticulation, and even hemicorpectomy.

V. NEUROLOGIC EVALUATION

In the conscious, cooperative patient without major extremity injury, determination of sensory and motor function may be straightforward. Confounding factors such as altered mental status, pulmonary insufficiency requiring mechanical ventilation, major organ damage, and long bone fractures may combine to limit definitive neurological evaluation. Every effort must be made to perform a thorough, accurate neurological assessment, which may reveal the presence of spinal shock, complete spinal cord lesion, or other pattern of SCI. Somato-sensory evoked potentials (SSEP) can be used to diagnose SCI in the unconscious trauma victim (35).

A. Spinal Shock

The loss of neurological function below the level of injury may represent physiological rather than anatomical interruption of spinal cord function. Flaccid paralysis and absent reflex activity below the level of the lesion are characteristic of spinal shock. Its duration is generally no more than 24–48 hours, but it may persist for 6 weeks. The return of the bulbocavernosus, anal wink, cremasteric and other reflexes below the level of the lesion indicates that the cord segment and nerve roots controlling that reflex are intact and functioning and marks the end of spinal shock. Absent any return of distal motor power or sensation, it indicates irreparable damage to the cord and isolation of the distal cord segments from the motor cortex. The longer the period of spinal shock lasts, the poorer the prognosis for ambulation.

B. Complete Spinal Cord Lesion

In complete spinal cord lesions, motor and sensory function are absent below the level of injury, which may be determined by the presence of a sensory level corresponding to the appropriate dermatome. Sensory overlap between adjacent dermatomes often limits precise determination of the anatomical location of the cord injury, which may extend over multiple levels.

C. Incomplete Spinal Cord Lesion

Partial motor or sensory function may be preserved below the level of the incomplete lesion, often without any specific pattern. These lesions have a much better prognosis for recovery of neurological function. The only indication that the lesion is incomplete may be the finding of "sacral sparing," the presence of voluntary anal sphincter control, perianal sensation, and great toe flexion. Its importance lies in the implication of at least partial structural continuity of the long tracts of the spinal cord (33).

D. Anterior Cord Syndrome

This is the most common of the incomplete SCI syndromes. Anteriorly directed trauma to the cord can be produced by fracture or subluxation of the spinal column or by traumatic herniation of a disc. Injury to the ventrally located corticospinal and spinothalamic tracts produces paralysis with loss of pain and temperature perception, but with preserved position and vibratory sensation. There is usually sacral sensory sparing in the perianal region and some distal motor function.

E. Posterior Cord Syndrome

Isolated injury to or compression of the posterior portion of the spinal cord may result in the interruption of the dorsal columns with loss of position and vibratory sensation caudal to the lesion. Although motor and sensory functions are generally preserved, the loss of proprioceptive feedback may prove to be as disabling as frank paralysis. Posterior element disruption with laminar fracture or hematoma formation may produce isolated posterior cord injury.

F. Central Cord Syndrome

Most often resulting from a cervical hyperextension injury in the setting of preexisting spondylosis, this syndrome is characterized by quadriparesis affecting mainly the distal upper extremities, with a variable sensory pattern. Like the motor loss, the sensory deficits are most profound in the distal upper extremities. Bowel and bladder control are often preserved but may be affected as well. As in posterior cord syndromes, the loss of proprioceptive input from the lower extremities may limit ambulatory potential despite motor recovery.

G. Brown-Séquard Syndrome

Hemisection of the spinal cord is most often produced by penetrating trauma such as a gunshot wound or stabbing. Motor loss and dorsal column sensory deficits are ipselateral to the lesion, whereas pain and temperature loss are contralateral. The partial transection of the cord is usually functional rather than anatomical, and the prognosis for good functional recovery in these cases is very good.

H. Conus Medullaris Syndrome

Injury to the terminal portion of the cord results in the clinical picture of pain, loss of perineal sensation, and incontinence with loss of anal sphincter tone on physical examination. The prognosis for recovery of sphincter control in such cases is poor.

I. Mixed Cord and Root Lesion

Noting the variation in neurological deficits resulting from fractures at the same level, Holdsworth proposed the combination of cord and root lesions (33). A lesion of the caudal portion of the cord may be accompanied by injury to adjacent lumbar nerve roots that arise from the cord proximal to the site of greatest injury, giving the appearance of a higher lesion. This would account for the fact that some patients with apparent incomplete lesions recover function of some lumbar motor groups without regaining distal lumbar or sacral cord function.

VI. RADIOGRAPHIC EVALUATION

The occurrence of multiple noncontiguous spinal injuries in as many as 15% of spinal trauma patients has been well documented (31,49). The entire spine must therefore be evaluated radiographically before immobilization may be discontinued.

A. Plain Radiographs

Good quality plain films of the cervical, thoracic, and lumbar spine are often sufficient to exclude the presence of a fracture, but there are many clinical situations in which further imaging is needed. In an emergency room setting, it may be extremely difficult to perform optimal radiographs, particularly if the patient is unconscious, uncooperative, or has associated injuries. If there is suspicion of a fracture on plain films, or if neurological evaluation suggests the possibility of SCI, further imaging of the spinal cord and spinal column must be undertaken. The cervicothoracic junction is difficult to evaluate due to the surrounding anatomy, and plain films may not reveal injuries in this area. Once a fracture is identified, further detail of the injury is usually needed to determine subsequent management. In these situations, conventional tomography, computed tomography (CT), magnetic resonance imaging (MRI), or myelography may yield important details concerning the injury.

B. Tomograms

The advent of axial, sagittal, and coronal plane imaging by CT and MRI has diminished the usefulness of conventional tomography, but it continues to have important, if limited application in spinal trauma. Laminar fractures are often best demonstrated with polytomography, as are flexion-distraction injuries, in which the fracture plane coincides with that of axial CT images.

C. CT

Axial imaging helps to define injury to the vertebral body or posterior elements, encroachment on the spinal canal, and when combined with myelography, helps to visualize the spinal cord and thecal sac (40). These determinations are vital in the assessment of spinal stability and preoperative planning. When there is retropulsion of bone into the canal, disc herniation, laminar fracture, or hematoma formation, axial imaging is used to assess the need for spinal cord decompression (62.) Computed tomography is also useful in postoperative evaluation of the adequacy of decompression of the spinal canal (30,52). As the technology improves, sagittal and coronal reconstructions of the spinal column gain increasing importance in the definition of injuries (65). One patient treated at the authors' institution suffered traumatic paraplegia from a T1-T2 fracture dislocation that escaped detection by plain films, axial CT, and MRI. The sagittal plane displacement at that level was clearly visualized by reconstructed CT images.

D. MRI

Magnetic resonance imaging is easily the best imaging technique available for the evaluation of SCI (9,19,20,49,56). The MRI characteristics of the acutely injured cord reflect the clinical symptoms. If the injury is mild, with transient neurological dysfunction, the cord may appear normal. With increasing injury and neurological deficits, MRI may reveal edema and hemorrhage. Long TR (T2) images are the most sensitive in showing cord edema, which is seen as areas of high signal intensity within the substance of the cord. Areas of hypointensity with subsequent evolution to hyperintensity are typical of hemorrhage. The presence of hemorrhage is associated with a poor prognosis (57). Newer techniques that may expand the clinical utility of MRI include the use of contrast agents such as gadolinium, fat suppression techniques, 3-D imaging, and magnetic resonance angiography (MRA) (48). The usefulness of MRI in determining the extent of skeletal injury is limited because it does not adequately visualize cortical bone. Disruption of the anterior and posterior longitudinal ligaments may be demonstrated, however, and may aid in the assessment of spinal stability and the need for stabilization.

E. Myelography

In many centers, myelography has been largely replaced by advances in MRI. Although it provides little information concerning injury to the spinal cord, myelography demonstrates extrinsic compression of the dural sac as well as or better than MRI. In combination with axial CT, its visualization of bony impingement on the neural structures is superior to that of MRI. Dural tears may be revealed by extravasation of contrast material from the sac (44).

VII. SKELETAL INJURIES

Sir Frank Holdsworth classified thoracolumbar fractures according to the structural integrity of the vertebral column (33). His two-column biomechanical concept of the spine, which emphasized the anterior column and the "posterior ligamentous complex," was subsequently modified by Denis to include a third column, the middle column (16). The currently accepted biomechanical model of the spine includes the anterior column (anterior vertebral body, anterior longitudinal ligament, and anterior annulus fibrosus), the middle column (posterior vertebral body, posterior longitudinal ligament, and posterior annulus fibrosus), and the posterior column (posterior elements and posterior spinal ligaments). Denis described and classified each fracture type according to the status of each of the three columns.

A. Compression Fractures

The anterior column fails under axial load during anterior flexion of the spinal column. There is loss of height of the anterior vertebral body on a lateral film, but the height of the posterior vertebral body, which constitutes the middle column, is preserved. These fractures are distinguished from other types by the preservation of height of the posterior vertebral body. Except in severe compression, there is no disruption of the posterior ligaments, and no increase in the distance between the spinous processes is seen on the lateral x-ray. A lateral compression variant of this injury was also described. The compressive load is applied along with lateral flexion of the trunk and spinal column, and the lateral portion of the vertebral body fails. An AP film reveals the lateral loss of height of the vertebral body.

B. Burst Fractures

These injuries occur by axial loading of the spinal column with little or no spinal flexion. They occur generally only in those flexible portions of the spine in which the normal curvature (lordosis or kyphosis) can be straightened to allow axial compressive loading. Cervical burst fractures are well described as are those of the lumbar spine, whereas thoracic burst fractures are unusual. Both the anterior and middle columns fail under compression and the vertebral body "bursts," usually propelling bone fragments posteriorly into the spinal canal. Lateral films demonstrate loss of height of the entire vertebral body, including the posterior cortex. An AP film shows widening of the interpedicular distance due to greenstick fracture of the anterior cortex of the lamina. The association of dural tears with burst fractures accompanied by fractures of the lamina is well established (12). An axial CT scan through the fracture demonstrates the bursting of the body with retropulsion of fragments into the canal. The spinal canal is often compromised to a variable degree by the retropulsed bone, with or without neurological deficits, and anterior surgical decompression may be warranted.

In the absence of neurological injury, the indications for decompression are controversial. A 40–50% reduction in the sagittal diameter of the canal is often cited as an indication for decompression, but the correlation between the degree of canal compromise and the incidence of subsequent pain, neurological injury or canal stenosis is not well established (27). There is some evidence that retropulsed bone fragments will eventually be resorbed, but this remains controversial (63).

Burst fractures were further subclassified by Denis according to radiographic features indicating variations in the mechanism of injury. Subtypes include pure axial injuries, flexion-burst injuries, lateral flexion-burst injuries and rotation-burst injuries.

C. Fracture-Dislocations

The presence of any significant anteroposterior or lateral translation between adjacent vertebral bodies suggests fracture dislocation. These are the most unstable thoracolumbar fractures and are most often associated with neurological injury, including paraplegia (27). Biomechanically, they are characterized by failure of all three columns under compression, tension, rotation, shear, or combinations thereof, resulting in subluxation or dislocation. Subtypes are distinguished by the mechanism of injury: flexion-rotation, shear, and flexion-distraction. The flexion rotation type is by far the most common.

D. Flexion-Distraction ("Seat Belt") Injuries

Holdsworth did not include this fracture type in his classification, although it had been reported by Chance in 1948, and by Bohler years earlier. This injury, also known as a "Chance fracture," is most often sustained by an automobile passenger restrained by a lap seat belt. With sudden deceleration of the motor vehicle, the trunk is sharply flexed, particularly if the seat belt is worn improperly about the abdomen. Ecchymoses are often present over the abdomen, and the combination of intra-abdominal injury and spinal fracture, the so-called "seat belt syndrome," may create diagnostic confusion (57). These fractures usually occur in the upper lumbar spine near the transition between the relatively mobile lumbar spine and the relatively inflexible thoracic spine, which is stabilized by the thoracic cage. As the trunk flexes, the spine flexes about an axis that is thought to lie anterior to the spinal column. There is some disagreement as to the precise mechanism of injury. Smith and Kaufer, White and Panjabi, and others state that this injury involves the failure of all three columns under tension; Denis described the anterior column as failing under compression or not at all (16,17,28,60).

The injury may be osseous, passing through the vertebral body and posterior elements, or may occur as a "Chance equivalent," through soft tissue structures including the disc and posterior ligament complex. Bony injuries are thought to be more stable than their soft tissue counterparts and are less likely to need surgical stabilization. Plain x-rays show little displacement but often demonstrate a fracture line passing through the vertebral body and spinous process. If any signigicant translation is found, either on the lateral or AP films, a fracture dislocation should be suspected.

E. "Minor" Injuries

Denis separated the above four "major" injuries from another group of fractures, none of which resulted in any acute instability, but which might be found in combination with a major injury at another level. Isolated fractures of the transverse process, articular process, pars interarticularis, or spinous process were considered partial column injuries. The greater importance of these injuries lies perhaps in their association with specific neurological injuries: (1) brachial plexus or lumbosacral plexus injuries with transverse process fractures in those regions or (2) contusion of the conus with thoracolumbar spinous process fractures.

F. Sagittal Slice Fracture

This fracture occurs when the vertebra above slices in the sagittal plane through the vertebra below, displacing half of the lower vertebra laterally. The spine appears telescoped on the lateral x-ray, with one vertebra overlapping on the other. On the anteroposterior view, the upper vertebra is displaced to the side of the shear fracture (4).

G. Pediatric Injuries

Unique to the pediatric population is the entity of spinal cord injury without radiographic abnormality (SCIWORA) (46,64). The mechanism by which these injuries occur is not known, but it is believed that the increased elasticity of the child's spine permits sufficient displacement to injure the cord without fracture. Others have proposed a vascular etiology. Children who sustain paraplegia are at extremely high risk to develop paralytic scoliosis and must be observed through skeletal maturity. Broadly speaking, the younger the child and the higher the spinal level of injury, the greater is the risk of deformity developing.

VIII. MANAGEMENT OF NEUROLOGIC INJURY

Fernandez, et al. reviewed 157 experimental studies on SCI published in neurosurgery journals between 1975 and 1989 (24). The focus of most of this work was the development of an ideal animal model of SCI rather than on methods of preventing neural injury or reversing established injury. Although considerable progress has been made in limiting the morbidity and mortality of acute SCI, the prognosis for neurological recovery remains largely unchanged. A few agents show promise in limiting neurological deterioration or enhancing recovery and have gained some acceptance. Currently, considerable research is based on the belief that a period of delayed, progressive injury (secondary injury) occurs after the initial insult, although this remains unproven. The prevention of secondary injury and preservation of white matter tracts by pharmacological means or other modalities may improve the outlook for neurologic recovery.

A. Pathophysiology of SCI

Within minutes of injury, small hemorrhages appear in the central gray matter, followed by the leakage of erythrocytes into the perivascular spaces. These small hemorrhages soon coalesce to form a central hemorrhagic necrosis and progress in a centrifugal pattern to involve the surrounding white matter. Vasogenic edema develops, peaks in a few days, and may last as long as 15 days.

Subarachnoid and subpial hemorrhage develops on the surface of the cord directly under the point of injury. Hemorrhages are first seen in the corticospinal tracts at about 4 hours. Eight hours after injury, white matter tracts are characterized by a nonhemorrhagic necrosis associated with edema. The edema obliterates the subarachnoid space and compresses pial veins, spreading over several segments in either direction from the initial lesion. Histological studies suggest that small hemorrhages at the site of initial injury result from shear forces exerted on the microvasculature by mechanical trauma. There is no initial change in the axons or myelin sheaths, but the process progresses ultimately to extensive tissue necrosis and shrunken axons.

Additional information has been derived from autopsy studies of patients who survived variable periods after SCI. The segmental vessels and anterior spinal arteries were always intact, casting doubt on the possibility of a major spinal infarct. In patients surviving a few hours, central hemorrhagic necrosis was apparent, and the spinal cord was markedly edematous. After 48 hours, the spinal cord tissues become soft and liquified as the myelin is degraded to neutral fat. Macrophages enter the lesion shortly to clean up the necrosis. In autopsies performed after 5 or 6 days, glial cells had laid down astrocytic fibers between necrotic and viable tissue. After several weeks, fully developed cavities had formed, and after 3 to 6 weeks, the central cavity was completely cleared of debris. The primary lesion, which extended over several segments, appeared as a multiloculated cyst containing glial fibers and surviving white matter tracts. Rarely was the cord transected (55).

B. Secondary Injury

Ischemia, edema, and hemorrhage are responsible for much of the delayed injury thought to take place after SCI. Ischemia results from microvascular injury sustained at the time of the injury as well as the release of vasoactive substances resulting in local vasoconstriction. The inflammatory response that accompanies any injury is responsible for the edema. The edema causes compression of the neurological structures and adds to the compromise of the spinal microvasculature, perpetuating the cycle and advancing the neurological deficit. Cell death, the degradation of cell membranes, and the liberation of arachadonic acid increase the production of free radicals and mediators of the inflammatory response. A complex biochemical sequence of events ensues that promotes injury to neurons, glial cells, and other supportive elements. It is these events which are often the target of pharmacotherapy (55).

1. Methylprednisolone

The subject of extensive study, methylprednisolone appears to enhance neurological recovery when used promptly and in appropriate dosage (6,13). One-year follow-up data from a large multicenter, randomized, controlled trial showed that patients who received methylprednisolone (30 mg/kg bolus and 5.4 mg/kg/hr for 23 hours) within 8 hours of injury demonstrated increased neurological recovery as compared with patients receiving placebo (6). This difference was apparent at 6 weeks, 6 months, and at 1 year, but only patients who received the drug within 8 hours of injury benefited from treatment. Although not established, the basis for this effect of methylprednisolone is believed to be the inhibition of lipid peroxidation and perhaps an increase in blood flow through the injured cord.

2. GM-1 Ganglioside

Gangliosides, which are complex glycolipids present in high concentrations in central nervous system cells, form a major component of the cell membrane. Although their function is not well understood, there is experimental evidence that they augment neurite outgrowth in vitro and induce regeneration, sprouting, and restoration of neuronal function after injury in vivo. In trials involving SCI victims at Maryland Shock Trauma Center, significantly greater motor recovery was observed after administration of GM-1 than with placebo (26). The clinical effects of the drug were interpreted by the authors as representing enhanced survival of axons traversing the zone of injury, permitting neurological recovery of distal motor groups.

Thyroid releasing hormone (TRH), opiate antagonists such as naloxone, dimethyl sulfoxide (DMSO), and osmotic diuretics are among the agents that have showed some promise in the treatment of SCI (10,55). Other modalities, including spinal cord cooling, hyperbaric oxygen, and myelotomy, have proven beneficial (42,55).

IX. SURGICAL MANAGEMENT

Eighteenth century English surgeons performing the earliest laminectomies for traumatic paraplegia defended the procedure on the basis that "it is difficult to see that further harm can come of it, and possibly some good might ensue" (33). Bohlman and others have shown that laminectomy performed acutely in many cases has resulted in further harm and there is a significant trend away from its use in acute SCI (1,5,32).

The management of thoracic and thoracolumbar fractures involves consideration of two major issues: (1) The stability of the spinal column, and (2) Preservation and restoration of neurological function when possible. White and Panjabi define clinical instability as "the loss of the ability of the spine under physiological loads to maintain its pattern of displacement so that there is no initial or additional neurological deficit, no major deformity, and no incapacitating pain" (60). Thus the issues of spinal stability and neurological function are closely related.

Compression fractures of the thoracic spine are usually very stable and may be treated with a brief period of bed rest and early ambulation in an extension orthosis. Surgical stabilization is only indicated when there is severe collapse of the vertebral body (more than 50% loss of height of the anterior column), severe angulation at one level (more than 20 degrees), or multiple adjacent compression fractures. In these situations, the potential for instability is significant and posterior compression instrumentation and fusion are indicated (43).

In the absence of neurologic deficits, most burst fractures do not require surgical stabilization. A period of bed rest of 4 to 6 weeks in a hyperextension orthosis is acceptable. To achieve early ambulation and avoid the morbidity associated with prolonged recumbency, many surgeons are now recommending surgical stabilization by posterior instrumentation and fusion.

When complete SCI has occurred, a decompressive procedure is usually not indicated. In the presence of incomplete lesions, when bony encroachment on the spinal canal can be demonstrated by axial CT, decompression of the dural tube is indicated. Primary anterior decompression by retroperitoneal, transperitoneal, or transthoracic vertebrectomy, bone grafting, and fusion is currently the method of choice of most surgeons (7,8,18,37,38,39,59). Decompression can result in neurological improvement even when performed months or years after incomplete SCI. Some authors believe that decompression may be accomplished by posterior instrumentation (45). If the posterior longitudinal ligament (PLL) is intact, instrumentation can accomplish reduction of the posteriorly displaced fragment. The PLL can be visualized by MRI and, in many burst fractures, is shown to be disrupted (9). Although posterior surgery can decompress the canal of retropulsed bony fragments, the extent and reliability of this decompression is probably inferior to that offered by anterior decompressive surgery (22). When there is insufficiency of the anterior and middle columns, posterior instrumentation alone will not adequately stabilize the spinal column and should be supplemented with anterior bone graft and possibly instrumentation (29). Postoperative CT scanning is used to assess the adequacy of decompression. If significant canal compromise remains, anterior decompression is indicated.

Fracture-dislocations always require reduction and stabilization, usually with posterior instrumentation. These injuries are frequently so unstable that postural reduction can be used to obtain adequate reduction. When open reduction is necessary, reduction and stabilization may be readily accomplished with Cotrel-Dubousset instrumentation (21) or with the A-O internal fixator (23). Because the majority are associated with complete SCI, decompression is seldom necessary. Although the outlook for neurological recovery is poor, early surgical stabilization allows early mobilization to decrease morbidity and hasten rehabilitation.

Flexion-distraction injuries do not always require surgical stabilization. Those that are purely osseous injuries are generally stable and may be treated with a hyperextension orthosis, but associated intra-abdominal injury complicates brace treatment. Variants of this fracture, which involve failure of the posterior ligamentous complex, must be stabilized by posterior compression instrumentation. If the injury is combined with a burst fracture with middle column failure, it will not be stable under compressive instrumentation. Therefore, the middle column must be carefully evaluated.

Despite the advances in instrumentation and surgical stabilization procedures, it is generally advisable to support patients postoperatively with an appropriate orthosis. A total contact orthosis and the Jewett hyperextension brace are preferred spinal orthoses for postoperative immobilization (3).

X. LONG-TERM MANAGEMENT OF SCI

The long-term care and rehabilitation of the patient with SCI requires a multidisciplinary team approach. Orthopedists, neurosurgeons, urologists, physiatrists, psychologists, occupational therapists, and social workers are among the specialists whose services are needed.

A. Rehabilitation

The goal of rehabilitation is the restoration of the individual to the highest possible level of function and productivity. In this regard, social workers, occupational therapists, and vocational rehabilitation counselors assume a central role. Paraplegic patients routinely gain functional independence with the use of mobility aids and modifications of their homes.

Mobility aids include wheelchairs, walking aids, and orthoses. Ambulation is possible for many paraplegics with the use of Lofstrand (elbow) crutches and long leg braces, but requires tremendous energy expenditure. A broad range of wheelchair models are available to meet the individual needs of the patient. The ability to drive is essential to attaining the goal of functional independence and is possible with automobile modification.

B. Spasticity

The management of spasticity requires consideration of its beneficial effects as well as its better known adverse ones. Some paraplegics use their spastic lower extremities to mechanical advantage for transfers. Spasticity of sphincter muscles can improve bowel or bladder continence, and the increased bulk and strength of spastic muscles may help prevent osteopenia (47). Treatment should therefore only be instituted when the advantages of spasticity are outweighed by the disadvantages. Paroxysmal spasms can be painful and sleep may be disturbed. Hip adductor spasm can impair perineal hygiene; urethral sphincter spasm can lead to stasis, hydronephrosis, and renal insufficiency. Joint contractures are a disabling and disfiguring result of spastic hypertonicity, and abnormal postures resulting from spasticity can promote pressure ulceration.

Treatment may include active and passive range-of-motion therapy, splinting, functional electrical stimulation, heat and cold, and pharmacologic agents. Benzodiazepines, Baclofen, dantrolene, clonidine and Thorazine are among the agents routinely used to control disabling spasticity, but each has a tendency to cause drowsiness. Surgical alternatives such as tendon releases, neurectomies, and rhizotomies have met with limited success.

C. Syringomyelia

An increase in pain, neurological deterioration, increased spasticity, and autonomic dysreflexia are suggestive of syringomyelia. Traumatic myelomalacia with cystic degeneration results in the formation of a syrinx, which may or may not communicate with the cerebrospinal fluid. The syrinx may extend cranially or caudally within the cord, with neurological deterioration. The MRI clearly shows a sharp interface between the syrinx and normal cord. The syrinx itself is often well defined and smooth, but occasionally septa are present. Syringoperitoneal or syringopleural shunting is usually necessary, although myelotomy alone is effective in some cases. Approximately half of patients will experience neurological improvement after surgery.

D. Neuropathic Spinal Arthropathy

The deafferented motion segments below the level of injury may develop neuropathic arthropathy in 10–25% of patients after SCI (34). Aging, duration of paraplegia, spinal level of injury, and surgical intervention are among the factors that may contribute to this lesion (11,36,41,54). The advanced "Charcot spine" is characterized by instability, difficulty with sitting and, in some cases, deformity. Although nonoperative treatment may be effective in some cases, anterior and posterior fusion is the optimal treatment for unstable, symptomatic lesions (34,50,51,53).

REFERENCES

1. Ahn JH, Ragnarsson MD, Gordon WA, Goldfinger G, Lewin HM. Current trends in stabilizing high thoracic and thoracolumbar spinal fractures. Arch Phys Med Rehabil 1984; 65:366–369.
2. Apple DF, Hudson LM, eds. Spinal cord injury: The model Proceedings of the National Consensus Conference on Catastrophic Illness and Injury. Atlanta, GA: Dec 1989. The Georgia Regional Spinal Cord Injury Care System, Sheperd Center for Treatment of Spinal Injuries, 1990.
3. Benzel EC, Larson SJ. Postoperative stabilization of the posttraumatic thoracic and lumbar spine: A review of concepts and orthotic techniques. J Spinal Disord 1989; 2(1):47–51.
4. Bohlman HH. Current concepts reviews. Treatment of Fractures and dislocations of the thoracic and lumbar spine. J Bone Joint Surg 1985; 67-A:165–169.
5. Bohlman HH, Freehafer A, Dejak J. The results of treatment of acute injuries of the upper thoracic spine with paralysis. J Bone Joint Surg 1985; 67-A:360–369.
6. Bracken MB, Shepard MJ, Collins WF, Holford TR, Baskin DS, Eisenberg HM, Flamm E. Methylprednisolone or naloxone treatment after acute spinal cord injury: One year follow-up data. Results of the Second National Acute Spinal Cord Injury Study. J Neurosurg 1992; 76(1):23–31.
7. Bradford DS. Thoracic and lumbar spine fractures. Decompression and anterior approaches. AAOS Instructional Course Lecture #313, Las Vegas, 1989.
8. Bradford DS, McBride GG. Surgical management of thoracolumbar spine fractures with incomplete neurologic deficits. Clin Orthop 1987; 218:201–216.
9. Brightman RP, Miller CA, Rea GL, Chakeres DW, Hunt WE. Magnetic resonance imaging of trauma to the thoracic and lumbar spine. Spine 1992; 17(5):541–550.
10. Brooks ME, Ohry A. Conservative versus surgical treatment of the cervical and thoracolumbar spine in spinal trauma. Paraplegia 1992; 30(1):46–49.
11. Brown CW, Jones B, Donaldson DH, Akmakjian J, Brugman JL. Neuropathic (Charcot) arthropathy of the spine after traumatic spinal paraplegia. Spine 1992; 17(6S):S103–S108.
12. Cammisa FP, Eismont FP, Green BA. Dural laceration occurring with burst fractures and associated laminar fractures. J Bone Joint Surg 1989; 71-A:1044–1052.
13. Collins WF. A review of the acute treatment of spinal cord injury. Resid Staff Phys 1992; 38(3):21–26.
14. Cotler HB. The treatment of cervical spine trauma: A century of progress. Orthopedics 1992; 15(3):279–283.
15. Cotrel Y, Dubousset J, Guillaumat M. New universal instrumentation in spinal surgery. Clin Orthop 1988; 227:10–23.
16. Denis F. The three-column spine and its significance in the classification of acute thoracolumbar spine injuries. Spine 1983; 8:817–831.
17. Denis F. Spine instability as defined by the three-column spine concept in acute spinal trauma. Clin Orthop 1984; 189:65–76.
18. Dunn HK. Anterior spine stabilization and decompression for thoracolumbar injuries. Orthop Clin N Am 1986; 17(1):113–119.

19. Edelman RR, Warach S. Magnetic resonance imaging (first of two parts). New Eng J Med 1993; 328(10):708–716.

20. Edelman RR, Warach S. Magnetic resonance imaging (second of two parts). New Eng J Med 1993; 328(11):785–790.

21. Engler GL. Cotrel-Dubousset instrumentation for reduction of fracture-dislocations of the spine. J Spinal Disord 1990; 3(1):62–66.

22. Esses SI, Botsford DJ, Kostuik JP. Evaluation of surgical treatment for burst fractures. Spine 1990; 15(7):667–673.

23. Esses SI, Botsford DJ, Wright T, Bednar D, Bailey S. Operative treatment of spinal fractures with the AO internal fixator. Spine 1991; 16(38):S146–S150.

24. Fernandez E, Pallini R, Marchese E, Talamonti G. Experimental studies on spinal cord injuries in the last fifteen years. Neurol Res 1991; 13(3):138–159.

25. Frankel HL, Hancock DO, Hyslop G, Melzak J, Michaelis LS, Ungar GH, Vernon JDS, Walsh JJ. The value of postural reduction in the initial management of closed injuries of the spine with paraplegia and tetraplegia. Paraplegia 1969; 7:179–192.

26. Geisler FH, Dorsey FC, Coleman WP. Recovery of motor function after spinal cord injury—A randomized, placebo-controlled trial with GM-1 ganglioside. N Engl J Med 1991; 324(26):1829–1839.

27. Gertzbein SD. Scoliosis research society multicenter spine fracture study. Spine 1992; 17(5):528–540.

28. Gertzbein SD, Court-Brown CM. Flexion-distraction injuries of the lumbar spine: Mechanism of injury and classification. Clin Orthop 1988; 227:52–60.

29. Gertzbein SD, Macmichael D, Tile M. Harrington instrumentation as a method of fixation in fractures of the spine. J Neurosurg 1983; 58(5):760–762.

30. Golimbu C, Firooznia H, Rafii M, Engler G, Delman A. Computed tomography of thoracic and lumbar spine fractures that have been treated with Harrington instrumentation. Radiology 1984; 151(3):731–733.

31. Henderson RL, Reid DC, Saboe LA. Multiple noncontiguous spine fractures. Spine 1991; 16(2):128–131.

32. Holdsworth FW, and Hardy A. Early treatment of paraplegia from fractures of the thoracolumbar spine. J Bone Joint Surg 1953; 35-B:540–550.

33. Holdsworth F. Fractures, dislocations and fracture-dislocations of the spine. J Bone & Joint Surg, 1970; 52-A:1534–1551.

34. Hoppenfeld S, Gross M, Giangarra C. Nonoperative treatment of neuropathic spinal arthropathy. Spine 1990; 15(1):54–56.

35. Houlden DA, Schwartz ML, Klettke KA. Neurophysiologic in uncooperative trauma patients: Confounding factors. J Trauma 1992; 33(2):244–251.

36. Kalen V, Isono SS, Cho CS, Perkash I. Charcot arthropathy of the spine in long-standing paraplegia. Spine 1987; 12(1):42–47.

37. Kaneda K, Abumi K, Fujiya M. Burst fractures with neurologic deficits of the thoracolumbar-lumbar spine. Results of anterior decompression and stabilization with anterior instrumentation. Spine 1984; 9(8):788–785.

38. Kostuik JP. Anterior fixation for fractures of the thoracic and lumbar spine with or without neurologic involvement. Clin Orthop 1984; 189:103–115.

39. McAfee PC, Bohlman HH, Yuan HA. Anterior decompression of traumatic fractures with incomplete neurological deficit using a retroperitoneal approach. J Bone Joint Surg 1985; 67-A:89–104.

40. McAfee PC, Yuan HA, Fredrickson BE, Lubicky JP. The value of computed tomography in thoracolumbar fractures. J Bone Joint Surg 1983; 65-A:461–473.

41. Main WK, Blades DA, Ahn JH, Errico TJ, Engler GL. Factors contributing to the development of the neuropathic spine after complete spinal cord injury. Presented at The Scoliosis Research Society, Annual Meeting, Dublin, Ireland, 1993.

42. Martinez-Arizala A, Green BA, Bunge RP. Experimental spinal cord injury: pathophysiology and treatment. In Herkowitz HN, Garfin SR, Balderston RA, Eismont FJ, Bell GR, Wiesel SW (eds). The Spine, 3rd ed. Philadelphia: WB Saunders, 1992.

43. Montesano PX, Benson DR. The thoracolumbar spine. In: Fractures in Adults. Green DP, Bucholz RW, Philadelphia JB Lippincott: eds. 1991.

44. Nussbaum ES, Sebring LA, Wolf AL, Mirvis SE, Gottlieb R. Myelographic and enhanced computed tomographic appearance of acute traumatic spinal cord avulsion. Neurosurgery 1992; 30(1):43–48.

45. Olerud S, Karlstrom G, Sjostrom L. Transpedicular fixation of thoracolumbar vertebral fractures. Clin Orthop 1988; 227:44–51.

46. Osenbach RK, Menezes AH. Pediatric spinal cord and vertebral column injury. Neurosurgery 1992; 30(3):385–390.

47. Parziale JR, Akelman E, Herz DA. Spasticity: Pathophysiology and management. Orthopedics 1993; 16(7):801–811.

48. Perovitch M, Perl S, Wang H. Current advances in magnetic resonance imaging (MRI) in spinal cord trauma: Review article. Paraplegia 1992; 30(5):305–316.

49. Powell JN, Waddell JP, Tucker WS, Transfeldt EE. Multiple-level noncontiguous spinal fractures. J Trauma 1989; 29(8):1146–1151.

50. Raynor RB. Charcot's spine with neurological deficit: Computed tomography as an aid to treatment. Neurosurgery 1986; 19(1):108–110.

51. Schwartz HS. Traumatic Charcot spine. J Spinal Disord 1990; 3(3):269–275.

52. Shuman WP, Rogers JV, Sickler ME, Hanson JA, Crutcher JP, King HA, Mack LA. Thoracolumbar burst fractures: CT dimensions of the spinal canal relative to postsurgical improvement. Am J Roentgenol 1985; 145:337–341.

53. Slabaugh PB, Smith TK. Neuropathic spine after spinal cord injury. J Bone Joint Surg 1978; 60-A:1005–1006.

54. Sobel JW, Bohlman HH, Freehafer AA. Charcot's arthropathy of the spine following spinal cord injury. J Bone Joint Surg 1985; 67-A:771–776.

55. Sonntag VK, Douglas RA. Management of spinal cord trauma. Neurosurg Clin N Am 1990; 1(3):729–750.

56. Sze G. MR imaging of the spinal cord: Current status and future advances. Am J Roentgenol 1992; 159(1):149–159.

57. Triantafyllou SJ, Gertzbein SD. Flexion distraction injuries of the thoracolumbar spine: A review. Orthopedics 1992; 15(3):357–364.

58. Tucci KA, Landy HJ, Green BA, Eismont FJ. Trauma and paraplegia. In: Diseases of the Spinal Cord. Critchley E, and Eisen A, eds., London. Springer-Verlag 1992.

59. Westfall SH, Akbarnia BA, Merenda JT, Naunheim KS, Connors RH, Kaminski DL, Weber TR. Exposure of the anterior spine. Techniques, complications, and results in 85 patients. Am J Surg 1987; 154:700–704.
60. White AA, Panjabi MM. Clinical biomechanics of the spine. Philadelphia; JB Lippincott 1990.
61. Wigglesworth EC. Motor vehicle crashes and spinal injury. Paraplegia 1992; 30(8):543–549.
62. Willen J, Lindahl S, Irstam L, Nordwall A. Unstable thoracolumbar fractures. A study by CT and conventional roentgenology of the reduction effect of harrington instrumentation. Spine 1984; 9(2):214–219.
63. Willen JAG, Gaekwad UH, Kakulas BA. Burst fractures in the thoracic and lumbar spine. Spine 1989; 14(2):1316–1323.
64. Yngve DA, Harris WP, Herndon WA, Sullivan JA, Gross RH. Spinal cord injury without osseous spine fracture. J Pediatr Orthop 1988; 8(2):153–159.
65. Zinreich SJ, Rosenbaum AE, Wang H, Quinn CB, Townsend TR, Kim WS, Ahn HS, Rybock JD, McAfee PC, Long DM. The critical role of 3-D CT reconstructions for defining spinal disease. Acta Radiol (Suppl) 1986; 369:699–702.

7

Birth Injuries

Kent Patrick
Spinal Surgeon, Private Practice, Sacramento, California

Injuries of the spine at the time of birth are not an uncommon event. Spinal cord injury has an incidence of up to 10% in all neonatal deaths (23,58,59). One investigator reported an incidence as high as 30–50% after a review of the literature (3). Patients who survive may go undiagnosed or misdiagnosed for years, with problems that range from minimal loss of function to major deficits including paraplegia or quadriplegia (23,30,47).

I. ANATOMY

At the time of birth, the spine is fully developed with bone, cartilage, and fair ligamentous stability. The ligaments do not develop completely until about 8 years of age (39). There is no wedging of the vertebral bodies as suggested by x-ray. The cervical musculature, so important in the adult cervical spine, is still poorly developed in the infant. The head is relatively large and heavy for the cervical spine. The occiput to C2 complex is stable with firm ligamentous fixation and an anatomically stable occiput-C1 joint (30). This includes the tectorial membrane and posterior atlanto-occipital membrane posteriorly, the antlanto-occipital joint capsules laterally, and anteriorly, the anterior antlanto-occipital membrane. The alar ligaments also provide support.

Hypermobility can be found in the upper cervical spine below C2. The pseudosubluxation is a combination of its proximity to the stable occiput-C2 complex and the horizontally oriented facets in the midcervical spine (14,17,55). The ligaments are not fully developed, and this contributes as well. At the cervical-thoracic junction, the facets become more vertical. The thoracic spine is further stabilized by the thorax. The junction between the mobile cervical spine and the stable thoracic spine is a high stress point and helps explain the occurrence of injuries here.

II. FUNCTION

Spinal cord injury at the time of birth may render the infant in immediate respiratory distress. Typically, there is a history of a difficult delivery with low Apgar scores and resuscitation being necessary. The child breathes inadequately and consequently is cyanotic. Death may occur within hours to days as a result of respiratory distress. Those who survive may exhibit a variety of deficits. Without a brachial plexus avulsion or midcervical injury, the paralysis of the trunk and lower extremities may pass unnoticed in the beginning until a more careful examination is done. The thorax may be retracted, with a prominent abdomen during inspiration controlled solely by the diaphragm. The extremities are usually atonic and areflexic. The bladder may exhibit overflow emptying or automatic emptying associated with a relaxed detrusor and closed sphincter (54). Early life is normally complicated by repeat urinary tract infections and pneumonia. These children may be misdiagnosed with infantile spinal muscular atrophy (Werdnig-Hoffmann disease) or amyotonia congenita (Oppenheim's disease). Allen found 18 cases of probable spinal cord injury at birth in 31 such cases (3). An infant who exhibits hypotonia with or without symmetrical paraplegia or quadriplegia from birth should be suspected of having a spinal cord injury. Children may exhibit varying amounts of anoxic brain injury associated with respiratory distress and resuscitation. This "cerebral palsy" is not a primary effect of the spinal cord injury but rather a secondary one associated with apnea.

III. PATHOLOGY

There are a number of pathological patterns seen in birth injuries to the cervical and thoracic spine. Fortunately, obvious vertebral fracture-dislocation and mangling transection of the cord is not frequently seen. Injuries that do not result in transection of the cord exhibit one of the following patterns of injury: meningeal lesions, spinal nerve root lesions, and cord lesions (58,59).

Meningeal lesions include dural laceration, dural hemorrhage, (epidural, subdural, and intramural), pia-arachnoidal congestion, and subarachnoid hemorrhage. The epidural hemorrhage in the spinal canal of a newborn may be the only significant finding. Hemorrhage may be found along the entire length of the canal, or it may be localized to one segment. The cervical and upper thoracic portions of the canal are most frequently affected. In Towbin's study of 170 autopsies, there were 30 in which there was evidence of spinal cord injury. Epidural hemorrhage of the cord proved to be the most frequent indication of spinal cord injury in the newborn (58).

Spinal nerve root lesions include laceration or avulsion of spinal roots and perineural hemorrhage. Klumpke's and Erb's palsy are examples of this.

Cord lesions include laceration, architectural distortion, edema, congestion, acute neuronal damage, and focal hemorrhage (focal malacia). With injury of intermediate anatomical severity, the damage is particularly prone to be most prominent in the gray columns. Reid reviewed postmortems of 48 cases of neonatal deaths. She found a 4% incidence of spinal cord damage, a 25% incidence of tearing and bruising of the cervical roots, and a 52% incidence of distortional damage to the cervical spine (46).

Injury to the spinal column ranges from undetected column damage through ligamentous disruption and dislocation and fracture dislocation (15,23,30,39,53) (Fig. 1). Fracture patterns include anterior dislocation with a fracture through the superior end plate of the inferior vertebral body and a more rare vertical fracture through the posterior part of the vertebral body (20,44,59) (Fig. 2). In Pierson's study of 38 cases of spinal and cranial injuries associated with breech deliveries, he noted 14 fractures (44). The most typical lesion was found to be a transverse separation of the upper epiphyseal plate (cartilage) of the sixth cervical vertebra. Only one of these fractures occurred outside of the cervical spine. This was a transverse fracture of T3. Other authors have found evidence of vertebral fractures in the newborn at autopsy (46,59).

Injuries may occur to the vertebral arteries, resulting in microscopically apparent intramural hematomas and thrombosis. This was found in 40% of 60 infants who died in the perinatal period regardless of route of delivery, including Cesarean section (62). In treating 204 children with "labor traumas" of the vertebral column, Saniukas found 41 patients with evidence of ischemias in the vertebrobasilar area (49).

IV. PATHOGENESIS

Birth trauma to the cervical and thoracic spine can occur with either breech or cephalic delivery. The act of birth, even under the best conditions, is potentially a traumatic crippling event for the fetus.

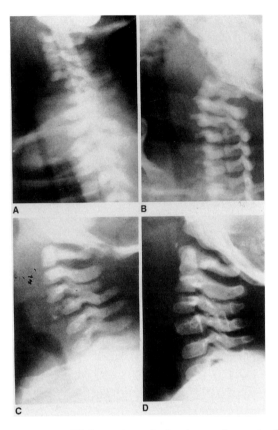

Figure 1 (A) Lateral cervical spine radiograph of forward dislocation of C3 on C4. (B) Oblique view: locking of inferior facet of C3 under superior facet of C4. (C) At 3 weeks, considerable callus anteriorly and superiorly at C4. There is still misalignment at C3–C4. (D) At 14 months, almost complete realignment and post-traumatic overgrowth of C4 body. (From Ref. 53.)

Spinal cord injury complicating breech deliveries is well known. Spinal cord and spinal column injury resulting from cephalic deliveries is only more recently appreciated (41,51). Injuries occurring during cephalic delivery are usually found in the mid to upper cervical spine. These include atlanto-occipital and atlanto-axial dislocations, fracture of the odontoid, and transection of the cord (51). These severe injuries occur as obstetrical complications of forceps delivery when the head may be rotated up to 180 degrees. These infants often die at the time of delivery. The upper cervical spine is not resistant to major torsional stresses, and injury occurs proximal to the tethering of the large bra-

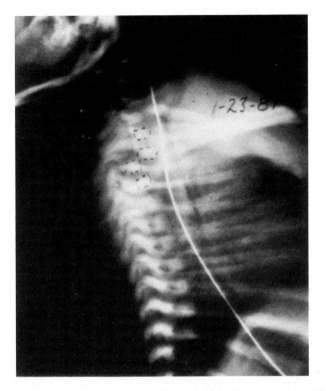

Figure 2 Lateral chest radiograph revealing complete C6–7 dislocation. (From Ref. 39.)

chial nerve roots (50). This can, however, occur with otherwise uneventful labor and cephalic delivery without forceps.

The association of breech deliveries and spinal injury was first described by Parrot in a well-documented case in 1870 (42). After that, a number of other reports appeared demonstrating the association of low cervical injuries with breech delivery (1,3,11,13,15,28,44,51,58,59). The exact mechanism of injury appears to be excessive longitudinal traction, particularly when combined with flexion. When this force is applied to the infant during the second stage of labor, the incidence of spinal cord injury greatly increases (4,15,28). There is a stretch injury to the cord and brainstem and compression of the head resulting from uterine contraction or direct suprapubic pressure by the operator or assistant (15). This best explains certain diffuse longitudinally oriented injuries, which can be seen to occur in many segments of the spinal cord from the cervical through the thoracic cord (59). This traction was studied by Duncan

(1874) who tested the tensile strength of the spinal column in a fresh human fetus. He concluded that traction of 90 lbs. could result in yielding of the vertebral column in the cervical spine and with 120 lbs. of force, decapitation occurred. The autopsy specimen showed that the vertebral column can be stretched 2 inches, and the cervical cord pulled only ¼-inch (19). With breech delivery, the after-coming head can be held tightly by uterine contractions. The entire spinal column can be stretched to the point of rupture of the meninges and cord (36). The cord with meninges is tethered by the brachial plexus and the cauda equina. The damage occurs to the cord more readily than to the skeletal structures (20). Brainstem injury can occur with traction when the brain is drawn into the foramen magnum with compression of the medulla (59).

Another mechanism during delivery, the change in axis of the fetal column during extraction-traction, requires consideration (54). This is even more important when these maneuvers are performed in haste to deliver an infant in distress.

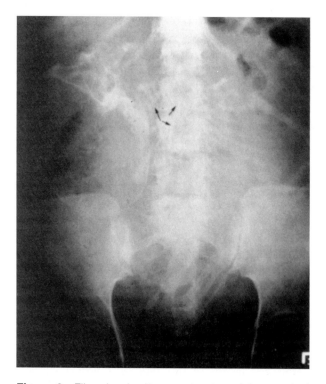

Figure 3 Film showing hyperextension of the cervical spine. Arrows point to the cervical, cervicothoracic, and thoracic spine. (From Ref. 11.)

A special consideration is intrauterine hyperextension of the head and neck in breech deliveries (Fig. 3). The presence of hyperextension in utero (stargazing fetus or flying fetus) is unlikely to be diagnosed without a roentgenogram or ultrasound (11). Hellström and Sallmander (26) discussed the relationship of hyperextension of the fetal head and neck and subsequent cervical cord injury with breech delivery. Their report of two cases and review of the literature found that 7 of 17 infants delivered vaginally sustained spinal cord injuries. Only two of these patients survived. The incidence of neurological deficit in this situation is reported to be as high as 25% (1,11). There is only one report of a patient delivered by Cesarean section where there was slight subluxation of a cervical vertebrae with a normal neurological picture (57). With this in mind, the current recommendations are for Cesarean delivery when hyperextension of the head and neck is recognized in breech presentations (1,5,11,26,35).

V. DIAGNOSIS

Cervical and thoracic spine injuries should be suspected in any neonate after a difficult delivery with a nonprogressive, nonfamilial, neurological, or "myopathic" disorder (floppy infant). Infants who exhibit symmetrical paraplegia or quadriplegia from birth are suspect. Typically there is a history of low Apgar scores and respiratory distress. If the infant survives, there may be a history of recurrent urinary tract infections or pneumonia. There are three main clinical groups of patients, with only group 3 showing long-term survival (58).

The first group is made up of neonates who die during the course of labor or immediately thereafter. Death is secondary to damage to the vital brainstem or core structures and injury occurs during descent or extraction of the fetus.

The second group is made up of infants with cord or brainstem damage who survive up to days. Respiratory depression or distress with intubation from the onset often points toward such an injury. Death occurs as the result of pulmonary disease including pneumonia or, more often, hyaline membrane disease.

The third group is made up of survivors with varying degrees of injury. Paraplegia or quadriplegia may be present. This may be transient or permanent. There may be evidence of anoxic brain injury. It is possible that a large number of mild injuries with minimal neurological symptoms that go unnoticed or misdiagnosed as cerebral palsy or clumsy children (22,28,58).

In the group of survivors with more significant injury, there are two primary neurological syndromes (3). The first group consists of infants who are flaccid and areflexic at birth and who develop hyperreflexia of the lower extremities in weeks to months after birth. This is most likely the result of a single lesion of the cervical or thoracic spinal cord. This is confirmed by a number of authors with such cases (4,15,51,59,62). The return of reflex activity after spinal shock depends on the status of the cord and roots distally. It has been suggested that children may have an earlier and more active return of reflex activity.

The second syndrome involves the infant who remains flaccid and areflexic without development of hyperreflexia. This could be secondary to infarction of the spinal cord in the distribution of the anterior spinal artery, or there could be multiple cord and root lesions.

With spinal cord injury, the newborn will lie with his or her thighs partly flexed and abducted in the frog-leg position. The abdomen will have a soft bulge. The infant will have a weak cry that may strengthen remarkably when abdominal compression is applied to aid in fixation of the muscles. There will be no voluntary motor power in the lower extremities. Depending on the level of involvement and if there is a brachial plexopathy, the upper extremities may or may not move. The chest is bell shaped (Fig. 4).

Reflex testing shows areflexia or hyperreflexia depending on the syndrome. Testing for a sensory level is done by watching the facial expression, not reflex movement of the extremities. There will be loss of sweating below the lesion. Priapism has been reported in a newborn with cord transection, and this is felt to be related to sympathetic vasopressor interruption, leading to penial engorgement (51).

The diagnosis of birth-related spine injury is made by first suspecting such an injury, whether the patient is seen shortly after birth or later when the child with some degree of involvement has been undiagnosed or misdiagnosed previously.

Studies include plain films of the spinal column to look for fracture dislocation or instability. The films are often normal, or they may show fracture and/ or dislocation of cervical and/or thoracic vertebrae. In a recent study of 40 newborns with total or subtotal "plexitis," Evtushenko and others showed computerized tomography (CT) was more informative than plain roentgenograms in evaluating trauma to the vertebral canal and spinal cord in this group of patients (21). Computerized tomographic scanning alone may be falsely negative.

These children will have had multiple chest x-rays with their respiratory distress problems. With the loss of the chest wall muscles of respiration due to cord injury (or other neuromuscular disease), the thorax becomes bell-shaped on the anteroposterior (AP) roentgenogram. The diameter of the upper chest is narrow, with a lateral bulge at the level of the diaphragm, and there is an associated inferior inclination of the rib cage (23) (Fig. 5). It is possible to pick up a fracture or dislocation of the spine on the chest roentgenogram.

Until the advent of the magnetic resonance imaging (MRI), a myelogram was often helpful in diagnosing these severe injuries. The myelographic find-

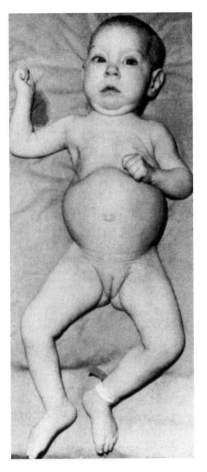

Figure 4   This infant shows a protuberant abdomen, intercostal paralysis, typical frog-leg position, and bell-shaped chest. (From Ref. 4.)

ings are usually that of an extradural or nonspecific block in the subarachnoid space; less frequently cord atrophy and/or incomplete block are noted (23). Adams et al. studied eight patients who presented with clinical features of spinal cord injury. All eight underwent myelography, and seven underwent CT after the myelogram (2). The authors felt that the presence of a block after the neonatal period usually is associated with an adherent dura or fibrous tissue with atrophic cords. The conclusion was that CT myelography is of value to confirm the clinical diagnosis and help exclude other diagnoses, such as neuromuscular disorders, severe hypoxic-ischemic encephalopathy (HIE), or a con-

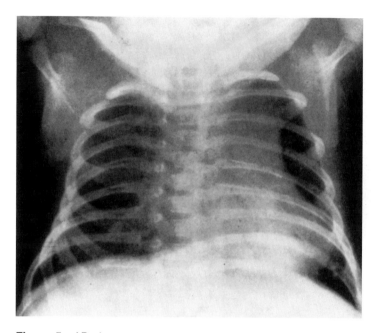

Figure 5 AP chest roentgenogram. The superior aspect of the thoracic cage is narrow, and there is a caudal pitch to the posterior ribs. There is a patchy atelectasis in the left lung base. (From Ref. 23.)

genital spinal cord tumor. It provides excellent information on nerve root injuries such as brachial plexus avulsion.

There are false-negative results reported, and the study is associated with a higher frequency of complications, does not define the underlying pathology, and the level of spinal cord block may not correspond to the lesion (33).

The advent of MRI has opened a new door to visualization and documentation of pathology of the spinal cord, the spinal canal, and the spinal column. Despite its high cost and unique logistics, it has been suggested as the investigation of choice because of its better soft tissue delineation, avoidance of radiation exposure, and its capacity to provide information on the spinal column (33) (Fig. 6).

Normals are being established for age groupings from birth through 2 years (56). A variety of pathological processes, including hemorrhage, hematoma, contusion, laceration, transection, and late sequelae of cord injury such as myelomalacia and spinal cord syrinx formation, can be beautifully visualized with avoidance of the risk of metrizamide myelography (61) (Fig. 7). After reviewing 23 patients with abnormalities identified by MRI, Bale et al. concluded that MRI should be the preferred screening technique for children or infants

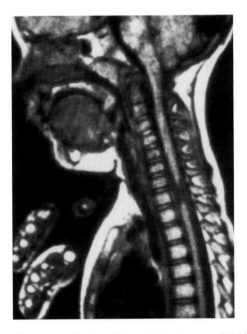

Figure 6 Sagittal T1-weighted image (500/40) reveals a complete transection of the cord at the level of C7–T1 with no associated skeletal injury at this level. (From Ref. 40.)

with suspected spinal cord disorders (8). In a review of 15 patients undergoing MRI scanning 12 hours to 2 months after injury using decoupled surface coils and ventilatory support, Davis et al. found that of seven patients with spinal cord neurological deficits, six showed evidence of hemorrhagic contusions, nonhemorrhagic contusions, and extensive infarction (16).

Eight patients without cord neurological deficit revealed no cord lesions on MRI (16). This group included epidural hematoma, ligamentous disruption, and bone compression. Several other reports document the usefulness of MRI in evaluating children and infants with a suspected cervical or thoracic cord birth injury (33,34,38,40). This is true whether they are evaluated acutely or years after the injury.

Bone scanning may be helpful, although many of the patients have no bony injury and would likely have a negative scan. This can be a screening tool for undetected musculoskeletal trauma in infants with traumatic cord injury, however (52).

The spinal column of neonates can be evaluated with ultrasonography (Fig. 8). It is very useful in the initial evaluation of neonates with suspected spinal cord injury. Incomplete ossification of the posterior vertebral arch allows visu-

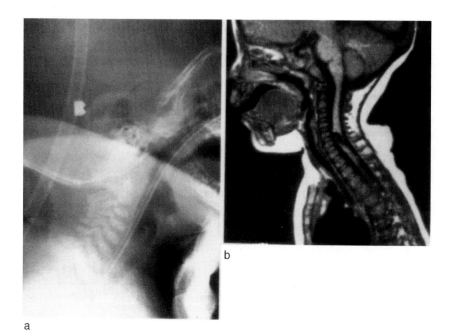

b

a

Figure 7   (a) Normal lateral cervical spine radiograph. (b) Sagittal T1-weighted image (500/40) shows cord transection at the C5–6 level with normal vertebral and soft tissue alignment. (From Ref. 40.)

alization of the neonatal spinal cord. Changes in the echo allow differentiation between initial edema, hematomyelia, and later, myelomalacia (Fig. 9). It is an easy, inexpensive, quick, reproducible, and noninvasive bedside investigation that allows frequent re-evaluation. Babyn et al. were able to assess pathology in all four cases of spinal cord birth trauma, and sonography was correlated with necropsy findings, which were evaluated in three of the cases (7) (Figs. 10 and 11). Two recent investigators recommended it as the imaging study of first choice (37,45).

Electrophysiological studies [electromyography, nerve conduction velocities, and somato-sensory evoked potentials (SSEP)] are relatively nonspecific, but they may provide supportive evidence for the suspected level of the lesion. However, they cannot localize or evaluate the type of lesion. The usefulness of SSEP in cervical cord lesions is limited, as cervical bioelectric potentials are typically small, and one-third of even normal-term neonates may fail to show scalp potentials overlying the somatosensory cortex (9). These electrical studies are felt to be an adjunct to the other imaging modalities including ultrasonography and MRI.

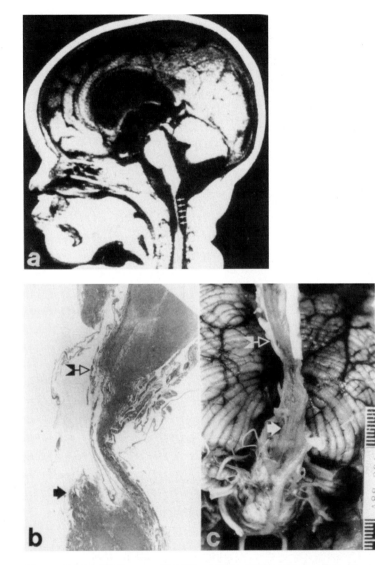

Figure 8 (a) Midline sagittal T1-weighted (TR, 500 ms; TE, 15 ms) MRI showing marked attenuation of cord caliber from the level of the caudal medulla to
the level of C3–4 (arrows). (b) Gross specimen demonstrating complete disruption between the lower medulla (solid arrow) and the upper cervical cord (open
arrow). (c) Microscopic section of upper cervical cord showing discontinuity between the lower medulla (solid arrow) and the upper cervical cord (open arrow).
The segment between the two arrows contains no neural elements, only leptomeninges and minimal scar tissue (Hematoxylin and eosm; original magnification ×1.5). (From Ref. 33.)

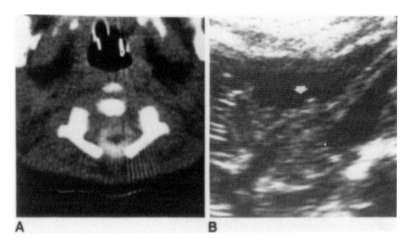

Figure 9 (A) Transverse CT myelogram with flattened upper cervical cord. (B) Sagittal sonogram showing small brain stem caused by cord degeneration. Note the widened CSF space (arrow). (From Ref. 7.)

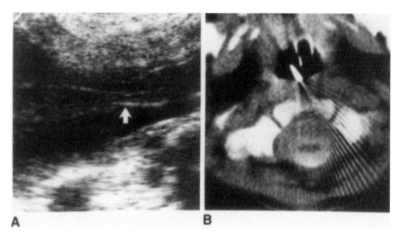

Figure 10 (A) Sagittal sonogram showing spinal cord narrowing at cervicomedullary junction with widened CSF space and increased echogenicity at age 3 months (arrow). (B) Axial CT myelogram showing marked flattening of upper cervical cord. (From Ref. 7.)

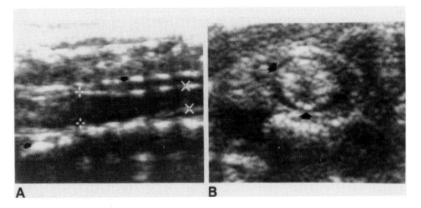

Figure 11 (A) Longitudinal sonogram of upper cervical cord shows widening of cord with increased echogenicity at cervicomedullary junction just to the left of the + signs. Extramedullary hemorrhage along outside of cord (arrows). Normal cord outlined by X's. (B) Transverse sonogram at level of + signs in (A) shows widening cervicomedullary junction with replacement of normal cord hypoechogenicity with markedly increased hyperechogenicity of cord (arrows). Central canal not seen. (From Ref. 7.)

A workup should include urinalysis and urine cultures and a cystometrogram; a voiding cystogram may be necessary to diagnose a neurogenic bladder. A lumbar puncture performed at the time of injury may show an acute hemorrhage or xanthochromia.

With a variety of diagnostic tests that may confirm the diagnosis, the choice may depend upon the local availability of these various modalities. Changes in health care and medical management may dictate which tests may be ordered. Rehan and Seshia proposed an algorithm to be used in the diagnostic workup of suspected neonatal spinal cord birth trauma (45) (Fig. 12). Acutely, they recommend an ultrasound scan of the neck. If abnormal, they recommend follow-up by serial scans in the acute stage, followed by MRI scanning subsequently at a few weeks of age. If the clinical index of suspicion is high and the initial ultrasound scan is normal, an MRI scan is recommended. Repeat MRI and ultrasound scans are recommended if both are initially negative in a suspect neonate. False-negatives can occur (48). Electrophysiological studies can be a good adjunct, and a post myelogram CT scan is useful in some cases.

The differential diagnosis includes distinguishing birth injury to the spinal cord that is nonfamilial and nonprogressive from familial and progressively deteriorating neuromuscular diseases such as spinal muscular atrophy (Werdnig-Hoffmann) and amyotonia congenita (Oppenheim's disease). One patient

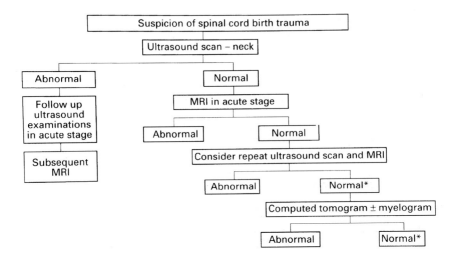

Figure 12 Algorithm proposed for use in diagnostic workup of suspected neonatal spinal and birth trauma (asterisks). Electrophysiological tests (electromyography, nerve conduction studies, and somatosensory evoked potentials) may be helpful. (From Ref. 45.)

was initially diagnosed as having Larsen's syndrome (30). If found, the single most important test is the demonstration of a sensory level (36). Presentation must be distinguished from cervical spine disease and myelopathy seen with instability in diastrophic dwarfism, Morquio's disease, and spondyloepiphyseal dysplasia congenita (31).

VI. TREATMENT

The greatest challenge in treatment of birth injuries to the spine is to recognize the situation and make the diagnosis. Only then can one begin treatment.

There are only a handful of cases in the literature in which acute care of these injuries is discussed and followed. Treatment is based on basic principles of spine and spinal cord injuries in children. Depending on the degree of neurological injury, the patient may require special care in positioning to prevent pressure sores and contractures. Mechanical ventilation may be necessary, either short term or indefinitely. Long term, these patients will need to be monitored, as would any spinal cord injury patient with appropriate physical therapy, bracing, urologic, and orthopedic management. General care is similar to that of other spinal cord injury patients, with the added factor that they are growing children. Because the patients are children, they need a proper education, support, and understanding from parents, siblings, and extended families; later, they will also need vocational guidance for ultimate independence (32).

A. Nonsurgical

The majority of the injuries to the spinal column can be treated nonoperatively if recognized at the time of injury. A newborn's ability to heal is tremendous, and simple immobilization after reduction of unstable or displaced injuries will usually suffice. For newborns with instability, halter traction can be used until there is sufficient healing to put the patient in a collar, brace, or even a Minerva brace or cast (27,39,43). Even if the injury is not recognized for weeks or months, it is still possible to improve alignment with or without traction, and ultimately this will allow healing with stability (39,53). Stability is restored by healing of bone and ligament tissue if the head and neck are held in a reduced position. Remodeling in this age group can be impressive.

There is some suggestion that pharmacological intervention early in acute spinal shock may be beneficial (10,18,25,60). This information is early in development, and the applicability in this age group is not yet established.

B. Surgical

If immobilization does not lead to stability, or if the injury is not recognized until the child is older, surgical stabilization and fusion may be required (30,43). Wire fixation with bone graft is recommended (24,29,30,50). At the time of fusion, care must be taken to avoid excessive stripping, which could lead to spontaneous fusion of adjacent levels in this age group. Jones and Hensinger reported improvement in neurological function in a 20-month-old child with a probable birth injury that was not recognized until late (30) (Figs. 13 and 14). There is no role for laminectomy in these young patients. This can lead to reduced cervical stability, resulting in severe swan neck deformity (14).

VII. PROGNOSIS

The prognosis for these injuries can be good if the injury to the spinal column is recognized before any damage to the spinal cord or roots has occurred. Nerve injury can be peripheral or central, and if central, either complete or incomplete. Distinguishing a complete vs. incomplete lesion in a newborn could be difficult. In cases of myopathy or incomplete lesions, there is potential for improvement in function with reduction and stabilization. In a series of 156 spinal injuries in children seen at the Mayo Clinic during a 28-year period, no com-

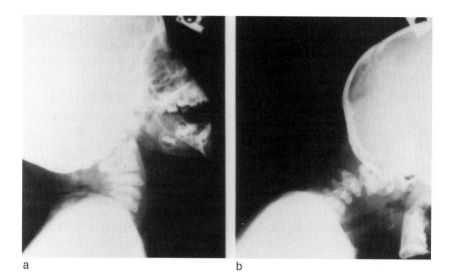

a   b

Figure 13   (a) Flexion and (b) extension lateral views of the cervical spine reveal anterior subluxation of C2 on C3 of greater than 1 cm. (From Ref. 30.)

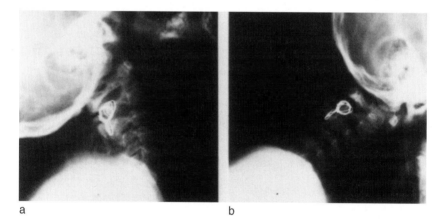

a   b

Figure 14   Following spine fusion of the case in Figure 13, (a) flexion and (b) extension lateral views of the cervical spine show no change in the position of C2 relative to C3 with flexion and solid posterior fusion. (From Ref. 30.)

plete lesion ever improved (6). If cervical hyperextension in utero is recognized, Cesarean section is indicated to reduce the 25% risk of spinal cord injury seen with vaginal delivery. There are no reports of these patients having neurological injury if delivered by Cesarean section (26). Prevention of the injury affords the best prognosis and result.

MacKinnon et al. looked at 22 patients in a retrospective case series to try to establish criteria, evident soon after birth, that predict long-term outcome of neonates with spinal cord injury at birth (37). They grouped patients according to breathing levels as follows: (1) Upper cervical spinal cord injury causing apnea (above C4, which is above the spinal roots of the phrenic nerve); (2) Cervical-thoracic spinal cord injury causing respiratory difficulty of varying severity (at C4 to T4, and involving the spinal roots of the phrenic nerve and innervation of the upper intercostal muscles); and (3) Thoracolumbar spinal cord injury not causing respiratory difficulty (at T11-L5, and involving no or little intercostal intervention). In patients with upper cervical spinal cord injuries who had no coexistent central nervous system abnormality associated with early death, long-term outcome and survivors (depending on mechanical ventilation and on aides for upper limb activity and for ambulation) were best predicted by age when breathing was first observed and by the rate of recovery of limb motor function in the first 3 months. The presence of breathing movements on day 1 was associated with mild disability. The absence of breathing movements on day 1 and little or no recovery of motor function in the first 3 months was associated with permanent total dependency on mechanical ventilation and severe quadriplegia. Apnea on day 1 and intermediate recovery rates in the first 3 months were associated with variable long-term prognoses. Survivors with cervicothoracic and thoracolumbar lesions ultimately became free of mechanical ventilation, except for one patient who remained dependent at night. All four patients who died in this group had recurrent pneumonia and chronic restrictive lung disease. It was the authors' opinion that patients with upper cervical spinal cord injuries who failed to manifest any breathing and spontaneous limb movements at a time when complete recovery from spinal shock is expected (by 3 weeks of age) should be considered for withdrawal of mechanical ventilation. Prognostic certainty will be strongly reinforced in most cases by 3 months of age. Failure to develop autonomous respiratory function while awake and establishment of only minimal motor function below the level of the lesion by this age will probably be associated with permanent mechanical ventilation dependency and severe quadriparesis. As available health care dollars shrink in future years and care becomes rationed, these prognostic criteria may have grave implications (Fig. 15).

Long-term prognoses with cervicothoracic spinal cord injury in neonates has been considered by several authors (2,12,32). Cervical lesions from C4 to T1 are compatible with life, but these patients will likely have recurrent respira-

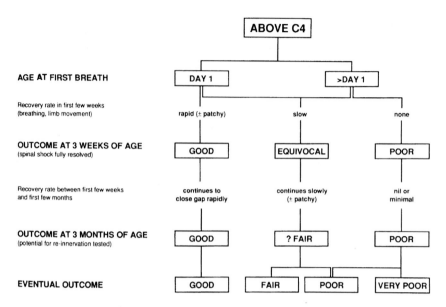

Figure 15 Recovery from upper cervical SCI. Schematic representation of outcomes of neonates with SCI based on level of lesion, timing of first observed breathing movements, and rates of recovery of breathing and limb movements. Caution is required in interpretation of clinical findings and course in other patients; this schema has not been validated in a test set of neonates with SCI. (From Ref. 37.)

tory and urinary tract infections. Bucher et al. deduced from their data that T4 is the approximate pivotal level, below which the outcome is relatively good—"walking with crutches" and "will be able to live independently" (12). These guidelines for prediction of outcome should be applied cautiously until validated by larger numbers of patients.

VIII. CONCLUSION

It is important to recognize these injuries early to minimize the risk of neurological injury or death. Cervical and thoracic spine injuries should be suspect in any neonate after a difficult or breech delivery with a nonprogressive, nonfamilial neurological or myopathic disorder (floppy infant). Mild cases of spinal injury must occur and are labeled cerebral palsy or clumsy children. Recognizing that some of these children may have a spinal injury, there may be a number of them who could benefit from treatment if identified.

REFERENCES

1. Abroms IF, Bresan MJ, Zuckerman JE, Fisher EG, Strand R. Cervical cord injuries secondary to hyperextension of the head in breech presentation. Obstet Gynecol 1973; 41:369–378.
2. Adams C, Babyn PS, Logan WJ. Spinal cord birth injury: Value of computed tomographic myelography. Pediatr Neurol 1988; 4:105–109.
3. Allen JP. Birth injury to the spinal cord. Northwest Medicine 1970; 69:323–326.
4. Allen JP, Myers GG, Condon VR. Laceration of the spinal cord related to breech delivery. JAMA 1969; 208:1019–1022.
5. Ameil GJ. Approach to the delivery of the hyperextended foetus. J Obstet Gynaec Brit Comm 1955; 62:102–105.
6. Anderson JM, Schutt AH. Spinal injury in children: A review of 156 cases seen from 1950 through 1978. Mayo Clin Proc 1980; 55:499–504.
7. Babyn PS, Chuang SH, Danemana, Davidson GS. Sonographic evaluation of spinal cord birth trauma with pathologic correlation. AJNR 1988; 9:765–768.
8. Bale JF, Jr, Bell WE, Val Dunn, Afifi AK, Menezes A. Magnetic resonance imaging of the spine in children. Arch Neurol 1986; 43:1253–1256.
9. Bell HJ, Dykstra DD. Somatosensory evoked potentials as an adjunct to diagnosis of neonatal spinal cord injury. J Pediatr 1985; 106:298–301.
10. Bracken MB, Shepard MJ, Collins WF, Holford TR, Young W, Baskin DS, Eisenberg HM, Flamm E, Leo-Summers L, Maroon J, Marshall LF, Perot PL, Jr, Piepmeier J, Sonntag VKH, Wagner FC, Wilberger JE, Winn HR. A randomized, controlled trial of methylprednisolone or naloxone in the treatment of acute spinal-cord injury. N Engl J Med 1990; 322:1405–1411.
11. Bresnan MJ, Abroms IF. Neonatal spinal cord transection secondary to intrauterine hyperextension of the neck in breech presentation. J Pediatr 1974; 84:734–737.
12. Bucher HU, Boltshauser E, Friderich J, Isler W. Birth injury to the spinal cord. Helv Paediatr Acta 1979; 34:517–527.
13. Burke DC. Spinal cord trauma in children. Paraplegia 1971; 9:1–12.
14. Cattell HS, Filtzer DL. Pseudosubluxation and other normal variations in the cervical spine in children. J Bone Joint Surgery (Am) 1965; 47:1295–1309.
15. Crothers B. Injury of the spinal cord in breech extraction as an important cause of fetal death and paraplegia in childhood. AM J Med Sci 1923; 165:94–110.
16. Davis PC, Reisner A, Hudgins PA, Davis WE, O'Brien MS. Spinal injuries in children: Role of MR. AJNR 1993; 14:607–617.
17. Donaldson JS. Acquired torticollis in children and young adults. JAMA 1956; 160:453–461.
18. Ducker TB. Treatment of spinal-cord injury. N Engl J Med 1990; 322:1459–1461.
19. Duncan JM. Laboratory note on the tensile strength of the fresh adult foetus. Brit Med J 1874; 11:763–764.
20. Ehrenfest H. Injuries of the vertebral column and spinal cord in birth injuries of the child. In: Ehrenfest H, ed. New York: Appleton, 1931.
21. Evtushenko SK, Iatsko VD, Momot NV. [Comparative analysis of the information

value of roentgenological diagnosis and computerized tomography of birth injuries of the cervical spine in newborn infants]. Pediatriia 1990; 10:50–52.

22. Ford FR. Breech delivery in its possible relations to injury of the spinal cord. Arch Neurol Psychiatry 1925; 14:742–750.

23. Franken EJ. Spinal cord injury in the newborn infant. Pediatr Radiol 1975; 3:101–104.

24. Gaufin LM, Goodman SJ. Cervical spine injuries in infants. J Neurosurg 1975; 42:179–184.

25. Geisler FH, Dorsey FC, Coleman WP. Recovery of motor function after spinal-cord injury—A randomized, placebo-controlled trial with GM-1 ganglioside. N Engl J Med 1991; 324:1829–1838.

26. Hellström B, Sallmander U. Prevention of spinal cord injury in hyperextension of the fetal head. JAMA 1968; 204:107–110.

27. Henrys P, Lyne ED, Lifton C, Salciccioli G. Clinical review of cervical spine injuries in children. Clin Orthop 1977; 129:172–176.

28. Hillman JW, Sprofkin BE, Parrish TF. Birth injury of the cervical spine producing a "cerebral palsy" syndrome. Am Surg 1954; 20:900–906.

29. Hubbard DD. Injuries of the spine in children and adolescents. Clin Orthop 1974; 100:56–65.

30. Jones ET, Hensinger RN. C2-C3 dislocation in a child. J Pediatr Orthop 1981; I:419–422.

31. Jones ET, Hensinger RN. Spinal deformity in individuals with short stature. Orthop Clin N Am 1979; 10:877–890.

32. Koch BM, Eng GM. Neonatal spine cord injury. Arch Phys Med Rehabil 1979; 60:378–381.

33. Lanska MJ, Roessmann U, Wiznitzer M. Magnetic resonance imaging in cervical cord birth injury. Pediatrics 1990; 85:760–764.

34. Lasker MR, Torres-Torres M, Green RS. Neonatal diagnosis of spinal cord transection. Clin Pediatr 1991; 30:322–324.

35. Lazar MR, Salvaggio AT. Hyperextension of the fetal head in breech presentation: Report of a case. Am J Obstet Gynecol 1959; 14:198–199.

36. Leventhal HR. Birth injuries of the spinal cord. J Pediatr 1960; 56:447–453.

37. MacKinnon JA, Perlman M, Kirpalani H, Rehan V, Sauve R, Kovacs L. Spinal cord injury at birth: Diagnostic and prognostic data in twenty-two patients. J Pediatr 1993; 122:431–437.

38. Mathis JM, Wilson JT, Barnard JW, Zelenik ME. MR imaging of spinal cord avulsion. AJNR 1988; 9:1232–1233.

39. McClain RF, Clark CR, El-Khoury GY. C6-7 dislocation in a neurologically intact neonate. Spine 1989; 14:125–127.

40. Mendelsohn DB, Zollars L, Weatherall PT, Girson M. MR of cord transection. J Comput Assist Tomogr 1990; 14:909–911.

41. Norman MG, Wedderburn, LCW. Fetal spinal cord injury with cephalic delivery. Obstet Gynecol 1973; 42:355–358.

42. Parrot J. Rupture of the spinal cord in the newborn. L'Union Med 1870; 9:137.

43. Pennecot GF, Leonard P, Peyrot Des, Gachons S, Hardy JR, Pouliquen JC. Trau-

matic ligamentous instability of the cervical spine in children. J Pediatr Orthop 1984; 4:339–345.

44. Pierson RN: Spinal and cranial injuries of the baby in breech deliveries. Surg Gynecol Obstet 1923; 37:802–815.

45. Rehan VK, Seshia MMK. Spinal cord birth injury—Diagnostic difficulties. Arch Dis Child 1993; 69:92–94.

46. Reid H. Birth injury to the cervical spine and spinal cord. Acta Neurochir Suppl (WIEN) 1983; 32:87–90.

47. Ross P. Neonatal spinal cord injury. Ortho Rev 1980; 9:97–97.

48. Rossitch E, Jr., Oakes WJ. Perinatal spinal cord injury: Clinical radiographic, and pathologic features. Pediatr Neurosurg 1992; 18:149–152.

49. Saniukas KA, Tamashauskeng LL, Algkseev EA. [Birth injuries of the spine]. Ve Stn Khir 1989; 143:78–81.

50. Sherk HH, Schut L, Lane JM. Fractures and dislocations of the cervical spine in children. Orthop Clin N Am 1976; 7:593–604.

51. Shulman ST, Madden JD, Esterly JR, Shanklin DR. Transection of spinal cord: A rare obstetrical complication of cephalic delivery. Arch Dis Child 1971; 46:291–294.

52. Sobus KM, Alexander MA, Harcke HT. Undetected musculoskeletal trauma in children with traumatic brain injury or spinal cord injury. Arch Phys Med Rehabil 1993; 74:902–904.

53. Stanley P, Duncan AW, Isaacson J, Isaaccson AS. Radiology of fracture-dislocation of the cervical spine during delivery. Am J Roetgenol 1985; 145:621–625.

54. Stern WE, Rand RW. Birth injuries to the spinal cord. Am J Obstet Gynecol 1959; 78:498–512.

55. Sullivan CR, Bruwer AJ, Harris LE. Hypermobility of the cervical spine in children: A pitfall in the diagnosis of cervical dislocation. Am J Surg 1958; 95:636–640.

56. Sze G, Baierl P, Bravo S. Evolution of the infant spinal column: Evaluation with MR imaging. Radiology 1991; 181:819–827.

57. Taylor JC. Breech presentation with hyperextension of the neck and intrauterine dislocation of cervical vertebrae. Am J Obstet Gynecol 1948; 56:381–385.

58. Towbin A. Latent spinal cord and brain stem injury in newborn infants. Dev Med Child Neurol 1969; II:54–68.

59. Towbin A. Spinal cord and brain stem injury at birth. Arch Pathol 1964; 77:620–632.

60. Walker MD. Acute spinal cord injury. N Engl J Med 1991; 324:1885–1887.

61. Yamano T, Fujiwara S, Matsukawa S, Aotani H, Maruo Y, Shimada M. Cervical cord birth injury and subsequent development of syringomyelia: A case report. Neuropediatrics 1992; 23:327–328.

62. Yates PO. Birth trauma to the vertebral arteries. Arch Dis Child 1959; 34:436–441.

8

Posttraumatic Syrinx
DIAGNOSIS AND TREATMENT

Noel I. Perin
Mount Sinai Medical Center, New York, New York

Spinal cord injury leading to paraplegia is no longer a fatal disease, especially in young adults, and is compatible with long survival. In spite of improvements in the overall management of these patients after spinal cord injury, many complications and posttraumatic sequelae occur. Significant among these is the syndrome of progressive ascending posttraumatic syringomyelia. In this chapter, the author discusses the incidence, presentation, diagnosis, possible mechanisms of origin, and treatment options.

Although cavitation in the spinal cord was first described in 1564 (6), posttraumatic syrinx formation was considered a rarity. With the increasing awareness of this entity in recent years and access to computed tomography (CT), myelography, and magnetic resonance imaging (MRI) techniques, more cases are now diagnosed. The incidence of posttraumatic syringomyelia is reported to be 0.3–2.3% (4), as opposed to the incidence of a true syringomyelia, which ranges from 0.01–0.4% (5,19). A review of the literature shows a wide variation in the time of symptom onset. Thus, progressive neurological deterioration as a sequel to posttraumatic cystic degeneration of the spinal cord has been reported from 9 months to 17 years after the injury, with a median of 4.5 years (26). The incidence of this complication as reported in the literature (12) shows that syrinx formation is higher in patients with paraplegia from thoracolumbar injuries than in patients with quadriplegia after high cervical injuries (paraplegia:quadriplegia, 9:1). No difference in the incidence of posttraumatic syringomyelia was noted in patients who had a complete neurological deficit at the time of admission vs. those who had incomplete deficits. Also, no relationship was noted between the occurrence of posttraumatic cavitation or the spinal level of injury and the latency period before the diagnosis of the syrinx.

I. SYMPTOMS AND SIGNS

The onset of symptoms in posttraumatic syringomyelia as in the other forms of syringomyelia varies greatly. Common initial symptoms are pain and numbness, followed several years later by muscle weakness. Patients usually report pain— its character may vary, often presenting as a dull ache, but less frequently as a stabbing or burning sensation.

Sensory disturbances occur at some stage in the progression of the disease. In most patients, sensory loss begins at the level of the injury and moves upward, often insidiously. Progression of the neurological deficit may be interrupted for months or years and then suddenly, after an episode of coughing or straining, may ascend a few more segments. The speed and direction of progression of the sensory deficit varies, in some patients taking years, but occasionally rapidly progressing within hours.

Dissociated sensory loss to pain and temperature typically occurs when the cyst forms at the base of the posterior horn of the gray matter in the spinal cord, thus interrupting the crossing fibers of the spinothalamic tract. However, a loss of both deep and superficial sensation sometimes occurs, as shown by the development of "Charcot" joints in these patients.

Motor involvement is an unusual initial presentation; the onset of weakness is usually subtle and insidious. Sometimes the wasting and weakness is so severe that peripheral neuropathy should be entertained in the differential diagnosis. In patients with a complete cord injury, the weakness appears above the level of primary injury in the upper limbs. However, in patients with incomplete injuries, the motor weakness from cavitation may appear below the level of the primary injury as well as above. The majority of patients at presentation have pain and unilateral sensory symptoms; the side presenting first remains the most severely affected.

II. PATHOGENESIS

The origin of the cavity that initiates the formation of the posttraumatic syrinx is poorly understood. The cavity may be formed by liquefaction of the initial cord hematoma or of the traumatized cord itself. Subsequent enlargement of

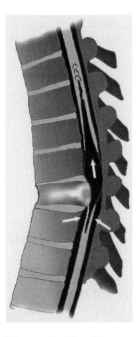

Figure 1 Possible mechanism of progression of the syringomyelic cavity. Coughing and straining produces compression on the lower end of the cyst cavity (see lower two arrows), forcing fluid within the cavity upwards, further dissecting into the rostral spinal cord.

the cavity and progression upward and downward within the spinal cord may be caused by the pulsatile action of the cerebrospinal fluid and its sloshing (24) within the cavity due to changes in intraspinal pressure (Figs. 1 and 2). In some posttraumatic cases, the cavity seems to arise away from the zone of maximal damage; in such cases, the above theory of cord cavitation after liquefaction of the initial cord hematoma and progression may not apply.

The spinal cord may become adherent to the overlying dura at the level of injury due to focal arachnoiditis (Fig. 3). Subsequently, a complete arachnoidal block may result when pressure differences occur above and below the site of cord adherence. Repetitive movement of the vertebral column above the fixed cord causes the cord to be stretched and compressed circumferentially at the site of the adherence, thus increasing the pressure within the cyst cavity and forcing disruption into adjacent cord tissue along the lines of least resistance. In these patients with obstruction of the arachnoidal pathways during periods of pressure differentials, cerebrospinal fluid may be forced into the cord from the subarachnoid space through minute pores in the wall of the spinal cord,

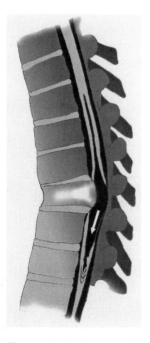

Figure 2 At the end of the coughing and straining, the returning fluid within the cavity tends to dissect into the spinal cord caudally (see arrow within cavity), but to a lesser extent.

initiating or propagating the cord cavitation. In some patients, significant improvement followed, but only after opening the pathways outside the cord. Finally, in the progressive phase of posttraumatic syringomyelia, cavitation fluid may come from the following sources: traumatized cells lining the cavity; the bloodstream by transudation; and cerebrospinal fluid pathways by either fistulae at the injury site or seepage along perivascular spaces.

III. DIAGNOSTIC STUDIES

Plain films occasionally show widening of the interpedicular distance in younger patients with long-standing cavitations. Computed tomographic myelography has been used extensively and accurately in the diagnosis of at least 90% of intramedullary cysts (12). Scans are taken through the level of the injury, extend cephalad at least to the highest level of clinical involvement, and extend caudally two vertebral segments below the injury level (Figs. 4 and 5).

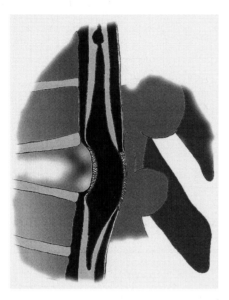

Figure 3   Arachnoiditis and adhesions of the cord to the adjacent spinal canal at the level of the fracture, obstructing the free communication of subarachnoid fluid.

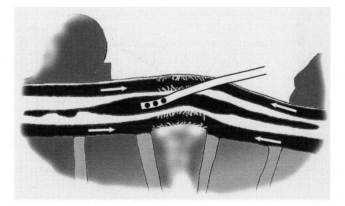

Figure 4   The syrinx is shunted to one of the body cavities and communication is re-established in the subarachnoid space.

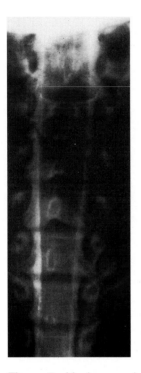

Figure 5 Myelogram showing the dilated cord in a patient with syringomyelic cavitation.

The sequence of scans is as follows: immediately, 5 to 8 hours after injection, and 24 hours after injection (Fig. 6). More recently, MRI scanning has been shown to be more specific in evaluating myelomalacia and cord cavitation. For example, sagittal T1-weighted images are most helpful in evaluating the spinal cord for cysts (Fig. 7). A well-defined area of low signal intensity within the cord, extending from the level of injury, is indicative of a posttraumatic syrinx.

IV. TREATMENT

Abbe in 1892 demonstrated the performance of a syringostomy at necropsy (1). Later, Elsberg first described syringostomy in two patients with syringomyelia (8). However, Freeman is credited for rationalizing surgical treatment of syringomyelia after performing experimental concussive injuries on the spinal cords of cats and dogs (10,11). By 1959, he had applied his experimental findings

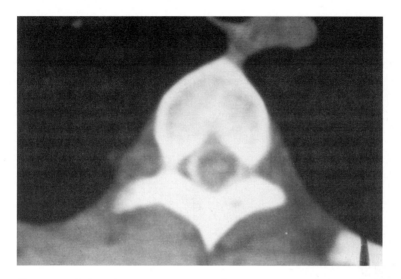

Figure 6   Delayed postmyelographic CT scan showing contrast within the syrinx cavity.

and used syringostomy to treat a patient with posttraumatic syringomyelia. A number of other surgical techniques have emerged over the years for the treatment of this condition. The basic principle in the treatment of patients presenting with progressive neurological symptoms related to posttraumatic syringomyelia is drainage of the cyst. The cyst can be drained into the subarachnoid space or into one of the body cavities (for example, pleural, peritoneal). Additionally, arachnoidal adhesions at the injury site must be lysed to establish free communication rostral and caudal to the injury site.

A.   Tube Syringostomy

Tube syringostomy involves the placement of a shunt tubing in the syrinx. One of the following techniques is used: syringosubarachnoid, syringoperitoneal, or syringopleural shunts. The syringosubarachnoid shunt is the least suitable in the treatment of posttraumatic cavitation and at best only equalizes the pressures between the syrinx and the subarachnoid space. It is more likely to become obstructed and cease to function with arachnoiditic scar tissue.

Syringoperitoneal and syringopleural shunts are preferred because the trend is to drain the cyst into a body cavity with lower pressure. The pleural cavity offers a negative pressure and thus facilitates drainage. Pleural shunts are technically easier because the patient does not have to be moved during the proce-

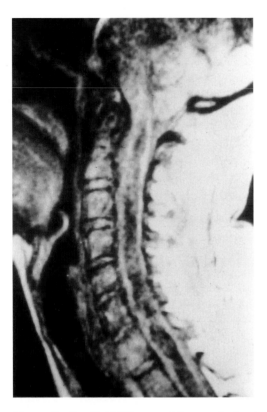

Figure 7 Sagittal MRI scan of the cervical spinal cord shows the syringomyelic cavity extending up to the medulla, with dilatation of the spinal cord.

dure. However, syringoperitoneal shunting is more effective with fluid absorption, particularly because the rate of fluid flow within syrinx shunts is unknown. The drainage tube may be introduced into the syrinx in the operating room with intraoperative ultrasonic guidance. The tube is placed either via a midline myelotomy in the paraplegic patient or via a dorsal root-entry zone myelotomy in the patient in whom preservation of the posterior columns is important.

Because drainage alone may not be enough, the cause of the cyst formation should also be addressed. If the filling mechanisms are still active or a sizable residual syrinx persists, propagation of the syrinx can occur. Thus, the abolition of the pressure differences by opening up the adhesions caused by arachnoiditis and correction of any significant gibbus deformity causing compression may be necessary (25). Occasionally leaving the dura open with a bypass drain from above the level of the obstruction to below it may be beneficial.

B. Transection

This technique is the most effective method for disabling the filling mechanisms in patients with complete lesions (7). Here the thinned cord through which cerebrospinal fluid most certainly enters as well as the zone of arachnoiditis are removed. A drainage tube is left in the remaining cyst and is brought out into the distal subarachnoid space through the funnel-shaped lower end of the syrinx, which is closed around the tubing.

C. Myelotomy

This technique is not often used. A midline or root-entry zone myelotomy is performed and left open. The residual elasticity in the cord may facilitate a myelotomy to deflate the cord. However, this opening allows both filing as well as deflating of the cyst at the same time, and will eventually close due to scarring.

D. Syrinx-Cisternal Shunt

In cervical and upper thoracic syrinxes, a laminectomy is performed at the level of the syrinx. Next, a Silastic catheter with a floppy guide wire is passed cephalad in the subdural space to reach and perforate the cisterna magna. Finally, the distal end of the catheter is placed in the syrinx cavity. This technique has not gained popularity, especially in syrinxes located in the lower spinal cord.

E. Endoscopy

In patients with extensive cavitation in the spinal cord with septae noted in the syrinx, we use a flexible endoscope to break down the septations to communicate the whole cyst. Thus, a more effective drainage of the whole syrinx occurs.

In summary, patients who present with ascending symptomatology should be evaluated with magnetic resonance imaging (MRI). If a posttraumatic syrinx is demonstrated, decompression is considered. Symptom onset may be sudden, caused by episodes of vigorous straining and may result in permanent neurological deficits. Although these patients may not recover their deficits, they should undergo surgical treatment to prevent worsening of the deficits. Most surgeons treat patients with progressive symptoms associated with a posttraumatic syrinx using one of the tube syringostomy techniques. A syrinx without neurological progression and detected incidentally should be followed up regularly with yearly MRI scanning.

Posttraumatic, noncystic myelopathy (a part of syringomyelia syndrome) is demonstrated on MRI scanning as a spectrum of microcysts and septate macrocysts. This process of ascending degeneration is indistinguishable from the cystic myelopathy and is unresponsive to surgical drainage.

V. PROGNOSIS

Vernon et al. reported that all untreated cases of posttraumatic syrinx ($n = 40$) progressed, either slowly or rapidly, and sometimes to severe disability (23). However, there is no way to predict from the extent, level, severity of injury, or etiology at what rate the condition will progress or to what extent. Remission, particularly sensory, can occur and last for several years. Surgical treatment does not always improve the patient's condition. Symptoms may worsen after manipulation; this worsening is usually temporary but it can be permanent. At best, successful surgery reverses some or most of the newer deficits but, for the most part, prevents further progression. Thus, early recognition of neurological deterioration and treatment offers the best protection against further progression. Overall treatment of posttraumatic syringomyelia remains unsatisfactory and further work is necessary to better understand the etiology and progression of this condition and methods to improve care for patients with this condition.

REFERENCES

1. Abbe R, Coley WB. Syringomyelia: Operation, exploration of cord, withdrawal of fluid, exhibition of patient. J Neurol, Dis 1892; 19:572.
2. Backe HE, Betz RR, Mesgarzadeh M, et al. Post-traumatic spinal cord cysts evaluated by magnetic resonance imaging. Paraplegia 1991; 29:607–612.
3. Barbaro NM, Wilson CB, Gutin PH, et al. Surgical treatment of syringomyelia: Favourable treatment with syringo-pleural shunting. J Neurosurg 1984; 61:531–538.
4. Barnett HJM, Jousse AT. Post-traumatic syringomyelia (cystic myelopathy). In: Vinken PJ, Bruyn EM, eds. Handbook of Clinical Neurology. Vol. 26. Amsterdam; North Holland Publishing Co., 1976; 113–157.
5. Brewis M, Poskanzer DC, Rolland C, Miller H. Neurological disease in an English city. Acta Neurol Scand 1966; 42:suppl 24.
6. Davis CHG, Symon L. Mechanism and treatment in post-traumatic syringomyelia. Brit J Neurosurg 1989; 3:669–674.
7. Durward QJ, Rice GP, Ball MJ, et al. Selective spinal cordectomy: Clinicopathological correlation. J Neurosurg 1982; 56:359–367.
8. Elsberg GA. The surgical treatment of intra-medullary affections of the spinal cord. Proceedings of the 17th International Congress of Medicine (London) (1913):Section XI.
9. Finlayson AI. Syringomyelia and related conditions. In: Baker AB, Baker LH, eds. Clinical Neurology. Hagertown, MD: Harper & Row, 1977:3:32.

10. Freeman G. Ascending spinal paralysis. J Neurosurg 1959; 16:120–122.
11. Freeman LW, Wright TW. Experimental observations of concussion and contusion of the spinal cord. Ann Surg 1953; 137:433–443.
12. Griffiths ER, McCormick CC. Post-traumatic syringomyelia (cystic myelopathy) Paraplegia 1981; 19:81–89.
13. La Haye PA, Batzdorf U. Post-traumatic syringomyelia. West J Med 1988; 148:657–663.
14. Lyons BM, Brown DJ, Calvert JM, et al. The diagnosis and management of post-traumatic syringomyelia. Paraplegia 1987; 25:40–350.
15. Mclean DR, Miller JDR, Allen PBR, Ezzedin S. A. Post-traumatic syringomyelia. J Neurosurg 1973; 39:485–492.
16. Peerless SJ, Durward QJ. Management of syringomyelia: A pathophysiological approach. Clin Neurosurg 1983; 30:531–576.
17. Rossier AB, Werner A, Wildi E, Berney J. Contribution to the study of late cervical syringomyelic syndromes after dorsal or lumbar traumatic paraplegia. J Neurol Neurosurg Psychiatry 1968; 31:99–105.
18. Rossier AB, Foo D, Shillito J. Post-traumatic cervical syringomyelia. Brain 1985; 108:439–461.
19. Schliep G. Problems der syringomyelie. Fortschr Neurol Psychiat 1979; 47:557–608.
20. Shannon N, Symon L, Logue V, Cull D, Kang J, Kendall BE. Clinical features, investigation and treatment of post-traumatic syringomyelia. J Neurol Neurosurg Psychiatry 1981; 44:35–42.
21. Suzuki M, Davis C, Symon L, Gentili F. Syringo-peritoneal shunt for treatment of cord cavitation. J Neurol Neurosurg Psychiatry 1985; 48:620–627.
22. Tator CH, Meguro K, Rowed DW. Favourable results with syringosubarachnoid shunts for treatment of syringomyelia. J Neurosurg 1982; 56:517–523.
23. Vernon JD, Silver JR, Symon L. Post-traumatic syringomyelia. Paraplegia 1983; 21:37–46.
24. Williams B. On the pathogenesis of syringomyelia: A review. J Royal Soc Med 1980; 73:798–806.
25. Williams B, Page N. Surgical treatment of syringomyelia with syringopleural shunting. Brit J Neurosurg 1987; 1:63–80.
26. Williams B, Terry AF, Jones HWF, McSweeney T. Syringomyelia as a sequel to traumatic paraplegia. Paraplegia 1981; 19:67–80.
27. Williams B. Post-traumatic syringomyelia: An update. Paraplegia 1990; 28:296–313.

9

Infections of the Spinal Cord

J. B. Peiris
University of Colombo, Colombo, Sri Lanka

S. B. Gunatilake
University of Kelaniya, Colombo, Sri Lanka

I. INTRODUCTION

The incidence and types of bacterial and viral infections of the spinal cord vary widely from country to country. Tuberculosis (TB), poliomyelitis, and rabies are important infections of the spinal cord in most developing countries but are rarities or do not occur in many developed countries. Infections of the brain and spinal cord have assumed a new importance in the present day, in view of the susceptibility of immune-suppressed patients, such as those with AIDS, an increasingly common disease in the world, including the developing countries.

II. SOURCES AND ROUTES OF INFECTION

The most common mode of infection is blood borne. The spinal cord can also be involved in infections of the adjacent vertebrae as in osteomyelitis, both pyogenic and tuberculous. Cerebrospinal fluid infections as in meningitis can affect the spinal cord, causing a myelitis, a radiculopathy, or abscess formation.

III. CLINICAL PRESENTATION

The clinical presentation, irrespective of organism, may be a pure myelopathy, pure radiculopathy, a radiculomyelopathy, or an arachnoiditis. As the spinal canal is rigid and nonyielding, an expanding disease process will eventually produce cord and/or root compression. Infections of the spinal cord usually present subacutely over days or a few weeks, but may present acutely in hours, or chronically over weeks or months. The possibility of an infective pathology is suggested mainly by the temporal profile of the presenting manifestation, whereas the etiology is often suggested by extraspinal manifestations, as for example, the presence of easily detectable pulmonary TB or septic focus elsewhere.

Viral infections of the spinal cord include poliomyelitis, rabies, (both still seen in developing countries), *Herpes zoster varicella,* coxackie virus, enteric cytopathic human orphan (ECHO) viruses, HTLV-1 and HTLV-3. The main bacterial infections of the spinal cord are pyogenic infections, tuberculosis, and syphilis. Myelitis and polyradiculopathies of unclear etiology may be postinfectious, postvaccinal, acute inflammatory polyradiculopathy (AIDP), and chronic inflammatory polyradiculopathy (CIDP).

These infections can be categorized into the following groups:

1. Myelitis due to viruses:
    Polio virus, coxsackie virus groups A and B, ECHO virus
    Herpes simplex and varicella
    Rabies
    HTLV-1, HIV
2. Myelitis due to bacterial, fungal, and parasitic infections:
    Spinal syphilis
    Spinal tuberculosis
    Pyogenic infections
    Parasitic and fungal infections
3. Myelitis of unknown etiology:
    Postinfectious
    Postvaccinal

IV. VIRUS INFECTIONS OF THE SPINAL CORD

Poliomyelitis and herpes zoster are two of the important virus infections of cord. The viruses of poliomyelitis have an affinity for neurons of the anterior horn and herpes zoster for the dorsal root ganglia.

A. Poliomyelitis

Polio virus, an RNA enterovirus, has three types. Major epidemics have been caused by type 1 while the other two types usually cause sporadic cases and small outbreaks. Polio vaccine is a most effective vaccine and mass immunization programs have drastically reduced the incidence worldwide. Small epidemics and outbreaks occur in poorer countries, a consequence of poor sanitation and difficulties encountered by immunization programs in reaching the masses. The World Health Organization (WHO) aims to eradicate polio worldwide by the year 2000 (1). The disease claimed about 120,000 victims in 1992. Although 80% of the world's children have been immunized against poliomyelitis, reaching the other 20% is a difficult task and WHO has formed the Polio Eradication Network (PEN) consisting of international health agencies and NGOs (Nongovernmental Organizations) to achieve this goal. Rotary International alone has contributed $240 million for the provision of polio immunization programs worldwide. The United Nations Children's Fund (UNICEF) estimates the cost of global polio eradication at $1.4 billion over the next 10 years. When polio is eradicated, immunization will no longer be necessary, and the world will be saving $500 million every year in vaccines and $3 billion by the year 2015.

In the developing countries, poliomyelitis occurs in infancy and childhood. Outbreaks and epidemics may still occur and are of two varieties. In nonimmunized children, it is due to wild polio virus (among Amish in the United States in 1979); in immunized subjects, it is due to polio virus type 3 (Finland 1984–1985, the Netherlands 1992–1993). Immunity to type 3 was low, and the virus responsible for the outbreak was antigenically different to that in vaccine. Small outbreaks were also reported in 1992/1993 in Jordan, Malaysia, and in the Netherlands.

1. Clinical Features

Four clinical groups can be recognized: asymptomatic, abortive, nonparalytic, and paralytic. Severity is determined by the immune response of the host. Asymptomatic cases only excrete the virus in the stools. The abortive cases manifest prodromal symptoms of a viral infection. Nonparalytic cases develop features of meningeal involvement but do not progress to paralysis. The paralytic cases reach the maximum weakness in 3 to 5 days, usually by 72 hours. Pain in the spine and the limbs precede the onset of weakness. The spinal and bulbar muscles are involved with varying degrees of severity. Weakness is usually asymmetrical and often patchy. Reflexes are lost in involved limbs and wasting appears early. There is no sensory loss and no upper motor neuron signs. In severe cases, bulbar palsy and respiratory failure can be life threatening. About 2 to 5% of children and 15 to 30% of adults with paralyzing infection die. As temporarily damaged neurons regain their function, recovery begins and may continue for as long as 6 months.

Some patients develop a progressive muscle weakness, usually 20 to 30 years after the initial infection and paralysis. This is called the postpolio syndrome or the postpoliomyelitis neuromuscular atrophy (2). Symptoms vary from mild to moderate deterioration of function, with fatigue, muscle pain, fasciculations, and weakness that may stabilize or progress to muscle atrophy. The limbs are often affected, and involvement of bulbar and respiratory muscles can sometimes lead to dysphagia, choking episodes, aspiration, or sleep apnoea (3). The pathogenesis is usually thought to be due to dysfunction of surviving motor neurons with slow disintegration of axon terminals, leading to late denervation of muscle. There is also evidence that reactivation of latent or persistent poliovirus may occur in some.

2. Differential Diagnosis

In endemic regions, any case of acute flaccid paralysis (AFP), including the Guillain-Barré syndrome (GBS), in a child younger than 5 years for which no other cause is apparent is considered as a probable case of poliomyelitis. If weakness progresses beyond 7 days it is very unlikely to be poliomyelitis. This is one of the most important factors in the differentiation of poliomyelitis from other causes of AFP. Fever at onset, meningism and lymphocytic CSF are useful pointers for a diagnosis of polio. Diagnosis is confirmed by isolation of the virus from stool specimens and detection of rising antibody titers in the serum and cerebro-spinal fluid (CSF). Other conditions in the differential diagnosis are acute intermittent porphyria, paralytic rabies, (in areas where rabies is prevalent), and botulism. Acute poliomyelitis-like syndrome may also be caused by other enteroviruses, such as coxsackie and ECHO viruses, although paralytic complications are very rare. Epidemic acute hemorrhagic viral conjunctivitis caused by enterovirus 70, seen in Asia and Africa, may cause an illness resembling poliomyelitis in a small percentage of cases (4).

3. Prevention and Treatment

Trivalent oral polio vaccine (OPV) is the vaccine of choice. All children in countries endemic for polio should receive four doses in the first year of life. The first dose should be given at birth or the first contact with four weeks between subsequent doses. Treatment in the acute stage is mainly symptomatic. Early detection of bulbar involvement and respiratory failure is important to prevent fatalities. Modern methods of treatment have not helped in preventing residual disability.

B.   Acute Hemorrhagic Viral Conjunctivitis

A polio-like illness with asymmetrical lumbosacral radiculomyelitis may follow AHVC, presenting as an AFP. Somewhat similarly a brachial radiculomyelitis with cranial and peripheral neuropathy or a GBS may occur. Recovery in the upper limbs is better than in the legs and sensory signs are rare. The CSF shows a lymphocytic picture, with raised protein, normal sugar, and chlorides. Half to two-thirds of the patients have a residual motor disability. As it is highly contagious and spreads rapidly, strict environmental and public health measures are indicated.

C.   Rabies

Rabies is caused by a number of different strains of highly neurotropic viruses. Most belong to a single serotype in the genus lyssavirus, family rhabdoviridae. Rates of human rabies are highest in Asia. In India there are about 15,000 to 20,000 deaths each year and 75% of cases occur in villages. Over 90% are due to dog bites, mostly stray dogs. Thailand, Indonesia, and Sri Lanka are other countries in Asia where rabies causes a significant number of deaths (5). In Africa, rabies is particularly common in Ethiopia and Nigeria.

1.   Rabies in Animals

Domestic and stray dogs are mostly responsible for human rabies in Africa and Asia, where canine rabies has not been adequately controlled. In Europe and the Americas, where it has been controlled, dogs account for less than 5%, and wildlife rabies is the important source of human infection. The principle wildlife vectors include mongoose and jackals in Africa, and the fox in Europe, Canada, arctic and subarctic regions, the wolf in western Asia, and the vampire bat in Latin America. Any warm-blooded animal can be infected by the rabies rhabdovirus. Practically all cases of rabies are the result of inoculation of the virus through the skin by an animal bite. The incubation period in animals varies from 5 days to 14 months but once symptoms appear, the animal usually dies within 10 days—a useful practical guide as to whether the animal had rabies.

2.   Human Rabies

Only 5 to 15% of unimmunized humans develop rabies after a bite by an infected animal. The susceptibility to infection depends on a number of factors: the infecting strain, the host's genetic background, the concentration of nicotinic acetylcholine receptors in skeletal muscle, size of the inoculum, degree of innervation of the bite site, and its proximity to the nervous system.

The virus spreads by retrograde axoplasmic flow at 8 to 20 mm per day until it reaches the spinal cord, when the first specific symptoms of the disease, pain or paresthesiae at the site of the wound, appear. The incubation period depends on the distance the virus has to travel to reach the central nervous system. The incubation period is usually 1 to 2 months, but can vary from 9 days to several years.

There are two varieties of rabies in humans, as in animals: (1) "furious variety" due to an encephalitis with affinity for bulbar and limbic neurones; (2), "paralytic or dumb" variety due to affection of the spinal cord.

Spinal or Paralytic Rabies

Although the paralytic variety is said to constitute 10% of all cases of human rabies, paralytic rabies after the bite of a rabid dog is rare. It is the variety more commonly seen after "bat bites." Rabies of the spinal cord appears to be more common after bites on the limbs and in vaccinated individuals for unknown reasons.

Clinical Features of "Spinal Rabies"

The incubation period is the same as for the classic "furious" variety. The bitten limb develops sensory disturbances (pain and numbness) and weakness, which then spread to involve the other limbs. Retention of urine and constipation develop as in myelitis. This is often followed by an ascending paralysis with involvement of the muscles of respiration and deglutition, which prevents the occurrence of spasms of these muscles. Paralysis of the throat muscles gives rise to the "dumb" features. Spasms of the throat muscles induced by attempts to swallow water (hence hydrophobia) and spasms of throat muscles induced by cold air (fan sign), characteristic features of furious rabies, do not occur in the paralytic variety. Respiratory paralysis may occur and the patient usually remains conscious till he dies of respiratory failure. The patient may survive for more than a month with intensive care and ventilatory assistance, when a terminal phase of encephalitic coma may ensue.

3. Diagnosis

The "paralytic" variety has to be differentiated from viral myelitis, post antirabies vaccine (ARV) encephalomyelitis, poliomyelitis, and GBS. Whereas human diploid cell vaccine has not been responsible for nueroparalytic complications, the less expensive goat brain or duck embryo vaccine more commonly available in developing countries can produce features similar to paralytic rabies. Post ARV encephalomyelitis develops as a hypersensitivity reaction to nervous tissue in the vaccine. Post ARV myelitis occurs 1 to 3 weeks after the first dose—earlier than the average onset of paralytic rabies of 1 to 2 months after a bite. During life, the diagnosis can be made by assessing the antibody titers and by examining a corneal smear for Negri bodies. An antibody titer of more than 1:5000 is seen only with the disease, the vaccine raising the level to less than 1:64.

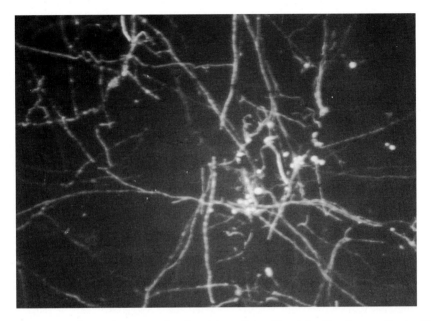

Figure 1 Corneal smear showing intracellular Negri bodies in a patient with rabies.

4. Corneal Smear

A corneal epithelial smear is obtained at the two ends of a glass slide by pressing firmly on the cornea. This is stained using the fluorescent dye, fluorescein isothiocyanate, conjugated with a high-titer rabies antibody. Immunofluorescence detects the intracellular Negri bodies (Fig. 1). When carried out properly the test is very specific and has a sensitivity of more than 70%. At present, this test is done only at the Medical Research Institute, Colombo, Sri Lanka.

5. Pathology

The disease is characterized by the presence of intraneuronal eosinophilic inclusion bodies (Negri bodies, lyssa bodies). In the brain, they are most profuse in Ammon's horn of the hippocampus, but they are also frequently seen in the pyramidal cells of the cerebral cortex and the Purkinje cell layer of the cerebellum. There is neuronal destruction with phagocytosis as opposed to the perivascular demyelination of ARV myelitis. After death, the diagnosis can be established by examination of the brain tissue. Fluoroscent antibody tests are rapid and accurate. Brain tissue is examined for Negri bodies. Virus particles are rarely seen. Negri bodies are seen in at least 70% of human cases and 90% of animals.

6. Treatment

Once the symptoms of the disease have appeared, there is no known successful treatment. It is generally believed that rabies is invariably fatal, but one recovery has been reported in a boy in whom the diagnosis appeared to be established (6) and a second in a woman in whom the diagnosis was less certain. The main hope of treatment is that intensive care may keep the patient alive until the disease process in the brain ceases and the brain recovers, if it ever does. In the absence of any effective treatment, prevention becomes very important.

7. Prevention

The prevention of rabies involves two approaches: (1) the control of the disease in animals to prevent it reaching man, and (2) the prophylactic treatment of human, both before and after exposure.

The first measure is a veterinary and social question, the second mainly a medical one.

Pre-Exposure Prophylaxis in Humans

Prophylaxis before exposure is recommended for persons who are at risk of frequent exposure to rabid animals. Animal handlers, laboratory workers, veterinarians, and persons spending a month or more in countries where canine rabies is common and medical care is difficult to obtain, should be immunized with the human diploid cell (HDC) vaccine (7).

Postexposure Prophylaxis in Humans

After a bite by a seemingly healthy animal, surveillance of the animal for a 10-day period is necessary as almost all animals develop signs of rabies during this period. If signs of illness appear in the animal, or if risk of the animal having the disease is high, the animal should be sacrificed and its brain sent under refrigeration to a laboratory for diagnostic tests. After severe bites, it is advisable to start the vaccine, preferably the HDC vaccine, without delay. Unprovoked bites by stray animals need to be considered as rabid unless proven to the contrary. Wild animal bites are considered to be rabid, unless determined otherwise.

Local Treatment of Bite.   Bites and scratches should be thoroughly washed with soap and water and, after all soap had been removed, cleansed with benzyl ammonium chloride or iodine 0.1% solution. These have been shown to inactivate the virus. Infiltration of antirabies serum around the wound is recommended for severe exposures and for bites on the face or close to the face.

Vaccination Schedule.   If the animal is found to be rabid or has escaped (stray dogs and wild animals), the patient should receive postexposure prophylaxis. Human rabies immune globulin, which avoids the complications of equine antirabies serum, is given in a dose of 20 u/kg of body weight, with one-half infiltrated around the wound and the other half given intramuscularly. This provides adequate immunization for 10 to 20 days, allowing time for active immunization. For active immunization nervous tissue vaccine, duck embryo vaccine and HDC vaccine are available. Serious allergic reactions, such as encephalomyelitis and ascending myelitis occur at the rate of 1 per 1000 with nervous tissue vaccine and 1 per 20,000 with duck embryo vaccine. The newer HDC vaccine is safe from these complications and has reduced the doses needed to five, given as 1 mL intramuscular injections on the day of the exposure and then on days 3, 7, 14, and 28 after the first dose. With nervous tissue vaccine and duck embryo vaccine, 23 doses, given daily, are necessary. The HDC vaccine provides a better antibody response.

D.   HTLV-1-Associated Myelopathy/Tropical Spastic Paraparesis

The HTLV-1-associated myelopathy (HAM) is also known as tropical spastic paraparesis (TSP). Tropical spastic paraparesis was first described in India in 1969 (8) and was found to be similar to the spastic form of Jamaican neuropathy (9). Since then, it has become evident that this syndrome has a wider geographical distribution, occurring endemically in South America and the Caribbean. It has also been reported from the southern United States, southern Japan, and Africa. In 1985, IgG antibodies to HTLV-1 were found in the sera of 59% of patients from Martinique with TSP (10), and antibodies to HTLV-1 were found in the CSF and sera of Jamaican patients with TSP (11). Around the same time, a myelopathy associated with HTLV-1 infection from an HTLV-1 endemic area in southern Japan was reported (12) and this syndrome is now known as HAM (13).

   The HTLV-1 is a type-C lymphotropic retrovirus that has a predilection for T4 lymphocytes. Lymphocytes that become infected are capable of indefinite growth and express specific surface viral antigens. The HTLV-1 is also associated with a form of adult T-cell leukemia (ATL). Both HAM and ATL have been described in the same patient. The HTLV-1 has been isolated from cultured peripheral blood and CSF mononuclear cells of patients with HAM. HTLV-1 nucleic acid sequences have been identified in blood and CSF cells, and viral antigens have been detected in CSF (14).

   There is distinct geographical variation in the incidence of HTLV-1 positivity and HAM. The disease tends to cluster, and adult black females appear to be the most vulnerable. It is found in southern Japan, the Caribbean, clusters in Panama, equatorial regions of Africa, the Pacific coast of Columbia, and other areas of South America (15). Studies of migrant populations demonstrate that infection is often acquired in early life and can travel with the individual to nonendemic areas and cause disease later (16).

The method of transmission is not known in most cases but it is known that transmission can occur sexually, the most common method being male to female. Other methods of transmission are in utero to the fetus, through breast milk to the child, via blood transfusions, and from intravenous drug abuse. The incubation period is not known in the naturally occurring form of the disease and may be as short as 6 months after infection in some cases (17).

The onset is usually before the fourth decade. The clinical picture is that of a slowly progressive paraparesis with peripheral sensory symptoms of painful paresthesiae and exaggerated tendon reflexes. Sphincter disturbance is common and is often an early feature. Sensory loss is variable and usually affects only the lower limbs; a sensory level in the trunk is rare. Some of the reported patients have an associated polyneuropathy. The upper limbs, brainstem, and cerebral hemispheres are usually spared. A diagnosis of HAM/TSP should be considered in all patients with a noncompressive myelopathy. Some cases have been described with lower motor-neurone features that may resemble amyotrophic lateral sclerosis clinically. In one such patient, the autopsy showed an atrophic spinal cord with degeneration of pyramidal tracts and anterior horn cells and thickened leptomeninges infiltrated with inflammatory cells. An HTLV-1 myelopathy appears to be the most common form of endemic TSP.

The diagnosis of HAM is suggested by the presence of a chronic progressive myelopathy in an adult who lives in an endemic area or who has migrated from an endemic area. Antibodies to HTLV-1 are found in the blood by enzyme-linked immuno-sorbent assay (ELISA) or Western blot. Using polymerase chain reaction (PCR), HTLV-1 can be distinguished from HTLV-2. Most patients have IgG antibodies to HTLV-1 in the CSF with oligoclonal bands. There may be CSF pleocytosis, with lymphocytes predominating and the protein content may be raised. Recently raised neopterin levels in the CSF had been suggested as a marker for HAM (18). Neopterin is released by macrophages under stimulation by T lymphocytes and is a marker for activation of cellular immunity. Raised levels of neopterin may help to distinguish HAM from other chronic myelopathies, including multiple sclerosis and motor neurone disease.

Dual infection with HIV and HTLV-1 has been found in AIDS patients with myelopathy, and the myelopathy is similar to that seen in HAM. It has been suggested that the presence of HIV increases the likelihood of HAM developing in a dually infected person (19).

1. Pathology

The pathological changes are not confined to the spinal cord but do predominate in it, particularly in thoracic region. The posterior columns and corticospinal tracts are the main sites of the disease. An inflammatory myelitis with focal spongiform demyelinative and necrotic lesions and perivascular and meningeal infiltrates occur. Neurones seem to be relatively spared.

2. Treatment

At present, treatment is supportive. Antiviral agents and immunomodulation may be potentially therapeutic, but as yet, there is no evidence of their efficacy in this disease. Oral prednisolone may have a transient beneficial effect in some patients. Intrathecal hydrocortisone, intravenous methylprednisolone, plasmapheresis, interferon alpha, and oral azathioprine have been shown to have transient effects (20). None of these treatments have been studied systematically in a controlled trial. There is a tendency for the condition to arrest so that it often ends in chronic disability rather than in death.

E. Acquired Immune Deficiency Syndrome

The HIV virus is neurotropic, and invasion of the nervous system occurs at an early stage. Neurological syndromes associated with the presence of the HIV virus are meningitis, encephalitis, dementia, myelopathy, neuropathy, and myositis. In addition to the changes in the brain, at least 30% of adult AIDS patients have a vacuolar myelopathy affecting the white matter of the lateral and posterior columns of the spinal cord in the thoracic region. The vacuoles arise within the myelin sheath, and in advanced cases, there is destruction of the myelin sheath (21). A myelopathy, without vacuoles has also been described (22). There is no correlation between the severity of the cerebral and spinal conditions. Commonly, spastic paraparesis develops, associated with sensory loss, then sphincter disturbance (23). Myelopathy and the AIDS-dementia complex may occur in the same patient. Spinal cord infection also can occur from opportunistic infection. Myelitis may be caused by varicella zoster, cytomegalovirus (CMV), and herpes simplex. Each of these syndromes may mimic or coexist with that produced by direct HIV infection, and treatment must be given to cover all possible diagnoses. Often the symptoms and signs of spinal cord disease are obscured by a neuropathy or one or more of the central nervous system disorders that complicate AIDS. The progressive radiculopathy that may be caused by CMV may improve after treatment with ganciclovir if started early (24). The interval between the onset of spinal cord symptoms and death was 4 to 6 months.

F. Acute Necrotizing Myelitis

The term "acute necrotizing myelitis" can be applied to patients developing severe inflammation of the spinal cord, in whom flaccid areflexic paraplegia with anesthesia and loss of sphincter control manifests rapidly over hours. Inflammation of the spinal cord affects both the gray and white matter. In acute viral encephalomyelitis, inflammation may lead to necrosis of the spinal cord. Clinical presentation is of an acute or subacute weakness of the lower extremities. The picture may be that of a transverse myelitis with symptoms or signs attributable to a transverse lesion at one level or an ascending weakness where the inflammation seems to spread up the cord. The inflammation is sufficient to cause severe pain with meningism and systemic symptoms including pyrexia. The course of acute necrotizing myelitis can be influenced significantly by high-dose intravenous methylprednisolone. Several organisms have been implicated in the etiology, and the recent literature has emphasized the role of herpes viruses, especially herpes simplex types 1 and 2, herpes zoster, and simian virus (25). Acute necrotizing myelitis has also been described as a complication of acute lymphocytic leukemias, lymphoma, hypernephroma, and AIDS.

G.   Herpes Zoster Radiculopathy

A painful vesicular eruption occurs in a dermatomal distribution most commonly in the thoracic area but can affect the cervical and lumbosacral nerve roots. The prodrome of 1 to 4 days comprises fever, malaise, and dysesthesiae. Radicular pain may be severe and may mimic an acute thoracic or abdominal emergency. Groups of vesicles appear on an erythematous base, becoming pustular in 3–4 days and crust in 7–10 days. Scarring is common.

Immunocompromised patients are more vulnerable, and in them dissemination may occur. In the immunocompromised patient, intravenous acyclovir therapy reduces complications and mortality. About a fifth to a quarter of patients develop postherpetic neuralgia, the prevalence increasing with age. In about 50%, the neuralgia resolves in a few months, whereas in others it may persist for many years. Particularly in these individuals, it is important to exclude a compressive lesion of the dorsal nerve root (DNR).

1.   Pathogenesis

It is presumed that the varicella zoster virus gains access to the dorsal nerve root ganglia during the primary skin infection and is later reactivated.

2.   Segmental Zoster Paresis

Although herpes zoster affects the dorsal root ganglion primarily; motor manifestations may occur. Inflammation of the ganglia probably spreads to the posterior horn, causing a unilateral segmental anterior and posterior polio myelitis and leptomeningitis. Contiguous spread may also occur to the ventral nerve root.

The neurological sequelae of varicella zoster virus (VZV), coxsackie and ECHO virus infection include meningoencephalitis with a cerebellar ataxic presentation, post infectious myelitis, encephalomyelitis, and a Guillain-Barré-type syndrome.

H. Postinfectious and Postvaccinal Myelitis

The characteristic features of these diseases are their temporal relationship to a virus infection such as varicella, rubeola and rubella, or a vaccination, the development of spinal cord signs over a period of a few days, and the monophasic temporal course without any further progression or recurrences. In most cases, the disease involves the brain as well as the spinal cord. The neurological symptoms progress for several days, after which they remain static and then recede slowly. The CSF contains lymphocytes and other mononuclear cells in the range of 20 to 200 cu mm with normal or slightly raised protein and normal glucose. Clinically, it may be difficult to differentiate between a postinfectious myelitis and myelitis of multiple sclerosis (MS), especially when the preceding infection is not apparent. The MS-associated myelitis shows spinal cord plaques on magnetic resonance (MR) scanning without swelling, whereas swelling is prominent with the parainfectious myelitis, which may also be associated with features of spinal shock. Oligoclonal bands are not seen in the CSF of the postinfectious variety. Once the symptoms develop, it is doubtful if any except supportive therapy is of value. Assuming the pathogenesis to be autoimmune, there is a tendency to administer high-dose intravenous steroids as soon as the diagnosis is made. There is no evidence that this practice alters the course of the illness.

V. BACTERIAL INFECTIONS OF THE SPINAL CORD

A. Spinal Epidural Abscess

The spinal epidural space is a true space containing fat and veins. It is widest in the midthoracic, lower lumbar, and sacral regions. The dura is unattached posteriorly, whereas anteriorly, it is attached to the vertebrae and ligaments.

The source of infection in this region may be hematogenous, arterial, or venous in about half the patients, or direct from the adjacent vertebrae or beyond from the thorax, abdomen, pelvis, retropharyngeal space, bed sores, or after spinal surgery. In many situations, the primary infection is mild, latent, or perhaps ignored.

1. Clinical Features

Systemic manifestations of infection may be present but they may be mild or masked by the acute presentation. Severe localized spinal pain with tenderness is followed by rapidly developing symptoms of root and cord compression. An acute root or cord lesion appearing over the course of a few days should alert the clinician to the possibility of an epidural inflammatory process requiring urgent confirmation and intensive management.

Root Compression

Root compression may produce both motor and sensory symptoms and signs. Root pain is severe, sharp, and shooting in the distribution of the root with aggravation by movement, laughing, straining, coughing, and sneezing. Overlap from adjacent roots often prevents the detection of sensory deficit or hyperesthesia. Lower motor neuron lesions with diminished or absent appropriate reflex may be seen with involvement of roots supplying the limb musculature (C5 to T1 and L1 to S2) but are seldom detected with root lesions above C5 and from T1 to T12.

Cord Compression

Rapidly progressive compressive lesions produce "spinal shock" with flaccid, areflexic, or hyporeflexic limbs and absent plantar responses. Then it may take days or weeks for the classic signs of spastic cord compression to appear. Although features may be initially unilateral, they rapidly become bilateral but asymmetrical. The final picture is that of an asymmetrical spastic paraparesis with hyperreflexia, extensor plantar responses and a sensory level. After initial difficulty in initiating micturition, there may be retention with automatic incomplete bladder emptying.

2. Management

Plain films of the spine are usually not helpful but may occasionally show evidence of an osteitis. Although spinal fluid examination may be considered useful for confirmation of an infective process or even in determining the organism at times, lumbar puncture (LP) may produce neurological deterioration. Hence LP/myelography should be avoided if computed tomography (CT) or magnetic resonance imaging (MRI) scanning is available. Computed tomography at the level of the compression is very useful to determine the extraspinal extent of the compression and to detect an associated or causative bony lesion (Fig. 2). Magnetic resonance imaging, while demonstrating the level of compression without the dangers of lumbar puncture, may not produce axial views of sufficient clarity. If scanning is not available or is inconclusive, LP should be combined with myelography, with the surgeon in readiness for emergency decompression.

The prognosis depends on the degree of deficit and how soon surgical decompression is achieved. Any patient with a suspected epidural abscess should be considered a surgical emergency and a diagnosis arrived at with minimum delay. If paralysis is complete (absence of even a flicker of movement, with retention of urine and loss of position sense), the prognosis is poor. Even with early surgery, prognosis is poor if there is a significant degree of vascular involvement. Urgent decompressive laminectomy with drainage of abscess with parenteral, bacteriologically appropriate or broad-spectrum antibiotic therapy

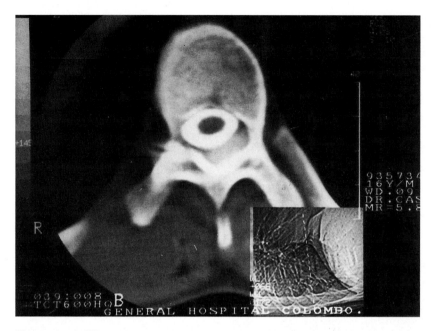

Figure 2 A CT myelogram showing an epidural abscess compressing the spinal cord.

usually proves gratifying if the diagnosis is not delayed and when vascular complications are not present.

B. Spinal Tuberculosis

Spinal TB is a disease of childhood and the young adult in developing countries (26,27). In the developed world, middle-aged immigrants from Asia and Africa are more likely to be affected. In countries where TB is common, vertebral TB accounts for more than 50% of bone and joint TB. Spinal cord involvement is seen in about 20% of vertebral TB, resulting in paraplegia. Although spinal TB is more common in the under-12-years age group, paraplegia is more common in the over-12-years age group. Paraplegia may occur in a patient with recognized Pott's disease of the spine, or it may be the first manifestation of the disease.

1. Pathology

Spinal manifestations can be divided into (1) primary spinal, (2) spinal secondary to tuberculous meningitis, and (3) spinal secondary to vertebral tuberculosis

(28,29). Tuberculous infection affects the vertebral bodies and the discs, commonly in the cervical and thoracic regions. The most common site is the mid-dorsal spine (nearly 50%), whereas 30 to 40% of the lesions occur in the lower dorsal and lumbar spine. Two adjacent vertebral bodies are often affected, with involvement of the anterior inferior angle of one and the adjacent anterior superior angle of the vertebra below (Fig. 3). The disc space collapses as the vertebral plate is destroyed. The infective process spreads throughout the vertebral body and may involve the pedicles and the facet joints subsequently (Fig. 4). Exuberant granulation tissue may spread for several segments.

2. Clinical Features

Systemic manifestations of weight loss, evening pyrexia, and night sweats may not always be present. Tuberculosis of the spine as a cause of persistent chronic backache has to be considered in the differential diagnosis, especially in developing countries. Symptoms of vertebral involvement are commonly insidious. The spine is stiff and painful on movement and tender over the affected region.

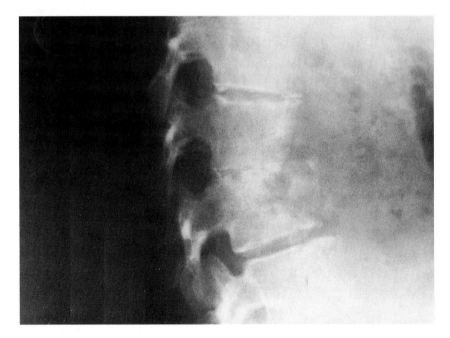

Figure 3 Plain lateral x-ray of the thoracic spine showing tuberculous infection of the anterior inferior angle of one vertebra and the anterior superior angle of the vertebra below.

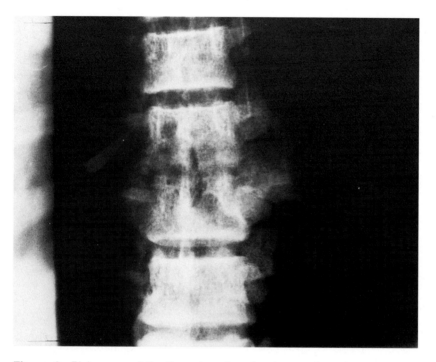

Figure 4   Plain x-ray of the thoracic spine showing a tuberculous process involving the body and the pedicles.

Spasm of the vertebral muscles is present. A history of tuberculosis in the patient or his family should raise the suspicion of possible spinal TB.

3. Neurological Presentation

Neurological complications are the most dreaded and crippling. In affluent, developed countries, it is extremely rare to see these complications. However, in developing countries, spinal TB and its complication, Pott's paraplegia, are still common. Patients present to hospitals late, after developing paraplegia. The disability is often irreversible by that stage. In certain parts of India, tuberculosis was the cause of compression paraplegia in nearly 50% of cases (30).

There are various types of presentation. In acute radiculopathy, there is fever, backache, and root pain. In acute polyradiculopathy of the Guillain-Barré type, TB may present like GBS with predominant sensory symptoms that may draw attention to the radicular component. Cerebrospinal fluid protein may be markedly elevated. Tubercle follicles and bacilli may be demonstrable in the nerve roots at autopsy (Fig. 5) with the CSF forming a coagulum around the cord (31).

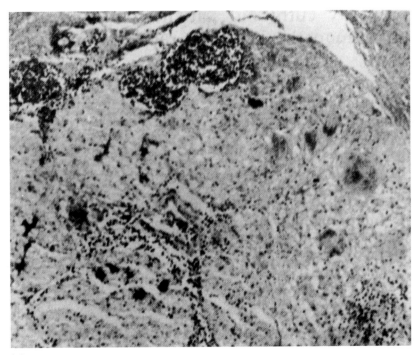

(a)

Figure 5   (a) Section of nerve root showing tuberculous granulomata, mononuclear cell infiltrate, swelling, and destruction of myelinated nerve fascicles with
lipid phagocytes. (b) High-power magnification of nerve root section.

Tuberculosis myelitis presents as an acute progressive paraparesis with
sphincter disturbance and a sensory level. Occasionally it presents in the ascending form. In the chronic form, a syndrome resembling progressive spinal cord
compression is seen. This occurs insidiously in about 20% of cases due to accumulation of caseous granulation tissue, or pus, commonly in the extradural space.

Typical signs of spinal cord involvement are clumsiness while walking,
exaggerated lower limb reflexes, extensor plantar response, sphincter disturbance, and sensory loss. Motor functions are affected to a greater extent than
the sensory functions because the tuberculous lesions are located anteriorly in
the spine. Position and vibration sense are the last to disappear. When there is
no discernible motor function and all sensations are lost, the prognosis for any
motor recovery after treatment is poor. Rarely, sudden complete paralysis may
occur due to collapse of vertebrae, infarction of the cord due to arterial thrombosis, or rapid expansion of a tuberculous abscess. There is evidence of verte-

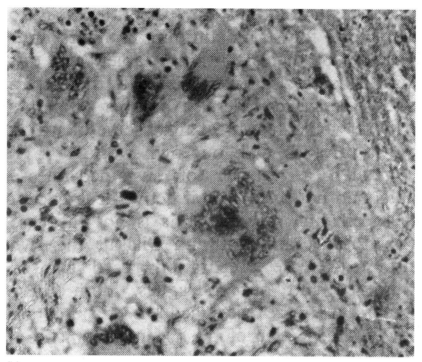

(b)

bral disease in the form of a painful tender kyphus with root pains. Tuberculosis elsewhere and a tracking cold abscess may be present.

Tuberculomas of the cord are rare. They could be intramedullary, subdural, or extradural. Extradural ones are mostly secondary to a bony lesion, although this may be apparent only at surgery. Extradural compression requires decompressive laminectomy with excision of granulation tissue. Intradural tuberculomas are hard, round, or oval lesions adherent to dura and cord. Intramedullry ones usually are single, hard, circumscribed lesions with central necrosis that enucleates easily. Lastly, arachnoiditis due to TB may present with features of cord compression or with predominantly sensory symptoms.

4. Diagnosis

A high index of suspicion is necessary for early detection of spinal TB.

Radiology

An x-ray of the chest may show evidence of disease in as many as 25 to 50% of patients with spinal TB and should be a routine investigation in spinal disease. Plain films of the spine at the appropriate level may show evidence of disease in relation to the disc but sometimes may fail to differentiate this from malignant conditions (32). Early radiological changes include reduction of intervertebral disc space and paradiscal erosions, seen more frequently anteriorly. If not treated at this stage, vertebral body destruction and collapse occur with development of an angular kyphus. Paravertebral abscesses may be seen on plain x-ray films of the spine. Myelographic findings are variable and include complete obstruction, partial obstruction with candle guttering, multiple filling defects, or arachnoiditis.

Computed tomographic scanning is a useful tool in assessing the destructive lesions of the vertebral column. It is especially useful in craniovertebral and cervicodorsal regions, where early lesions do not show up so well on plain x-rays. Computed Tomographic myelography will detect any tuberculous abscess that is pressing on the cord. Magnetic resonance imaging has been found to be extremely useful in detecting tuberculous infection of difficult areas.

Cerebrospinal Fluid

Color. Usually clear and colorless but may be xanthochromic and form a "cobweb" coagulum on standing. The CSF preferably should be left standing in a test tube and compared with a test tube of water.

Cells. It is rare for no cells to be present. Usually there is a mild pleocytosis with only 100–500 cells. The predominant cell is the lymphocyte. A mixed picture may be due to a pyogenic and tuberculous infection, requiring treatment for both initially, with review by repeat puncture.

Sugar. Often less than 50% of the blood sugar measured simultaneously. A rise in the sugar level on treatment with anti-TB drugs strengthens the diagnosis.

Protein. If there is a spinal block or polyradiculopathy, the protein may be markedly elevated and the CSF may not flow out, coagulating in the needle. If a syringe is used to suck out the fluid, it may coagulate in the syringe.

AFB. Seen in fewer than 25% of cases. Examination of a thick smear after centrifuging 10 mL and/or repeating the procedure may provide a higher yield.

Cultures. May be positive in 40 to 90%, but it takes several weeks to obtain the result.

As organism isolation is difficult, a simple, specific, rapid test is needed for confirmation of the diagnosis. Detection of antigen of the mycobacterium using a PCR technique in the CSF has allowed early diagnosis of meningeal TB and now can be used in the early diagnosis of these cases. In developing countries, a typical clinical picture and radiological appearances of tuberculosis may be sufficient to start treatment without biopsy. In cases of doubt, a small paravertebral abscess or a vertebral lesion may be biopsied using a core-biopsy needle under fluoroscopic control (33).

Tuberculous paraplegia has to be differentiated from cord compression due to primary and metastatic tumors, viral myelitis, TSP, and nutritional myelopathies such as lathyrism.

5. Treatment

The medical treatment of TB recommended in the United Kingdom is as follows (34). The first 2 months, in the initial phase after diagnosis: isoniazid, 200 mg (for patients weighing less than 40 kg) or 300 mg (patients at or more than 40 kg) once per day; rifampicin, 450 mg (less than 50 kg weight) or 600 mg (at or more than 50 kg); pyrazinamide, 1.5 g (less than 40 kg), or 2.0 g, (40–70 kg) or 2.5 g (more than 70 kg), once per day. Ethambutol or streptomycin may be added.

For the next 4 months, isoniazid and rifampicin are given as above, or isoniazid 15 mg/kg and rifampicin, 600–900 mg, three times per week or 2 times per week (if funds are insufficient). Though a total of 6 months therapy is adequate in pulmonary TB, a longer period up to 12 months may be neccessary in spinal TB.

Surgery is indicated if paraplegia develops while the patient is receiving anti-TB treatment, if the patient deteriorates while receiving treatment, for severe weakness or rapid progression, and for recurrence of weakness after initial improvement.

Surgery for Tuberculous Disease of the Spine

Laminectomy is contraindicated in those patients with lesions of the body but is ideal for spinal compressive lesions due to neural arch involvement. Anterolateral decompression is best for the thoracic region: granulation tissue and intraspinal abscesses can be removed better through this approach. The anterior approach gives a good exposure at all levels, and the compressive lesion is removed with immediate fusion by bone graft. Costotransversectomy is useful for poor risk cases with paraspinal abscesses, but is not suitable for intraspinal compressive lesions.

C. Sarcoidosis

Sarcoidosis is a systemic disease characterized by the formation of noncaseating granulomas containing macrophages, epithelioid cells, and multinucleate giant cells. The cause is unknown, but there is evidence of a defect in cellular immunity. The nervous system is involved in about 5% of patients with sarcoidosis (35). It may affect the central and the peripheral nervous system.

Sarcoidosis of the spinal cord is usually accompanied by obvious sarcoidosis elsewhere. Local granulomatous deposits may occur in the spinal cord, although involvement of the basal meninges and the adjacent brain are more common. The spinal cord may be compressed by extramedullary or intramedullary masses or may be the site of multiple parenchymatous granulomas. Spinal presentation may be as a myelitis or cord compression. Findings in the CSF depend on whether there is obstruction to the flow of CSF. The myelogram usually indicates the site of the main lesion but may be normal even in the presence of a greatly raised CSF protein level (36). Findings on the MRI include leptomeningeal enhancement, fusiform spinal cord enlargement, focal or diffuse intramedullary lesions, and spinal cord atrophy (37). Corticosteroids are the mainstay of therapy, the effective daily dose being approximately 60 mg or more. High-dose intravenous methylprednisolone may be effective in nonresponders. Cyclosporine and other immunosuppresants may enhance the response to steroids. Surgery has no place in the treatment of spinal cord lesions (38).

D. Spinal Neurosyphilis

The classic textbook picture of tabes dorsalis and general paresis of the insane is now rare and seems to be replaced by atypical and in-between forms (39). These conditions are, however, very rare and seen only very occasionally even in developing countries. More atypical cases are now being encountered due to the increasing incidence of syphilis in AIDS patients. The pathological forms are spinal pachymeningitis, meningomyelitis, spinal endarteritis, and radiculitis.

1. Spinal Pachymeningitis

Syphilitic inflammation of the spinal dura mater may follow syphilitic osteitis of the spine or may occur independently. The cervical region is usually involved and is termed pachymenigitis cervicalis hypertrophica. The dura mater is thickened and adherent to the arachnoid and pia. the vessels and nerve roots are involved and the cord becomes ischemic. Compression of long tracts leads to ascending and descending degeneration. The earliest symptom is pain due to compression of nerve roots. The pain radiates around the neck, shoulders, and down the upper limbs. Atrophy of the muscles supplied by these nerves then occurs. Ischemia and compression of the cord eventually lead to a progressive spastic paraplegia with sensory loss below the level of the lesion.

2. Meningomyelitis

The meninges and blood vessels are both involved, although often unequally (40). When the vessels are involved, thrombosis of a major vessel can lead to an acute or subacute transverse lesion of the cord. Microscopically, the vessels show endarteritis and perivascular cellular infiltration, and the meninges are also infiltrated. Within the cord, there is degeneration of both myelin and axons. Syphilitic myelitis usually involves the dorsal region and, although the leptomeninges may be extensively infiltrated, the area of softening on the cord is usually limited to two or three segments. Motor symptoms due to a dorsal lesion are generally preceded by pain in the back and in a girdle distribution. Weakness of the lower limbs develops from a few days and several weeks after the onset of pain.

Sometimes when the onset is more gradual, the patient develops a spastic paraplegia, bladder control is less severely affected, and the sensory loss may be slight (sometimes called Erb's spastic paraplegia). In some cases, a flaccid paraplegia may develop rapidly with retention of urine and impairment of all forms of sensation below the level of the lesion.

3. Spinal Endarteritis

Endarteritis of a spinal artery or of its branches may cause thrombosis, resulting in a localized area of softening within the cord. The picture of complete anterior spinal artery occlusion is rarely seen. When a lateral branch of the artery is occluded, there is a sudden onset of weakness, followed by wasting of muscles innervated by the affected spinal segment with involvement of the lateral spinothalamic tract. When thrombosis of a posterior spinal artery occurs, all forms of sensations are impaired in the corresponding cutaneous segments owing to destruction of the posterior horn of the gray matter. The posterior columns and the corticospinal tract on the same side are also infarcted, resulting in loss of position and joint sense below the level of the lesion and spastic paralysis also on the same side.

4. Radiculitis

The spinal roots may be involved in syphilitic meningeal inflammation. Inflammation of dorsal roots causes pain and hyperpathia in the corresponding segments. When the ventral roots are also affected, weakness and wasting in relevant muscles ensues.

5. Diagnosis

Serology should be done in selected cases, not routinely as in the past. The serum fluorescent treponemal antibody absorption (FTA-ABS) test is the most sensitive. Concurrent serum and CSF FTA-ABS may be of value in atypical neurosyphilis. Nontreponemal serological tests such as the VDRL are not sensitive enough and it can be negative in late stages of syphilis.

The CSF has an excess of cells ranging from 20 to 100 per mm^3. The cells are mononuclear. The protein content of the fluid is usually increased to between 0.5 and 1.5 g/L. An increase in gammaglobulin (IgG and IgM) is almost invariable, and oligoclonal bands may be present. In subacute meningomyelitis, there is often a considerable increase of protein and mononuclear cells. Meningeal adhesions may obstruct the subarachnoid space, resulting in spinal block.

6. Treatment

Penicillin is the drug of choice for all forms of neurosyphilis. Procaine penicillin G, 1200 mg daily intramuscularly for 14 days, with probencid 500 mg orally four times daily or aqueous penicillin 12 to 24 megaunits daily intravenously for 14 days are used. In patients allergic to penicillin, erythromycin, 500 mg four times daily for 10 to 15 days can be used. The Jarisch-Herxheimer reaction, which occurs usually after the first dose of penicillin and is a matter of concern in the treatment of primary syphilis, is usually of little concern in neurosyphilis and consists of a mild temperature elevation and leukocytosis.

In all forms of neurosyphilis, the patient should be re-examined every 3 months and the CSF should be re-tested after a 6-month interval. If after 6 months the patient is asymptomatic and the CSF abnormalities have been reversed (disappearance of cells, reduction in protein, gamma globulin, and serology titers), no further treatment is indicated. Further follow-up should include another clinical examination at 9 and 12 months and another CSF examination at the end of a year. Satisfactory response to treatment is judged by improvement in the CSF with reduction of serology titers. If at the end of 6 months, an increased number of cells and an elevated protein in the CSF are still apparent, another full course of penicillin should be given. Rapid clinical worsening in the face of a negative CSF suggests the presence of a nonsyphilitic disease of the brain or cord, such as MS.

E. Lyme Disease

This condition is named after the town of Lyme in Connecticut, USA, where outbreaks of arthritis accompanied by a characteristic skin lesion, erythema chronicum migrans, occurred in the 1970s. The causative organism is *Borrelia burgdorferi*. The vectors for the organism are the *Ixodes* ticks; namely, *Ixodes ricinus* in Europe and *Ixodes dammini* in the USA. Lyme disease occurs widely in the USA and northern and southern Europe. It has also been reported from Russia, the Far East, and Australia (41).

About 15% of infected patients develop neurological complications: a subacute lymphocytic meningitis, cranial nerve palsies, and a painful myeloradiculitis or peripheral neuritis. The myeloradiculitis is characterized by radicular pain followed by signs suggestive of spinal cord, brachial, or lumbosacral plexus involvement. A spastic paraparesis may occur in the late stages of the disease (42).

The organism is difficult to culture and evidence of infection depends on serological testing in blood and CSF. Indirect immunoflorescence tests or ELISA are available. Elevated antibody titers are seen in almost all patients after some weeks of infection, and evidence of an IgM response in acute and convalescent sera is diagnostic in a typical case. False-positive results may occur with syphilis and other spirochetal disorders.

Neurological complications of Lyme disease should be treated with parenteral antibiotics. Penicillin G, 20 megaunits daily in divided doses for 14 days is recommended. Other regimes are ceftriaxone, 2 g daily intravenously for 14 days or doxycycline, 100 mg orally twice daily for 30 days, or chloramphenicol. The value of antibiotics, with or without steroids, in chronic neurological disease remains unclear (43).

F. Acute Inflammatory Polyradiculopathies

Recognized infective causes of acute, generalized polyradiculopathies are rabies, diphtheria, Lyme disease, HIV infection, and GBS. The most common cause of acute generalized paralysis today is GBS. Other important causes to exclude are acute intermittent porphyria, botulism, paralytic rabies, poliomyelitis, and exposure to toxins (Table 1).

Table 1 Important Causes of Acute Generalized Paralysis

Acute intermittent porphyria	More in children but seen in adults. Recurrent episodes of abdominal pain and vomiting. Positive family history.
Botulism	Acute onset with colic abdominal pain. Pupillary and bulbar involvement are early features and the pattern of paralysis is descending.
Poliomyelitis	Occurs in small epidemics. Fever and meningeal symptoms are present. Paralysis is asymmetric, and sensory symptoms are absent.
Paralytic rabies	In endemic areas. Features of cerebral involvement may be present and some reflexes are retained.

1. Treatment

Plasmapheresis and intravenous gammaglobulin are the accepted treatment in acute GBS in adults and children. Intravenous gammaglobulins may be more suitable for children, as plasmapheresis can be difficult. For places without facilities for plasmapheresis and lacking finances to afford gammaglobulins, a modified form of plasma exchange can be used (4). In this method, 250 to 500 mL of blood is removed from the patient, the cells are separated from the plasma, the cells are reinfused, and plasma is discarded. Plasma, albumin or saline can be used to replace the lost volume of plasma. This cycle is repeated for about 7 to 10 days and the improvement seen is comparable to results of conventional plasmapheresis. Alternatively, the cycle can be repeated five to six times the same day for about 3 days. In children, infusion of 200 mL of fresh plasma, tested negative for HIV and hepatitis B, for 7 to 10 days has shown encouraging results (45).

G. Chronic Inflammatory Polyradiculopathies

This group consists of the inflammatory polyradiculopathies that progress beyond 4 weeks and those that relapse after improvement. It is important to exclude other causes of chronic neuropathies (Table 2).

The CSF protein is elevated in more than 90% of patients with chronic inflammatory polyradiculopathy and the motor nerve conduction velocities are considerably reduced.

Steroids have been found to be useful in treatment. The initial recommended doses are prednisolone 60 to 120 mg daily or 120 mg and 7.5 mg on alternate days for about a month, then reduction of the dose gradually at monthly intervals. Should steroid therapy prove unsuccessful, a course of azathioprine for about 3 months at a dose of 3 mg/kg daily may be tried. Plasma exchange and intravenous gammaglobulins are effective alternative forms of treatment, but the initial improvement is usually not maintained. These two methods may be useful in patients deteriorating rapidly and in those who respond poorly to steroids.

Table 2 Causes of Chronic Inflammatory Neuropathies

1. Toxic
2. Paraproteinemias
3. Hereditary motor sensory neuropathies
4. Infective: TB, HIV

H. Fungal and Parasitic Diseases

A variety of fungal and parasitic agents may involve the spinal meninges and the cord. However they are rare and are confined to certain geographic areas. *Actinomyces, Blastomyces, Coccidioides,* and *Aspergillus* may invade the spinal epidural space through intervertebral foramina or by extension from vertebral osteomyelitic focus. This can result in paraspinal abscess and cord compression. Hematogenous metastases to the spinal cord may occur in blastomycosis and coccidioidomycosis. *Cryptococcus* seldom leads to spinal lesions.

Schistosomiasis (bilharziasis) is a recognized cause of myelitis in the Far East, Africa, and South America. All three forms of *Schistosoma (S. haematobium, S. mansoni,* and *S. japonicum*) affect the spinal cord. Infection is acquired by swimming or bathing in contaminated water. The lesions in the spinal cord cause destruction of the gray and white matter, with *schistosoma* ova in arteries and veins resulting in ischemia (46, 47). Diagnosis is confirmed by positive serology. An ELISA test developed to indicate the presence of infection within the theca had been found to be sensitive, although not entirely specific. Conus medullaris and cauda equina lesions improve rapidly when treated with a combination of praziquantel and steroids. Treatment with praziquantel helps to arrest the course of the illness but may not reverse the disability if treatment was delayed.

A recurrent myelitis responding to diethylcarbamazine may occasionally occur with *toxocara canis.* There is a persistent eosinophilia in blood and CSF, and the specific serology tests are positive in blood and CSF.

VI. CONCLUSION

In the developed world, spinal cord infections are mostly due to AIDS, GBS and chronic inflammatory polyradiculopathy. In developing countries, a much wider spectrum of infections of the cord are seen. At a time when immunocompromised patients (due to HIV and chemotherapy) are increasing in the west, an awareness of these other infections is important, as these infections may occur in increasing numbers in the developed countries.

REFERENCES

1. Wright PF, Kim-Farley RJ, De Quadros CA, et al. Strategies for the global eradication of poliomyelitis by the year 2000. N Engl J Med 1991; 325:1774–1779.
2. Dalakas MC, Hallett M. The post polio syndrome. In: Plum F, ed. Advances in Contemporary Neurology. Vol 29 of the Contemporary Neurology Series. Philadelphia: F.A. Davis, 1988:51–94.

3. Sonies BC, Dalakas MD. Dysphagia in patients with the post-polio syndrome. N Engl J Med 1991; 324:1162–1167.

4. Wadia NH, Katrak SM, Misra V, et al. Polio-like motor paralysis associated with acute haemorrhagic conjunctivitis in an outbreak in 1981 in Bombay, India: Clinical and serologic studies. J Infect Dis 1983; 147:660.

5. Bogel K, Mostschwiller E. Incidence of rabies and post-exposure treatment in developing countries. Bull World Health Organ 1986; 64:883–887.

6. Hattwick MAW, Weis TT, Stechschulte CJ, et al. Recovery from rabies. A case report. Ann Intern Med 1972; 76:931–942.

7. Rabies prevention—United States, 1991 recommendations of the Immunization Practices Advisory Committee (ACIP). MMWR Morb Mortal Wkly Rep 1991; 40(3):1–19.

8. Mani KS, Mani AJ, Montgomery RD. A spastic paraplegic syndrome in south India. J Neurol Sci 1969; 9:179–199.

9. Cruickshank EK. A neurological syndrome of uncertain origin. West Indian Med J 1956; 39:592–595.

10. Gessain A, Barin F, Vernant JC, et al. Antibodies to human T-lymphotrophic virus type 1 in patients with tropical spastic paraparesis. Lancet 1985; ii:407–410.

11. Rodgers-Johnson PEB, Gajdusek DC, Morgan O, St. C, et al. HTLV-1 and HTLV-111 antibodies and tropical spastic paraparesis. Lancet 1985; ii:1247–1248.

12. Osame M, Usuke K, Izumo S, et al. HTLV-1 associated myelopathy, a new clinical entity. Lancet 1986; 1:1031–1032.

13. Bartholomew C, Cleghorn F, Charles W, et al. HTLV-1 and tropical spastic paraparesis. Lancet 1986; ii:99–100.

14. Bhagavati S, Ehrlich G, Kula RW, et al. Detection of human T-cell lymphoma/leukaemia virus type 1 DNA and antigen in spinal fluid and blood of patients with chronic progressive myelopathy. New Engl J Med 1988; 318:1141–1147.

15. Blattner WA. Epidemiology of HTLV-1 and associated diseases. In: Blattner WA, ed. Human retrovirology: HTLV. New York: Raven Press, 1990; 251–265.

16. Cruickshank JK, Richardson J, Newell A, et al. HTLV-1 and tropical spastic paraparesis in Caribbean migrants in Britain: Clinical and familial studies. In: Blattner WA, ed. Human Retrovirology: HTLV. New York: Raven Press, 1990; 221–223.

17. Kaplan JE, Litchfield B, Rouault C, et al. HTLV-1 associated myelopathy associated with blood transfusion in the United States: Epidemiological and molecular evidence linking donor and recipient. Neurology 1991; 41:192–197.

18. Nomoto M, Utatsu Y, Soejima Y, Osame M. Neopterin in cerebrospinal fluid: A useful marker for diagnosis of HTLV-1 associated myelopathy/tropical spastic paraparesis. Neurology 1991; 41:457–202.

19. Berger JR, Raffanti S, Svenningsson A, et al. The role of HTLV in HIV-1 neurologic disease. Neurology 1991; 41:197–202.

20. Osame M, Igata A, Matsumota M, et al. HTLV-1 associated myelopathy (HAM) revisited. In: Roman C, Vernant JC, Osame M, eds. HTLV-1 and the Nervous System. New York. Liss, 1989:213–223.

21. Petito CK, Navia BA, Cho ES, et al. Vacuolar myelopathy pathologically resembling subacute combined degeneration in patients with the acquired immunodeficiency syndrome. New Engl J Med 1985; 312:874–879.

22. Sharer LR, Kapila R. Neuropathologic observation in acquired immunodeficiency syndrome. Acta Neuropath (Berlin) 1985; 66:188–198.
23. McArthur JC. Neurologic manifestations of AIDS. Medicine 1987; 66:407–437.
24. Miller RG, Storey JR, Greco CM. Ganciclovir in the treatment of progressive AIDS-related polyradiculopathy. Neurology 1990; 40:569–574.
25. Wiley CA, van Patten PD, Carpenter PM, et al. Acute ascending necrotizing myelopathy caused by herpes simplex virus type 2. Neurology 1987; 37:1791.
26. Kemp H. Tuberculosis of the spine. Br J Hosp Med 1976; 15:39.
27. Gorse GJ, Pais MJ, Kusske JA, et al. Tuberculous spondylitis. Medicine 1983; 62:178–193.
28. Wadia NH, Dastur DK. Spinal leptomeningitides with radiculomyelopathy. Part 1. Clinical and radiological features. J Neurol Sci 1969; 8:239–260.
29. Dastur DK, Wadia NH. Spinal meningitides with radiculomyelopathy. Part 2. Pathology and pathogenesis. J Neurol Sci 1969; 8:261–297.
30. Tuli SM. Tuberculosis of the Skeletal System. New Delhi. Jaypee Brothers Medical Publishers (P) Ltd, 1991.
31. Peiris JB, Wickremasinghe HR, Chandrasekera MA. Tuberculous radiculopathy. Br Med J 1974; 4:107.
32. Kocen RS, Parsons M. Neurological complications of tuberculosis: Some unusual features. Q J Med 1970; 39:17–30.
33. Silverman JF, Larkin EW, Carney M, Weaver MD, Norris HT. Fine needle aspiration cytology of tuberculosis of the lumbar vertebrae (Pott's disease). Acta Cytol 1986; 30:538–542.
34. McNicol MW, Campbell IA, Jenkins PA. Clinical features and management of tuberculosis. In Brewis RAL, Corrin B, Geddes DM, and Gibson GL. Respiratory Medicine. 2d ed. London and Philadelphia: WB Saunders, 1995:822–823.
35. Stern BJ, Krumholz A, Johns C, et al. Sarcoidosis and its neurological manifestations. Arch Neurol 1985; 42:909–917.
36. Bogousslavsky J, Hungerbuhler JP, Regli F, et al. Subacute myelopathy as the presenting manifestation of sarcoidosis. Acta Neurochir 1982; 65:193–197.
37. Junger SS, Stern BJ, Levine SR, et al. Intramedullary spinal sarcoidosis: Clinical and magnetic resonance imaging characteristics. Neurology 1993; 43:333–337.
38. Martin CA, Murali R, Trasi SS. Spinal cord sarcoidosis. J Neurosurg 1984; 61:981–982.
39. Koffman O. The changing pattern of neurosyphilis. Can Med Assoc 1956; 74:807–812.
40. Adams RD, Merritt HH. Meningeal and vascular syphilis of the spinal cord. Medicine 1944; 23:181.
41. Steere AC. Lyme disease. New Engl J Med 1989; 321:586–596.
42. Kollowski HH, Schwendemann G, Schulz M, et al. Chronic Borrelia encephalomyeloradiculitis with severe mental disturbance: Immunosuppressive versus antibiotic therapy. J Neurol 1988; 235:140.
43. Dattwyler RJ, Halperin JJ, Volkman DJ, et al. Treatment of late Lyme borreliosis—Randomised comparison of ceftriaxone and penicillin. Lancet 1988; I:1191–1194.

44. De Silva HJ, Gamage R, Herath HKN, Karunanayake MGS, Peiris JB. The treat-
    ment of Guillain-Barre syndrome by modified plasma exchange—A cost effective
    method for developing countries. Postgrad Med J 1987; 63:1079–1081.
45. Peiris JB, Gunatilake SB, Ranasinghe PS, Thavakodirasah AS. Plasma infusion in
    childhood Guillain-Barré syndrome J Neurol Neurosurg Psychiatry 1991; 54:1120.
46. Queiroz L. de S, Nucci A, Facure NO, Facure JJ. Massive spinal cord necrosis in
    schistosomiasis. Arch Neurol 1979; 36:517.
47. Haribhai HC, Bhigjee AI, Bell PL A, et al. Spinal cord schistosomiasis—A clinical,
    laboratory and radiological study. Brain 1991; 2:709–726.

10

Guillain-Barré Syndrome and Postinfective Neuroradiculoneuropathies

John Winer

University Hospital Birmingham NHS Trust, Edgbaston, Birmingham, England

Disorders of the nerve roots are common in clinical practice and represent an important differential diagnosis of conditions in which the pathology is confined to the spinal cord, such as in poliomyelitis. In this chapter, I will discuss the inflammatory and immune-mediated disorders of roots and peripheral nerves. Our knowledge and classification of these disorders has improved greatly in recent years, although the pathogenesis remains incompletely understood. Guillain-Barré syndrome (GBS) remains the most frequent cause of acute neuromuscular paralysis in the developed world and is the most important condition within this group. Chronic inflammatory demyelinating polyneuropathy appears to be a closely related condition that differs most importantly in that it fails to follow a monophasic course. Other postinfective disorders included in the differential diagnosis of acute neuropathy include Lyme disease, Miller-Fisher syndrome, and the rare conditions of acute pandysautonomia and acute sensory neuronopathy.

I. GUILLAIN-BARRÉ SYNDROME

Guillain-Barré syndrome is now considered to be a clinical syndrome comprising a group of conditions with a similar clinical presentation but differing in their pathology and probably in their pathogenesis. These include acute demyelinating polyradiculoneuropathy (AIDP), acute motor axonal neuropathy (AMAN), and acute motor and sensory axonal neuropathy (AMSAN). The first, AIDP, is the most common and constitutes about 75% of cases of GBS. Acute motor axonal neuropathy is equivalent to chinese paralytic syndrome and differs from AIDP in that it is an entirely axonal process confined to motor nerves, whereas in AMSAN motor and sensory nerves appear damaged by a primarily axonal process.

A. History

In 1916, George Guillain, Jean Alexandre Barré, and Andre Strohl described two soldiers presenting to the sixth army neurological unit with a rapidly progressive paralyzing illness associated with sensory symptoms. They correctly deduced by careful measurements of tendon reflexes that the disorder affected the peripheral neuromuscular system. Both soldiers recovered quickly and completely. They published their findings (1), and the disorder subsequently became known as the Guillain-Barré syndrome (Strohl's omission from the eponymous name for the disorder is unfair and unexplained).

Guillain and Barré's account emphasized two important features of the disorder: the absence of tendon reflexes and the increase in cerebrospinal fluid (CSF) protein without pleocytosis. Since that time, diagnostic criteria have been developed to define the disease more carefully (Table 1). Progressive weakness in more than one limb, absent reflexes, and exclusion of other known causes of a neuropathy are required for diagnosis. Some authors would suggest that the neuropathy must not progress for more than 4 weeks to qualify as GBS (2). Variants of the syndrome in which purely sensory symptoms and signs are present are conventionally excluded. Many of these variants of the disorder may prove to share a similar etiology but were felt to be sufficiently different from the core syndrome to justify exclusion until a clear understanding of the pathogenesis of the syndrome was available. These variants can be labeled as postinfective neuroradiculopathies and include the Miller-Fisher syndrome (3) and the sensory neuronopathy syndrome (4). They will be discussed briefly later in this chapter. The incidence of GBS varies between 0.7 and 1.9 per 100,000 of the population (5,6). No reliable figures are available to estimate the prevalence of the disease. There is no clear seasonal variation, although there does seem to be a gradually increasing frequency in older patients (7). There may also be a minor peak in incidence in the second and third decades. Guillain-Barré syndrome has been reported from all regions of the world and among all races. It is slightly more common in men than women. Although Guillain and Barré's patients did not experience any recognized antecedent event, subsequent studies have confirmed the clinical impression that approxi-

Table 1 Diagnostic Criteria for Guillain-Barré Syndrome

Required	Supportive
Progressive weakness of at least two limbs due to neuropathy	Relatively symmetrical weakness
Arreflexia	Mild sensory signs
Progression less than 4 weeks	Cranial nerve involvement, especially facial nerve
Absence of other causes of neuropathy, e.g., porphyria, toxins, diphtheria	Absence of fever with neuropathic symptoms
CSF protein increased and cell count normal	Autonomic dysfunction
	Electrophysiological evidence of demyelination

Source: Adapted from Ref. 39.

mately 75% of cases of GBS are associated with an antecedent event of possible etiological importance in the 1 to 2 months prior to the onset of the neuropathy. In many cases the patients have experienced an upper respiratory tract infection or infection of the gastrointestinal tract with diarrhea and vomiting. In 1966 Leneman (8) reviewed the reported associations of GBS recorded in the literature and found some 1100 possible triggering events. It is difficult to know how many of these are coincidental and how many are definitely linked to the onset of neuropathy. There is good evidence, however, that swine flu vaccination can increase the incidence of GBS (9) and that rabies vaccination is probably associated with an increased incidence of the disease (10). The mechanism by which these two immunizations precipitate the disease is unknown.

Serological evidence of a precipitating infection is obtained in only about 25% of patients (11). Among these patients, the two most often identified organisms are *Campylobacter jejuni* and cytomegalovirus. The incidence of *Campylobacter* infection preceding GBS varies according to the method of detection and the country in the world in which the study is being performed. An average incidence of *C. jejuni* infection of about 15% is obtained from several studies. A further 10–15% of patients have serological evidence of recent cytomegalovirus infection (12). Good studies also incriminate mycoplasma and Epstein Barr virus as being organisms linked with the onset of GBS (12, 13). A number of well-documented cases of GBS have been triggered by HIV infection (14), but this association has not yet been confirmed by a controlled study. Several lines of evidence suggest that GBS takes 2–3 weeks to begin after the antecedent event responsible for its initiation. The risk of developing GBS after swine flu vaccination falls to a background level after about 6 weeks. There is no clear human leukocyte antigen (HLA) link with the disease, although patients who develop GBS after *Campylobacter infection* appear to have an excess of certain HLA types (15).

B. Clinical Features

The diagnosis of GBS is usually relatively straightforward in a patient with rapidly progressive weakness and absent reflexes. Sensory symptoms occur in approximately 50% of patients, whereas sensory signs on examination are much less frequent. Weakness that may be proximal or distal is characteristically severe in elbow extension and hip flexion. The cranial nerves are frequently involved, with facial weakness being the most common abnormality. Weakness of intercostal and diaphragmatic muscles leads to reduced vital capacity in most patients, although only about 25% of patients require assisted ventilation. Monitoring of vital capacity is essential in the progressive phase of the disease, and an increase in vital capacity is often the first objective measure of improvement. Abnormalities of eye movements are common, and there is a variant of GBS called the Miller-Fisher syndrome in which ophthalmoplegia, ataxia, and areflexia coexist.

Pain is a relatively frequent feature of the acute disease and usually occurs in the back or loin. Patients may also be severely frightened and anxious because of the severity of their weakness. It is not infrequent for patients with GBS to be labeled as hysterical because of the severe weakness and considerable anxiety they experience, as well as the absence of any sensory abnormality. Some patients do not lose all reflexes but have absent reflexes distally in the legs or arms. Patients seen very early in the course of the disease may simply have reduced reflexes that can easily be discounted. The differential diagnosis of patients presenting in this acute way includes botulism. This is a rare disease, but several patients included in trials of GBS have subsequently turned out to have botulism, and the diagnosis is difficult in a rapidly progressive neurological picture with cranial nerve involvement. Porphyria and poisoning with acute toxins can also cause diagnostic confusion. A toxin screen together with measurement of urinary and, if possible, fecal porphyrins can be helpful diagnostically. A CSF analysis typically shows a very high CSF protein, which may be of the order of several grams per liter. The CSF cell count is typically normal or only minimally raised, and a CSF cell count higher than 50 per mL should raise considerable diagnostic doubt. The CSF often contains oligoclonal bands. These, however are also usually present in serum suggesting peripheral synthesis of immunoglobulin as a consequence of immune stimulation. About one in 100 patients with GBS develop benign intracranial hypertension (BIH) with headaches, vomiting, and papilledema (Fig. 1) (16). This rare complication of the disease is thought to arise from cerebral edema rather than as a manifestation of the high CSF protein. There does not appear to be a good correlation between the rise in CSF protein and the incidence of BIH (17). In most patients symptoms begin in the legs, although occasionally, patients are encountered in whom the symptoms begin and are more severe in the upper limbs.

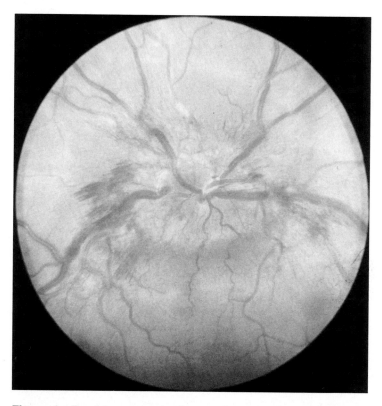

Figure 1 Fundal appearance in a patient with Guillain-Barré syndrome who developed headaches during the third week of his illness. The figure shows gross papilloedema, which gradually settled without treatment.

C. Investigation

Investigation of patients with GBS should include detailed nerve conduction and electromyographic studies. In the acute phase of the disease, abnormalities on standard nerve conduction studies may be minimal. It is frequently reported that nerve conduction studies can be entirely normal in GBS. In my experience this is rare and the normal values are usually encountered when electrophysiological studies are limited. In the acute demyelinating form of the syndrome, the most frequent abnormalities in the early stage of the disease are a reduced muscle action potential and some decrement between nerve stimulation distally and proximally (18). F-wave values are frequently prolonged (19) and distal motor latencies may be increased. As the disease progresses, there may be abnormalities in sensory amplitude and conduction velocity and after a few weeks, denervation is commonplace. Denervation is characteristically very severe in the acute axonal forms of the disease in which the pathology suggests primary axonal damage. Cases of acute motor axonal neuropathy of the Chinese paralytic type characteristically show only motor abnormalities. Lumbar puncture is desirable in the majority of patients with GBS: the typical features have been mentioned. The CSF protein may not rise within the first week of the disease and therefore it may be necessary to repeat CSF sampling at a later date if the diagnosis remains in doubt.

Measurements of urinary porphyrins together with lead concentrations are important in the distinction of other conditions in the differential diagnosis. It is conventional to look for other causes of neuropathy, and such tests should exclude a paraprotein and a vitamin B_{12} level. Serum electrolytes, liver function tests, and erythrocyte sedimentation rate may be abnormal. Inappropriate antidiuretic hormone (ADH) secretion has been described (20).

D. Pathology

Guillain-Barré syndrome is predominantly a demyelinating condition of the peripheral nerves. In recent years it has been recognized that neurophysiological tests and pathological examination can divide GBS into subtypes. Until recently, all cases of GBS were considered to show scattered areas of primary demyelination maximal in the nerve roots (21). This pathological picture, however, appears to be characteristic of the majority of, but not all cases of GBS. Such cases have been termed AIDP to emphasize the demyelinating pathology.

A small number of GBS patients reaching autopsy show an apparently primarily axonal picture, and this subtype of GBS is frequently associated with a much worse prognosis (22). Another small group of patients develop an acute motor neuronopathy in which sensory function is entirely spared. This disorder has been labeled the Chinese paralytic syndrome (23). The pathological findings in AIDP have been reported by several authors. Patchy areas of demyelination are seen throughout the peripheral nerves, but particularly in the nerve roots with evidence of a periventricular lymphocytic infiltrate. A variable amount of axonal damage is seen secondary to the demyelination. The earliest pathological change appears to be the lymphocytic infiltration (Fig. 2), although there has been some controversy surrounding the early pathological features of GBS. Many original studies were based on postmortem studies of nerves with considerable artifactual changes including vesicular dissolution. On electron microscopy, macrophages can be seen in close proximity to axons undergoing active demyelination. The concept of macrophage-mediated demyelination has arisen (24) and is assumed to be the primary pathological process underlying AIDP. Pathological studies have also confirmed that autonomic nerves are frequently involved in the disease.

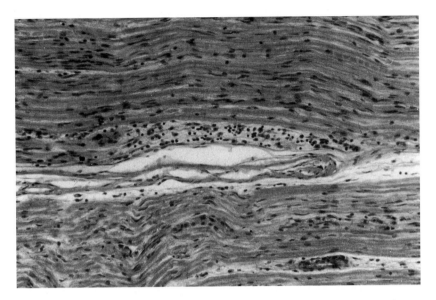

Figure 2   Longitudinal section of a motor nerve taken at post mortem in a patient who died from Guillain-Barré syndrome in the acute stage of the illness.

E. Etiology

The relationship of the disease to infection and the natural history of the disorder suggests that it might be an immune-mediated response to a preceding infection or immunological trigger. There is evidence that the immune system is disturbed in GBS and activated lymphocytes circulate in the peripheral blood (25). Oligoclonal bands are common, implying immune stimulation. Furthermore, plasma exchange appears to be effective in improving outcome (26), and this has been interpreted as suggesting that antibodies may have a role in causing the disease. A number of animal models exist for GBS, of which the most studied is experimental allergic neuritis (EAN). This is a peripheral neuropathy induced by injecting peripheral nerve myelin, together with Freunds' adjuvant into Lewis rats or other susceptible species. The disorder resembles GBS pathologically with macrophage-mediated demyelination. Experimental allergic neuritis can be induced with T cells that recognize the P2 protein of peripheral nerve. Anti-P2 antibodies may play a role in mediating disease, and damage to the blood-nerve barrier seems to be important (27). Both humoral and cellular immunity to other peripheral nerve proteins also appears to influence the degree of demyelination obtained in EAN.

There have been extensive studies of antibody and cellular responses to peripheral nerve constituents in the human disease. Unfortunately such studies have been largely negative. The only reliably identified antibody in patients with GBS appears to be antibodies against peripheral nerve gangliosides (28). This does to some extent correlate with *Campylobacter* serology, suggesting that *Campylobacter* infection may somehow precipitate an antiganglioside response. Whether this antiganglioside response is a primary or secondary phenomenon has been the subject of much debate. It is possible that GBS is a heterogeneous condition and that within the syndrome are a number of disorders with different etiological mechanisms. One unifying hypothesis suggests that infection with either a viral or bacterial organism leads to an immune response directed against antigenic determinants on the infecting organism that cross react with similar host antigens. Thus, both cellular and humoral immunity might be generated against host peripheral myelin leading to a rapid demyelinating illness. T-cell control of this response is then regained and the disorder gradually recovers. In a small proportion of patients with the appropriate genetic background, this process may continue and lead to a chronic demyelinating disorder. The exact nature of the cross reacting epitopes remains to be elucidated. This may involve gangliosides (29) in the case of *Campylobacter,* but this is far from certain. The extent of demyelination or axonal damage may in part be determined by the nature of the antigen inducing the autoimmune response.

F. Management and Treatment

Management of GBS can be divided into supportive medical care and active treatment designed to alter the course of the disorder.

Supportive medical care was the only management option available until a decade ago and was responsible for the considerable improvement in the natural history of the disease in the early part of this century. The advent of assisted ventilation, together with appropriate intensive care management of infections and complications, is largely responsible for this improvement. In the acute progressive phase of the disease, it is important to continue monitoring vital capacity in order to institute assisted ventilation at the appropriate moment. It is generally considered that a vital capacity at or approaching 1 L is an indication for instituting assisted ventilation. Clearly, the degree of change in the vital capacity is more important than the absolute value. Patients with GBS frequently do not show typical signs of dyspnea and so many develop respiratory arrest without warning. It is far better to institute elective ventilation than to try intubating the patient at the time of a respiratory arrest. Although peak flows and blood gases are frequently performed in these patients, the most important parameter is the amount of gas that is transferred into and out the lungs; therefore, the vital capacity is the most appropriate measurement. Blood gases may remain entirely normal until respiratory arrest occurs.

Patients with severe tetraplegia may develop profound autonomic disturbance. Electrocardiographic (ECG) changes resembling an infarct are well described and the most life-threatening disorder is a sudden brady-arrhythmia. Sudden disturbances of cardiac rate may be induced by maneuvers that increase vagal tone such as sucking out the trachea. It is my practice to electively pace patients who show significant brady arrhythmias. Patients should be followed up with continuous ECG monitoring so that serious cardiac rhythm disturbances can be identified. Such autonomic disturbances probably arise from demyelinating lesions within autonomic nerves.

If ventilation becomes necessary, then strict attention should be given to chest physiotherapy to reduce chest infections. The incidence of such infections can also be improved by the use of end expiratory pressure ventilation. Frequent turning and passive physiotherapy are important to prevent contractures from occurring. In the later stages of the disease, more active physiotherapy, together with intensive rehabilitation, is essential. Careful positioning of patients in the intensive care unit is important to prevent deformities of posture that make subsequent rehabilitation difficult.

Patients with GBS frequently develop venous thromboembolism and it is conventional to use subcutaneous heparin in an effort to prevent venous thrombosis and pulmonary emboli. Patients who require anticoagulation for a long period may be more conveniently managed with warfarin. Longer acting heparin is also desirable to reduce the number of injections required per day. The prognosis of patients with GBS is difficult to predict, but patients who require ventilation usually do so for a long period. It is, therefore, desirable to instigate tracheostomy fairly early on in the course of the illness to prevent vocal cord damage from prolonged intubation.

Treatments designed to alter the course of the disease have been tried with GBS for many years. Initial enthusiasm for the use of oral steroids was subdued by the publication of a small control trial in the late 1970s suggesting that they were not effective (30). A recent trial using intravenous methylprednisolone has confirmed this impression (31). Plasma exchange, however, has been shown to be beneficial in three large control trials (26,32,33). Two other smaller control trials have also shown a trend toward improvement with plasma exchange (34,35). It is conventional to perform five or six exchanges and to exchange approximately 50 mL. The nature of the replacement fluid does not seem to be important, nor does it seem to matter whether continuous or intermittent plasma exchange is carried out. Plasma exchange is most beneficial within the first 2 weeks of the illness and seems to be less effective after that. Plasma exchange is not without complication and morbidity. There may be problems with venous access and the complication of pneumothorax associated with inserting a central venous line. In addition, the rapid change in circulating fluid volume may exacerbate any autonomic disturbance or precipitate heart failure. Bleeding complications and infections at the site of venesection can occur rarely. Controlled trials have shown that the time taken to improve one grade on a six-step functional scale is reduced by half in treated patients (26). Patients with the most severe disease requiring ventilation seem to benefit the most. There seems relatively little indication for plasma exchange in patients who stabilize and still retain the ability to walk.

Although plasma exchange is effective in GBS, there is still a proportion of patients that do not respond to plasma exchange. Other more effective treatments are clearly needed and a Dutch controlled trial has suggested that intravenous gammaglobulin (IVIg) infusions may be at least as effective and possibly better (36). This treatment consists of giving infusions of intravenous gammaglobulin, which was used originally in the treatment of idiopathic thrombocytic purpura. This disorder has many similarities with GBS and is frequently triggered by antecedent infection. Intravenous gammaglobulin is effective in improving thrombocytopenia in this condition and is thought to be effective by virtue of anti-idiotypic antibodies. As a result, intravenous gammaglobulin was tried in GBS and found anecdotally to be beneficial. A multicenter trial comparing IVIg with plasma exchange (37) has recently confirmed the Dutch experience and will almost certainly be influential in changing opinion into using IVIg as the preferred first line treatment for GBS rather than plasma exchange. The dose of gammaglobulin is 0.4 g/kg/day and it is usually given over a period of 5 consecutive days. It is possible that its mode of action could include blockage of macrophage receptors or even reduction in circulating tumor necrosis factor levels. Occasionally, patients develop allergic responses to gammaglobulin. Gammaglobulin has the advantage in that it is available in many smaller hospitals and does not require transfer of the patients to specialized units that can perform plasma exchange.

G. Prognosis of GBS

Approximately 3–5% of patients with the acute disease will develop a chronic demyelinating disorder. Of the remainder patients, approximately 5–10% of patients will die in the acute stage of the disease. Death usually arises as a result of cardiac rhythm disturbances, but also may occur from pulmonary emboli and infection. Guillain-Barré Syndrome is a very severe, life-threatening disease, and one that frequently produces psychiatric disturbance. In most studies of GBS, one or two patients per hundred have committed suicide. Data from the preplasma exchange era suggest that approximately 15% of patients who survive the acute stage of the disease will remain quite severely disabled and be unable to return to normal activity, even after several years. Little long-term follow-up data from patients treated with plasma exchange are available to determine whether persistent deficit from GBS has been reduced. A major cause of disability is wasting and weakness in the legs, together with foot deformity and contracture. Some patients with severe GBS remain tetraplegic and require long-term ventilation. Minor symptoms of sensory disturbance are not uncommon in patients that have recovered from GBS.

II. CHRONIC INFLAMMATORY DEMYELINATING POLYNEUROPATHY

Patients pursuing a chronic course with progression of motor deficit for longer than 8 weeks are considered separately from acute GBS and given the diagnostic label of chronic inflammatory demyelinating polyneuropathy (CIDP). Included within this diagnostic label are the small number of GBS patients identified at an early stage who continue to progress, and those patients with a relapsing demyelinating polyneuropathy. The distinction of this group of patients seems justified in view of their clear response to steroid therapy, which is ineffective in GBS (37). The name is a misnomer, because a very small number of patients have a significant inflammatory infiltrate on nerve biopsy.

A. Clinical Features

Like GBS, CIDP is more common in men than women and there is evidence of an HLA association with DR3 and B8 (38). The disease usually presents with both weakness and sensory symptoms, aching pain in the muscles, and tendon areflexia. Cranial nerve involvement is less frequent than in GBS, with facial weakness occurring in about 15% and bulbar symptoms in only 6% of patients. Tremor occurs in some patients and about 11% exhibit thickening of the peripheral nerves. A small number of patients have some associated upper motor neurone signs and magnetic resonance imaging (MRI) scans have shown abnormalities in rare patients that appear to have both central and peripheral nerve demyelination (39).

Electrophysiology shows evidence of conduction block or severly slowed velocities. Electrophysiological criteria for demyelination have been defined (40). Nerve biopsy reveals demyelination with typically little, if any, inflammatory infiltrate; onion bulb formation from chronic demyelination and remyelination is not infrequently found.

B. Treatment

Controlled trials have demonstrated the efficacy of steroids (41), plasma exchange (42,43), and IVIg (44) in improving muscle strength in CIDP. Steroids at a dose of about 60 mg of prednisolone daily have been the mainstay of treatment, and some authors advocate a gradual increase in dose to prevent occasional worsening of the weakness with start of therapy. Intravenous gammaglobulin represents an alternative initial treatment that has fewer side effects but is both more difficult to deliver and more expensive. Maintenance of therapy is usually accomplished by the use of azathioprine, but other immunosupressants such as cyclosporin and cyclophosphamide have been used succesfully.

The prognosis with treatment is good, with an average 80% response to treatment and only a small percentage of patients severely disabled at 10 years (45).

C. Etiology

Some patients with CIDP have antibodies against gangliosides, but the possible relevance of these to the demyelination is unknown. The efficacy of plasma exchange in the treatment of CIDP argues for a role for circulating factors in the etiology of the disease, but studies so far have been confusing and the relative role of cell-mediated and humoral immunity remains to be determined.

III.   MILLER FISHER SYNDROME

In 1956, Miller Fisher described three patients with ophthalmoplegia, ataxia, areflexia, and sluggish pupillary reflexes (3). In view of the similarity of this condition to GBS, Miller Fisher proposed that this condition was similar in etiology. A similar clinical presentation may be seen in cases of brainstem encephalitis, but such patients almost invariably have associated drowsiness and CSF pleocytosis. Cases of pure Miller Fisher syndrome are relatively rare and many patients with ophthalmoplegia appear to have GBS with only mild limb weakness.

Antibodies to the ganglioside GQ1b are associated with more than 90% of cases of Miller Fisher syndrome, whereas such antibodies are much less frequent in GBS as a whole (46,47). A recent report has suggested that serum from patients with Miller Fisher syndrome produces neuromuscular block in experimental preparations, providing a possible mechanism for the neurological syndrome (48). Electrophysiological studies of patients with Miller Fisher syndrome are relatively few but these suggest a sensory axonal neuronopathy is the basis for the initial symptoms (49).

IV.   LYME DISEASE

Descriptions of neurological disease as a result of tick bites were described in Europe in the first half of the twentieth century(50), but convincing epidemiological studies were not available until the late 1970s after observations in the region of Old Lyme, Connecticut (51). Diagnostic criteria have recently been agreed upon by the American Academy of Neurology (52). Diagnosis requires:

1. Possible exposure to the tick vector
2. One of the following:
   a. Erythema migrans
   b. Immunological evidence of exposure [Western blot or enzyme-linked immunosorbent assay (ELISA)]
   c. Demonstration of spirochete [polymerase chain reaction (PRC) or culture/histology]
3. One or more of the following:
   a. Lymphocytic meningitis, cranial neuritis, radiculoneuritis
   b. Encephalomyelitis
   c. Peripheral neuropathy
   d. Encephalopathy

Only about three-quarters of patients have the classical erythema migrans rash, which consists of a red macule or papule that extends to form a red ring with central clearing. The rash usually resolves even without treatment in a few weeks. During the second phase of the illness, the spirochete spreads through the blood stream and patients may show secondary skin rashes and develop migratory joint pain. Neurological symptoms begin after several weeks and consist of a radiculoneuritis or an encephalitis. Six months after onset of the disease, some patients develop an asymmetrical arthritis.

A. Treatment

Oral antibiotics are recommended for localized disease; for example, 3 weeks of doxycycline, 100 mg twice a day or amoxicillin, 500 mg four times a day (53).

In patients with central nervous system (CNS) disease, intravenous antibiotics are usually suggested, such as ceftriaxone 2 g/per day or ceftriaxone 6 g/per day.

V. ACUTE SENSORY NEURONOPATHY

This syndrome was described in 1986 in three adults who developed an acute sensory syndrome of numbness ataxia and painful paraesthesiae after an infection treated with antibiotics (54). Sensory action potentials were absent and Sterman et al. suggested an acute problem in the cell bodies of the dorsal root ganglia affecting large myelinated sensory afferents. In these patients, motor nerve function was normal as was small myelinated and unmyelinated sensory nerves. Subsequent to this description, several similar cases have been described (55–57). The syndrome has also been described associated with carcinoma and in patients with ovarian carcinoma who have been given *Cis*-platinum in high doses.

Although extraordinarily rare, such patients have enabled considerable research on their residual motor functions without touch or movement and positional feedback (without visual control (58). Their prognosis is variable: most of these patients have remained wheelchair bound, living full and active lives, although one has successfully learned to walk again and live independently. A similar clinical presentation occurs in association with the sicca syndrome (59).

VI. ACUTE PANDYSAUTONOMIA

Guillain-Barré syndrome is frequently accompanied by an autonomic neuropathy. However, autonomic disturbance in the absence of weakness is exceptionally rare but has been described as presumed postinfectious phenomena. This syndrome is known as acute pandysautonomia (60,61). In one well-documented example, postural hypotension, blurred vision, dry eyes, and sphincter disturbance evolved over a few weeks. The pathology of this rare syndrome is unknown. In one case, there was evidence of improvement with gammaglobulin treatment.

REFERENCES

1. Guillain G, Barré JA, Strohl A. Sur un syndrome deradiculo-nevrite avec hyperalbuminose du liquide cephalorachidien sans reaction cellulaire. Remarques surles caracteres cliniques et graphiques des reflexes tendineux. Bull Soc Med Hop Paris 1916; 40:1462–1470.
2. Hughes RAC, Winer JB. Guillain-Barre syndrome. In: Mathews WB, Glazer GH, eds. Recent Advances in Clinical Neurology 4. Churchill Livingstone, 1984; 19–50.
3. Fisher CM. An unusual variant of acute idiopathic polyneuritis (syndrome of ophthalmoplegia, ataxia and areflexia). New Engl J Med 1956; 273:57–65.
4. Sterman AB, Schaumberg HH, Asbury AK. The acute sensory neurononopathy syndrome: A distinct clinical entity. Ann Neurol 1986; 7:354–358.
5. Gudmundson KR. Prevalence and occurrence of some rare neurological diseases in Iceland. Acta Neurol Scand 1969; 45:114–118.
6. Bremen SG, Hayner NS. Guillain-Barré syndrome and its relationship to swine influenza vaccination in Michigan. Am J Epidemiol 1984; 119:880–889.

7. Kaplan JE, Katona P, Hurvitz ES, Schonberg LB. Guillain-Barré syndrome in the United States 1979–1980 and 1980–1981. Lack of an association with influenza vaccination. JAMA 1982; 248:698–700.

8. Leneman F. The Guillain-Barré syndrome. Definition etiology and review of 1000 cases. Arch Intern Med

9. Langmuir AD, Bregman DJ, Kurland LT, Nathanson N, Victor M. An epidemiological and clinical evaluation of GBS reported in association with administration of swine influenza vaccines. Am J Epidemiol 1984; 119:841–879.

10. Hemachadha T, Phanauphak P, Johnson RT, Gritten DE, Ratanvongsiri J, Siripramsomsap W. Neurologic complications of Semple-type rabies vaccine: Clinical and immunologic studies. Neurology 1987; 37:550–556.

11. Winer JB, Hughes RAC, Anderson MJ, Jones DM, Kangro H, Watkins RPF. A prospective study of acute idiopathic neuropathy. II. Antecedent events. J Neurol Neurosurg Psychiatry 1988; 51:613–618.

12. Dowling PC, Cook SD. Role of infection in Guillain Barré syndrome: Laboratory confirmation of Herpes viruses in 41 cases. Ann Neurol 1981; Suppl 9:44–45.

13. Goldschmidt B, Menonna J, Fortunato J, Dowling P, Cook S. Mycoplasma antibody in Guillain-Barré syndrome and other neurological disorders. Ann Neurol 1980; 7:108–112.

14. Cornblath DR, Griffin DE, Chipp M, Griffen JW, McArthur JC. Mononuclear cell typing in inflammatory demyelinating polyneuropathy nerve biopsies. Neurology 1987; 37:253–254.

15. Yuki N, Satos Hoh T, Migatake T. HLA B35 and acute axonal polyneuropathy following *Campylobacter* infection. Neurology 1991; 41:1561–1563.

16. Winer JB, Hughes RAC, Osmond CA. A prospective study of acute idiopathic neuropathy. Clinical features and their prognostic value. J Neurol Neurosurg Psychiatry 1988; 51:613–618.

17. Morley JB, Reynolds EH. Papilloedema and the Guillain Barré syndrome. Brain 1966; 89:205–222.

18. Feasby TE, Brown WF, Gilbert JJ, Hahn AF. The pathological basis of conduction block in human neuropathies. J Neurol Neurosurg Psychiatry 1985; 48:239–244.

19. Kimura J, Butzer JF. F wave conduction velocity in Guillain-Barré syndrome. Arch Neurol 1975; 32:524–529.

20. Posner JB, Ertel NH, Kossman RJ, Scheinberg LC. Hyponatraemia in acute polyneuropathy. Arch Neurol 1967; 17:530–541.

21. Asbury AK, Arnason BG, Adams RD. The inflammatory lesion in idiopathic polyneuritis. Its role in pathogenesis. Medicine 1969; 48:173–215.

22. Feasby TE, Gilbert JJ, Brown WF, et al. An acute axonal form of Guillain Barre polyneuropathy. Brain 1986; 109:1115–1126.

23. McKhann GM, Cornblath DR, Griffin JW, et al. Acute motor axonal neuropathy: a frequent cause of acute flaccid paralysis in China. Ann Neurol 1993; 33:333–342.

24. Prineas JW. Acute idiopathic polyneuritis. An electron microscope study. Lab Invest 1972; 26:133–147.

25. Taylor WA, Hughes RAC. T lymphocyte activation antigens in Guillain Barre syndrome and chronic demyelinating polyradiculoneuropathy. J Neuroimmunol 1989; 24:33–39.

26. Guillain-Barré Syndrome Study Group. Plasmapheresis for acute Guillain-Barré syndrome. Neurology 1985; 35:1096–1104.
27. Spies JM, Westland KW, Bonner JG, Pollard JD. Cytokines of activated T cells open the blood nerve barrier. 1993 11th Biennial Peripheral Nerve Study Group, Boppard Germany.
28. Kuroki S, Saida T, Nukima M, Haruta T, Yoshika M, Kobsayashi Y, Nakanishi H. Campylobacter jejuni strains from patients with Guillain-Barré syndrome belong mostly to Penner serogroup 19 and contain Beta-N-acetylglucosamine residues. Ann Neurol 1993; 33:243–247.
29. Yuki N, Taki T, Ihagaki F, Kasama T, Takahashi M, Saito K, Handa S, Miyatake T. A bacterium lipopolysaccharide that elicits Guillain Barre syndrome has a GM1 ganglioside structure. J Exp Med 1993; 178:1771–1775.
30. Hughes RAC, Newsom Davis JM, Perkin GD, Pierce JM. Controlled trial of prednisolone in acute polyneuropathy. Lancet 1978; ii:750–753.
31. Guillain-Barré Syndrome Steroid Trial Group. Double-blind trial of intravenous methylprednisolone in Guillain-Barré syndrome Lancet 1993; 341:586–590.
32. French Cooperative group in plasma exchange in Guillain-Barre syndrome. Efficiency of plasma exchange in Guillain-Barré syndrome: role of replacement fluids. Ann Neurol 1987; 22:753–761.
33. Osterman PO, Lundemo G, Pirskanen R, et al. Beneficial eff,ects of plasma exchange in acute inflammatory polyradiculoneuropathy. Lancet 1984; ii:1296–1299.
34. Greenwood RJ, Hughes RAC, et al. Controlled trial of plasma exchange in acute inflammatory polyradiculoneuropathy. Lancet 1984; i:877–879.
35. Mendell JR, Kissel JT, Kennedy MS, et al. Plasma exchange and prednisone in Guillain-Barré syndrome. A controlled randomised trial. Neurology 1985; 35:1551–1555.
36. Van der Meche FGA, Schnitz PIM, and the Dutch Guillain-Barré Study Group. A randomized trial comparing intravenous immunoglobulin and plasma exchange in Guillain-Barré syndrome. N Engl J Med 1992; 326:1123–1129.
37. The Plasma Exchange/Sandoglobulin Guillain-Barré Syndrome Trial Group. Ann Neurol 1996; 40(3):551.
38. Feeney DJ, Pollard JD, Mcleod JG, Stewart GJ, Doran TJ. HLA antigens in chronic inflammatory demyelinating polyneuropathy. J Neurol Neurosurg Psychiatry 1990; 53:170–172.
39. Thomas PK, Walker RWH, Rudge P, et al. Chronic demyelinating peripheral neuropathy associated with multifocal CNS demyelination. Brain 1987; 110:53–76.
40. American Academy of Neurology AIDS Task Force. Research criteria for diagnosis of chronic inflammatory demyelinating polyneuropathy (CIDP). Neurology 1991; 41:617–618.
41. Dyck PJ, O'Brien PC, Oviatt KF, et al. Prednisone improves chronic inflammatory demyelinating polyradiculoneuropathy more than no treatment. Ann Neurol 1982; 11:136–141.
42. Dyck PJ, Daube J, O'Brien P, Pineda A, Low PA, Windebank AJ, Swanson C. Plasma exchange in chronic inflammatory demyelinating polyneuropathy. New Engl J Med 1986; 314:461–465.
43. Hahn AF, Bolton CF, Pillay N, Chalk C, Benstead T, Bril V, Shumak K, Vander-

voort MK, Feasby TE. Plasma exchange in chronic inflammatory demyelinating polyneuropathy (CIDP). A double blind sham-controlled, cross over study. Brain 1996; 119:1055–1066.

44. Hahn AF, Bolton CF, Zochodne D, Feasby TE. Intravenous immunoglobulin treatment in chronic inflammatory demyelinating polyneuropathy. A double-blind placebo controlled cross over study. Brain 1996; 119:1067–1077.

45. McCombe PA, Pollar JD, Mcleod JG. Chronic inflammatory demyelinating polyneuropathy. Brain 1987; 110:1617–1630.

46. Chiba A, Kusonoki S, Shimizu T, Kanazawa I. Serum IgG antibody to ganglioside GQ1b: A possible marker for Miller Fisher syndrome. Ann Neurol 1992; 31:677–679.

47. Willison HJ, Veitch J, Paterson G, Kennedy PGE. Miller-Fisher syndrome is associated with serum antibodies to GQ1b ganglioside. J Neurol Neurosurg Psychiatry 1993; 56:204–206.

48. Roberts M, Willison H, Vincent A, Newsome-Davis J. Serum factor in Miller Fisher variant of Guillain-Barré syndrome and neurotransmitter release. Lancet 1994; 343:454–455.

49. Guillof RJ. Peripheral nerve conduction in Miller Fisher syndrome. J Neurol Neurosurg Psychiatry 1977; 40:801–807.

50. Bannwarth A. Zur Klinic und Pathogenese der "chronischen lymphocytaren meningitis." Arch Psychiatr Nervenkr 1944; 117:161–185.

51. Steere AC, Malawista SE, Snydman DR, et al. Lyme arthritis: An epidemic of oligoarticular arthritis in children and adults in three Connecticut communities. Arthritis Rheum 1977; 20:7–17.

52. Halperin JJ, Logigian EC, Finkel MF, Pearl RA. Practice parameters for the diagnosis of patients with nervous system Lyme borreliosis (Lymes disease). Neurology 1996; 46:619–627.

53. Steere AC. Lyme disease. N Engl J Med 1989; 321:586–596.

54. Sterman AB, Schaumberg HH, Asbury AK. The acute sensory neuropathy syndrome: A distinct clinical entity. Ann Neurol 1980; 7:354–358.

55. Cole JD, Sedgwick EM. The perceptions of force and of movement in a man without large myelinated sensory afferents below the neck. J Physiol 1992; 449:503–515.

56. Forget R, Lamarre Y. Rapid elbow flexion in the absence of proprioceptive and cutanoeous feedback. Human Neurobiol 1987; 6:27–37.

57. Sanes JN, Mauritz KH, Dalaka MC, Evarts EV. Motor control in humans with a large-fibre peripheral neuropathy. Human Neurobiol 1985; 4:101–114.

58. Cole J. Pride and a Daily Marathon. Boston and London: MIT Press, 1995.

59. Kennett RP, Harding AE. Peripheral neuropathy associated with the sicca syndrome. J Neurol Neurosurg Psychiatry 1986; 49:90–93.

60. Young RR, Asbury AK, Corbett JL, Adams RD. Pure pandysautonomia with recovery—Description and discussion of diagnostic criteria. Brain 1975; 98:613–636.

61. Heafield MTE, Gammage MD, Nightingale S, Williams AC. Idiopathic dysautonomia treated with intravenous gammaglobulin. Lancet 1996; 347:28–29.

11

HIV Disease of the Spinal Cord and Nerve Roots

Hadi Manji
*National Hospital for Neurology and Neurosurgery, London,
and Ipswich Hospital, Suffolk, England*

I. INTRODUCTION

After the first cases of the acquired immunodeficiency syndrome (AIDS) were reported in 1981, it was soon apparent that the nervous system was frequently involved. Initially, most of these neurological complications were considered a consequence of the immunosuppressive effects of the human immunodeficiency virus (HIV), resulting in opportunistic infections such as toxoplasmosis, cryptococcal meningitis, and progressive multifocal leukoencephalopathy (PML) or to tumors including primary central nervous system lymphoma (PCNSL). However, as the epidemic unfolded, it became obvious that these presentations, at best, accounted for up to 60% of the neurological problems encountered (1). In particular a progressive decline in cognitive function and motor deficits, which in some cases were associated with a myelopathy, were observed, especially in the later stages of the disease.

There is now a substantive body of evidence to suggest that HIV itself, by direct or indirect mechanisms, results in damage that may affect all areas of the neuraxis including the spinal cord and nerve roots.

In some patients, HIV seems to enter the nervous system early in the course of the disease. The evidence for this lies in the primary HIV seroconversion illnesses such as encephalitis (2); cerebrospinal fluid (CSF) studies performed on asymptomatic individuals in the Centre for Disease Classification

(CDC) II and III reveal abnormalities of white cell count, protein levels, and the presence of oligoclonal bands. The human immuno-deficiency virus may be cultured from the CSF in one-third of such patients. These features need to be taken into consideration when interpreting the results of diagnostic CSF examinations (3).

This review will discuss the various spinal cord and nerve root complications encountered during the primary seroconversion phase (CDC I), the asymptomatic phase (CDC II/III), and the symptomatic phase (CDC IV) (Table 1).

II. THE SEROCONVERSION PHASE

Involvement of the spinal cord and nerve roots occurs rarely, with occasional case reports in the literature. It is however, important to consider HIV disease in the differential diagnosis as a cause of a number of relatively common neurological syndromes.

Anecdotal case reports have described a transverse myelitis as a manifestation of an HIV seroconversion illness (4). During this period, serum HIV antibody tests may be negative and therefore, in cases in which the history suggests that an individual may be at high risk of HIV infection, it may be necessary to perform HIV antibody tests on the CSF. Furthermore, measurement of the viral p24 antigen can also be undertaken in both the blood and the CSF (5). Sero-

COMPLICATION	SERO CONVERSION	ASYMPTOMATIC	AIDS RELATED COMPLEX	AIDS
MENINGITIS	ACUTE	CHRONIC		
DEMYELINATING NEUROPATHY				■ ■ ■ ■ ■
DISTAL SYMMETRICAL PERIPHERAL NEUROPATHY		? ■ ■ ■		
VACUOLAR MYELOPATHY			■ ■ ■	
MYOPATHY	POLYMYOSITIS			? ZIDOVUDINE RELATED
ENCEPHALOPATHY	SEROCONVERSION ENCEPHALITIS	? ■ ■ ■ ■		

Table 1   HIV complications according to the stage of infection.

logic studies may need to be repeated in the convalescence phase about 12 weeks later.

Nerve roots may also be involved at the time of seroconversion. Zeman and Donaghy reported a patient who presented with urinary retention and altered perineal sensation but with normal lower limbs. In the initial serum sample, p24 antigen, but not HIV antibody, was detected (6).

An acute inflammatory demyelinating polyradiculopathy may also be the manifestation of seroconversion in some individuals (7) but more commonly occurs during the asymptomatic phases of the HIV disease spectrum. The clinical presentation and management are discussed below.

III. THE ASYMPTOMATIC PHASE

During this phase, the length of which may vary, sometimes lasting years, patients remain physically well, often with no inkling of their HIV infection. There are no documented cases of spinal cord disease during this period, in particular the vacuolar myelopathy that occurs in a significant proportion of patients with stage CDC IV disease. For instance, serial clinical studies in cohorts of CDC II and III homosexual or bisexual men have found no evidence of the development of a myelopathy.

Some workers have, however, found neurophysiological abnormalities in this group: Smith et al. (8) found an increased latency from the gluteal crease to T12 in response to tibial nerve stimulation when compared to age-, height-, and sex-matched controls in a study of 12 neurologically normal HIV infected individuals from CDC groups II and III. Because the mean conduction from T12 to cortex was not significantly different from that in the control group, and peripheral nerve conduction was normal, it was concluded that the site of pathology lay either within the dorsal root ganglia or the lumbar spinal cord. With the development of AIDS, the latency from T12 to the cortical foot area also increased significantly. As the latency from C7 to the contralateral hand area remained stable, the thoracic cord was implicated as the site of pathology. More recent and larger studies have, however, failed to confirm these findings (9).

Acute inflammatory polyradiculoneuropathies, similar to the Guillain-Barré syndrome and chronic inflammatory demyelinating polyradiculoneuropathy (CIDP), although well documented in the literature, occur rarely and usually in the asymptomatic phases. Distal muscle weakness that progresses proximally is associated with progressive areflexia. Sensory signs and symptoms are variable in severity.

Examination of the CSF may reveal an elevated protein level and, in contrast to the demyelinating neuropathies in non-HIV patients, the cell count may be elevated. In the largest published series, Cornblath found a mean cell count of 23 cells/mm^3 (range, 1–43) in contrast to a mean of 1.8 cells/mm^3 (range, 0–6) in non-HIV patients with a similar presentation (10). This raised cell count may be an additive effect of the changes found in the CSF of asymptomatic HIV infected individuals, together with the changes that may be found due to the inflammatory radiculoneuropathy per se.

Nerve conduction tests show a demyelinating pattern of changes with slowing of motor and sensory conduction velocities, evidence of conduction block, and prolonged distal motor latencies. Sural nerve biopsies reveal axonal loss, areas of demyelination, and an infiltrate of mononuclear cells (10).

A number of factors suggest that these demyelinating neuropathies have an underlying autoimmune mechanism. Most reported cases have occurred early in the course of HIV disease when a hypergammaglobulinemia due to polyclonal B-cell stimulation has been identified. Associated autoimmune phenomena also described at this stage include a thrombocytopenia and polymyositis. Anecdotal reports of treatment with plasmapheresis and corticosteroids have been shown to be successful (10).

The clinical course is variable—in some cases there is a slow progression and in others spontaneous improvement can occur, making it difficult to assess treatment protocols without a prospective randomized study. The therapeutic options lie between plasmapheresis and corticosteroids (10). Each form has its own advantages and disadvantages, although practically, there may be difficulties in obtaining the use of HIV-dedicated plasmapheresis equipment. The procedure has its own complications, with the necessity of central lines and the risk of infection. High-dose corticosteroid therapy may, theoretically, result in further immunosuppression. Recent evidence in non-HIV cases of Guillain-Barré syndrome and CIDP suggests that intravenous immunoglobulin is effective treatment (11, 12). It is unclear whether this data can be extrapolated to patients with HIV, but it is clearly another option to be considered.

IV. THE SYMPTOMATIC PHASE

A. Opportunistic Infections

1. Toxoplasmosis

Toxoplasma gondii is an obligate intracellular parasite that is ubiquitous in the human population. The cat is the definitive host. Transmission is mainly by the fecal-oral route, by eating under cooked meat infected with the cysts. After the primary infection, which is usually asymptomatic, the organism encysts in all tissues including the brain and spinal cord. Immunosuppression, as found in HIV disease, results in reactivation of the cysts. Toxoplasmosis is the most common cause of focal cerebral deficits in patients infected with HIV. The incidence of toxoplasmosis varies between 5% and 30%, reflecting the background seroprevalence: 20% of British adults and 90% of French adults have antibodies to *T. gondii*. This large variation may be attributed to dietary differences.

Clinically, the features of toxoplasmosis result from multifocal brain abscesses with or without a diffuse meningoencephalitis. On rare occasions, patients present with a meningoencephalitis without focal symptoms or signs. The diagnosis is usually made from the typical radiological findings on cranial tomography (CT) of multiple contrast enhancing lesions that have a predilection for the basal ganglia or for straddling the corticomedullary junction in the frontoparietal and occipital lobes. Magnetic resonance imaging (MRI), being more sensitive, may demonstrate multiple lesions after only a single lesion had been visualized on CT. This may influence management because the finding of multiple lesions makes toxoplasmosis more likely, whereas a single lesion on MRI is most probably lymphoma (13).

Toxoplasmosis of the spinal cord, although reported in neonates with congenital toxoplasmosis, is distinctly rare in HIV neurological practice. Case reports in the literature have described toxoplasma myelitis, diagnosed postmortem, mimicking an intramedullary spinal cord tumor. Empirical treatment with radiotherapy resulted in a rapid deterioration (14). A further, open biopsy-proven case, presented with a cauda equina syndrome that responded to antitoxoplasma treatment. In the latter, gadolinium enhanced-MRI identified an intramedullary lesion at the conus (15).

More than 90% of cases of toxoplasmosis in HIV infection are due to reactivation of latent cysts. Hence, specific IgM indicating de novo infection is rarely detected. Most patients with toxoplasmosis will be seropositive for IgG antibody, consistent with previous exposure, but the fourfold rise in an acute infection, which is diagnostic in an immunocompetent individual, does not occur. A positive titer, therefore, simply indicates that a person is at risk of developing toxoplasmosis but gives no guide as to presence of active disease. The risk of developing toxoplasmosis in an HIV-infected individual with positive toxoplasma serology had been estimated at 12–30%. A negative IgG test does not exclude the diagnosis, given that with increasing immunosuppression antibody production may decline, but does make it less likely. In view of this, it has been recommended that all HIV-positive patients should have their toxoplasma titers measured at the time of diagnosis.

It is important to diagnose toxoplasmosis because it is eminently responsive to appropriate chemotherapy and should be considered in any HIV-positive patient, as well as any individual who is at high risk whose HIV status is unknown, with cerebral or spinal cord mass lesions. The empirical protocol now accepted as standard is to treat such patients with antitoxoplasmosis therapy for up to 2 weeks. In nonresponders, consideration is then given to performing a stereotactic biopsy.

Standard regimens of treatment in the acute illness include pyrimethamine (day 1, 75 mg, followed by 25–50 mg/day, by mouth) plus sulphadiazine (6–8 g/day, by mouth) plus folinic acid (10 mg/day by mouth) for up to 6 weeks. The latter drug reduces the bone marrow toxic side effects of pyrimethamine. Clindamycin (2400 mg/day, by mouth) is an alternative to sulphadiazine. Life-long maintenance therapy is mandatory because the drug treatment is active against the proliferative but not the cyst form of *T. gondii*. Generally, reduced doses of the primary therapy medication are used.

2. Progressive Multifocal Leukoencephalopathy

Progressive multifocal leukoencephalopathy, caused by the reactivation of the JC papovavirus, results in widespread cerebral demyelination. There are increasing reports of extensive gray matter involvement clinically, radiologically, and on histology. To date, there have been no reports of spinal cord involvement.

3. Herpes Viruses

In view of the frequency of symptomatic infection with herpes simplex virus with mucocutaneous lesions and shingles due to herpes varicella—zoster, it is not suprising that occasional cases of a transverse myelitis have been described (16) (Fig. 1).

More than 90% of HIV-infected patients have serological evidence of infection with cytomegalovirus (CMV). Within the central nervous system, it is responsible for an encephalitis. One case of a combined myelitis due to CMV and herpes simplex virus has also been described (17). Cytomegalovirus is also the most common cause of blindness in AIDS patients, causing a retinitis. In the peripheral nervous system, it has been etiologically linked to a multifocal neuropathy and to a lumbar polyradiculopathy syndrome.

Cytomegalovirus lumbar polyradiculopathy is now a well-recognized syndrome in AIDS patients, with an estimated incidence of 2% in AIDS patients presenting with neurological problems (18). At presentation, patients are generally in the late stages of their AIDS illness, having had at least one AIDS-defining condition.

Characteristically, the presentation is with back pain followed by a rapidly progressive cauda equina syndrome with lower motor neurone weakness in the legs associated with sphincter disturbance. Sensory symptoms and signs are usually mild, although there is often evidence of diminished perineal sensation.

Myelography or MRI scanning with gadolinium enhancement, which is essential to exclude a mass lesion such as a metastatic deposit, is usually normal but may sometimes reveal nonspecific nodules or thickening of the nerve roots (19).

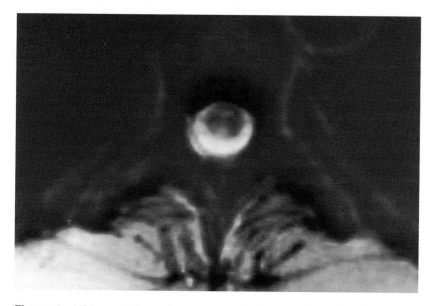

Figure 1   MRI scan with high signal at the T4 dorsal root level in a patient presenting with a transverse myelitis. 24 hours later he developed shingles over the appropriate dermatome.

Examination of the CSF is helpful inasmuch as characteristically, there is a polymorphonuclear cell leucocytosis (PML), which is unusual in a viral infection. It is postulated that an initial monocyte response results in a secondary neutrophil chemotaxis due to the release of cytokines (18). It is essential to check the CSF venereal disease research laboratory (VDRL) and *Treponema pallidum* hemagglutination (TPHA), because one differential is a syphilitic polyradiculopathy (20). Cytological examination is also necessary to exclude lymphomatous infiltration of the nerve roots, especially if the cell population is mainly lymphocytic in nature (21).

Neurophysiological studies are helpful in localizing the lesion. Some patients may have small or absent sensory nerve action potentials, implying dorsal root ganglia or peripheral nerve involvement. However, the neurophysiological data may be difficult to interpret because up to 30% of AIDS patients may have additional evidence of a distal symmetrical peripheral neuropathy (22).

Without treatment, there is usually a progression of the neurological deficit with death occurring in 2 or 3 months. In 1989, the first reports of treatment with 9-(1,3,-dihydroxy-2-propoxymethy (DHPG, gancyclovir) were published; subsequent reports in two small series suggested that with earlier recognition of the syndrome, when the neurological deficit is milder, treatment with DHPG results in better outcome (18, 23), (24). There have been no trials comparing the efficacy of DHPG with the other anti-CMV drug, trisodium phosphonoformate hexahydrate (Foscarnet). Most patients will, nevertheless, be left with some neurological deficit and in spite of maintenance therapy, which is essential, relapses may occur.

In the largest series of acute lumbosacral polyradiculopathy in AIDS to date, So et al. described a group of patients who presented with a less aggressive clinical picture than is found in cases of CMV polyradiculopathy and with a CSF mononuclear pleocytosis. In some cases spontaneous improvement occurred. It is postulated that these may represent an atypical host response to CMV or alternatively may be due to another pathogen (22). It would seem prudent to perform repeat CSF examinations, looking for an increase in polymorphonuclear cell count and attempting culture of CMV. If there is any evidence of deterioration in the neurological signs, treatment with anti-CMV therapy should be initiated.

4. Mycobacterium Tuberculosis

Individuals with evidence of previous exposure to *M. tuberculosis* seem to be more likely to develop active disease if coinfected with HIV. Most cases are due to reactivation of latent disease rather than to new acquired infection. In one retrospective study, tuberculous infection occurred in up to 6% of AIDS patients (25).

In HIV-infected individuals, tuberculosis usually occurs before other opportunistic infections such as *Pneumocystis carinii* pneumonia, which is indicative of its higher virulence. The mean CD4 count is higher in patients with disseminated tuberculosis when compared to those with *P. carinii* pneumonia or disseminated *Mycobacterium avium-intracellulare* infection (26). Thus, tuberculous infection should be considered in the differential diagnosis of a relatively immunocompetent HIV-infected individual and conversely, HIV infection should be considered in a patient presenting with tuberculous disease.

A striking feature of *M. tuberculosis* infection in HIV is the high frequency of extrapulmonary infections. In the less advanced stages, this may occur in up to 45% of cases but rises to 70% in patients with AIDS (27). In the central nervous system, this may present as tuberculous meningitis and intracerebral tuberculomas, which are indistinguishable from toxoplasma abscesses on CT scans. Spinal cord disease results from extradural abscesses whose main differential diagnosis is metastatic deposits.

Generally, the response rate to standard triple or quadruple therapy in all HIV groups is satisfactory, with few reported cases of treatment failure (28). Recently however, a nosocomial outbreak of multiresistant tuberculosis was reported in a group of AIDS patients in New York City (29).

5. Syphilis

The clinical manifestations of neurosyphilis are protean and enter within the differential diagnosis of most of the neurological complications encountered in HIV disease. This includes focal lesions within the brain and spinal cord as well as in cases of lumbosacral polyradiculopathy.

There are reports suggesting that in patients coinfected with HIV, *Treponema pallidum* may be more aggressive and may present with atypical signs (30). Furthermore, altered B-cell function may result in the suppression of serological markers that may remain negative or be delayed in the presence of active neurosyphilis. Most cases of active neurosyphilis will, however, have a positive CSF VDRL. As noted previously, routine CSF cytochemical parameters are invalid markers for active treponemal infection because the abnormalities may result from infection with HIV itself.

B. Tumors

The most common neoplasm to involve the central nervous system in HIV disease is PCNSL, with an incidence in patients with AIDS of about 2.6%. It is the second most common cause, after toxoplasmosis, of mass lesions within the brain. Pathologically, these are multicentric tumors derived from high grade B cells. The Epstein Barr virus has been implicated as a possible trigger mechanism. There have been no reports of this lesion within the spinal cord.

Since the beginning of the AIDS epidemic, there has been a gradual increase in the frequency of non-Hodgkin's lymphoma. Patients infected with HIV tend to present with high-grade tumors, with wide spread disease involving extranodal sites. In one study, 42% of patients had evidence of central nervous system disease at presentation (31).

Clinically, leptomeningeal infiltration presents with cranial nerve palsies or spinal root involvement. Occasionally, extradural metastases will present with spinal cord compression or a cauda equina syndrome (Fig. 2).

Treatment of central nervous system complications is by the intrathecal or ventricular reservoir route with methotrexate and/or cytosine arabinoside. The acute compressive myelopathies are best treated with radiotherapy. Because occult involvement of the central nervous system occurs at presentation and particularly at relapse, prophylaxis with intrathecal methotrexate or cranial irradiation has been recommended (32). In spite of these drug regimens, the prognosis remains poor.

C. HIV-Related Vacuolar Myelopathy

During the later stages of their AIDS illness, patients may, during a period of a few weeks or months, develop increasing leg weakness and ataxia, sphincter

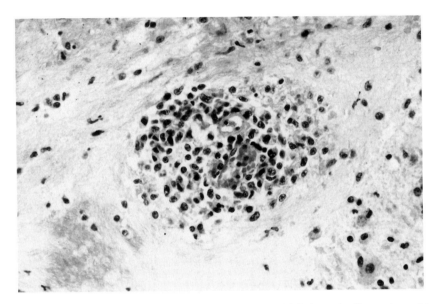

Figure 2 Extradural lymphoma of B-cell origin which is typically angiocentric at magnification × 300.

disturbance, impotence, and distal sensory symptoms. There is usually no evidence of a sensory level. This myelopathic syndrome commonly occurs in conjunction with a decline in cognitive function and motor deficits due to HIV encephalopathy. At this stage of the illness, there may also be evidence of a distal symmetrical peripheral neuropathy, making it difficult to disentangle the different clinicopathological entities at the bedside.

The vacuolar myelopathy, found in up to 30% of AIDS patients at postmortem, was described by Petito et al. in 1985 (33). Microscopically, the myelopathy is defined as vacuolation associated with lipid-laden macrophages (Figs. 3 and 4). The predominant sites affected are the lateral and posterior columns in the middle and lower thoracic levels. The pathological changes resemble those found in subacute, combined degeneration of the cord due to vitamin B_{12} deficiency and, rarely, folic acid deficiency.

To date, no neuroradiological correlates on MRI have been demonstrated. There is also no evidence of improvement with antiretroviral drug treatment such as zidovudine.

Although evidence of productive HIV infection has been demonstrated within the vacuolar areas using in situ hybridization and immunohistochemical staining techniques, the mechanisms underlying the myelin damage and conse-

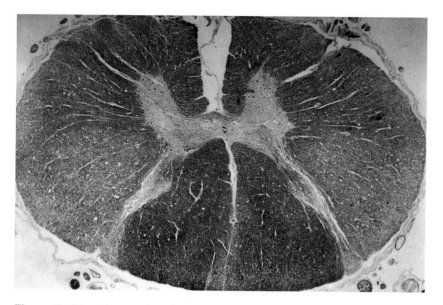

Figure 3 Vacuolar myelopathy at × 12 magnification showing pallor in the corticospinal tracts.

quent vacuole formation remain unanswered (34). Tyor et al. (35) found activated macrophages in the posterior and lateral columns of AIDS patients, regardless of the presence or absence of vacuolar myelopathy. They postulate that myelin damage may be initiated by these macrophages by the release of toxins such as tumor necrosis factor-alpha and interleukin-1 (35).

An important consideration in trying to unravel the pathogenic mechanisms is that this vacuolar myelopathy is, however, not restricted to patients with AIDS. Kamin et al. reported similar findings in a group of 21 patients who were immunosuppressed for reasons other than HIV infection. These included prolonged corticosteroid therapy, system carcinoma, cirrhosis, and diabetes with end-stage renal failure (36).

In view of the pathological similarities between subacute combined degeneration of the cord and the vacuolar myelopathy found in association with immunosuppression, the numerous attempts at correlating B_{12} and folate blood levels have produced disparate results. Low vitamin B_{12} levels have been found in up to 35% of AIDS patients. In some cases, this has been ascribed to a malabsorption syndrome (37) It is debated whether the levels found are low enough to account for the neurological complications seen.

An alternative explanation to account for the similarities with subacute combined degeneration, in spite of normal B_{12} and folate levels, is to propose

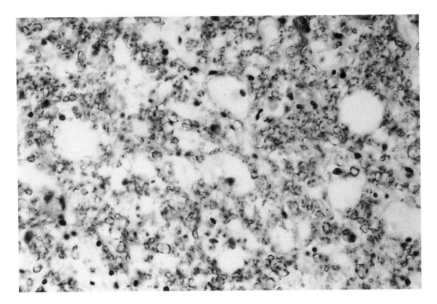

Figure 4 Vacuolar myelopathy at magnification × 400 showing vacuoles within the spinal cord. Some vacuoles contain macrophages.

deficits within the B_{12} and methionine pathways, as encountered in prolonged exposure to nitrous oxide, which also produces a similar picture (38).

Infection with other viruses has also been postulated to play a role in the development in the vacuolar myelopathy of AIDS. Although occasional cases of dual infection with HIV and the human T-lymphotrophic virus type 1 (HTLV-1) have been described, a retrospective study looking for serological evidence of HTLV-1 in 23 autopsy proven cases of vaculolar myelopathy failed to find any such evidence (39).

In view of the similarities in the transmission of HTLV-1 to HIV by sexual intercourse and blood transfusion, it is recommended that HTLV-1 serology be performed in high-risk patients or those with a predominant myelopathic presentation. Anecdotal reports in dually infected patients suggest a benefit with corticosteroid treatment (40).

ACKNOWLEDGMENTS

To Professor F. Scaravilli, for his help with the photographs of the pathological specimens; to Dr. K. Chong for use of the MRI scans.

REFERENCES

1. Snider WD, Simpson DM, Nielson S, et al. Neurological complications of Acquired Immune Deficiency Syndrome: Analysis of 50 patients. Ann Neurol 1986; 14:403–418.
2. Carne CA, Smith A, Elkington SG, et al. Acute encephalopathy coincident with seroconversion for anti-HTLV-III. Lancet 1985; 2:1206.
3. McArthur JC, Cohen BA, Homayoun F, Cornblath DR, Selnes O. Cerebrospinal fluid abnormalities in homosexual men with and without neuropsychiatric findings. Ann Neurol 1988; 23(Suppl):534–535.
4. Denning DA, Anderson J, Rudge P, et al. Acute myelopathy associated with primary infection with human immunodeficiency virus. BMJ 1987; 294:143–144.
5. Kessler HA, Blauw B, Spear J, et al. Diagnosis of HIV infection in seronegative homosexuals presenting with an acute viral syndrome. JAMA 1987; 258:1196–1199.
6. Zeman A, Donaghy M. Acute infection with human immunodeficiency virus presenting with neurogenic urinary retention. Genitourin Med 1991; 67:345–347.
7. Riette AM, Russeau F, Mignon D, et al. Acute neuropathy coincident with seroconversion for anti LAV/HTLV III. Lancet 1989; i:852.
8. Smith T, Jakobsen J, Trojaborg W. Myelopathy and HIV infection. AIDS 1990; 4:589–591.
9. McAllister RH, Herns M, Harrison MJG, et al. Neurological and neuropsychological performance in HIV seropositive asymptomatic individuals. J Neurol Neurosurg Psychiatry 1992; 55:143–148.
10. Cornblath DR, McArthur JC, Kennedy PGE, Witte AS, Griffin JW. Inflammatory demyelinating peripheral neuropathies associated with human T cell lymphotrophic virus infection. Ann Neurol 1987; 21:32–40.
11. van der Merche FGA, Schmitz PIM, Dutch Guillain—Barré Study Group. A randomised trail comparing intravenous immune globulin and plasma exchange in Guillain-Barré syndrome. N Engl J Med 1992; 326:1123–1229.
12. Cornblath DR, Chaudhry V, Griffin JW. Treatment of chronic inflammatory demyelinating polyneuropathy with immunoglobulin. Ann Neurol 1991; 30:104–106.
13. Cirillo J, Rosenblaum D. Imaging of solitary lesions in AIDS (letter). J Neurosurg 1991; 74:1029.
14. Mehren M, Burns DO, Mamani F, Levy CS, Laureno R. Toxoplasmic myelitis mimicking intramedullary spinal cord tumor. Neurology 1988; 38:1648–1650.
15. Overhage J, Greist A, Brown D. Conus medullaris syndrome resulting from Toxoplasma gondii infection in a patient with the acquired immunodeficiency syndrome. Am J Med 1990; 89:814–815.
16. Devinsky O, Cho ES, Petito CK, Price RW. Herpes zoster myelitis. Brain 1991; 114:1181–1196.
17. Tucker T, Dix RD, Katzen C, et al. Cytomegalovirus and herpes simplex virus ascending myelitis in a patient with acquired immunodeficiency syndrome. Ann Neurol 1985; 18:74–79.

18. de gans J, Tiesens G, Portegies P, et al. Predominance of polymorphonuclear leucocytes in the cerebrospinal fluid of AIDS patients with CMV polyradiculomyelitis.
J AIDS 1990; 3:1155–1158.

19. Brazan C, Jackson C, Jinkins JR, et al. Gadolinium-enhanced MRI in a case of
cytomegalovirus polyradiculopathy. Neurology 1991; 41:1522–1523.

20. Lanska MJ, Lanska DJ, Schmidley JW. Syphilitic polyradiculopathy in an HIV
positive man. Neurology 1988; 38:1297–1301.

21. Leger J, Henin D, Belec L. Lymphoma induced polyradiculopathy in AIDS: two
cases. J Neurol 1992; 239:132–134.

22. So YT, Olney RK. Acute lumbo sacral polyradiculopathy in acquired immunodeficiency syndrome: experience in 23 cases. Ann Neurol 1994; 35:53–58.

23. Graveleau P, Perol R, Chapman A. Regression of cauda equina syndrome in AIDS
patients being treated with ganciclovir. Lancet 1989; ii:511–512.

24. Miller RG, Storey JR, Greco CM. Ganciclovir in the treatment of progressive
AIDS related polyradiculopathy. Neurology 1990; 40:569–574.

25. Helbert M, Robinson D, Buchanon D, et al. Mycobacterium infection in patients
infected with the human immunodeficiency virus (HIV). Thorax 1990; 45:45–48.

26. Crowe SM, Carlin JB, Stewart KI, Lucas CR, Hoy JF. Predictive value of CD4
lymphocyte numbers for the development of opportunistic infections and malignancies in HIV infected persons. J AIDS 1991; 4:770–776.

27. Barnes PF, Bloch AB, Davidson PT, Snider DEJ. Tuberculosis in patients with
human immunodeficiency virus infection. N Engl J Med 1991; 324:1644–1650.

28. Small PM, Goodman PC, Sande MA, Chaisson RE, Hopewell PC. Treatment of
tuberculosis in patients with advanced HIV infection. N Engl J Med 1991;
324:289–294.

29. Edlin BR, Tokars JI, Grieco MH. An outbreak of multi drug resistant tuberculosis
among hospitalised patients with AIDS. N Engl J Med 1992; 326:1514–1521.

30. Munscher DM, Hamill RJ, Baughn RE. Effect of HIV infection on the course of
syphilis and on the response to treatment. Ann Intern Med 1990; 113:872–881.

31. Ziegler JL, Beckstead JA, Volberding PA, et al. Non-Hodgkins lymphoma in 90
homosexual men. N Engl J Med 1984; 311:565–570.

32. Krown SE. treatment of AIDS associated malignancy. Cancer Detection and Prevention 1990; 14:405–409.

33. Petito CK, Navia BA, Cho ES, et al. Vascual myelopathy pathologically resembling sub acute combined degeration in patients with the acquired immunodeficiency syndrome. N Engl J Med 1985; 312:874–879.

34. Eilbott DJ, Peress N, Burger H, et al. Human immunodeficiency virus type 1 in
spinal cords of acquired immunodeficiency syndrome patients with myelopathy:
Expression and replication in macrophages. Proc Natl Acad Sci USA 1989;
86:3337–3341.

35. Tyor WR, Glass JD, Baumrind N, et al. Cytokine expression of macrophages in
HIV-1 associated vacuolar myelopathy. Neurology 1993; 43:1002–1009.

36. Kamin S, Petito CK. Idiopathic myelopathies with white matter vacuolation in non
acquired immunodeficiency syndrome patients. Hum Pathol 1991; 22:816–824.

37. Kieburtz K, Giang D, Schiffer R, Vakil N. Abnormal vitamin B12 metabolism in
HIV infection. Arch Neurol 48:312–314.

38. Keating JN, Trimble KC, Mulcahy F, Scott JM, and Weir D. Evidence of brain methyltransferase inhibition and early brain involvement in HIV positive patients. Lancet 1991; 337:935–939.

39. Brew B, Hardy W, Zuckerman E, et al. AIDS related vacuolar myelopathy is not associated with co infection by human T-lymphotrophic virus type 1. Ann Neurol 1989; 26:679–681.

40. McArthur JC, Griffin JW, Cornblath DR, et al. Steroid responsive myeloneuropathy in a man dually infected with HIV-1 and HTLV-1. Neurology 1990; 40:938–944.

12

Pathology of Spinal Tumors

Roy O. Weller

University of Southampton Medical School, Southampton, Hampshire, England

I. INTRODUCTION

Interpretation of the signs and symptoms of spinal tumors, their effective management, and appropriate treatment depend upon an understanding of the anatomy and pathology of the spine, spinal cord, and its coverings. The spinal canal is a confined space, and expanding tumors within this space may have a devastating effect upon the function of the spinal cord and nerve roots.

This chapter includes a description of the types of tumor that occur within the spinal canal, the structures from which they arise, and their effects upon the spinal cord and nerve roots. A full account of primary intramedullary spinal cord tumors will be found in Chapter 14, so this section will concentrate more on the extramedullary tumors of the spinal canal.

II. SPINAL TUMORS

Tumors of the spine and spinal canal produce neurological signs and symptoms mainly from damage and functional disturbance of the spinal cord and spinal nerve roots (Fig. 1). Destruction of the bones by tumor may cause instability of the spine with collapse of vertebrae and compression of nerve roots or the spinal cord itself. Metastatic tumors in the extradural space and primary or

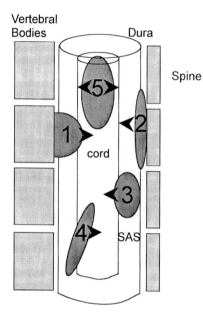

Figure 1 A diagram of the spinal canal to illustrate the position of tumors affecting the spinal cord and nerve roots. SAS – subarachnoid space. (1) Metastatic carcinoma expanding from a vertebral body, remaining extradurally but compressing the spinal cord. (2) Extradural metastatic carcinoma or lymphoma remaining outside the dura but compressing the spinal cord within the spinal canal. (3) Subdural meningioma attached to the inner aspect of the dura compressing the cord. (4) Schwannoma arising on a dorsal nerve root compressing the spinal cord. (5) Intrinsic astrocytoma expanding the spinal cord.

metastatic tumors growing within the spinal cord and its meningeal coverings result in compression or ischemia of nerve roots and the spinal cord. Diffuse invasion of the subarachnoid space by primary or metastatic tumor cells may result in local infiltration of nerve roots or spinal cord, which may also produce neurological signs and symptoms.

A. Classification

The classification set out in Table 1 is based not only on tumor type but also on the anatomical position of the tumor. In this way, it is easier to visualize the effects of each tumor upon the spinal cord and nerve roots.

Table 1 Classification of Spinal Tumors

A. Vertebral Column—Tumors of Bone
    Primary
        Chordoma
        Osteosarcoma
        Osteoclastoma (giant cell tumor of bone)
        Hemangioma
        Myeloma
    Secondary
        Carcinoma—bronchus, prostate, and breast
        Lymphoreticular tumors
B. Extradural Tumors
    Metastatic carcinoma and malignant melanoma
    Lymphoma
C. Intradural Tumors
    Extramedullary—primary
        Meningioma
        Schwannoma
        Neurofibroma
        Hemangioblastoma
        Malignant melanoma
        Lipoma
        Epidermoid and dermoid cysts
    Extramedullary—metastatic
        Astrocytoma
        Primitive neuroectodermal tumor (PNET—medulloblastoma)
        Ependymoma
        Metastatic carcinoma—seedlings
        Spinal cord deposits—rare
        Carcinomatous meningitis
D. Leukemias
    Invasion of nerve roots and spinal cord
E. Intramedullary Tumors
    Astrocytoma
    Anaplastic astrocytoma
    Glioblastoma multiforme
    Ependymoma—including myxopapillary ependymoma
    Primitive neuroectodermal tumor (PNET)
    Gangliocytoma
    Neurocytoma
    Lipoma
    Epidermoid cyst
    Hemangioma

B. Incidence

It is estimated that some 15% of all primary tumors of the central nervous system and its coverings occur in the spine, with an average annual incidence of between 0.8 and 2.5 per 100,000 (average 1.3) (4). Slooff et al. (5) estimated that primary tumors of the spine occur in the following proportions: 29% schwannomas, 25.5% meningiomas, 22% gliomas (63% of which are ependymomas), and 12% sarcomas.

Most spinal tumors occur in adults and, apart from the specific sites of chordomas in the sacral region and myxopapillary ependymomas at the lower end of the spinal cord, both primary and metastatic tumors may occur at any level in the spine. There is little noticeable sex difference between the incidence of the various types of spinal cord tumor, except that spinal meningiomas are more common in elderly women, reflecting the pattern of incidence of meningiomas generally (6, 7). Metastatic tumors are also more common in older age groups. Lipomas and epidermoid cysts, on the other hand, usually present early in life, often due to tethering of the lower end of the spinal cord.

C. Tumors Involving Bones in the Spine

Primary bone tumors involving the spine are less common than metastatic tumors (4). Chordomas derived from tissue similar to the notochord arise almost exclusively in the sacral regions of the spine and in the clivus of the skull. In the sacrum, chordomas destroy bone and expand as a gelatinous mass into the spinal canal to compress the cauda equina or the lower end of the cord. They may also extend anteriorly into the pelvis or posteriorly to present behind the sacrum itself. Compression of the nerve roots at the lower end of the cord may produce pain, abnormal sensations, or denervation and weakness of leg muscles. Ideally, chordomas are treated by radical excision and radiotherapy (8).

Primary osteogenic sarcomas and osteoclastomas of the spine are uncommon, but they may also destroy bone and cause compression of the spinal cord or cauda equina due to collapse of vertebrae or extension of the tumor into the spinal canal. Vascular tumors such as hemangiomas within vertebral bones cause problems not only by the bony destruction of vertebrae but also because of enlargement of the venous channels in the spinal canal that drain the hemangioma. This causes aberrant blood flow in the spinal cord, which may destroy cord tissue and result in paraparesis. Most hemangiomas occur in the thoracic or lumbar region, and treatment by excision of the lesion in the bone may arrest or alleviate the circulatory problems within the cord.

Metastatic tumors may involve any part of the vertebral column. They destroy bone and result in vertebral collapse, or the metastasis may extend into the spinal canal causing cord or cauda equina compression (Fig. 1). Virtually any carcinoma may metastasize to the spine—carcinomas of the bronchus, breast, lung, and prostate are the most common. Lymphoreticular tumors, particularly plasmacytoma or myeloma, also involve bones of the spine.

D. Tumors of the Extradural Space

Metastatic carcinomas are the most common tumors to involve the extradural space in the spinal canal. Tumor cells invade and replace extradural fat (Fig. 1) and may form a complete and constricting collar around the dura and spinal cord. In this position, metastatic tumors may cause back pain and, subsequently, paraparesis and paraplegia from spinal cord compression (Fig. 1). Carcinomas of the bronchus, adenocarcinomas of the lung, breast, and prostate are the most common tumors to be found at this site, but metastatic carcinomas from colon and thyroid are also found in this region. When extradural compression of the spinal cord occurs with no obvious primary tumor elsewhere in the body, high-grade non-Hodgkin's lymphoma is frequently found at biopsy (7).

Laminectomy with removal of the extradural metastases may alleviate the spinal cord compression, but the ultimate prognosis often depends upon the progress of the primary tumor.

Enterogenous cysts containing elements of tissues derived from the gut may also involve the spine; they are often associated with defects of vertebral bodies. Excision of the cyst and its lining and repair of severe bony defects is the treatment of choice. They are benign lesions and should not recur if completely excised.

E. Intradural Tumors

Tumors within the confines of the dural sleeve or sac may either arise outside the spinal cord—extramedullary tumors—from leptomeninges (meningiomas from the arachnoid), from nerve roots (schwannomas and neurofibromas), or from adipose tissue (lipomas) or remnants of epidermal tissue (epidermoid cysts). Metastatic extramedullary intradural tumors also occur. The majority of tumors within the spinal cord—intramedullary tumors—arise from glial or neuronal tissue (Table 1) and are only very occasionally metastatic in origin.

1. Extramedullary Intradural Tumors

Meningiomas and schwannomas are the most common intradural tumors in the spine (5); neurofibromas, primary malignant melanoma, lipomas, and epidermoid cysts are less common.

Meningiomas

Arising from the arachnoid on the surface of the spinal cord and histologically resembling cells of the arachnoid, meningiomas are usually slowly growing tumors. They are firmly attached to the dura and sometimes to the nerve roots but are usually well encapsulated, globular or ovoid in shape with a lobulated surface and a rubbery or hard consistency. Meningiomas in the spinal canal most frequently occur in elderly women. They present with back pain and occasionally with spinal cord compression and leg weakness or nerve root compression and pain. Such tumors often have a gritty consistency due to the presence of large numbers of psammoma bodies—literally, grains of sand formed from small granules of calcification within the tumor. Other meningiomas may be softer and less stone-like than psammomatous meningiomas. Because they are usually single and easily accessible, meningiomas can be adequately treated by local excision and they rarely recur at this site.

Tumors Arising on Nerve Roots

The most common tumor arising from nerve sheaths in the spinal canal is a schwannoma composed of sheets of tightly packed, elongated, spindle-shaped Schwann cells and areas of loosely packed tumor cells (9). Like meningiomas, they are well encapsulated but may be stuck firmly to one or more nerve roots. Schwannomas usually have a firm consistency and are ovoid or globular in shape. They may compress either the spinal cord or nerve roots in the cauda equina (Fig. 1), resulting in back pain or neurological signs of root or cord compression. Such tumors arise most commonly on the posterior spinal roots, and surgical excision is rarely followed by a recurrence.

Unlike schwannomas, which are well-circumscribed tumors that remain distinct from the nerve roots from which they arise, neurofibromas infiltrate nerve roots (9) and, on occasion, may infiltrate and destroy bones of the vertebrae. Typically, neurofibromas arise within the nerve roots and may extend medially to involve the spinal canal and laterally along the nerve as it passes into the intervertebral foramen. They not only cause symptoms of root pain and motor and sensory disturbances due to compression of the associated nerve roots, but they also damage nervous tissue through infiltration. At surgery, neurofibromas are often difficult to separate from surrounding tissue and, when viewed as a pathological specimen after surgery, the spindle-shaped cells of the neurofibroma are seen to expand nerve roots and infiltrate dorsal root ganglia, destroying nerve fibers and nerve cells alike. Total excision may be difficult to attain surgically and, when incompletely removed, they may recur.

Quite apart from the difficulty in completely removing neurofibromas, these tumors may have two further associated complications. Von Recklinghausen's neurofibromatosis is associated with multiple tumors. In the less ag-

tomeninges on the surface of the cord, but they frequently invade both cranial and spinal nerve roots. The diagnosis can be made by isolating metastatic carcinoma cells in centrifuge (cytospin) deposits of cerebrospinal fluid (7,9). Malignant melanomas, whether primary from the meninges or metastatic, may also coat the leptomeninges and invade the surface of the brain, spinal cord, and nerve roots, producing a chocolate-brown icing over all these structures.

2. Spinal Cord–Intramedullary Tumors

Primary tumors in the spinal cord are less common than those in the brain; nevertheless, they form the majority of intramedullary tumors. Astrocytomas and anaplastic astrocytomas cause enlargement of the spinal cord as the tumor cells diffusely invade both gray and white matter elements within the cord. Such tumors may be slowly growing and the spinal canal may enlarge progressively to accommodate the tumor until its final stages. Astrocytomas and the more aggressive anaplastic astrocytomas usually occur in children or young adults. The typical anaplastic tumor of older adults—glioblastoma multiforme—is rare in the spinal cord.

The most common primary intrinsic tumor of the spinal cord is ependymoma. Such tumors show a range in their activity. Very slowly growing lesions may be present for many years before there is significant neurological deficit. Others are less well-differentiated, more aggressive tumors that spread widely and cause neurological signs and symptoms due to spinal cord compression (Fig. 1), infiltration of tracts and damage to nerve roots early in the course of the disease. A particularly favorable prognosis for ependymomas is seen in the myxopapillary type, which occurs at the lower end of the spinal cord (4,7). Such tumors may be circumscribed and it may be possible to remove them without damage to cord and spinal roots and without leaving remnants of the tumor behind. Gangliogliomas and slowly growing neurocytomas occasionally occur at the lower end of the cord, but the more aggressive primitive neuroectodermal tumors usually spread from the cerebellum rather than arising primarily in the spinal cord.

F. Effects of Tumors on the Spinal Cord and Nerve Roots

There are three major forms of damage to the spinal cord and nerve roots induced by tumors: compression, ischemia, and infiltration by neoplastic cells.

Compression and ischemia are often difficult to separate as mechanisms of spinal cord damage, so they will be described together.

1. Spinal Cord Compression and Ischemia

Sudden, catastrophic compression of the spinal cord has the same effect whether it is due to fracture dislocation of spinal vertebrae, an acute extradural hematoma, or the sudden collapse of a vertebra destroyed by primary or metastatic bone tumor. As the cord is compressed, a central area of hemorrhage occurs, not only at the site of compression but also extending above and below it. Neurons and axons within the region of compression are destroyed either by direct compression or by occlusion of the blood vessel supplying the cord tissue with infraction in the affected area. If the damage is severe, immediate paraplegia or quadriplegia may ensue, depending on the level of involvement of the cord.

Microscopic examination of the damaged cord reveals interruption of axons in the long corticospinal tracts and sensory dorsal columns of the cord. This change will be permanent as little, if any, regeneration occurs within damaged tracts in the spinal cord or elsewhere in the central nervous system. If the damage is very severe and the patient survives, a fluid-filled cyst will eventually form at the site of damage as necrotic tissue is removed by macrophages.

Spinal nerve roots are vulnerable to compression not only within the spinal canal but also in the intervertebral foramina (Fig. 1). Tumors, prolapsed intervertebral discs, and even hematomas from torn vertebral ligaments may compress nerve roots, resulting in pain and eventually sensory disturbance, muscle denervation and muscle weakness. Again, the cause of the damage may be partly due to mechanical compression of the nerve roots with axonal damage, or partly to ischemia of the nerve, also causing axonal degeneration. Despite the brisk and effective regeneration capacity exhibited by peripheral nerves, regeneration from damaged spinal nerve roots is frequently ineffective due to the distances involved from the nerve roots to their effector, sensory, or motor organs in the limbs.

2. Infiltration of Nerve Roots and Spinal Cord by Tumor Cells

Infiltration of spinal nerve roots often occurs when the leptomeninges and subarachnoid space are invaded by tumor cells. Metastatic carcinomas and melanomas may coat nerve roots and the spinal cord; leukemias and lymphomas behave in a similar way. Carcinoma cells have differing capacities to invade neural tissue, and the major symptoms are usually due to invasion of peripheral nerves. Pathologically, tumor cells invade between peripheral nerve fibers or they may invade along perivascular spaces within the spinal cord itself, but usually they only affect the surface tracts of the spinal cord and not the major corticospinal tracts or dorsal columns.

Primitive neuroectodermal tumors—medulloblastomas—and, less commonly, astrocytomas and ependymomas, also spread through the spinal subarachnoid space and invade nerve roots and spinal cord.

G. Clinical Investigation as a Guide to Pathology of Spinal Cord Tumors

Radiology, including plain x-rays of the vertebral column, myelography, computed tomography (CT) and magnetic resonance imaging (MRI) may give a firm indication of the pathological diagnosis of a tumor in the extradural, intradural, extramedullary, or intramedullary compartments. However, nothing is ever certain until a firm histological diagnosis is made.

X-rays of the spine provide valuable information for the pathologist in cases of primary and metastatic bone tumors. Magnetic resonance imaging has proved to be particularly useful for the localization and diagnosis of tumors within the spinal canal (13). By the use of MRI and gadolinium enhancement, which reflects the absence of a blood-brain barrier in tumors such as meningiomas, schwannomas, and metastatic tumors, the tumor cannot only be localized, but its identity can be defined by its radiological appearance. Well-differentiated primary glial tumors, such as astrocytomas, usually fail to enhance with gadolinium due to an intact blood-brain barrier, but primitive neuroectodermal tumors and ependymomas frequently enhance.

Cerebrospinal fluid cytology may allow the diagnosis of carcinomatous meningitis or involvement by PNET through the detection of tumor cells in centrifuge preparations of the cerebrospinal fluid.

With regard to treatment of intraspinal tumors, only a minority of tumors are really sensitive to irradiation or chemotherapy. Plasmacytomas or myelomas arising in the bones of the vertebral column or lymphomas in the extradural space or in the cerebrospinal fluid, leukemic involvement of the cerebrospinal fluid spaces, and primitive neuroectodermal tumors spreading from the cerebellum down into the spinal subarachnoid space are examples of tumors that can be treated effectively by irradiation or chemotherapy. Malignant tumors metastasizing to the bones of the vertebral column or to the extradural space can usually only be treated symptomatically by excision to relieve the spinal cord or nerve root compression. Schwannomas and meningiomas, on the other hand, may be very effectively treated by excision and some ependymomas may also be treated in this way.

III. CONCLUSION

A wide variety of tumors involving the spine may cause signs and symptoms as a result of compression, ischemia, or invasion of the spinal cord or nerve roots. Damage to nerve tracts within the spinal cord or nerve fibers within peripheral nerves may be reversible in the early stages but rapidly become irreversible if compression is severe. An understanding of the anatomy and pathology of the spinal canal may help to appreciate the sequences of events that lead to neurological damage and may assist in the planning of management and treatment schedules for such disorders.

REFERENCES

1. Nicholas DS, Weller RO. The fine anatomy of the human spinal meninges. J Neurosurg 1988; 69:276–282.
2. Weller RO. Fluid compartments and fluid balance in the central nervous system. In: Williams PL et al, ed. Gray's Anatomy. 38th ed. Edinburgh: Churchill Livingstone, 1995; 1202–1224.
3. Dolan RA. Spinal adhesive arachnoiditis. Surg Neurol 1993; 39:479–484.
4. Russell DS, Rubinstein LJ. Pathology of Tumours of the Nervous System. London: Edward Arnold, 1989.
5. Slooff JL, Kernohan JW, MacCarty CS. Primary Intramedullary Tumours of the Spinal Cord and Filum Terminale. Philadelphia: WB Saunders, 1964.
6. Barker DJP, Weller RO, Garfield J. The epidemiology of primary tumors of the brain and spinal cord: A regional survey in Southern England. J Neurol Neurosurg Psychiatry 1977; 39:209–296.
7. Weller RO. Tumors of the nervous system. In: Weller RO, ed. Systemic Pathology. Volume 4. Nervous system, muscle and eyes. Edinburgh: Churchill Livingstone, 1990: 427–503.
8. Burger PC, Scheithauer BW. Tumors of the Central Nervous System. Washington: Armed Forces Institute of Pathology, 1994.
9. Weller RO. Colour Atlas of Neuropathology. Oxford: Harvey Miller and Oxford University Press, 1984.
10. Shu HH, Mirowitz SA, Wippold FJ, II. Neurofibromatosis: MR imaging findings involving the head and spine. AJR Am J Roentgenol 1993; 159–164.
11. Barker D, Wright E, Nguyen K, et al. Gene for von Recklinghausen neurofibromatosis is in the pericentromeric region of chromosome 17. Science 1987; 2361:1100–1102.
12. Seizinger BR, Rouleau G, Ozelius LJ, et al. Common pathogenetic mechanisms for three tumor types in bilateral acoustic neurofibromatosis. Science 1987; 2363:317–319.
13. Bradley WG, Bydder G. MRI Atlas of the Brain. London: Martin Dunitz, 1990.

13

Benign Spinal Tumors

Ali R. Rezai and Mark Lee
New York University Medical Center, New York, New York

Rick Abbott
Beth Israel Medical Center, North Division, New York, New York

I. INTRODUCTION

Spinal neoplasms can be classified into primary or secondary tumors. Primary lesions are usually benign, arising locally from the bony spinal column, the meningeal coverings of the spinal cord, or from the spinal cord parenchyma itself. Secondary or metastatic spinal tumors are more common than primary lesions. They can arise from any solid tumor or systemic cancer within the body. This chapter primarily deals with benign spinal tumors, their clinical presentation, diagnosis, pathology, treatment, and outcome.

II. STRUCTURE

A. Anatomy

A comprehensive knowledge of the anatomy and the vascular supply of the spinal cord and the spinal column is essential for the diagnosis and treatment of patients with spinal tumors (6, 48, 71, 77, 78). The vertebral column encloses and protects the spinal cord while providing structural support for the trunk, head, and the extremities. The spinal canal extends from the foramen magnum to the coccyx. The spinal cord is covered with dura, a tough fibrous membrane that extends from the foramen magnum to the S2 level. The spinal cord is structurally anchored via the nerve roots and the laterally placed dentate ligaments. The dentate ligaments arise from the pia and attach to the dura, hence anchoring the spinal cord to the dura (6, 48, 71, 77, 78). Thus, lesions that mechanically displace the spinal cord can result in stretching, torsion, and tethering of the cord.

B. Spinal Deformity

Spinal tumors can be associated with spinal deformities such as scoliosis and kyphosis (10, 13, 37, 44, 52, 77–78). These deformities can be a direct result of intrinsic lesions of the spinal column causing bony destruction and deformity, or they may be due to chronic pressure effects on the spine (10, 37, 44). Spinal deformity can also be the only presenting finding in a patient with a spinal tumor (10). Magnetic resonance imaging (MRI) analysis of 28 pediatric patients with scoliosis demonstrated two spinal cord tumors, seven tethered spinal cords, and five syringomyelias (52). In general, those with left-sided scoliotic curves have an associated increase in the incidence of spinal neoplasms, whereas right-sided scoliotic curves are more commonly idiopathic. Certain spinal tumors, however, have a high degree of associated spinal deformities. For example, bony tumors of the spinal column, such as osteoblastoma and osteoid osteoma, can cause scoliosis in up to 70% of the cases (13, 37, 44, 57, 77, 78).

Spinal surgery or radiation therapy can also cause spinal deformity and instability (36, 47, 49). This is particularly important in the pediatric population, where progressive skeletal growth can magnify the deformity. Radiation therapy has been shown to increase the incidence of spinal deformity in children, with higher radiation doses more frequently causing kyphoscoliotic deformities (47). Thus all children treated with radiation for spinal tumors should be monitored carefully during their period of skeletal growth (36, 47). The incidence of spinal deformity after multilevel laminectomy is also higher in children than in adults, with the highest incidence occurring in those having cervical laminectomies (23, 49, 79).

III. CLINICAL PRESENTATION

The clinical presentation of benign spinal tumors is often indolent, with neurological dysfunction being a late manifestation. Patients may remain asymptomatic for long period. Symptoms arise from progressive involvement of the bony spinal column and paravertebral soft tissues, as well as from the spinal cord, its covering (meninges), and nerve roots.

Spinal tumors can present with any constellation of symptoms and signs including pain, weakness, sensory loss, autonomic (bowel, bladder, sexual) dysfunction, gait disturbance, hyperreflexia, spinal deformity (kyphosis and/or scoliosis), and spinal masses.

A. Pain

Pain is the most common presenting symptom of patients with spinal tumors, being present in 85–100% of patients (7, 43, 50, 66, 67, 77, 78). The diagnosis of a spinal tumor can often be delayed due to the similarity between neoplastic and degenerative spinal pain. However pain associated with a spinal neoplasm is characteristically unrelenting, not related to activity, not relieved by rest or recumbency, and most prominent at night (43, 50, 66, 71, 77, 78). Night-time pain can be so severe that some patients sleep upright in chairs for relief.

The characteristics and the quality of the pain are variable, depending on the area of involvement (43, 50, 71, 77, 78). Tumors causing bony destruction result in localized spinal pain and tenderness. Pain is worsened by movement in those with spinal deformity and instability. Pain secondary to spinal cord compression can be worsened by coughing, sneezing, or any maneuver that increases the intraspinal pressure. Radicular pain from compression of the nerve roots causes burning parasthesias or sharp lancinating pain. Intramedullary tumors, on the other hand, will frequently present with weakness or numbness rather than pain, although dysesthetic pain can occur.

B. Motor Deficits

The second most common complaint of patients with spinal tumors is motor weakness (43, 71, 77, 78). Weakness is usually the first sign of spinal cord compression, but this may not occur until tumor growth has become relatively advanced. Primary spinal tumors present with weakness in approximately 40% of the patients (43). Initially, patients complain of fatigue during ambulation, which gradually progresses to a spastic paraparesis. This is characteristic of slow-growing lesions such as meningiomas or neurofibromas. In contrast, rapidly progressive lesions can present with acute cord compression and myelopathy resulting in a flaccid paralysis and areflexia (43, 77, 78). In addition, tumor-induced skeletal deformity (kyphotic angulation) can occur acutely, thus resulting in rapid onset of motor deficits.

C. Sensory Deficits

Sensory deficits can include numbness, tingling, parasthesias, proprioceptive loss, and dysesthetic pain. Initially, sensory complaints are subjective. Objective sensory loss does not appear until later in the disease process (43). Sensory loss may be restricted to a dermatomal pattern, may be patchy or diffuse in distribution, or may involve one sensory modality more than the other, depending on the spinal cord region and tract most affected.

D. Symptoms Specific to Tumor Compartment

In addition to nonspecific symptoms, there are characteristics symptoms specific to the different compartments involved (extradural, intradural-extramedullary, and intramedullary) that can aid in the differential diagnosis of the lesion. Extradural or intradural-extramedullary lesions are usually eccentric and result in a focal, asymmetric compression of the spinal cord. This results in a high incidence of asymmetric signs and symptoms, such as the Brown-Séquard syndrome (ipsilateral motor and posterior column deficit along with contralateral pain and temperature deficit). Conversely, intramedullary tumors cause diffuse spinal cord expansion with a dissociated sensory loss due to the interruption of the crossing spinothalamic tracts (impaired pain and temperature sensation with sparing of the posterior columns (7, 71, 77, 78).

High cervical tumors usually present with headaches (in the greater occipital nerve distribution), and neck pain (more severe with neck motion). Low cervical tumors characteristically produce pain in the shoulders mimicking symptoms of cervical spondylosis, and can also present with atrophy of the upper extremities, in particular the hand muscles. When the extent of cervical involvement is diffuse and bilateral, respiratory distress can result. History of recurrent upper respiratory infections and aspiration pneumonia should increase the suspicion of a cervical lesion. Thoracic lesions produce motor and sensory disturbances, hyperreflexia, and myelopathy. Conus and cauda equina lesions characteristically give rise to early bowel and bladder dysfunction (urinary retention, overflow, constipation, difficulty with evacuation, and bowel incontinence) and sexual dysfunction (impotence) with a symmetrical saddle anesthesia (25, 43, 50, 71, 77, 78). Conus lesions will typically cause bladder dysfunction, hyperreflexia and spasticity prior to pain, whereas cauda equina lesions produce pain before bowel and bladder symptoms and hyporeflexia. Patients can also present with isolated sphincter dysfunction as the initial symptom (25, 43, 71, 77, 78).

E. Special Consideration in Children

Spinal tumors can present differently in children than adults. Young children are frequently unable to complain of symptoms. In addition, the early signs of spinal cord dysfunction are often attributed to poor progression toward developmental milestones. Children with spinal tumors can present with loss of developmental milestones, growth deformities (scoliosis, kyphosis), weakness, foot deformities (pescavus), gait dysfunction, and enuresis (in a previously toilet-trained child). Often these patients are first seen by orthopedic surgeons for their foot deformity or kyphoscoliosis.

IV. DIAGNOSIS

Radiological evaluation of spinal tumors consists of plain spine radiographs, computerized tomography (CT), MRI, and myelography.

A. Plain Spine Radiographs

Plain spine roentgenograms [anterior-posterior (AP), lateral, and oblique views] are inexpensive, easily obtained, and can rapidly provide valuable information. Plain radiographs can demonstrate a widened spinal canal, a widened neural foramen (best seen on oblique views), vertebral body scalloping, and flattening. In addition, vertebral body collapse, pedicular erosion, and pathological fractures can be identified easily (7, 77, 78). A classic sign of early vertebral body involvement is unilateral pedicular destruction from tumor infiltration (the "winking owl" sign) on AP view (78). Disc space evaluation is also important for the differential diagnosis of spinal lesions. Pyogenic osteomyelitis of the spine causes vertebral body destruction as well as disc space involvement, whereas neoplastic processes frequently spare the disc space because of their high resistance to tumor invasion.

It should be noted that plain radiographic evidence of bony destruction may not be evident until 30–50% of the trabecular bone has been destroyed (18). Thus early lesions can be difficult to detect by plain radiographs.

B. Computerized Tomography

Computerized tomographic scanning is particularly useful for assessing bony lesions. It can detect bone density changes, bone destruction, and osteolytic or osteoblastic lesions.

C. Myelography

Until the advent of MRI, myelography combined with postmyelogram CT was the study of choice in assessing the subarachnoid space, spinal canal, spinal cord, and nerve roots (78). Myelography identifies the level, the rostral and caudal extension, and the anatomical compartment of the lesion. In addition, it can be particularly useful in showing the relationship between a bony lesion and the dural sac.

D. Magnetic Resonance Imaging

Magnetic resonance imaging has become the imaging modality of choice for spinal lesions (7, 9, 41, 43, 53, 75, 77, 78). The advantages of MRI over other imaging modalities includes multiplanar imaging (sagittal, axial, and coronal planes), and superior soft tissue resolution. In addition, MRI is noninvasive with no exposure to ionizing radiation.

An optimal MRI study should include at the least sagittal and axial views utilizing T1- and T2-weighted images with and without gadolinium intravenous contrast. Any patient with a predominantly nonbony spinal column lesion should have a preoperative MRI, as this will be the imaging modality most likely used postoperatively to assess the extent of resection, and to follow-up with the patients.

V. SPECIFIC ENTITIES

Benign spinal tumors can be classified according to the anatomical compartment that they occupy. The most common benign spinal neoplasms are intradural-extramedullary (50–60% of the cases), followed by extradural in 28–30%, and intramedullary in 7–22% (21, 67, 68, 77, 78)

A. Extradural Tumors

1. Osteoid Osteoma and Osteoblastoma

Osteoid osteoma and osteoblastomas are benign bony lesions that can involve the spinal column in approximately 10% and 40% of the cases respectively. These lesions have a high predilection for the posterior elements of the spine (1, 38, 42, 57, 74, 77). There is a higher prevalence among males. Patients usually present in their second or third decade of life, complaining of persistent back pain that is unrelated to activity, and most noticeable at night (38, 44, 77, 78). This pain characteristically responds well to aspirin. Significant spinal deformity can be associated with these benign bony lesions. Scoliosis can be present in 50–60% of these patients with tumors of the thoracolumbar spine (1, 37, 42, 57). Radiologically, on axial CT scans, osteoid osteomas exhibit thickened, sclerotic bone surrounding a lucency. Osteoblastomas appear as well-defined expansile lesions.

Osteoid osteomas and osteoblastomas have similar gross appearances and are histologically identical (38, 42, 44, 57, 77). They can be distinguished by size. Osteoid osteomas are well-defined lesions with limited growth potential and are less than 2 cm in diameter. Osteoblastomas are larger than 2 cm in diameter and can involve more than one vertebrae. Grossly, these tumors can be cystic, consisting of dense bone separated by a hypervascular tissue. There can also be an expansile, homogenous, granular mass. The highly vascular tissue can easily hemorrhage and rupture through the cortical bone extending into the epidural space or paraspinous soft tissue. Microscopically, these tumors have a chaotic arrangement of woven bony spicules with surrounding ostoblasts and a rich fibrovascular stroma and intervening connective tissue. There may be areas of hemorrhage and cyst formation. The cortical bone can be resorbed to the extent that only trabecular-like remnants are visible.

Treatment for ostoid osteomas and osteoblastomas is excision and radical curettage of the surrounding bone. This results in symptomatic pain relief, and the spinal deformity can also be corrected (37, 44, 57).

2. Aneurysmal Bone Cyst

Aneurysmal bone cysts of the spine are rare, benign lesions that occur in young individuals aged 5 to 20 years (34, 77, 78). They are more common in females. Aneurysmal bone cysts are usually located in the lumbar region and most often involve the posterior elements.

Radiographically the lesions are expansile and osteolytic, with a soft bubbly appearance and thinned-out surrounding cortex (Fig. 1). Grossly, they consist of anastamosing cavernous spaces filled with blood. Aneurysmal bone cysts are expansile lesions with a cystic cavity lined by a rubbery, fleshy vascular tissue. Microscopically, there are long delicate spicules of woven or lamellar bone separating fibrous tissue and large vascular spaces. There can be lakes of blood in spaces lined by flattened cells. Treatment consists of resection of the cyst and curettage, which usually is curative. There is a recurrence rate of 25% after incomplete resection (34, 77, 78).

3. Hemangiomas

Spinal hemangiomas are relatively common lesions, being present in 10–11% of autopsies (2, 13, 22, 77, 80). They are often asymptomatic (approximately 60%), and are more common in females with a peak incidence in the fourth to sixth decades of life. Hemangiomas become symptomatic after a pathological compression fracture or epidural extension (usually from acute hemorrhage). Spinal hemangiomas are predominantly located in the vertebral body, most commonly involving the thoracic spine. These benign bony lesions may be solitary or multiple, and have been associated with spinal deformities. Infrequently, hemangiomas can present with spinal cord compression (2, 13, 80).

Hemangiomas have a characteristic plain radiographic appearance of vertical striations in the vertebral bodies secondary to the abnormally thickened trabeculae from the reactive ossification around the hemangioma. This produces a character-

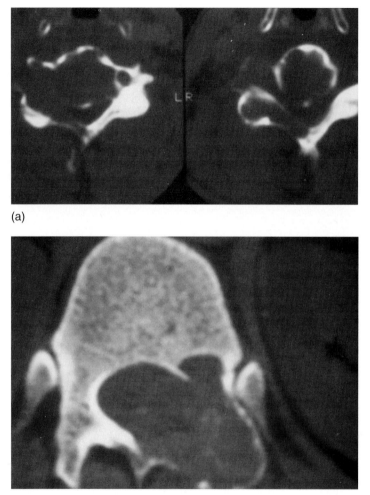

(a)

(b)

Figure 1   Aneurysm bone cyst of the cervical and thoracic spine. (a) Axial CT scans of the cervical spine demonstrating bubbly appearing, lytic, expansile mass involving the anterior and posterior elements. (b) Axial CT scan of the thoracic spine demonstrating a lytic, scalloped, expansile mass of the posterior elements. Note the thinned-out cortical bone.

istic "honey-combed" or "polka dot" appearance seen on axial CTs. In addition, paravertebral soft tissue masses can be seen, representing a paravertebral hematoma, or expansion of the hematoma into the soft tissue space (2, 80).

Grossly, hemangiomas arise in the bone marrow or the periosteum. There is resorbtion of the underlying bone that produces the characteristic honeycomb appearance. Histologically, they consist of capillaries, cavernous and venous blood vessels. There is an abundance of capillary channels and large dilated vascular spaces lined by endothelial cells. The intervening stroma is fibrous. There are occasional, larger feeding vessels, and there can be significant fatty replacement of the bone marrow.

Hemangiomas are radiosensitive lesions. However, in a symptomatic patient with neurological deficit or spinal deformity, surgical treatment becomes necessary.

4. Chordoma

Chordomas are rare, midline tumors arising from the embryonal remnants of the primitive notochord (3, 14, 55, 63, 73, 77, 78). Chordomas are slow growing, indolent but locally invasive tumors with the capacity to cause extensive bone destruction. They can reach large sizes before detection. Chordomas occur in all age groups but are commonly seen in the fifth or sixth decades of life.

Approximately 50% of chordomas arise in the sacrococcygeal region, 35% in the clivus and spheno-occipital regions, and 15% in the true vertebrae above the sacrum (14, 73, 77, 78). Symptoms depend on the location of involvement. Sacral chordomas usually present with pain or a sacral mass (often detected by rectal examination) causing bowel and/or bladder dysfunction. Clivus chordomas present with cranial nerve and brainstem dysfunction. Radiographically, chordomas appear as destructive, lytic bony lesions (Fig. 2). Mixed inhomogenous solid and cystic components are frequent, and calcification can occur in 30–70% of the cases. Spread to adjacent vertebrae is also commonly seen (14, 73, 77, 78).

Grossly, chordomas are lobulated and have cystic and solid components. They can resemble cartilaginous tumors. Tumor consistency varies from soft and gelatinous to ossified and calcified. The bony periosteum forms a pseudocapsule around the tumor. Microscopically, chordomas are separated into lobules by fibrous connective tissue septa. There is an extensive mucopolysaccharide basophilic matrix within which there are single, trabecular, or cord-like arrangements of cells containing mucin. These are polygonal, vacuolated, physaliphorous (soap bubble) cells with a clear cytoplasm that is divided by delicate septa into compartments (3, 55, 63).

Treatment of chordomas is surgical resection. In most cases, extensive surgical removal with a generous tissue margin is the goal. The overall prognosis, however, is poor because these tumors are locally invasive and frequently not

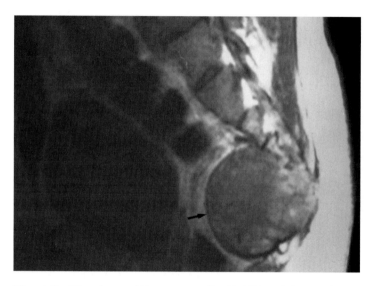

Figure 2 Chordoma of the sacrum. Sagittal T1-weighted MRI showing a large, destructive sacral mass (arrow) with a mixed signal intensity.

amenable to complete surgical resection. Adjuvant radiation and chemotherapy have not been found to be very effective. Chordomas can eventually metastasize in up to one-third of the patients (73, 77, 78, 14). The invasive characteristic of this tumor frequently prevents complete surgical excision.

5. Ganglioneuroma

Ganglioneuromas are slow-growing, benign tumors arising from mature sympathetic ganglion cells. They are the benign counterparts of neuroblastomas (the most common systemic malignant tumor in infancy). In contrast to neuroblastomas, which present during infancy, ganglioneuromas present during adolescence and early adulthood. Because of their slow growth, ganglioneuromas can reach large sizes before becoming symptomatic. Paravertebral ganglioneuromas can grow into the spinal canal and cause cord compression. Grossly, they are well delineated and encapsulated and can extend epidurally across several spinal levels. Histologically, ganglioneuromas are made of mature but architecturally abnormal neurons (multiple nuclei with irregular processes), fibroblasts, and Schwann cells. The treatment for ganglioneuromas is surgical resection (76).

B. Intradural-Extramedullary Tumors

The most common intradural-extramedullary tumors—nerve sheath tumors (neurofibromas and schwannomas) and meningiomas—comprise 80–90% of the cases, followed by congenital lesions (dermoids, epidermoids, teratoma, enteric cysts, and arachnoid cysts) (7, 67, 71, 77, 78).

1. Schwannomas and Neurofibromas

Schwannomas (neurilemoma, neurinoma) and neurofibromas are the most common types of intradural-extramedullary tumors. They are benign, slow-growing nerve sheath tumors arising from neoplastic Schwann cells. They most often arise from the dorsal sensory roots. Multiple lesions are common. Although these lesions are predominantly intradural-extramedullary, up to 15% can be extradural, and 15% can have both extradural and intradural components (41, 59, 67). The latter pattern gives rise to the characteristic "dumbbell" shape, as the tumor grows through the neural foramen and into the paravertebral tissues. Significant spinal cord or nerve root compression occurs late in the disease. Symptoms are usually radicular secondary to compression of the nerve roots. The sensory roots are usually involved first. As the tumor enlarges, spinal cord compression can occur.

Neurofibromas of the spine are associated with the type I (NF-I/Von Recklinghausen's) and type II (NF-2) neurofibromatosis syndromes (67, 78). Neurofibromas are relatively evenly distributed throughout the spinal canal, with 39% in the thoracic, 32% in the lumbar, and 23% in the cervical region.

Radiographically, neural foramen enlargement and pedicular erosion are common findings with dumbbell-shaped lesions. Schwannomas and neurofibromas enhance with contrast, and can have a more intensely enhancing surrounding as compared to the center of the lesion (Fig. 3). In addition, schwannomas can also exhibit cystic components (41, 46, 67).

Schwannomas and neurofibromas are distinguishable from one another by their morphological and histological features. They are both firm and rubbery on their surfaces. Grossly, schwannomas are well-encapsulated, well-circumscribed, round or oval lesions that displace the nerve roots they are associated with. They grow eccentrically and can exhibit cystic degeneration. In contrast, neurofibromas engulf and enclose the nerve roots they are associated with. In addition, neurofibromas are less well delineated and encapsulated and lack cystic degeneration and necrosis (3, 55, 63, 69).

Histologically, schwannomas have a mixture of two distinctive patterns of organization described as Antoni A and Antoni B. The tumor is devoid of any axons or functional neural tissue. Antoni A regions are characterized by a densely packed array of fusiform, spindle-shaped cells arranged in compact, interlacing bundles. Antoni B areas are less densely populated with cells and are accompanied by delicate reticulin and collagen fibers (3, 55, 63, 69). Neurofibromas contain a mixture of proliferative Schwann cells and fibroblasts growing between dispersed nerve fibers, along with numerous strands of collagen and reticulin fibers. Neurofibromas have a histological organization similar to Antoni B areas seen in schwannomas (3, 55, 62, 63, 69).

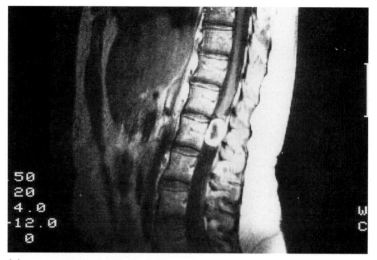

(a)

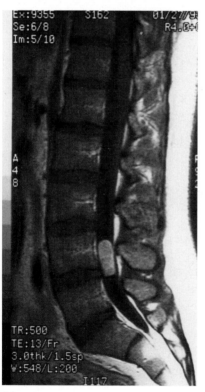

(b)

Figure 3 Lumbar schwannoma and neurofibroma. (a) Sagittal T1-weighted MRI with gadolinium enhancement demonstrating a well-circumscribed cauda equina schwannoma. Note the preferential enhancement of the periphery of the lesion. (b) Sagittal T1-weighted MRI with gadolinium enhancement showing a well-circumscribed, uniformly enhancing cauda equina neurofibroma.

Surgery with the goal of total resection is the treatment of choice for both neurofibromas and schwannomas. With neurofibromas, the involved nerve root is always sacrificed during attempts at gross total resection. With schwannomas, if an important nerve root is involved, it may be possible to preserve it by dissecting the tumor off the root using microsurgical technique in conjunction with intra-operative electrophysiological monitoring.

2. Meningiomas

Meningiomas are the second most common intradural-extramedullary tumors. Meningiomas are slow-growing, benign lesions predominantly occurring in older individuals (usually females), with a peak incidence in the fifth and sixth decades of life. Meningiomas have a high predilection for the thoracic region, occurring there in approximately 80% of the cases. The incidence in the cervical region is 15–16% and 3% in the lumbar area (7, 51, 67, 70, 74).

Meningiomas are extra-axial lesions arising from the arachanoid cells. They are well circumscribed and are usually located laterally or ventrolaterally to the spinal cord, being firmly attached to the dura with a broad base. Meningiomas can be extradural in up to 15% of the cases. Multiple spinal meningiomas are rare (7, 67, 70).

Radiographically, meningiomas can be calcified and are relatively isointense to the spinal cord on T1- and T2-weighted imaging. They uniformly enhance with contrast (Fig. 4), and most have a broad-based dural attachment with occasional dural tails (46, 70).

Meningiomas are classified into several important histological patterns, most commonly consisting of meningothelial (syncytial), fibrous, or mixed (transitional) patterns (3, 55, 63). All types of meningiomas have a tendency for the cells to form whorls or balls that can calcify, thus forming psammoma bodies. The most common histological type of meningioma is meningotheliomatous (syncytial), characterized by a lobulated arrangement composed of uniformly compact tumor cells without clearly defined cellular membranes, giving the appearance of a syncytium. A sharply defined, fibrous stroma separates these cells. The fibrous pattern of meningiomas has elongated spindle cells with closely interwoven and abundant bundles of collagen and reticulin fibers separating individual cells. The transitional form of meningiomas contains a mixture of meningothelial and fibrous types of pattern. The treatment for spinal meningiomas is gross total excision and duraplasty when necessary.

3. Dermoids, Epidermoids, and Teratomas

These are congenital lesions arising from the maldevelopment and displacement of tissues during the early period of neural tube closure in the embryo (third to fifth weeks of gestation). These lesions are far more common in children than adults (4, 24, 55).

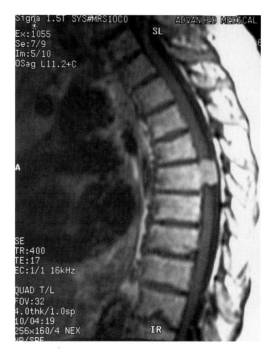

Figure 4 Thoracic meningioma. Sagittal T1-weighted post gadolinium MRI demonstrating a uniformly enhancing, well-circumscribed mass with a broad-based attachment to the ventral dura.

Epidermoids

Epidermoids most commonly arise from congenital epidermal cell rests or occasionally iatrogenically, via a lumbar puncture that carries with it a portion of viable epidermis (28, 29, 67, 68). Epidermoids arise eccentrically in the leptomeninges. They can comprise up to 10% of intraspinal tumors in children (5). Congenital spinal epidermoids usually occur in the conus or cauda equina, whereas acquired lesions occur in the lower lumbar region.

Radiographically, there can be apparent associated bony defects such as spina bifida. Epidermoids have a signal intensity that is isointense or slightly hyperintense compared to the cerebrospinal fluids (CSF) on CT scans.

Grossly, epidermoids consist of a smooth, glistening, nodular cyst capsule containing white flaky keratinous debris generated by the keratinocytes that arise from the proliferating epithelium. Histologically, the epidermoid cyst contains layers of stratified squamous epithelium resting on a thin connective tissue layer (55, 63). Cyst spillage in situ can cause aseptic meningitis (64). Treatment of epidermoids is surgical resection. Cyst recurrence can result if some of the epithelial rests are left behind.

Dermoids

Spinal dermoid cysts are more common in females and have a tendency to occur in the midline along the craniospinal axis (4, 24, 28). Dermoids usually occur in the lumbar spine, with 25% occurring in the sacrococcygeal region. The underlying pathogenesis occurs during embryogenesis and is most likely secondary to abnormal separation of the ectoderm from the neural tube. Dermoids are usually intradural-extramedullary but at times can extend extradurally. They can comprise up to 20% of intradural tumors seen during the first years of life (4, 24).

Spinal dermoids frequently communicate with the skin through dermal sinus tracts. There can also be an associated spina bifida. It is not always true, however, that a patient with a dermoid cyst also harbors a dermal sinus tract. In fact, less than one-third of patients with dermoid cysts have a dermal sinus tract, whereas approximately one-half of patients with a dermal sinus tract have a dermoid cyst. The presence of a dermal sinus tract predisposes the patient to the risk of meningitis. Recurrent meningitis should alert the clinician to the possibility of a dermal sinus tract. Radiographically, dermoids have a variable signal intensity pattern (Fig. 5), including fat signal intensity due to their content of fatty tissue.

Grossly, dermoids are smooth-appearing, well-defined, lobulated, cyst-like structures containing thick, yellow (buttery, cheesy) sebaceous fluid, desquamated epithelium, and at times hair. Histologically, skin adnexal structures and appendages such as sweat glands, hair follicles, sebaceous glands, and nerve twigs can be apparent beneath a stratified squamous epithelial lining of the cyst. Islands of cartilage and teeth may also be present (3, 55, 63). Furthermore, in contrast to epidermoids, up to 20% of dermoids can have calcification (28). Dermoids can also be caused iatrogenically via a lumbar puncture that carries elements of the skin intrathecally.

The treatment of dermoids is surgical excision. If a dermal sinus tract is present, it should be completely excised. Every attempt should be made at complete removal of the dermoid cyst in whole, because if contents spill into the subarachnoid space, a chemical meningitis or arachanoiditis can occur.

Teratomas

Teratomas are complex tumors containing elements of more than one component of the germ layer at various stages of maturation. Teratoma is the most common tumor of the sacrococcygeal region in children (45). They are three times more common in females. Teratomas are often cystic and can be histologically mature or immature. Immature teratomas are composed of primitive (em-

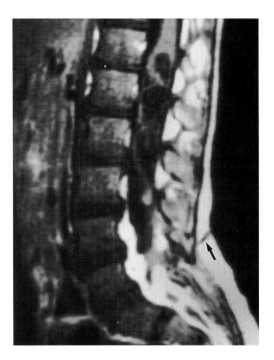

Figure 5 Lumbar dermoid and dermal sinus. Sagittal T1-weighted MRI show-ing a lumbar lesion of variable signal intensity, as well as the presence of a dermal sinus tract (arrow).

bryonic/fetal) ectoderm, endoderm, and mesoderm. Mature teratomas consist of differentiated tissue resembling adult tissues, including areas with organ differ-entiation and formation. In addition, teratomas can exhibit malignant features and grow very rapidly. The ectodermal remnants can be represented by skin, adnexa, and neural tissue. The mesodermal derivatives can include cartilage, bone, fat, fibrous tissue, and smooth muscles. Endodermal elements include respiratory and gastrointestinal tract epithelium, and other gastrointestinal tis-sues (3, 55, 56, 63). Treatment of teratomas includes surgical resection, chemo-therapy, radiation, or combinations thereof, depending on the histological evi-dence of malignant features.

4. Neurenteric Cyst

Neurenteric cysts are embryologically derived from endodermal tissue that is displaced dorsally into the spinal canal (35). Thus, abnormalities of the anterior vertebrae such as anterior spina bifida are common, whereas the posterior elements are usually intact. They can extend dorsally to compress or involve the spinal cord These cysts arise from the endodermal tissue of the foregut region that also gives rise to the esophagus and respiratory system.

Intraspinal neurenteric cysts are located ventral to the spinal cord in the thoracic (50%), cervical (40%), and cervicothoracic region (10%). These cysts are most commonly intradural-extramedullary but at times can be intramedullary. The presenting features include neurological deficits from cord compression and meningitis. In addition, a mediastinal mass often can be seen. Radiographic evaluation usually demonstrates an anteriorly located cystic mass that is slightly hyperintense as compared to the CSF (Fig. 6).

The cyst fluid has been described as brown to black, chocolate, coffee-ground, mucoid, or occasionally colorless. Histologically, the cyst is lined with simple or pseudostratified columnar epithelium with an underlying muscle layer in some cases. The epithelial linings are mucin secreting, similar to those of the respiratory and gastrointestinal tract (55, 63). Neurenteric cysts communicate with a mediastinal cyst via an anterior defect in the vertebral body in 69% of the patients.

Treatment includes drainage of the cyst and conservative resection of the cyst wall that is adherent to the spinal cord. In addition, the anterior dural defect should be repaired. The approach to the cyst is usually anterior (transthoracic). Posterior or lateral approaches via laminectomy or costotransversectomy, respectively, can also be performed. The prognosis depends on the severity of the preoperative neurological defect, with the deficits arresting or improving after the operation.

5. Arachnoid Cysts

Intradural spinal arachnoid cysts are rare lesions arising from the arachnoid of the spinal cord. The etiology of arachnoid cysts is unclear. They are believed to be caused by developmental abnormalities, inflamation, or trauma. The cysts usually become clinically apparent in the fifth decade of life (17, 58). They become symptomatic when cord compression occurs. Arachnoid cysts are usually intradural and have a predilection to be located posteriorly or posterolaterally in the thoracic region (Fig. 7). Males and females are equally affected. The signal intensity of arachnoid cysts is similar to that of CSF and because they communicate with the subarachnoid space, they can become filled with contrast dye after myelography. Grossly, the cysts are translucent, containing clear CSF-like fluid. Histologically there are arachnoidal cells lining the cyst cavity. Treatment includes operative excision or fenestration of the cysts, thus relieving the mass effect. This results in the resolution of symptoms in the majority of patients. Arachnoid cysts, however, can recur.

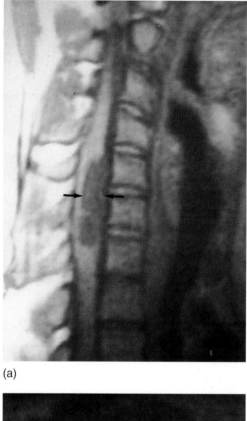

(a)

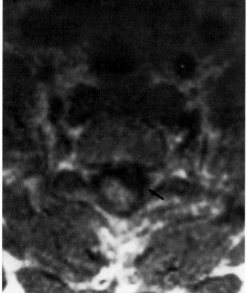

(b)

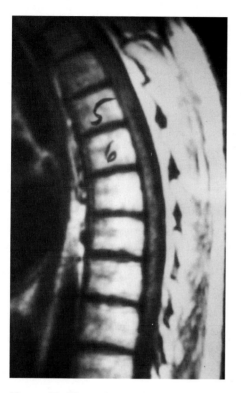

Figure 7 Thoracic arachnoid cyst. Sagittal T1-weighted MRI of the thoracic spine showing a posteriorly located arachnoid cyst extending across several spinal segments.

VI. TREATMENT AND PROGNOSIS

A. Surgery

In 1887, Victor Horsley performed the first successful operation for a spinal cord tumor (27). It was not until the 1920s that Charles Elsberg reported on the first series of intradural spinal operations (19). Today, the morbidity and mortality of spinal surgery has decreased as a result of the advances in surgical technique and instruments along with improved monitoring capabilities. Important

Figure 6 Thoracic neurenteric cyst. (a) Sagittal T1-weighted MRI showing an anteriorly located cystic lesion (arrows) with signal intensity that is slightly hyperintense as compared to CSF. (b) Axial T1-weighted MRI of the thoracic spine demonstrating an anteriorly located cystic lesion (arrow).

advances in the diagnosis and therapeutic modalities of spinal neoplasms include: (1) Improved imaging modalities such as MRI for accurate localization and diagnosis of the lesion; (2) Development of the operative microscope and microsurgical instrumentation; (3) Intraoperative ultrasound to accurately delineate the extent of the tumor, demonstrate tumor characteristics, and critique the extent of resection; (4) The ultrasonic cavitron aspirator (CUSA) (20) and the surgical laser; and (5) Intraoperative evoked potential monitoring including somatosensory and motor evoked potentials.

B. Surgical Indications and Rationale

The indications for surgery include neurological deficit, intractable pain, tissue diagnosis, unresponsiveness to other therapeutic modalities, and spinal deformity and instability. The goal of surgery includes decompression of the spinal cord, tumor resection or debulking, tissue diagnosis, correction of spinal deformity, and stabilization of the spine.

The preoperative neurological status of the patient is usually a good indicator of postoperative neurological function and recovery. A patient with a severe neurological dysfunction such as paraplegia usually does not recover, whereas patients with mild dysfunction can often recover in part or completely. Thus, early surgical management before the onset of significant neurological dysfunction is critical.

1. Surgical Approach and Technique

The selection of an approach is dependent on the rationale and goal of the operation, the accessibility of the lesion, its predominant location (anterior, posterior, cervical, thoracic, lumbar), the extent of involvement, and the presence of spinal deformity. There are numerous approaches to the spine but the most commonly used include the posterior laminectomy approach, the anterior approaches consisting of anterior cervical as well as transthoracic, transabdominal, or retroperitoneal for thoracic and lumbar lesions, and posterolateral (costotransversectomy) approaches (11, 31–33, 39, 40).

Posterior Approach

Laminectomy is the most commonly used posterior procedure. It is particularly useful for intradural lesions. Laminectomy provides easy access for tumor resection, debulking, and tissue diagnosis. Osteoplastic laminotomies using high-speed air drills have become increasingly prevalent. This allows for replacement of the bone with subsequent osteogenesis and posterior fusion, which may be beneficial in preventing subsequent spinal deformity (60).

Laminectomy, however, is not as useful for anteriorly located lesions (in particular bony lesions), where access to the anterior columns would be limited and difficult. In addition, with significant involvement of the anterior elements by the tumor, laminectomy can cause disruption of all three spinal columns (16), resulting in further spinal deformity and instability. Furthermore, post laminectomy spinal instability can be a possible iatrogenic complication of multi-level laminectomy (23, 49, 79).

Posterolateral Approach (Costotransversectomy)

Costotransversectomy can be particularly useful for upper thoracic lesions (39). It provides access to the posterior column and the lateral aspect of the vertebral body. The patient is placed in the lateral position. For a more rostral thoracic lesion, the scapula may need to be mobilized. Once the costotransverse ligaments and joints are visualized, the ribs are resected. Removal of the transverse processes can also enhance access to the intervertebral foramen. The approach is usually extrapleural, and if extended, the anterior part of the vertebral body can also be accessed.

Anterior and Anterolateral Approaches

With the advent of the anterior and anterolateral approaches, anteriorly located lesions in the thoracic and lumbar region have been approached safely and effectively. These approaches include transthoracic for thoracic lesions and transabdominal and retroperitoneal for lumbar lesions (11, 39). For anterior approaches, patients are placed in the full lateral decubitus position. The side of the exposure is determined by the location of the bony involvement. If the involvement is symmetrical, then the exposure is usually performed from the left side.

Using the transthoracic approach, the spine can be exposed from T2 to T12 (11, 31–33, 39, 40). Exposure of the thoracic region can be accomplished using a posterolateral thoracotomy incision with transection of the latissimus dorsi muscle and anterior reflection of the serratus anterior muscles. The lateral aspect of the chest is opened two interspaces above the involved vertebral bodies. This provides exposure of the involved vertebral bodies because of the caudal angulation of the ribs in the middle and lower thoracic spine. Once the tumor and/or the involved vertebral bodies are identified, biopsy and resection using standard surgical techniques can be accomplished. Briefly, the normal disc spaces above and below the affected area are resected using sharp dissection and curettes. The junction between the ipsilateral pedicles and the respective vertebral bodies is identified to locate the anterior border of the spinal canal. All affected bone is resected using curettes, rongeurs, and a high-speed air drill. Enough bone should be resected to remove all compression of the posterior longitudinal ligament. Rostrally and caudally, the adjacent cartilaginous end plates are removed to allow for autologous bone grafting. After bony resection, the posterior longitudinal ligament is resected to expose the dura and to further resect the lesion compressing the neural tissue.

Subsequent to resection, vertebrectomy, and decompression, reconstruction of the vertebrae is performed. The choice of material for reconstruction after vertebrectomy depends on the type of tumor and the patients' life expectancy. Allograft or autografts are favored for vertebral body reconstruction in benign tumors. Methylmethacrylate can also be used, but in general only for patients with malignant tumors and short life expectancies (11).

Exposure of lumbar lesions can be accomplished using a retroperitoneal or transabdominal approach. In the retroperitoneal approach, an oblique incision from the tip of the twelfth rib into the lower abdomen allows forward mobilization of the peritoneum, abdominal contents, and psoas muscle as described (11).

The necessity for instrumentation depends on the level and extent of bony destruction by the tumor (11, 12, 32, 33, 39, 40, 61, 72). There are many devices for posterior or anterior instrumentation. For the most part, these perform similar functions and the choice usually depends on the surgeon's preference. In general, tumors with minimal or no bony involvement do not require further instrumentation in addition to bone grafting, unless the laminectomy has caused spinal instability. The thoracic spine above T11 is inherently stable because of fixation by the rib cage. Therefore, if there is only anterior and middle bony column involvement, as defined by Denis (16), then vertebral body replacement by bone without instrumentation is sufficient to restore stability. With three-column involvement, supplemental instrumentation becomes necessary. The thoracolumbar and lumbar spines are less stable than the thoracic spine due to the absence of ribs. Thus one-column or two-column destruction should have vertebral reconstruction with supplemental anterior instrumentation. If there is three-column involvement, then additional posterior stabilization should be utilized.

2. Intraoperative Monitoring

Intraoperative electrophysiological monitoring has greatly evolved over the past several years and is now an important adjunct to spinal surgery. Continuous somatosensory evoked potential (SSEP) monitoring and motor evoked potential (MEP) monitoring are helpful for continuous real-time analysis of the electrophysiological status of the spinal cord (15, 54). Somatosensory evoked potential monitoring can be carried out using stimulation of the posterior tibial nerve (at the ankle) and median nerve (at the wrist) while recording from subdermal scalp electrodes, or epidural electrodes rostral to the lesion. Motor evoked potential monitoring is carried out via stimulation of scalp electrodes overlying the motor cortex and recording from epidural electrodes caudal to the lesion. A decrease in the amplitude of the MEP or SSEP potentials by more than 50% of baseline, or acute changes in the potential, are considered significant changes, which are immediately conveyed to the surgeon who can then modify the procedure accordingly.

3. Radiotherapy and Chemotherapy

Radiotherapy does not appear to have a significant role in the treatment of most benign spinal tumors. This is in contrast to metastatic spinal lesions which have been shown to have some response to radiation. Most benign spinal tumors are amenable to surgical resection, and every attempt at total resection should be made. In addition, radiation-induced transverse myelitis of the spinal cord and possible neurological deterioration are potential complications that can be avoided. Radiation therapy may be of certain benefit in radiosensitive tumors such as hemangiomas. In addition, it may be of some benefit in cases where only biopsy or partial resection is possible (8, 26, 67, 68).

Chemotherapy, like radiation, appears to have a limited role in the treatment of benign spinal lesions. Of the lesions described, teratomas and chordomas may respond to chemotherapy, in particular to alkylating agents (30).

VII. CONCLUSION

In this chapter, we have provided an overview of the clinical presentation, diagnosis, imaging, pathology, and treatment of benign spinal tumors. There has been a great deal of progress in the diagnosis and management of spinal tumors since Victor Horsley first operated on a spinal tumor more than 100 years ago. The introduction of MRI and high resolution CT scanning has resulted in improved imaging capabilities, and thus allowing earlier diagnosis and better operative planning and localization. Advances in surgical technique, the development of new technical devices, and intraoperative elecrophysiological monitoring have significantly improved surgical outcome and survival while decreasing morbidity and mortality. In addition, the advancement in spinal instrumentation and stabilization has enhanced the ability to correct spinal deformities and prevent iatrogenic deformities.

Unlike metastatic spinal tumors, surgery is the treatment of choice for benign spinal tumors. Early diagnosis and good preoperative neurological status are important factors for a more favorable outcome. With continuous advances in imaging and surgical capabilities, along with the further development of adjuvant therapies, the management of benign spinal tumors can continue to have a better prognosis in the future.

REFERENCES

1. Amacher AL, El Tomeg A. Spinal osteoblastoma in children and adolescents. Childs Nerv Syst 1985; 1:29–32.

2. Baker ND, Greenspan A, Neuwirth M. Symptomatic vertebral hemangiomas: A report of 4 cases. Skeletal Radiol 1986; 15:458–463.
3. Berger PC, Scheithauer BW, Vogel. Surgical Pathology of the Nervous System and Its Coverings. New York: Churchill Livingston, 1991.
4. Carmel PW. Brain tumors of disordered embryogenesis. In: Youmans JR, ed. Neurological Surgery. Philadelphia: WB Saunders, 1990; 3241–3244.
5. Caro PA, Marks HG, Keret D, et al. Intraspinal epidermoid tumors in children: Problems in recognition and imaging techniques for diagnosis. J Ped Orthopaed 1991; 11:288–293.
6. Carpenter MD, Sutin J. Human Neuroanatomy. Baltimore: Williams & Wilkins, 1983.
7. Cassidy JR, Ducker TB. Intradural neural tumors. In: Frymoyer, JW ed. The Adult Spine: Principles and Practice. New York: Raven Press, 1991; 889–903.
8. Chun HC, Schmidt-Urlich RK, Wolfson A, et al. External beam radiotherapy for primary spinal cord tumors. J of Neuro-Oncol 1990; 9:211–217.
9. Chamberlain C, Sandy AD, Press GA. Spinal cord tumors: Gadolinium-DTPA-enhanced MR imaging. Neuroradialogy 1991; 33:469–474.
10. Citron N, Edgar MA, Sheehy J, Thomas DGT. Intramedullary spinal cord tumors presenting as scoliosis. J Bone Joint Surg 1984; 66B:513–517.
11. Cooper PR, Errico TJ, Martin R, Crawford B, Dibartolo T. A systemic approach to spinal reconstruction after anterior decompression for neoplastic disease of the thoracic and lumbar spine. Neurosurgery 1993; 32:1–8.
12. Cotrel Y, Dubousset J, Guillaumat M. New universal instrumentation in spine surgery. Clin Orthop 1988; 227:10–23.
13. Dagi TF, Schmidek HH. Vascular tumors of the spine. In: Sundaresan N, ed. Tumors of the Spine. Diagnosis and clinical mangement. Philadelphia: Saunders, 1990: 181–185.
14. Dahlin DC, McCarty CS. Chordoma. A study of 59 cases. Cancer 1952; 5:1170–1178.
15. Deletis V. Intraoperative monitoring of the functional integrity of the motor pathways. In: Devinsky O, Beric A, Dogali M, eds. Electrical and magnetic stimulation of the brain and spinal cord. New York: Raven Press, 1993: 201–214.
16. Denis F. The three column spine and its significance in the classification of acute thoracolumbar spine injuries. Spine 1983; 8:817–831.
17. Di Rocco C. Arachnoid cyst. In: Youmans JR, ed. Neurological Surgery. Philadelphia: WB Saunders, 1990: 1299–1325.
18. Edelstyn GA, Gillespie PJ, Grebell ES. The radiologic demonstration of osseous metastasis: Experimental observations. Clin Radiol 1967; 18:158–164.
19. Elsberg CA. Tumors of the spinal cord and the symptom of irradiation and compression of the spinal cord and nerve roots. In: Pathology, Symptomatology, Diagnosis, and Treatment. New York: Pzb Hoverg 1925: 206–239.
20. Epstein FJ. The cavitron ultrasonic aspirator in tumor surgery. Clin Neurosurg 1983; 31:497–505.
21. Fetell MR, Stein BM. Spinal tumors. In: Rowland LP, ed: Meritt's Text Book of Neurology. Philadelphia: Lea & Febiger, 1989: 350–364.

22. Fox MW, Onfrio BM. The natural history and management of symptomatic and asymptomatic vertebral hemangiomas. J Neurosurgery 1993; 78:36–45.

23. Fraser RD, Paterson DC, Simpson DA. Orthopaedic aspects of spinal tumors in children. J Bone Joint Surg 1977; 59B:143–151.

24. French BN. Midline fusion defects and defects of formation. In: Youmans JR, ed. Neurological Surgery. Philadelphia: WB Saunders, 1990: 1081–1235.

25. Fricke RD, Romine JS. Thoracic spinal cord tumors presenting with dysautonomic diarrhea. Gastroenterology 1977; 73:1152–1156.

26. Garcia DM. Primary spinal cord tumors treated with surgery and postoperative irradiation. Int J Radiat Oncol Biol Phys 1985; 11:1933–1939.

27. Gowers WR, Horsley V. A case of tumor of the spinal cord: removal, recovery. Medical Chirurgical Transactions (London) 1888; 71:377–430.

28. Guidetti V, Gagliardi FM. Epidermoid and dermoid cyst. Clinical evaluation and late surgical results. J Neurosurg 1977; 47:12–18.

29. Gutin PH, et al. Cerebral convexity epidermoid tumor subsequent to multiple percutaneous subdural aspirations. Case Report. J Neurosurg 1980; 52:574–577.

30. Harmon DC. Chemotherapy. In: Sundaresan N, ed. Tumors of the Spine: Diagnosis and clinical management. Philadelphia: WB Saunders, 1990: 93–98.

31. Harrington KD. The use of methylmetacrylate for vertebral body replacement and anterior stabilization of pathologic fracture. Dislocation of the spine due to metastatic malignant disease. J Bone Joint Surg 1981; 63A:36–46.

32. Harrington KD. Metastatic disease of the spine. In: Harrington KD, ed. Orthopaedic management of metastatic bone disease. St Louis. CV Mosby Company, 1988: 309–383.

33. Harrington KD. Current concepts review. Metastatic disease of the spine. J Bone Joint Surg 1986; 68A:1110–1115.

34. Hay MC, Paterson D, Taylor TK. Aneurysmal bone cysts of the spine. J Bone Joint Surg (Br) 1978; 60:406–411.

35. Jackson FE. Neurenteric cysts. Report of a case of neurenteric cyst with associated chronic meningitis and hydrocephalus. J Neurosurg 1961; 18:678–682.

36. Katzman H, Waugh T, Berdon W. Skeletal changes following irradiation of childhood tumors. J Bone Joint Surg 1969; 51A:825–842.

37. Keim HA, Reina EG. Osteoid-osteoma as a cause of scoliosis. J Bone Joint Surg 1975; 57A:159–163.

38. Klein MH, Shankman S. Osteoid Osteoma: A radiologic and pathological correlation. Skeletal Radiol 1992; 21:23–31.

39. Kostuik JP. Surgical approaches to the thoracic and thoracolumbar spine. In: Frymoyer JW ed. The Adult Spine: Principles and Practice. New York: Raven Press, 1991: 1243–1265.

40. Kostuik JP, Errico TJ, Gleason TF, Errico CC. Spinal stabilization of vertebral column tumors. Spine 1988; 13:250–256.

41. Li MH, Holtas S, Larsson E-M. MR imaging of intradural-extramedullary tumors. Acta Radiol 1992; 33:207–212.

42. Lichtenstein L, Sawyer WR. Benign osteoblastoma: Further observations and report of 20 additional cases. J Bone Joint Surg 1964; 46A:755–765.

43. MacDonald DR. Clinical manifestations. In: Sundaresan N, ed. Tumors of the spine: Diagnosis and Clinical Management. Philadelphia: WB Saunders, 1990: 6–20.

44. Marsh BW, Bonfiglio M, Brady LP, Enneking WF. Benign osteoblastoma: Ranges of manifestations. J Bone Joint Surg (AM) 1975; 57:1–9.

45. Mahour GH, Walley MM, Trivedi SN, et al. Teratomas in infancy and childhood: Experience with 81 cases. Surgery 1974; 76:309–318.

46. Matsumoto S, Hasu K, Uchinio A, et al. MRI of intradural-extramedullary spinal neurinomas and meningiomas. Clin Imaging 1993;17:46–52.

47. Mayfield JK, Riseborough EJ, Jaffe N, Nehem ME. Spinal deformity in children treated for neuroblastoma. J Bone Joint Surg 1981; 63A:183–193.

48. McCormick PC, Post KD, Stein BM. Intradural extramedullary tumors in adults. Neurosurg Clin N Am 1990; 1:591–608.

49. Mikawa Y, Shikata J, Yamamuro T. Spinal deformity and instability after multilevel cervical laminectomy. Spine 1987; 12:6–11.

50. Nicholas JJ, Christy WC. Spinal pain made worse by recumbency: A clue to spinal cord tumors Arch Phys Med Rehab 1986; 67:598–600.

51. Nittner K. Spinal meningiomas, neurinomas, neurofibromas, and hourglass tumors. In: Vinken PJ, Bruyn BW, ed. Handbook of Clinical Neurology. Amsterdam, New York: North Holland Publishing Company, 1978: 172–322.

52. Nokes SR, Murtagh FR, Jone JD, et al. Childhood scoliosis: MR imaging. Radiology 1987; 164:791–797.

53. Norman D, Mills CM, Brant-Zawadzki M, Yeates A, Crooks LE, Kaufman L. Magnetic resonance imaging of the spinal cord and canal: Potentials and limitations. AJR 1984; 141:1147–1152.

54. Nuwer MR. Electrophysiologic evaluation and monitoring of spinal cord and root function. Neurosurg Clin N Am 1990; 1:533–549.

55. Okazaki H. Chordoma. In: Fundamentals of neuropathology. Morphologic Basis of Neurologic Disorders. New York: Igaku Shoin, 1989.

56. Parisi JE, Mena H. Nonglial tumor. In: Nelson JS, JE Parisis, Schochet SS, eds. Principles and Practice of Neuropathology. Philadelphia: Mosby, 1993: 226–257.

57. Pettine KA, Klassen RA. Osteoid-osteoma and osteoblastoma of the spine. J Bone Joint Surg 1986; 68A:354–361.

58. Pau A, Viale-sehrbundt E, Turjas S. Spinal intradural arachnoid cysts. Neurochirurgia 1982, 25:19–21.

59. Post MJD. Primary spinal and cord neoplasms. In: Categorical course on spinal and cord imaging. Am Soc of Neuroradiol 1988: 58–70.

60. Raimondi J, Gutierez FA, Di Rocco. Laminotomy and total reconstruction of the posterior spine in childhood. J Neurosurg 1976; 45:555–560.

61. Roy Camille R, Saillant G, Mazel C. Internal fixation of the lumbar spine with pedicle screw plating. Clin Orthop 1986; 203:7–17.

62. Rubinstein LJ. The malormative central nervous system lesions in the central and peripheral forms of neurofibromatosis: A neuropathological study of 22 cases. Ann NY Acad Sci 1986; 486:14–29.

63. Russel DS, Rubinstein LJ. Pathology of the Tumors of the Nervous System. Baltimore: Wiliam & Wilkins, 1982.
64. Schwartz JF, Balentine JD. Recurrent meningitis due to an intracranial epidermoid. Neurology 1978; 28:124–129.
65. Scotti G, Scialfa G, Colombo N, Landoni L. MR imaging of intradural extramedullary tumors of the cervical spine. J Comput Assist Tomogr 1985; 9:1037–1041.
66. Sim FH, Dahlin DC, Stauffer RN, Laws ER. Primary bone tumor simulating lumbar disc syndrome. Spine 1977; 2:65–74.
67. Simeone FA. Intradural tumors. In: Simeone FA, Rothman, ed. The Spine. Philadelphia: WB Saunders, 1992: 1515–1528.
68. Simeone FA. Spinal cord tumors in adults. In: Youmans JR, ed. Neurological Surgery. Philadelphia: WB Saunders, 1990: 3531–3547.
69. Smith D, Schmider HH. Tumors of the nerve sheath involving the spine. In: Sundaresan N, ed. Tumors of the Spine: Diagnosis and Clinical Management. Philadelphia: WB Saunders, 1990: 226–228.
70. Solerdo CL, Fornari M, Giombini S, et al. Spinal meningiomas. Review of 174 operated cases. Neurosurgery 1989; 25:153–160.
71. Stein BM. Spinal intradural tumors. In: Wilkins RH, Renagachary SS. Neurosurgery. New York: McGraw-Hill, 1985: 1048–1061.
72. Steffee AD, Biscup RS, Sitkowski DJ. Segmental spinal plates with pedicle screw fixation: A new internal fixation device for disorders of the lumbar and thoracolumbar spine. Clin Orthop 1986; 203:45–53.
73. Sundaresan N, Rosenthal DI, Schiller AL, Krol G. Chordoma. In: Sundaresan N, ed. Tumors of the Spine: Diagnosis and Clinical Management. Philadelphia: WB Saunders, 1990: 192–213.
74. Sypert GW. Osteoid-osteoma and osteoblastoma of the spine. In: Sundaresan N, ed. Tumors of the Spine: Diagnosis and Clinical Management. Philadelphia: WB Saunders, 1990: 117–128.
75. Takemoto K, Matsumura Y, Hashimoto H, Inooue Y, Fukuda T, Shakudo M. MR imaging of intraspinal tumors–capability in histological differentiation and compartmentalization of extramedullary tumors. Neuroradiology 1988; 30:303–309.
76. Tomita T. Special considerations in surgery of pediatric spine tumors. In: Sundaresan N, ed. Tumors of the Spine: Diagnosis and Clinical Management. Philadelphia: WB Saunders, 1990: 267–269.
77. Weinstein JN. Differential diagnosis and surgical treatment of primary benign and malignant neoplasms. In: Frymoyer JW, ed. The Adult Spine: Principles and Practice. New York: Raven Press, 1991: 829–860.
78. Weinstein JN, Mclain RF. Tumors of the spine. In: Simeone FA, Rothman RH, ed. The Spine. Philadelphia: WB Saunders, 1992: 1279–1318.
79. Yasuoka S, Peterson HA, MacCcarty CS. Incidence of spinal column deformity after multilevel laminectomy in children and adults. J Neurosurg 1982; 57:441–445.
80. Yochum TR, Lile RL, Schultz GD, et al. Acquired spinal stenosis secondary to an expanding thoracic vertebral hemangioma. Spine 1993; 18:299–305.

14

Primary Intramedullary Spinal Cord Tumors of Children and Adults

Shlomi Constantini
Tel-Aviv-Sourasky Medical Center and Dana Children's Hospital, Tel Aviv, Israel

Fred Epstein
Beth Israel Medical Center, North Division, New York, New York

I. INTRODUCTION

Intramedullary spinal cord tumors (IMSCT) are relatively uncommon neoplasms accounting for only 4–10% of central nervous system tumors. Whereas ependymomas of the cauda equina region have long been successfully removed, intramedullary astrocytomas and other gliomas have not been viewed with surgical optimism. There has been little impetus to modify the approach of biopsy, dural decompression, and radiation therapy despite the recognition that after a relatively short remission, serious disability or death ensues. This "traditional" attitude was based on the assumption that it is not feasible to carry out extensive removal of tumors from within the center of the spinal cord without a great likelihood of inflicting additional neurological injury (5,14). This is particularly unfortunate as most of these neoplasms are low-grade gliomas that are microscopically identical to their "sister" tumors that occur in the cerebellum and are surgically curable (2,13).

This chapter will address the overall approach to patients with intramedullary spinal cord tumors. We will direct most of our attention to astrocytomas and ependymomas. The content of this chapter is based on the experience of the senior author, Dr. Epstein, with radical excision of more than 350 intramedullary spinal cord tumors from 1980–1992 (4,7,8,11).

II. INCIDENCE AND PATHOLOGY

Spinal cord tumors are relatively rare neoplasms. Whereas in adult life intramedullary tumors comprise only about 25% of all intraspinal neoplasms, most of the pediatric spinal cord tumors are intramedullary (1, 20, 24). The glioma family accounts for the vast majority of IMSCT.

Among 226 patients of all ages with IMSCT operated on in our service between 1985–1992, there were 30% with astrocytomas, 29% with ependymomas, 14% with gangliogliomas, 7% with other gliomas and 20% with other lesions (among them hemangioblastoma, peripheral neuroectodermal tumors [PNETs], lipomas, and ganglioneurocytomas). Astrocytomas and gangliogliomas were especially prevalent in the young age group, whereas ependymomas are more frequent in the older age groups. The incidence of malignant vs. benign tumors was quite stable at about 30% throughout the different age groups.

III. SYMPTOMS AND SIGNS

In most cases, the clinical evolution was indolent and, almost invariably in children, parents became aware of the problem long before there were objective signs of neurological dysfunction. In a significant number of patients, the onset of symptoms was related to some apparently trivial injury, whereas in others, parents described exacerbations and remissions.

Weakness of the lower extremities was usually first noticed as an alteration of a previously normal gait. This was often extremely subtle and only obvious to a parent who noted a tendency in the child to fall more frequently or walk on the heels or toes. In young children, there was commonly a history of being a "late walker," and in the youngest (under 2 years), there was often a history of motor regression, i.e., starting to crawl again instead of walking, or refusing to stand.

Seventy percent of patients experienced severe pain along the spinal axis. It was most acute in the bony segments that were directly over the tumor. Characteristically, the pain was worse in the recumbent position, as venous congestion further distended the dural tube and resulted in typical night pains. It was common to discover that patients had been taking analgesics for a long time, including narcotics, after a nondiagnostic orthopedic evaluation. Radicular pain occurred in about 10% of cases and was usually limited to one or two cervical, thoracic, or lumbar dermatomes, similar to root pain from a variety of disease processes. Painful dysesthesias occurred in about 10% of cases and were generally described as painful hot or cold sensations in one or more extremities. In rare circumstances, this was the primary symptom and not associated with objective signs of neurological dysfunction. Paresthesias were occasionally associated with the dysesthetic pain, and both of these symptoms were more common with neoplasms in the cervical cord than in the thoracic spinal cord. Sensory abnormalities were generally limited to one upper extremity, and a discrete sensory level was only noted very late in the course of the disease, and then only in association with severe neurological disability. Cervical ependymomas characteristically present with bilateral and symmetrical dysesthesias.

Mild spasticity, increased reflexes and extensor plantar signs, with or without clonus, occurred relatively early in the neurological course with both cervical and thoracic tumors. Head tilt with torticollis is a common sign with cervical tumors. Neoplasms in the caudal cervical spinal cord typically caused weakness and atrophy of the intrinsic muscles of the hand. Mild scoliosis was the most common early sign of an intramedullary thoracic cord neoplasm. Pain and paraspinal muscle spasm often occurred before there were objective signs of neurological dysfunction and were usually assumed to be secondary to the evolving scoliosis.

Sphincter laxity was a very late sign, except for tumors that originated in the conus/cauda area. Higher tumors, even with cystic components extending into the conus, rarely present with sphincter abnormalities.

In the relatively rare malignant astrocytomas of childhood, symptoms were similar in quality but had a shorter duration and increased intensity.

IV. NEURODIAGNOSIS

Intramedullary spinal cord tumors may be either focal or diffusely elongated (Figs. 1 and 2). Holocord widening occurred in about 60% of pediatric patients and was usually manifest by expansion of the entire spinal cord from the medulla or cervicomedullary junction to the conus. Neoplasms extending for such long distances were most often cystic astrocytomas in which the solid component of the neoplasm spanned a variable length of the cord; they were associated with huge nonneoplastic rostral and caudal cysts that expanded the central canal above and below the tumor (Fig. 2).

A. Plain Films

Plain spinal x-rays often disclosed a diffusely widened spinal canal with relatively localized erosion or flattening of pedicles. Scalloping and scoliosis were also common manifestations of holocord IMSCT on plain films.

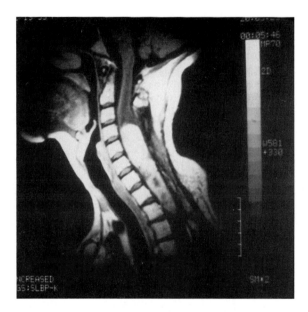

Figure 1 T1-weighted image (with contrast) of a cervical ependymoma. Note the homogenous enhancement and the sharp borders.

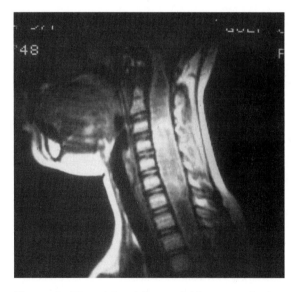

Figure 2 T1-weighted image (with contrast) of a cervical astrocytoma. Note the inhomogenous enhancement and the rostral and caudal cysts.

B. Computed Tomographic Scan and Myelography

Myelogram and computed tomography (CT) scans represented a primary investigational tool for a number of years. Two major problems were associated with the interpretation of these examinations. First, in cases of a complete block (majority of tumors), a C1-C2 puncture was usually indicated to verify the rostral extent of the tumor. The second interpretation problem was that holocord expansion caused by a spinal cord tumor or cyst may be confused with hydromyelia. This differential diagnosis needs to be firmly established prior to surgery. Intratumor cysts (as opposed to rostral and caudal cysts) were rarely present in the previously unoperated and nonradiated patient.

C. Magnetic Resonance Imaging

Magnetic resonance imaging (MRI) scanning has relegated most invasive neurodiagnostic studies to history (16). The MRI scan provides an excellent image of intramedullary neoplasms, and it is usually unnecessary to carry out other studies. The only case in which it is still necessary to perform a myelogram is in the rare situation when it is not impossible to visualize the entire expanded segment of the spinal cord. This is invariably a result of severe scoliosis, which may make it impossible to obtain the mandatory midsagittal images.

The T1-weighted image is the most informative (Figs. 1 and 2), disclosing the presence of rostral and caudal cysts, intramedullary cysts, and the solid component of the tumor. The T2-weighted image gives a myelographic appearance to the cerebrospinal fluid (CSF) and cysts. This is particularly important as it allows discernment between tumor-associated cysts and hydromyelia. Injection of gadolinium is mandatory for all spinal cord tumors (18,22). Gd-DTPA usually enhances the solid component of the tumor and helps delineate it from surrounding edema.

In the presence of a very focal expansion of the spinal cord (one to two segments), the tumor was more likely to be an ependymoma than an astrocytoma. In patients with very diffuse spinal cord widening, with or without associated cysts, astrocytoma was present in 90% of the cases and ependymoma in 10%. It is important to recognize, however, that in children under 10 years of age, an intramedullary spinal cord tumor above the conus has a 75% likelihood of being either an astrocytoma or a ganglioglioma and only a 10% likelihood of being an ependymoma. This is in contradistinction to patients older than 20 years of age in whom there is an approximate 60% chance of finding an ependymoma.

All ependymomas enhance brightly and homogeneously, whereas gliomas may or may not enhance heterogeneously. The symmetrical location, combined with their enhancement pattern, are quasipathognomonic for spinal cord ependymomas.

V. SURGERY

Spinal cord astrocytomas are relatively firm, occasionally contain microscopic foci of calcium, and only rarely have a cleavage plane to facilitate an en bloc resection. In the overwhelming majority of cases, it is necessary to remove the tumor from inside out until the almost invariably present "gliatumor interface" is recognized as a change in color and consistency between the tumor and adjacent normal neural tissues (Fig. 3). The principle of an initial central debulking applies also for ependymomas, although they invariably have a discrete cleavage from the surrounding white matter.

A. The Ultrasonic Aspirator and the CO_2 Laser

In the past, neurosurgeons were limited to traditional suction-cautery techniques for removal of neoplasms and, whereas that was often satisfactory for brain

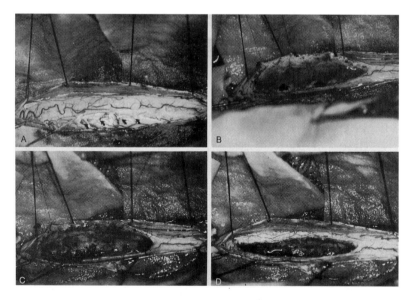

Figure 3   Operative exposure. (A) Initial view following dural opening of a swollen spinal cord. Note rotation of the cord. (B) Myelotomy completed and pial traction sutures in place (small arrows). The tumor (large arrows) and a caudal cyst (open arrow) are exposed. (C) Large intramedullary cavity after tumor resection. Note the cysts on both ends. (D) Subarachnoid space restored after removal of pial traction sutures.

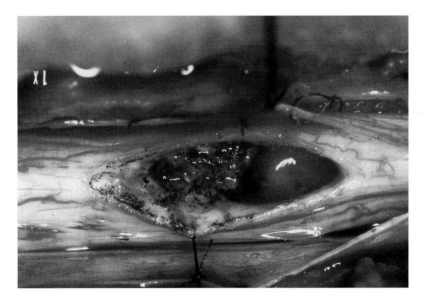

Figure 4 Tumor-cyst interface. Note the char produced by the CO_2 laser at the superficial aspect of the tumor and the pial traction sutures.

tumors, it was extremely hazardous in the spinal cord. This was because of the transmitted heat and movement through the tumor to the adjacent normal spinal cord, which was invariably firmly adherent. As a result of these technical limitations, there was a significant morbidity associated with IMSCT surgery. The development and application of the Cavitron Ultrasonic Aspirator (CUSA) system offered a significant improvement over the conventional system and made a major contribution to spinal cord surgery (10,12). The ultrasonic aspirator is the ideal instrument to rapidly debulk and remove all but residual fragments of a spinal cord neoplasm.

The neurosurgical laser is equally ideal to remove residual fragments, as it may be used with great precision along the length of the glia-tumor interface. Although the laser may be used in place of the CUSA, it is extremely tedious and time consuming when directed toward a very voluminous intramedullary neoplasm. In addition, the resulting laser char makes it difficult to recognize the glia-tumor interface and mandates frequent interruptions of the ongoing dissection as the blackened tissues are gently removed with a small-caliber suction (Fig. 4).

B. Surgical Technique

It is desirable to carry out a limited opening over the solid component of the neoplasm, but not to unnecessarily extend it rostrally or caudally. In our first surgical experience with holocord widening, a total laminectomy from C1-T12 was carried out. It was subsequently recognized that it was not necessary to expose the spinal cord over the rostral and caudal cysts. For this reason, it is important to define as accurately as possible the location of the solid component of the neoplasm vis-a-vis the cysts.

Even after careful consideration of the clinical and neuroradiological examination, it is not possible to ascertain that the laminectomy is of sufficient length to expose entirely the solid component of the neoplasm. For this reason, transdural ultrasonography is used to define further the location of the tumor vis-a-vis the bone removal (9). Therefore, after laminectomy is carried out, the wound is filled with saline and the head of the transducer probe is placed into gentle contact with the dura. Using this technique, the spinal cord is viewed in both sagittal and transverse sections. The rostral and caudal limits of the tumor, as well as the presence or absence of associated cysts, are immediately obvious. Ependymomas are commonly homogeneously hyperechogenic vis-a-vis adjacent tissues and, for this reason, the tumor mass may be completely visualized. In the presence of astrocytomas, the cord and tumor usually have the same acoustic property but the cord appears diffusely widened over the bulk of the tumor with tapering at the rostal and caudal poles. If the laminectomy is not sufficiently long to expose the entirety of the solid component of the neoplasm, it is lengthened, segment by segment, until the ultrasound discloses that the entire tumor mass is exposed.

In patients who have not been previously operated and who need bony opening of more than two segments, we use the high speed drill instrument to perform an osteoplastic laminotomy. This permits replacement of the bone, which is a nidus for subsequent osteogenesis, posterior fusion, and protection against future local trauma (see section on "Postoperative Spine Deformity").

At this juncture, the dura is opened, and this is limited to overlay the expanded spinal cord—it is not extended rostrally or caudally over normal spinal cord. In addition, it is not necessary to open the dura widely over the rostral or caudal cyst, because these are easily drained as the solid component of the neoplasm is excised.

After the cyst is entered, inspection of the cavity will localize the rostral or caudal neoplasm that extends into it (Fig. 4). It is not necessary, in most cases, to extend the myelotomy over the cyst, because it is easily drained as either pole of the neoplasm is identified and removed. Because the cyst fluid is produced by the tumor, it is unlikely to reaccumulate after gross total excision of the neoplasm. After identifying the rostral and caudal cyst-tumor junction, the myelotomy is continued over the midline of the cord between the pre-viously placed incisions. After completion of the myelotomy, there is usually 1–2 mm of white matter overlying the neoplasm that is removed with the laser or bipolar cautery and a very fine suction. The normal tissue is now splayed to the sides using the plated bayonette (Fig. 5). Most astrocytomas are gray and may be distinguished from adjacent white matter. Ependymomas are red or very dark gray and have a clear margin around the tumor. Pia traction sutures are used to open the myelotomy incision and further expose the intramedullary tumor (Figs. 3 & 4). It must be emphasized that in the presence of an astrocy-toma, there must be no effort to define a plane of cleavage around the tumor. These neoplasms must be removed from inside out until a glia-tumor interface is recognized by the change in color and consistency of the adjacent tissues. There is rarely a true plane of dissection, and futile efforts to define its presence only result in unnecessary retraction and manipulation of functioning neural tissue.

The excision of the solid noncystic astrocytoma is initiated in the midpor-tion rather than the rostral or caudal pole of the neoplasm. This is because there is no clear rostral or caudal demarcation of the tumor such as occurs when there are rostral and caudal cysts. In addition, the poles of the neoplasm are the least voluminous; for this reason, removal of this part of the neoplasm may be the most hazardous because normal neural tissue may be easily disrupted. It is

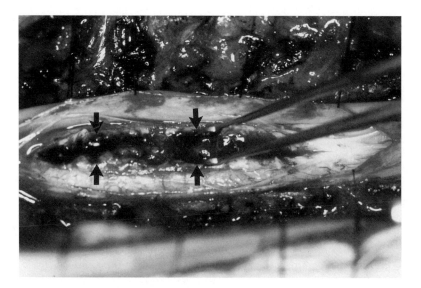

Figure 5 After midline myelotomy, the posterior columns (arrows) are dis-placed gently by the platted bayonette.

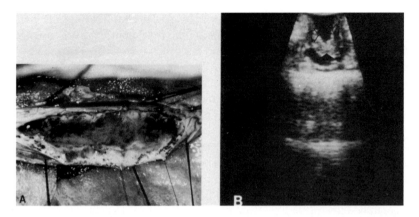

Figure 6 (A) Operative view at the end of tumor removal. (B) Simultaneous ultrasonography demonstrates the cavity and the remaining normal cord anteriorly (arrow).

very helpful to use intraoperative ultrasound to monitor progress and to clearly identify the rostral and caudal extent of the tumor. There are many cases in which the surgeon will have the impression that the anterior pia is visible and that tumor excision must be abandoned. In these situations, ultrasound may be invaluable in cross-section because it conveys a very precise image of the tumor cavity and its relationship to the anterior subarachnoid space (Fig. 6).

Ependymomas almost invariably have a true cleavage plane between the tumor and adjacent neural tissue. Although this contributes to total excision of these neoplasms, it is also a potential hazard, as it encourages the surgeon to attempt an en bloc resection and to remove the entire mass in one or two large pieces. If this is attempted, there will be excessive and unnecessary manipulation of normal neural tissue. It is essential to emphasize that under no circumstances should this be permitted. Rather, the ependymoma must be debulked as an astrocytoma, and only when the center of the tumor has been removed should the surgeon develop the plane of cleavage between the tumor and adjacent tissues. This may be accomplished by retracting the remaining tumor tissue into the residual cavity—not by retracting the spinal cord from the tumor. There is usually an area of variable length along the anterior extension of the tumor where it is adherent to the anterior median raphe. These tumor fragments must be removed in bits and pieces, under high magnification and with sharp dissection (no pulling or tugging), to avoid injury to the anterior spinal artery.

C. Conus, Filum Terminale, and Cauda Equina

In the most common case, these tumors expand the filum terminale, which appears much like a sausage-shaped mass that displaces the normal nerve elements of the cauda equina circumferentially (Fig. 7). In these cases, it is relatively simple to remove the tumor en bloc by dividing the distal filum terminale caudal to the tumor, displacing the entire mass out of the cauda equina, then incising the remainder of the tumor just below the conus. In many cases, the entire mass is within the filum, making it unnecessary to pursue tumor fragments rostrally into the conus. Occasionally this may be mandatory in an effort to obtain a surgical cure; however, it is essential that no neural tissue in the conus be manipulated in any way and that the tumor fragments be extracted from below.

A few ependymomas of the cauda equina seem to have grown from the region of the conus and to have erupted out of the filum, with tumor tissue filling the entire thecal sac below the conus. In these cases, the normal neural elements of the cauda equina are not displaced circumferentially around the mass, rather they run through the tumor tissue. In these cases, it is necessary to remove the tumor bit by bit by working between and around the neural ele-

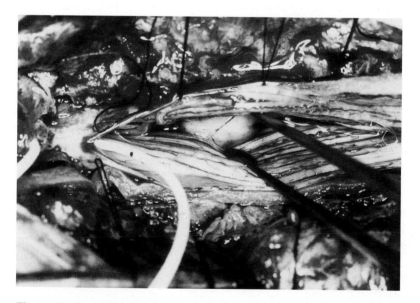

Figure 7 Operative view of a conus ependymoma displacing the normal elements of the cauda equina. Note the epidural and subdural electrodes for intraoperative monitoring.

ments until all of the neoplastic tissue is removed. In these cases, it is also usually necessary to extract remaining tumor fragments from the conus. It is again important that the neural tissue be undisturbed and that tumor fragments be removed by working through that area throughout which the tumor has grown into the thecal sac.

D. Wound Opening and Closure

Patients who have been previously radiated are at high risk for wound dehiscence and spinal fluid fistula. We, therefore have used plastic surgical expertise in wound closure in these patients.

There are several principles to closure after tumor removal (25,26). First, at least one layer must be CSF-tight. Second, permanent colored sutures are always used for the CSF-tight layers. Third, drainage is always used for the subcutaneous space. Finally, the skin is usually closed in three layers. We pay special attention to the fascia because this is usually the water-tight layer. The fascia and muscle are released, both superficially from the subcutaneous tissues and deeply from the bony elements. If this is not enough to achieve closure with no tension, relaxing incisions are performed.

E. Evoked Potentials Monitoring

The information provided by somatosensory evoked potentials (SSEP) is sufficient to assess the functional integrity of the motor system in procedures in which insults usually affect sensory and motor pathways simultaneously. During operations for IMSCT, the motor tract may be damaged independently of the sensory system. In addition, the SSEPs are often lost after midline myelotomy. We, therefore, routinely monitor motor evoked potentials (MEP) (6). We use the Sentinel-4 evoked potential/EEG analyzer (Axon Systems, Inc., Hauppauge, New York) as a mobile unit for recording, analyzing, and storing all operative evoked potentials. After laminectomy, rostral and a caudal epidural electrodes are placed (Fig. 7). The electrode proximal to the stimulus serves as a control and the distal one monitors the operation. For anesthesia, we use a combination of propofol and narcotics. Some basic principles apply for both methods. First, information needs to be immediately available and used by the surgeon to modify the operative dissection. Second, data should be continuously updated and communicated to the surgeon. Third, criteria for significant changes should be set and tailored for each patient according to the pathology and the baseline potentials.

Several clinical correlations have been made. Midline myelotomy and the placement of pia traction sutures commonly result in transient decrements in the amplitude of SSEPs, which probably occur as a result of movement of the posterior columns. Usually, the potential recovers within a few minutes. If it does not, the suture is removed and placed in another location under less tension. When the laser is used for more than 20 seconds at one time, there is often an adverse, probably thermal, effect that is manifest by a decrease in amplitude and increase in latency. When this occurs, the dissection is temporarily interrupted and the cord is irrigated with cool Ringer's solution. In most cases, electrical activity returns to baseline within 30 to 90 seconds.

In some cases, there is deterioration of evoked potentials as the dissection is directed toward tumor removal in specific locations. When this occurs, the manipulation is temporarily interrupted, and the electrical activity is permitted to recover. It is common to start and stop the procedure many times during the course of the tumor removal.

Perhaps the most important observation has been that if the dissection is inadvertently extended beyond the poles of the tumor, as is possible to do when there is no rostral caudal cyst, there is a dramatic decrease in amplitude and increase in the latency of the evoked potential. This has occurred over the caudal and rostral poles of the neoplasm and is indicative of tapering. It warns the surgeon against extending the myelotomy. This is most likely secondary to manipulation of the posterior columns, which are in their normal anatomical position, and indicates that a normal cord is being disrupted.

Improved electrical conductivity after tumor removal was invariably associated with a benign postoperative course. Impaired activity as compared to the preoperative baseline was not uncommon, and it was not necessarily associated with neurological morbidity. Nevertheless, the majority of patients with deteriorated activity have had transiently greater neurological dysfunction although, in most circumstances, this has ultimately recovered. In patients with impaired proprioception preoperatively, it was rarely possible to obtain baseline SSEPs for monitoring.

In several cases, the baseline SSEPs were normal or near normal and disappeared completely and permanently as the tumor dissection continued. Although this inevitably causes the surgeon great anxiety, it must not be construed as an indication for abandoning the surgery. The sensory pathways that conduct the SSEPs are via the dorsal columns and, therefore, not always correlated with motor function. Whereas the surgeon may be reassured and encouraged by stable or improving SSEPs, he or she must not be discouraged by the reverse.

For MEPs, we use transcortical electrical stimulation (23) and epidural recordings. This is a very reliable intraoperative technique that monitors the upper motor neuron without synapses on the way. It has the disadvantage of not differentiating between left and right.

The MEPs were most helpful during the removal of tumor at the most anterior and lateral aspects of the tumor cavity. Although the threshold for motor recovery has never been scientifically determined in such a setup, it is our routine not to push dissection beyond a 50% fall in MEPs. If and when such a decline would occur, we would stop manipulating the cord in this area and wait for the recovery of potentials.

VI. SURGICAL COMPLICATIONS

A. Increased Neurological Dysfunction

Patients with malignant tumors are at much greater risk of sustaining a surgical injury. It is also recognized that patients with severe preoperative disability and extensive noncystic tumors are very likely to deteriorate from surgery. Our incidence of a significant motor morbidity in intact patients is less than 5%. This experience mandates that patients with known IMSCT will not be followed up without treatment until severe symptoms appear, but rather will be referred early for surgery.

Impaired position sense, even in the presence of normal motor function, is a serious functional disability that requires the patient to undergo extensive physical therapy to learn to compensate. On the basis of our experience, we emphasize this potential complication in our preoperative discussion with patients and parents.

The only cases in which surgery was beneficial in the presence of advanced quadriparesis was when there were rostral, caudal, or intratumor cysts that were drained with little manipulation of neural tissue. In these patients, there was minor but significant improvement in upper extremity function. It is important to point out, however, that a similar degree of improvement in the lower extremities had much less functional significance. For this reason, there is rarely an indication to evacuate a cystic thoracic tumor in the presence of advanced disability in the lower extremities.

It is not uncommon for patients to inquire concerning the removal of a thoracic tumor in the presence of paraplegia. The fear that is usually expressed is that the tumor will grow rostrally and ultimately result in quadriplegia and death. This concern directed us to an analysis of patients with long-standing tumors, to make some assessment of whether the tumor ascended the neural axis over an extended period. It now seems clear that benign, noncystic astrocytomas caudal to T4 do not usually extend rostrally—they expand and destroy the spinal cord locally but do not seem to threaten upper extremity function. The same tumor that occurs above T4 is more likely to threaten upper extremity function, as it does not require a great deal of rostral extension to impair function in the hands. Therefore, tumors closer to the cervical-thoracic junction should be removed in an effort to preserve function in the hands and arms. All thoracic tumors with a rostral cyst extending into the cervical cord must also be removed, as expansion of the cyst (syrinx) will ultimately result in significant deterioration in motor function in the upper extremities.

B. Correlation of Postoperative Neurological Morbidity and Segmental Location

Postoperative neurological morbidity may be correlated with segments of the spinal cord that are involved with neoplasm. Whereas an extensive dissection may be carried out with little risk in those segments of spinal cord that are largely white matter, this does not seem to be the case in the lowest segments where gray matter is most abundant. Dissections within the cervical spinal cord are associated with little morbidity, although it is not uncommon to note some anterior horn cell dysfunction as manifested by atrophy of one or more muscle groups of an upper extremity. When this occurs, it is permanent. Dissections extending from the junction of the cervical and thoracic regions to T9 are also associated with remarkably little neurological morbidity.

Tumors that are located in the lower spinal cord segments from T9 to T12 have the greatest incidence of significant postoperative neurological morbidity. This is because neoplasms in the conus or just above it compress or infiltrate gray matter. Tumors that occur in more rostral regions of the spinal cord compress white matter tracts; therefore, the resultant signs and symptoms are based on pathological anatomy and pathophysiology that are specific to the segmental location of the neoplasm. Significant preoperative sphincteric dysfunction suggests that the tumor is extending into the conus, as this rarely occurs if the tumor is rostral to T12. Conversely, the absence of bowel and bladder problems suggests that the tumor does not extend into the conus, although it may be asymptomatically expanded by a caudal cyst. If there is no preoperative bowel and bladder dysfunction, it will occur postoperatively if the conus is disrupted. It is, therefore, essential that the myelotomy not be extended over the conus, as this will invariably result in sphincter dysfunction which may be permanent. It is important that the patient be advised that at least a temporary increase in neurological dysfunction is to be expected with surgery in this area. We would also assume that the long-term or permanent morbidity will also be significant.

C. Postoperative Spine Deformity

Scoliosis and kyphosis commonly evolve after surgery. In some cases of kyphosis, the deformity was of sufficient magnitude to cause spinal cord compression and progressive myelopathy (24). In these patients, a diagnosis of a recurrent tumor was always considered before the deformity was identified as being responsible for the neurological dysfunction. It is essential that this entity be understood, as treatment and prognosis are obviously very different. Scoliosis usually does not cause spinal cord compression, although it obviously potentiates an existing neurological disability.

It is essential that all children be closely followed up by an orthopedic surgeon who is experienced in caring for kyphosis and scoliosis. It is our recommendation that the surgical indication for spinal fusion be regarded as more urgent in this group of patients than in those with idiopathic deformity.

In a recent retrospective study of 45 patients who have had surgery for IMSCT, we looked at the influence of performing an osteoplastic laminotomy (OL) vs. a simple laminectomy (lam) on the incidence of progressive postoperative kyphoscoliosis (PPOKS) in children. The incidence of PPOKS, in a mean follow-up time of 3.4 years, was 3 of 20 patients in the OL group and significantly higher, 9 of 25 in the lam group. All three patients in the OL group who developed PPOKS experienced recurrent disease. We therefore concluded that replacement of the bone in OL is superior to a simple laminectomy, although it does not prevent the postsurgical evolution of spinal deformity if the tumor recurs.

D. Hydrocephalus

Fifteen patients developed hydrocephalus, and it was occasionally fulminating in its presentation (19,21). Twelve of these patients had an astrocytoma and/or associated rostral cyst, and in each case, the tumor extended into the cervical cord. There was obvious thickening of the leptomeninges overlying the cervicomedullary junction. It seems likely that this caused obstruction of the outlets of the fourth ventricle. The presence of hydrocephalus associated with an astrocytoma caudal to the cervicothoracic junction is strongly suggestive of a malignant tumor with secondary dissemination and obstruction of spinal fluid pathways. The hydrocephalus that occurred in patients with an astrocytoma was not associated with a significantly elevated CSF protein rostral to the block.

This was in contradistinction to the hydrocephalus that was associated with ependymomas (three patients), in which cases the tumors were commonly in the thoracic cord and were associated with massively elevated CSF protein rostral to the block. It, therefore, seems that in the presence of an ependymoma, the protein-rich viscous fluid, by some mechanism, obstructs the spinal fluid circulation.

E. Malignant Tumors

Most malignant astrocytomas and ependymomas had an atypical clinical course as compared to benign neoplasms (3,15). Whereas children with low-grade neoplasms were symptomatic for a minimum of many months and often years, those with malignant tumors became symptomatic over a few weeks. In addition, patients with low-grade tumors had relatively trivial symptoms vis a vis the MRI scan or myelogram, which disclosed massive spinal cord expansion. In contradistinction to this, patients with malignant tumors had rapidly evolving and advanced disability often associated with less dramatic expansion of the spinal cord.

The sole exception to this clinical pattern was the occasional patient with a nonmalignant ependymoma that had hemorrhaged. In these cases, the neurological disability evolved over a few days or weeks and was indistinguishable from the clinical course of the malignant tumors. In two of these cases, the MRI scan disclosed the area of hemorrhage. All patients with malignant tumors died within 12 months of surgery from neuraxis dissemination. In addition, the malignant neoplasms ascended the spinal cord rostrally, caudally, and through the subarachnoid space, resulting in paraplegia, quadriplegia, and death. On the basis of these observations, all of these patients should be treated with neuraxis radiation therapy as well as chemotherapy.

VII. DISCUSSION

A number of important observations are clearly relevant in terms of understanding the biology of this group of neoplasms, as well as for recommending proper surgical management. The lack of significant neurological dysfunction relating to spinal segments distended with cyst fluid is probably directly related to the anatomical location of the cyst. Apparently the primordial central canal of the cord was expanded as compared to the solid component of the neoplasm, which is more asymmetric in location. The presence of cysts that were similar in appearance to those associated with the cystic astrocytoma of the cerebellum suggests that many of these neoplasms are congenital tumors that have their inception during gestation. The fluid produced by the tumor extends up and down the spinal cord in the region of least resistance, that is, the central canal. One might also speculate that in some cases, the classic symptoms of syringomyelia may, in fact, be a late manifestation of such a cyst in which the tumor has either involuted or is not anatomically obvious. Perhaps the centrally located cyst may gradually expand over many years and compress the surrounding cord. In this regard, it is significant that a few patients with holocord widening had exceedingly small neoplasms, between 1.5 and 3 cm, and syringomyelia or hydromyelia was mistakenly diagnosed. Our experience would suggest that the presence of xanthochromic cyst fluid is pathognomonic of an associated neoplasm, whereas clear fluid is diagnostic of hydromyelia.

It is our perspective that the presence of a widened spinal cord from the cervicomedullary junction to the conus, which is associated with a relatively slowly evolving neurological deficit, is indicative of a very slowly growing neoplasm that has a good long-term prognosis and should be treated aggressively.

Nevertheless, it must be emphasized that despite a gross total tumor excision, it would be naive to assume that residual tumor fragments have not been left in situ. We have hypothesized that these remaining fragments may remain dormant, or involute, similar to what has been noted to occur in many astrocytomas of the cerebellum (2,13). However, whether this is reality or wish fulfillment will only be known many years from now after long-term follow-up and retrospective analysis.

In most cases of holocord tumor, the initial complaint was a weak arm or a mildly weak leg with associated pain somewhere along the spinal axis. The signs and symptoms were consistently relatively minor when compared to the apparently diffuse nature of the pathological process. It is perfectly understandable why neurosurgeons faced with this clinical dilemma have been most concerned about inflicting a greater neurological deficit as a result of extensive dissection within a rather well-functioning spinal cord. This rationale has encouraged a temporizing surgical approach consisting of a limited laminectomy and biopsy, then relying on radiation therapy to control tumor growth. Unfortunately, the natural history of these tumors with radiation therapy is slow deterioration and eventual severe neurological disability or death.

The outcome after radical resection of these tumors was directly related to the preoperative neurological status. Although a transient increase in weakness or sensory loss was commonly present in the immediate postoperative period, only a few patients had a significant, permanent increase in neurological deficit after operation. Patients with paraparesis or quadriparesis who were ambulatory before surgery had neurological improvement over several weeks. The group with severe deficits preoperatively rarely made any significant improvement, although their downhill course abated.

There is no evidence that radiation will cure benign astrocytomas of the spinal cord, and there is abundant evidence that it has a deleterious effect on the immature developing nervous and osseous systems. Spinal cord tumors should be recognized as potentially excisable lesions, with radiation therapy reserved for possible adjunctive use if there is a recurrence. At that time, it might be used after a second radical surgical resection.

REFERENCES

1. Alter M. Statistical aspects of spinal cord tumors. In: Vinken PJ, Bruyn GH, eds. Handbook of Clinical Neurology. Amsterdam: North-Holland publishing, 1975.
2. Bucy P, Theiman PW. Astrocytomas of the cerebellum. A study of a series of patients operated on over 28 years ago. Arch Neurol 1968; 18:14–19.
3. Cohen AR, Wisoff JH, Allen JC, Epstein F. Malignant astrocytomas of the spinal cord. J Neurosurg 1989; 70:50–74.
4. Cooper PR. Outcome after operative treatment of intramedullary spinal cord tumors in adults: Intermediate and long term results in 51 patients. Neurosurg 1989; 25:855–859.

5. Coxe WS. Tumors of the spinal canal in children. Am J Surg 1961; 27:62–73.

6. Deletis V. Intraoperative monitoring of the functional integrity of the motor pathways. In: Devinsky O, Beric A, and Dogali M, eds. Advances in Neurology. Vol. 63, New York: Raven Press, 1994; 201–214.

7. Epstein F, Epstein N. Surgical treatment of spinal cord astrocytomas of childhood. A series of 19 patients. J Neurosurg 1982; 57:685–689.

8. Epstein F, Farmer JP, Freed D. Adult intramedullary astrocytoma of the spinal cord. J Neurosurg 1992; 77:355–359.

9. Epstein F, Farmer JP, Schneider SJ. Intraoperative ultrasonography: an important adjunct for intramedullary tumors. J Neurosurg 1991; 74:729–733.

10. Epstein F, Raghavendra NB, John RE. Spinal cord astrocytomas of childhood: Surgical adjuncts and pitfalls. In: S. Karger, ed. Concepts in Pediatric Neurosurgery, American Society of Pediatric Neurosurgery, Salt Lake City, Utah, 1985; 224–237.

11. Epstein F, Wisoff J. Intra-axial tumors of the cervicomedullary junction. J Neurosurg 1987; 67:483–487.

12. Flamm ES, Ransohoff J, Wuchinich D, et al. A preliminary experience with ultrasonic aspiration in neurosurgery. Neurosurg 1978; 2:240–245.

13. Geissinger JD, Bucy PC. Astrocytomas of the cerebellum in children: Long-term study. Arch Neurol 1971; 24:125–135.

14. Guidetti B, Mercuri S, Vagnozzi R. Long term results of the surgical treatment of 129 intramedullary spinal gliomas. J Neurosurg 1981; 54:323–330.

15. Kopelson G Linggood RM. Intramedullary spinal cord astrocytoma versus glioblastoma. The prognostic importance of histologic grade. Cancer 1982; 50:732–735.

16. Li MII, Holtas S. MR imaging of spinal intramedullary tumors. Acta Radiol 1991; 32(6):505–513.

17. Merton PA, Morton HB. Stimulation of the cerebral cortex in the intact cerebral cortex. Nature 1980; 285:227.

18. Parizel PM, Baleriaux D, Rodesch G, et al. Gd-DTPA. Am J Radiol 1989; 8:339–346.

19. Rifkinson-Mann S, Wisoff JH, Epstein F. The association of hydrocephalus with intramedullary spinal cord tumors: A series of 25 patients. Neurosurgery 1990; 27:749–754.

20. Russell DS, Rubinstein LJ, eds. Pathology of tumours of the nervous system. Baltimore; Williams & Wilkins, 1989.

21. Schijman E, Zuccaro G, Monges JA. Spinal tumors and hydrocephalus. Child's Brain 1981; 8:401–405.

22. Shoshan Y, Constantini S, Ashkenazi E, et al. Intramedullary spinal cord renal carcinoma metastasis diagnosed by gadolinium enhanced MRI. Neuro-orthopedics 1991; 11:117–123.

23. Sim FH, Svien HJ, Bicket WH, et al. Swan neck deformity following extensive laminectomy. J Bone Joint Surg 1974; 56:564–580.

24. Slooff JL, Kernohan JW, MacCarty CS. Primary Intramedullary Tumors of the Spinal Cord and Filum Terminale. Philadelphia, WB Saunders, 1964.

25. Zide BM. How to reduce the morbidity of wound closure following extensive and complicated laminectomy and tethered cord surgery. Pediatr Neurosurg 1992; 18:157–166.

26. Zide BM, Wisoff JH, Epstein F. Closure of extensive and complicated laminectomy wounds. J Neurosurg 1987; 67:59–64.

15

Metastatic Disease of the Spine

Kenneth J. Paonessa
Norwich Orthopedic Group, Norwich, Connecticut

Michael J. Halperin
William W. Backus Hospital, Norwich, Connecticut

I. GENERAL

A. Incidence

Metastatic disease involving the spine is by far the most common skeletal tumor seen by orthopedic surgeons or those physicians involved in the care of the spine. The spine is the most common skeletal bone involved in metastatic disease (1). Of approximately 1 million new cases of cancer diagnosed annually, almost two-thirds of the patients will develop skeletal metastases (2). This number may be as high as 85% of all women with breast carcinoma (3). Symptomatic metastatic spinal cord involvement has been estimated to occur in 18,000 new patients a year (4). Metastatic disease is much more prevalent than primary bone cancer, accounting for skeletal lesions in 40 times as many patients as are affected by all other forms of bone cancer combined (5). Many of the patients with metastatic involvement go unnoticed; 60% of all skeletal lesions (6) and 36% of vertebral lesions are asymptomatic (7).

Skeletal metastases are produced by almost all malignant diseases, they are most often secondary to breast, lung, and prostate disease and less frequently due to renal, thyroid, or gastrointestinal carcinoma (8). Schaberg found in reviewing 322 patients with documented metastatic bone disease that 80% of carcinomatous metastases came from breast, prostate, lung, or renal carcinoma (7).

The estimated prevalence of metastatic disease for each tumor type has varied greatly depending on whether autopsy studies of metastatic disease or data from clinical reviews of treated patients are compared. The clinical behavior of each primary tumor type can also determine the perceived prevalence and its clinical importance. For example breast and prostate cancer patients tend to live longer, and treatment of spinal metastases is more likely to be needed. Pulmonary carcinoma patients tend to live a shorter time after diagnosis and therefore usually need only supportive care. Gastrointestinal carcinoma tends to metastasize to the liver and lungs before the spine and so is less likely to require treatment for spinal metastases (8,9). There have been several excellent reviews of the relative prevalence of each type of carcinoma in spinal metastatic disease. These are summarized in Table 1 (4,10–14). Multiple myeloma and lymphoma are the most common sources of disseminated skeletal lesions but whether they are considered metastatic or primary lesions has varied from author to author, making accurate assessment of their relative importance difficult to discern (8,9).

Brihaye and coworkers (15) (Table 2) in a literature review of 1,477 total cases with epidural involvement found that 16.5% were from the breast, 15.6% from the lung, 9.2% were from the prostate, 6.5% were from the kidney, and 4.6% were from gastrointestinal sources. A primary site was unable to be found in 12.5% of the cases. Among women breast is by far the most common primary tumor. It has been estimated that between 65 and 85% of women with breast cancer develop skeletal metastatic disease prior to death (16). Among men, lung and prostatic carcinomas are by far the most common primary sites (3).

Table 1 Location of Primary Tumors Producing Metastatic Disease of the Spinal Column (Summary of 2,748 Cases)

Primary neoplasm	Number	Percent
Breast	576	21.0
Lung	377	14.0
Prostate	211	7.5
Thyroid	73	2.5
Kidney	154	5.5
Lymphoma	180	9.0
Gastrointestinal	134	5.0
Other		35.5
Total	2,748	100.0

Data from Refs. 4,10–14.
Source: Ref. 8.

Table 2 Location of Primary Tumors

	Arseni 1959	Barron 1959	White 1971	Constans 1973	Paillas 1973	Chade 1976	Baldini 1979	Kretschmer 1979	Dunn 1980	Brihaye 1987	Total	%
Lung	39	31	31	4	12	27	20	11	19	37	231	15.6
Breast	27	20	37	30	8	23	24	10	7	58	244	16.5
Kidney	9	12	13	2	8	25	9	10	8		96	6.5
Prostrate	16	6	23	5	4	19	16	5	21	22	137	9.2
Thyroid	2	3	8	11	2	20	5	3			54	3.6
Gastrointestinal	15	6	11	3	6	10	11	1	6		69	4.6
Hematosarcoma		29	35	35	3			20	16	21	159	10.8
Miscellaneous	81	18	59	29	5	7	33	13	17	66	302	20.5
Unknown	42	6	9	15	12	16		32	10	14	185	12.5
% Unknown	18.18	4.7	3.98	11.19	20	10.88	26.40	30.47	9.61	6.4		
Total	231	127	226	134	60	147	125	105	104	218	1,477	

Source: Ref. 15.

The location for metastatic disease to the spine has also been studied. The prevalence of symptomatic vs. asymptomatic lesions has varied by location studied. Brihaye reported on 1,585 cases of symptomatic epidural metastases and found that the thoracic and thoracolumbar spine were involved in 70% of all cases, the lumbar and sacral areas in 22% of cases, and the cervical and cervicothoracic areas in 8% of cases (15). This report agreed with others that even though lumbar spine involvement is more common, most patients who develop neurologic dysfunction have disease in the thoracic area (13,17–22).

B. Tumor Biology

The route of tumor metastasis dictates its ultimate location. This may account for its presenting symptoms and can often affect treatment. The biological behavior of the primary tumor will determine, for example, if rapid vertebral erosion with fracture and acute spinal cord compression will develop, or if a slow and stable growth will occur. Understanding the tumor type and its biology will help predict when and if a specific tumor will endanger the neurologic structures (8).

Harrington (12) has stated that symptoms usually develop due to one or more of the following 5 reasons:

1. Expansion of the cortex of the vertebral body by tumor mass with a resultant pathological fracture with invasion of the paravertebral soft tissue
2. Compression or invasion of adjacent nerve roots by the expanding tumor
3. Pathological fracture due to vertebral destruction with pain
4. Development of spinal instability with pain
5. Compression of the spinal cord by epidural mass.

The distribution of metastatic lesions appears to be a function of both the number of metastatic emboli that are produced and the rate of survival of each emboli (23–25). Kostuik (8) has stated that this distribution is influenced by three main factors:

1. Tumor emboli enter the blood stream and arrest in the natural filters of the vascular tree: the capillary beds, the liver, lungs, and the bone marrow (26). There are several ways that metastatic emboli can spread by special lymphatic or venous channels. Lung carcinomas may spread to bone by means of direct segmental arteries. Breast and prostate carcinomas may spread by way of the paravertebral venous plexus of Batson (27) (Fig. 1) (28), which connects the intra-abdominal venous supply with the epidural and paravertebral venous supply. The azygous

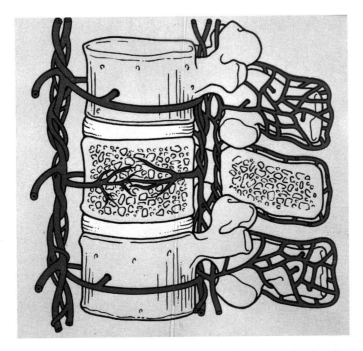

Figure 1 Batson's plexus. The veins of the vertebral column form intricate plexuses around the spinal column and freely communicate with the segmental systemic veins and the portal system. (From Ref. 28.)

vein, which is the main venous drainage of the breast, communicates with the paravertebral venous plexus of the thoracic region. The prostate drains through the pelvic plexus, which communicates in the lumbar region. During a valsalva maneuver, there may be retrograde flow from these organs to the vertebral spine.

2. The tumor distribution involves some aspect of tissue receptivity. Certain tissue provides a more favorable environment for survival of tumor emboli. Red marrow of bone provides a biochemically suitable environment for the proliferation of tumor cells. Harrington (12) used this "sead and soil" analogy to show how the capillary network provided an easier area for growth than other less suitable areas.

3. There are some intrinsic factors inherent to each specific tumor cell line that give it a particular advantage in surviving and growing in the medullary space. Specifically, prostaglandins and osteoclast activating factors by breast carcinomas have been associated with the establishment of lytic metastases in bone (29,30).

Within the vertebrae the vertebral body is the most common site of metastatic seeding (31) and is involved twenty times more often than the posterior elements (32). The cancellous bone is almost always invaded prior to the cortical bone (33). This is consistent with the finding that the pedicle, which is mostly cortical bone is rarely affected alone and is usually the result of direct extension and invasion from either the vertebral body or the posterior elements (32) (Figure 2). Fischer (34) has suggested that tumor cells lodge at sites of skeletal trauma and, because the vertebral body trabeculae develop microfractures routinely (35), this may provide a microenvironment necessary for metastatic seeding.

The pathogenesis of neurological injury with metastatic disease has also been studied. The thoracic spine area has a higher chance of neurological injury with metastatic disease. Dommisse (36) has described the area of T4 to T9 as a "critical vascular zone of the spinal cord" and has suggested that interference

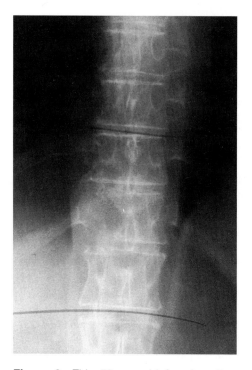

Figure 2 This 50-year-old female with a previously treated upper thoracic metastasis of metastatic breast carcinoma presented with increasing lower thoracic pain. Anteroposterior radiograph revealed a lesion of the T12 vertebrae with loss of the left pedicle and vertebral body and a second metastatic focus.

here to the spinal cord would most likely lead to paraplegia. This feeling has been refuted by injection studies by Crook (37) and Louis (38) that show a better developed segmental blood supply than previously appreciated.

The higher rate of neurological dysfunction with thoracic metastases may be due in part to biomechanical factors (20). The normal thoracic kyphosis is thought to predispose the thoracic vertebral bodies to fracture. The presence of an excessive spinal kyphosis deformity may compound the neurological dysfunction precipitated by neoplastic epidural compression (Fig. 3) (39). To define the natural history of metastatic spinal deformity, Asdorian et al. reviewed MRI on 27 patients with breast carcinoma metastases and analyzed the progression of disease (40). They found four stages of disease (Fig. 4), as follows:

Stage I-A. This early stage was characterized by only a small isolated deposit in the vertebral body.

Stage I-B. This stage had complete replacement of the bone marrow by tumor but no "collapse" or fracture.

Stage II-A. This stage had a single end plate fracture.

Stage II-B. This had a fracture of both endplates. The intervertebral disc

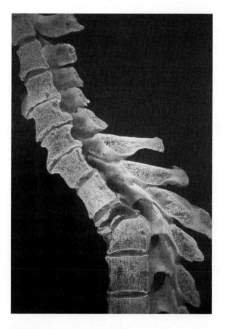

Figure 3 Photograph of a sagittal section of the macerated spine of a 58-year-old male with a lung carcinoma, who shortly before death developed paraplegia. The specimen shows a complete collapse of T2, with forward subluxation of T2 on T3, and a kyphotic deformity. (From Ref. 51.)

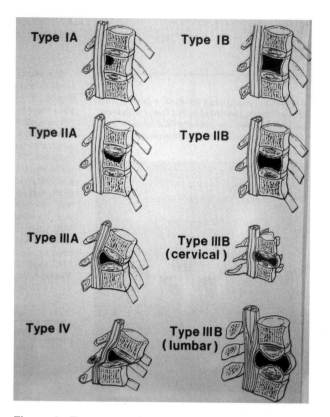

Figure 4 The stages of vertebral deformity. (From Ref. 40.)

was found to have imploded into the vertebral body. With progressive collapse, the posterior wall of the vertebral body and a portion of the superior and inferior end plate coalesce to create a "delta sign." Spinal canal compromise will come from the pressure of the bulging posterior wall of the vertebral body.

Stage III-A. There is collapse in the thoracic spine with increased localized kyphosis.

Stage III-B. In the lumbar or cervical spine, a more symmetrical collapse occurs.

Stage IV. With three-column involvement or disease, a subluxation or dislocation of the spine can occur.

The rate of neurological deterioration may also be determined by the specific type of tumor that is present, as well as by the degree of vascular compression or disruption that it causes. The venous congestion may occur from both metastatic infiltration with venous thrombosis (41) or from mechanical compression resulting from the vertebral body collapse with retropulsion of tumor debris. The vascular changes that occur have been shown to result in a wide spectrum of histological changes from only minimal cord edema (42) to extensive changes with massive hemorrhagic necrosis of the spinal cord (41).

C. Prognosis

The literature is often contradictory when reporting the success of various treatment protocols of metastatic disease of the spine. This is due to the lack of a standardized method of evaluating neurological dysfunction and treatment success and a lack of understanding of the natural history of metastatic disease itself (43). The treatment may include radiation, hormonal manipulation, chemotherapy, brace treatment, or surgical intervention; most often, it is a combination of two or three options. In addition there have been some who have advocated a pessimistic, almost nontreatment of these conditions.

Survival and outcome in metastatic disease are dependent on several factors; the most important seems to be tumor type. Although sex, age, location in the spine, interval between diagnosis of disease, and appearance of metastases have all been correlated with differences in outcome, they are all dependent on the nature of the primary (8). For example when comparing breast vs. lung carcinoma, breast cancer is more common in women and lung cancer is more common in men. If thoracic spinal metastases are compared, men have a worse prognosis than woman, primarily because lung carcinoma is more aggressive than breast cancer (44).

Because there is no current uniform approach to treatment in these patients, comparisons of treatment protocols are difficult and can result in challenging therapeutic choices. In appropriately selected patients, surgical treatment can offer a reasonable likelihood of functional improvement, pain relief and, in some cases, a cure of disease (9).

II.   DIAGNOSIS OF METASTATIC DISEASE

A.   Symptoms

As more patients with carcinoma survive longer, the proper diagnosis and treatment of metastatic spinal disease within an appropriate time frame becomes more important. Fortunately, the progression of neurological dysfunction can be halted if treated expeditiously and in many cases may be totally reversed. Some of the difficulty lies in the patient with previously undiagnosed carcinoma who presents with spinal involvement very early in their disease process. Usually the progression of disease in a patient who has known carcinoma will be self evident. It may be less obvious in the patient in whom cancer has not been previously diagnosed. Usually the symptoms of neurological compression remain constant (45). In order of appearance, they most prominently are: back or neck pain, radicular pain, weakness of the lower limbs, sensory loss, and loss of sphincter control.

Pain is the most common complaint of a patient with a spinal column neoplasia. It is the presenting symptom in up to 96% of patients (4,14,18,46–58). This local pain may begin as an insidious onset in the midline of the spine that is worse at night. It will usually increase in intensity over time and develop into either a burning or boring type of sensation (43). This pain usually does not have the close association with activity of mechanical back pain (9). The patient may associate onset of symptoms with a minor trauma but usually this is a tenuous relationship. Because many of these patients are elderly, they may be treated for may weeks or months for arthritis and may see several physicians before the correct diagnosis is made (8) (Fig. 5). Patients who experience severe mechanical pain preventing their performance of normal daily activities may have extensive bony destruction with resultant spinal instability (59). Radicular symptoms are less commonly seen but still occur frequently, especially in patients with cervical or lumbar involvement. Radicular pain in the thoracic region may result in "girdle pain" with a belt of dysethesia and paresthesias circumferentially from the level of the vertebral body involvement (9,47). This root pain can be either unilateral or bilateral and can be aggravated by coughing, sneezing, or movements of the trunk (43). Irritation of an intercostal nerve may falsely suggest thoracic or abdominal disease. Occasionally, diffuse pain is present below the level of the metastatic lesion. Patients with cervical or thoracic spinal cord compression may have pain in their legs that is thought to be due to irritation of the spinothalamic tracts of the spinal cord (43). Cervical and lower lumbar spinal metastases are often symptomatic, with pain occurring up to 6 months before neurological deterioration, whereas thoracic metastases are more typically associated with neurological findings shortly after symptoms begin (42). Gilbert's review of 130 patients (47) with spinal cord compression showed that only 10 patients (8%) presented with neurological involvement as the first symptom. Weinstein (9) felt that up to 70% of patients will have clinical weakness by the time the correct diagnosis is made. This would emphasize the importance of maintaining a high index of suspicion when treating patients with persistent back or radicular pain and particularly those with a history of known systemic malignancies (4,47,60). Radicular symptoms similar to a herniated disc may be seen and confusion may occur in the correct differential diagnosis. Sim (61) found 38 patients with bone tumors simulating herniated disc symptoms. Twenty-three had lumbar or sacral neoplasms. Pain was usually unremitting and progressive and was not relieved by rest or recumbency as opposed to the symptoms of a herniated disc.

It is unusual for sphincter dysfunction to be the first sign of neurological deterioration, except when the metastatic lesion is at the level of the conus.

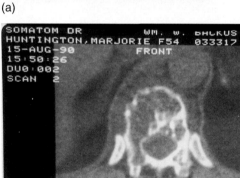

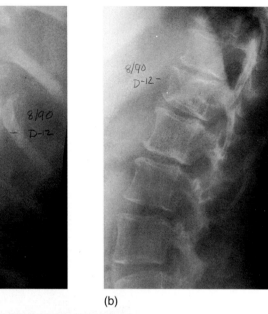

(a) (b)

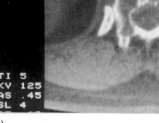

(c)

Figure 5 (a) A 54-year-old female presented with a 2-month history of increasing lower thoracic back pain made worse when working as a waitress. She had received several weeks of chiropractic care with no x-ray of the thoracic spine ordered. An anteroposterior radiograph, when seen in an emergency room, revealed an abnormality with sclerosis and collapse of T-12. (b) A lateral radiograph centered at the area of pain revealed a compression fracture of T-12 with a lytic lesion. (c) A CT scan showed a lytic lesion with partial erosion of the right pedicle. A biopsy revealed metastatic throid carcinoma. The patient had been treated for thyroid carcinoma with complete thyroidectomy 30 years earlier.

Constans (49) reported that only 3.2% of patients had this as their presenting complaint, and he stated that bowel and bladder dysfunction was usually the last event to occur in a progressive dysfunction. Unfortunately, this may develop in as many as 50% of the patients by the time the correct diagnosis is made (47). Bladder dysfunction may present in different ways (62). Above the conus level, an automatic (reflex) bladder with autonomic retention is seen with urinary retention and then overflow incontinence. At the conus or sacral root area, an autonomic (neurogenic) bladder is seen with dribbling incontinence due to flaccid detrusser muscles.

B. Neurological Status/Classification

There have been several attempts to classify patients through neurological presentation combined with the degree of bone involvement in metastatic disease of the spine. One of the most widely used methods was suggested by Harrington (50). This was based on the extent of neurologic dysfunction and bone compromise.

Class I. No neurological involvement or only minor sensory changes and very minor bone involvement;

Class II. Bony involvement without collapse or instability.

Class III. Major neurological involvement (sensory or motor) without significant bony involvement;

Class IV. Vertebral body collapse with mechanical pain or instability but no neurological compromise;

Class V. Vertebral body collapse or instability combined with major neurological impairment.

This classification has been widely used and quoted because it combines a concern for both the bony stability of the spine and the degree of neurological impairment caused by the metastatic process.

The degree of neurological involvement is extremely important in the possible treatment of spinal metastases, because if left untreated, it may be both devastating and irreversible. The patient's pretreatment neurological status is clearly correlated with the posttreatment outcome with regard to the degree and likelihood of recovery, the ability to maintain or regain ambulation, and the preservation or loss of bowel and bladder function (8,9). The rate of neurological deficit also has a clear prognostic significance. If a neurological deficit progresses from a minor to a major deficit in less than 24 hours, the prognosis for recovery is poor. A slow progression of neurological involvement has a more favorable prognosis for neurological recovery after treatment (12). Between 60 and 95% of patients who are ambulatory at the time of diagnosis will retain that ability after treatment. Only 35 to 65% of patients with paraparesis at presentation will regain the ability to walk and less than 30% of paraplegic patients will regain the ability to ambulate (4,5,13,45,50,63–65). Patients with complete neurological loss or complete paraplegia or quadraplegia, regardless of etiology, are generally not candidates for decompression and major surgery to regain motor function again. Patients with metastatic carcinoma of the lung, especially oat cell carcinoma with widespread metastases, should also be considered as nonoperative candidates inasmuch as many of these patients will survive less than 2 to 3 months (8,9).

C. Imaging

1. Plain Radiographs

In any patient being evaluated for the possibility of metastatic disease involving the spine, the plain radiograph should be the first test ordered. This is a useful "quick screening" test that can provide an early idea of the location and severity of involvement. Occasionally plain films are difficult to interpret because of the presence of severe osteopenia that may mimic metastatic disease.

The classic early finding finding is the "winking owl" sign, which is seen on the anteroposterior (AP) view of the involved spinal area (Fig. 6). This is seen as a loss of the pedicle ring unilaterally and is the result of the destruction of the cortex of the pedicle, usually by tumor invading from the vertebral body. The second most common finding on plain radiographs is vertebral collapse, usually secondary to erosion of bone by tumor or from acute fracture (Fig. 7). This may be difficult to differentiate from an acute osteopenic compression fracture. Two findings that should alert the clinician to consider a pathological fracture due to tumor is: 1. A periosteal reaction that seems too old or developed for the acute trauma; or 2. The presence of soft tissue calcifications or a soft tissue mass around the involved vertebrae (9).

The lesion in the vertebrae may produce either a lytic or blastic appearance. Early on a lytic lesion may be difficult to see, because radiographic evidence of bone destruction is not seen until 30–50% of the trabecular bone has been destroyed (66). The type of lytic bone destruction may also implicate either a benign or malignant lesion (Fig. 8). A geographical pattern with sclerotic borders suggests a slow-growing benign lesion; a rapidly growing tumor produces a more moth-eaten pattern, and highly malignant aggressive lesions produce a permeative pattern of destruction (67). Most metastatic carcinomas will produce a moth-eaten or permeative pattern, but a well-circumscribed benign lesion might be more suspicious for a benign primary bone tumor.

Osteoblastic lesions are most often seen with prostate and some breast carcinomas; they are seen less commonly with bladder, thyroid, gastrointestinal, lung, or malignant testicular tumors (68, 69). Osteoblastic lesions can be hard

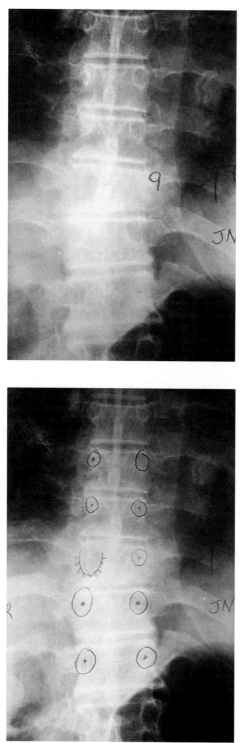

(a)

(b)

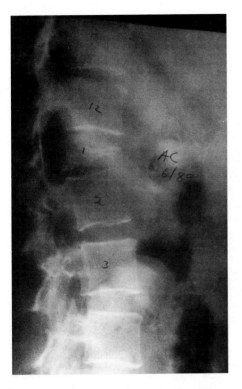

Figure 7 Lateral radiograph of a 45-year-old female with known uterine carcinoma presenting with severe back pain and weakness of the lower extremities and a collapse of L1, with a large lytic lesion that was a metastatic uterine tumor.

to see on plain radiographs, and up to 50% of osteoblastic lesions may be missed.

Using plain radiographs, it may be difficult at times to differentiate neoplasm from pyogenic osteomyelitis. With neoplasms, the disc space tends to be preserved even with severe destruction of the vertebral body as opposed to infection, where the disc is frequently destroyed along with the adjacent verte-

---

Figure 6 (a) A 62-year-old male presented with a several-day history of increasing weakness of gait and numbness to the lower extremities. An anteroposterior radiograph shows loss of definition of the right T9 pedicle shadow. (b) The loss of a unilateral pedicle shadow has been called the "winking owl" sign, because the pedicles look like the eyes of an owl when seen face on.

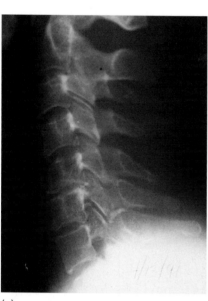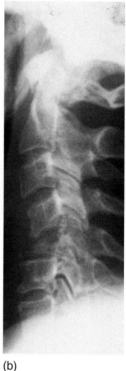

(a)   (b)

Figure 8   (a) A 49-year-old female with a history of both a previous primary lung carcinoma and a recent mastectomy for breast carcinoma presented with neck and shoulder pain. A lateral cervical radiograph was read as showing degenerative disc disease of C-5/C-6. (b) Four weeks later, after an MRI showed a large metastatic lesion, a lateral radiograph was repeated preoperatively. This showed rapid destruction of C5 from a very malignant breast metastasis.

brae (4). Sometimes tuberculosis of the spine can be difficult to differentiate from neoplasm, because the disc space may still be intact even with vertebral body collapse (Fig. 9).

2.   Bone Scan

Bone scans using technetium 99m are sensitive tests for neoplastic disease. They can detect lesions as small as 2 mm and are sensitive for any area of osteoid formation. They may predate radiographic changes of osteolytic or osteoblastic disease by 2–18 months (70–72). Radionucleotide uptake at sites of metastatic disease occurs by two mechanisms (73–75):

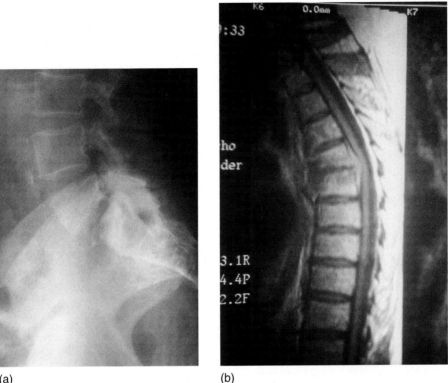

(a)   (b)

Figure 9 Many times it may be difficult to differentiate infection from metastatic disease by radiographic workup. (a) Lateral radiograph of a 52-year-old female with lower back pain and right leg pain. A typical destructive pattern for pyogenic discitis of L5-S1 is seen, with collapse of disc and erosion of the vertebral endplates. A biopsy revealed streptococcus infection. (b) Sagittal MRI of a 39-year-old male with thoracic back pain and mild weight loss. This shows a lesion more typical of tuberculosis infection with erosion of vertebrae but sparing of the disc space, along with a large epidural and anterior vertebral abscess. Initial needle biopsy was interpreted as possible lymphoma due to many small cells, but open biopsy and treatment showed an obvious tuberculous abscess.

1. Tumors with large fibrous stroma, such as prostate carcinoma, form new bone by intramembranous ossification.
2. More commonly, immature osteoid or new reactive bone is formed in response by the host bone to repair the injury produced by the neoplastic lesion. This is similar to the fracture callous commonly seen after injury.

A problem with bone scans is their lack of specificity, with false-positive and false-negative examinations being found. False negatives may occur with aggressive, rapidly growing metastatic lesions, such as renal or lung carcinomas, or with myeloproliferative disorders such as lymphoma, leukemia, multiple myeloma, reticulum cell sarcoma or Ewing's sarcoma (70). In isolated lesions, false positives can include fractures, infections, local soft tissue inflammations, and degenerative bony changes. Another frequent source of false-positive scans is osteoarthritis, which is commonly seen in an older population (76). Although these false positives can occur, the sensitivity of bone scanning makes it helpful in assessing a symptomatic patient with negative or equivocal plain radiographs, or as a method of determining the extent of dissemination in patients with systemic metastatic disease (77,78).

A pattern of uptake with multiple areas of skeletal involvement is virtually diagnostic of metastatic disease if a patient has a known primary malignancy (Fig. 10). If a primary malignancy has not been identified, such a pattern of uptake is still suggestive and enables the surgeon to choose the most accessible lesion for biopsy (9) (Fig. 11).

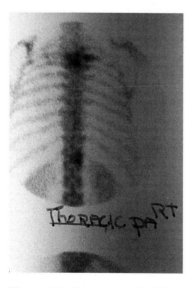

Figure 10 Bone scan of a 50-year-old female several years after a mastectomy for breast carcinoma who presented with upper thoracic back pain and weakness climbing stairs. This showed an area of intense uptake involving the T3 and T4 vertebrae and the left third rib. A smaller area of uptake was also present at the T12 area. On biopsy and treatment, this was a metastatic breast carcinoma.

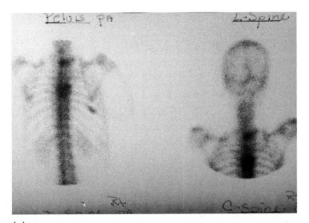

(a)

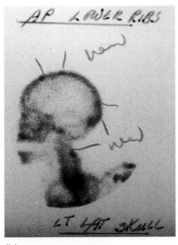

(b)

Figure 11 (a) A 60-year-old female presented with a several-week history of increasing weakness to the lower legs and a breast mass that she had refused biopsy of. X-rays showed an obvious fracture of the upper thoracic spine. A bone scan showed a pattern consistent with metastatic disease with multiple uptake in the T1, T5, and T6 vertebrae, the left sixth rib, and possibly the skull. (b) Several months later after treatment of her spinal metastasis, she presented with increased neck and skull pain. A repeat bone scan now shows definite lesions in the skull and midcervical spine despite chemotherapy, radiation, and hormonal therapy.

3. Computed Tomography and Myelography

Unenhanced Computed Tomography (CT) has an improved sensitivity in the detection of spinal neoplasms compared to plain radiographs and can be a very helpful tool for surgical preparation (79, 80). Computed Tomography is much more useful when combined with myelography (Fig. 12).

Myelography was once the only reliable way to assess spinal cord and nerve compression but now shares this ability with magnetic resonance imaging (MRI). It still may give some dynamic information, in that a complete block

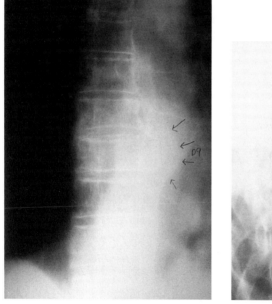
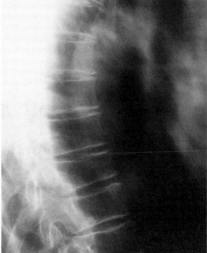

(a)   (b)

Figure 12   (a) Anteroposterior radiograph of a 76-year-old male with a 1-week history of hip pain and increasing weakness of gait and loss of urinary control. There is loss of the left pedicle shadow of T9, with a large, left soft tissue shadow. (b) Lateral radiograph shows no obvious compression or lytic processes. (c) Plain CT scan shows a large destructive process of T9, with soft tissue apparently in the canal and destruction of the left pedicle. (d) On myelography the anteroposterior view shows a complete blockage at T9. (e) Patient was treated with an anterior vertebrectomy of T9 with methylmethacrylate replacement and placement of a Cotrel-Dubousset single rod. The tumor was a metastatic hepatoma from the liver. Anteroposterior radiograph. (f) Lateral postoperative radiograph.

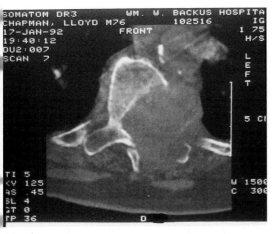

(c)

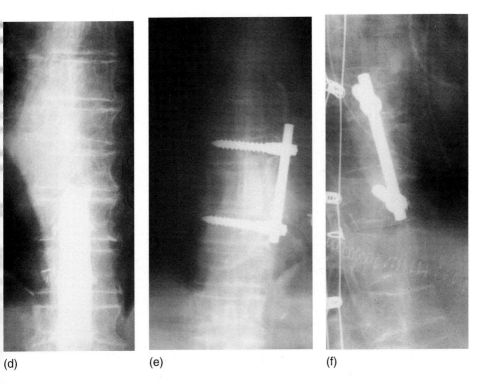

(d)   (e)   (f)

conclusively demonstrates pressure on the neural structures, which can only be inferred by an MRI (Fig. 13). In addition, cerebrospinal fluid (CSF) can also be removed and analyzed for cell content and for protein and glucose analysis. There are several drawbacks to myelography; it is an invasive procedure that can be uncomfortable; also, if a complete block is found, a second injection of contrast is necessary to demonstrate the proximal or distal extent of the tumor (9).

Rodichok, in 1981 (81), before MRI was widely available, recommended that myelography be performed if radiographic studies were positive in any patient with a history of carcinoma and spinal pain or in one who had an abnormal neurological examination even in the presence of negative radiographs. In a prospective study of 127 patients studied with myelography, 60% of patients who presented with back pain and evidence of metastatic disease but with a normal neurologic examination still had positive epidural disease.

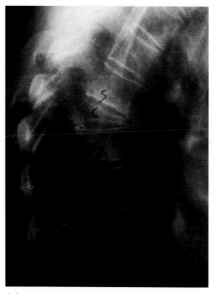

(a)

Figure 13 60-year-old female with metastatic breast carcinoma (same patient as Figure 11). (a) Lateral radiograph shows collapse of T6 and involvement of T7. (b) Plain CT of T6 showing lytic lesion of vertebral body. (c) Sagittal plain CT reconstruction showing collapse of T6 with kyphosis. (d) Lateral myelogram showing complete block at lower body of T6. (e) Anteroposterior myelogram showing complete block that correlated with severe myelopathy clinically. (f) Sagittal postmyelogram CT reconstruction showing area of dye cutoff at inferior T6.

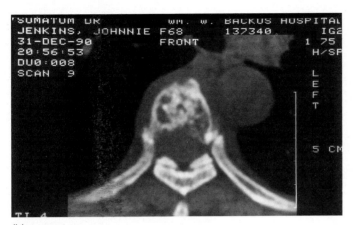

(b)

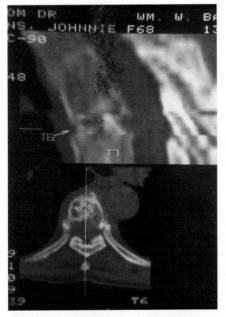

(c)

(*Fig. continues*)

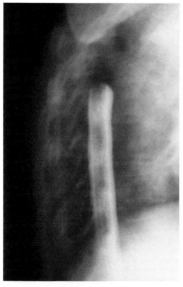

(d)

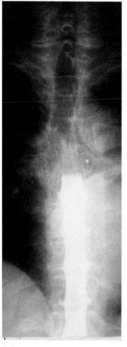

(e)

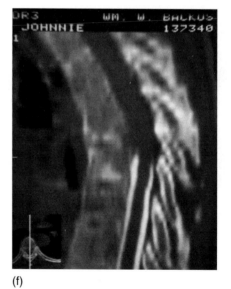

(f)

Figure 13 Continued

Sixty percent of the patients with abnormal neurological exam with negative radiographs had epidural disease. If a patient had an abnormal radiographic exam and an abnormal neurologic exam, then 90% had epidural disease.

There is great variability in the degree of neurological dysfunction seen with the degree of block, but usually a complete block will be likely to present with myelopathy (82). Acute neurological deterioration can occur after myelography especially with a complete block. Hollis (83) reviewed 100 patients with a complete block who had either a C1-C2 or lumbar injection. Fourteen percent of patients with complete myelogram blocks after lumbar puncture developed neurological deterioration, whereas none of the patients after C1-C2 puncture had deterioration. This may have been due to the pressure difference on the CSF after removal of fluid. Usually myelography is combined with a post-contrast CT scan to provide the maximum amount of information from the study.

4. Magnetic Resonance Imaging

Magnetic resonance imaging has proven very useful in evaluating metastatic disease in the spine. It can provide good soft tissue contrast, multiplanar images can be obtained and it can depict the spinal cord directly without the need for intrathecal contrast (84). When MRI was compared to myelography, MRI showed superior delineation of soft tissue, more clearly demonstrated the length of the lesion, and demonstrated anterior vs. posterior compression (84, 85). The T1 images usually show spinal cord compression best; the T2 images show the subarachnoid space better (84, 85) (Fig. 14).

Magnetic resonance imaging does have some disadvantages. It has a potential for decreased resolution in the thoracic spine due to respiratory and heart motion and some patients cannot withstand it because to claustrophobia. In addition there is an inability to scan patients with ferromagnetic material in their eyes, or with certain vascular clips in the brain or other locations in the body. Magnetic resonance imaging also does not visualize cortical bone involvement well (43) (Fig. 15). However, even with these disadvantages, MRI has added much to the evaluation of metastatic disease and probably has surpassed myelography.

D. Biopsy

Many times a known primary malignancy is not clearly defined or a patient presents with spinal involvement as their first sign of cancer. In these cases a biopsy may need to be done to make a definitive diagnosis and to plan for possible treatment options. A percutaneous biopsy may be performed in most cases before definitive surgical treatment is undertaken. Usually this is done under CT or fluoroscopic guidance with either a large special needle, such as a

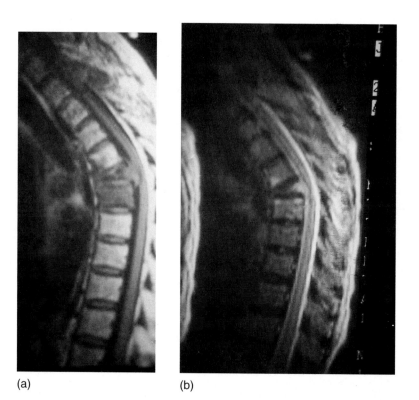

(a)   (b)

Figure 14 Same patient as Figures 11 and 13. (a) A T1 sagittal MRI shows involvement of T7 with tumor and large amount of tumor in epidural space well. (b) T2 sagittal MRI scan shows the involved vertebrae as lighter colored but does not show as much distinction between epidural tumor and CSF.

Turner, Ackerman, or Craig needle, or a small 22- or 23-gauge spinal needle (Fig. 16). In the cervical and thoracic spine, smaller needles are necessary compared to the lumbar spine (86). The accuracy rate for percutaneous bone biopsy can vary greatly. Tehtanzadeh (87) had a 75% success rate in diagnosis of metastatic disease and Mink (88) had a 95% success rate. Usually an osteolytic lesion will have a higher probability of providing enough tissue for a definitive diagnosis. Osteoblastic lesions may only provide a diagnosis in 20–25% of percutaneous biopsies, so that several larger specimens obtained with multiple biopsy passes may be necessary (48). The complication rate is usually low, with rates reported at 0.7% (88) and 0.2% (89). At times, if a rapidly developing neurological process is occurring, the biopsy must be done at the time of definitive surgical treatment.

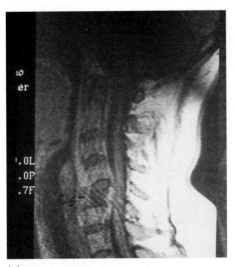

(a)

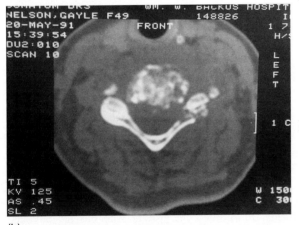

(b)

Figure 15 (a) Sagittal MRI (T1) of 49-year-old female with metastatic breast carcinoma (see Figure 8 for plain radiographs). This shows involvement of C5 vertebral body with kyphosis. (b) A CT scan at C5 shows fracture of left facets from involvement with tumor in addition to anterior vertebral body.

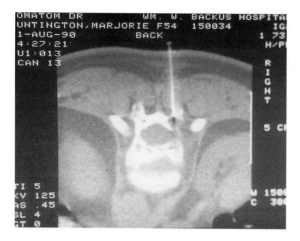

Figure 16 A CT-guided biopsy of metastaic thyroid carcinoma in a T12 verte-bral body in a 54-year-old female (see Figure 5). This is performed under intra-venous sedation with a 22-gauge chiba needle.

III. TREATMENT OF METASTATIC DISEASE

Once a diagnosis of metastatic disease to the spine has been established or is strongly considered, the options for the best treatment plan are considered. This is usually best done by a team approach involving an oncologist or an internist experienced in the treatment of advanced carcinomas, a spinal surgeon experienced with the possible surgical and nonsurgical options, possibly a radiation therapist, and possibly an interventional radiologist who may be able to do selective embolization. The medical evaluation of the patient with spinal metastases may be more complicated than the patient with isolated malignancies. These patients may have advanced disease and suffer from anemia, gastrointestinal, or pulmonary problems. In addition the patient who has recently had irradiation or chemotherapy may have altered immune and hematological systems that make surgical treatment difficult. Their skin healing may also be affected by any previous radiation scarring. In these patients with severe health problems, the risk of surgical morbidity or mortality must be weighed against the risk of incapacitating pain, neurological damage, including paralysis and a shortened life expectancy if surgical treatment is withheld (8, 9). There are several options for treatment of metastatic disease including brace treatment, medical treatment including radiation therapy and chemotherapy and surgical treatment.

A. Stability in Metastatic Disease

One of the concerns in the treatment of metastatic disease to the spine is whether spinal instability exists. A spinal column that is weakened due to destructive erosion is possibly at risk for neurological damage. Tumor location is helpful in predicting which lesions will develop vertebral body collapse and segmental instability. Tumors of the anterior one-third and middle one-third will develop profound neurological injury more frequently (8). Kostuik and Errico (64) attempted to base the stability of the spinal column on a model dividing the vertebrae into an anterior and posterior part with separate left and right halves (Fig. 17). The anterior column was then further divided into four parts defined as the anterior left, anterior right, middle left, and middle right, giving a total of six segments. If one or two segments were destroyed by tumor, the spine was considered stable; if three or four segments were destroyed, it was considered unstable; if more than four segments were destroyed, it was markedly unstable. Any kyphosis or angulation of a vertebral segment of more than 20 degrees was also considered a sign of instability because of the abnormal forces put on that segment (64). In addition it should be remembered that unlike a nonpathologically fractured spine, a spine involved with metastatic disease will usually not become more stable as healing occurs and will most likely suffer more bone erosion over time.

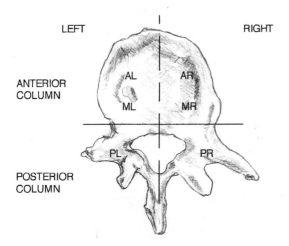

Figure 17 The vertebral body can be divided into six areas to determine the amount of instability present. (Modified from Kostuik, J. P., Errico, T. J., Gleason, T. F., Errico, C. C. Spinal stabilization of vertebral column tumors. Spine 1988; 13(3):250–256, Ref. 79.)

B. Brace Treatment

Plastic spinal braces or devices such as the halo vest are very useful in the treatment of metastatic disease involving the spine. In most cases, this will be combined with some other modalities of treatment such as radiation therapy, chemotherapy, or possibly after surgical treatment. It is somewhat rare that a brace will be used as an isolated treatment. The halo vest has been suggested as treatment for a neurologically intact patient with cervical spine metastases with pain or minimal instability. When used with radiation therapy, pain relief and sometimes bony healing can occur (8). This has been described a treatment option in two patients with multiple myeloma (90) and also in three patients with prostatic carcinoma (91). The halo vest in these cases was continued until there appeared to be bony healing and normal motion on flexion/extension radiographs. In addition, it was stressed that radiographs of the skull need to be evaluated to rule out skull involvement that would preclude use of skeletal pin fixation (90) (Fig. 18). A thoracolumbar orthosis is also an important part of the treatment of thoracic and lumbar metastatic disease but usually only as an adjunct to surgical treatment and not as a primary treatment modality. It can be used for patients who have pain but no deformity or neurological deficeit. The pain may be self limited if bracing is combined with radiation treatment.

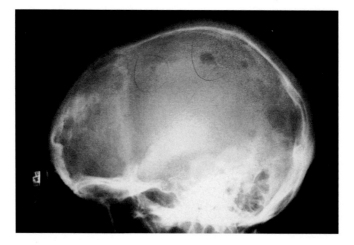

Figure 18 Lateral radiograph in a female with metastatic breast carcinoma showing lytic lesions of the skull. A lateral skull radiograph should be done in any patient who is to be placed into skeletal tong traction or a halo to determine if skull metastases are present.

C. Radiotherapy

Radiotherapy has historically been the treatment of choice and is still an important option in treatment of spinal metastases. This is particularly true in a patient with spinal pain or neurological compromise without vertebral body collapse. These patients will receive significant benefit from radiotherapy alone but their pre-existent neurological status will usually dictate what their likely outcome will be (8). Up to 70% of patients who are ambulatory will retain that functional ability after radiotherapy. Rarely will a patient who has lost the ability to walk become ambulatory again after radiotherapy alone (92). The type of metastases is very important given the significant difference in radiosensitivity between different tumor types. Prostatic and lymphoreticular tumors are quite radiosensitive, and excellent results are usually found with radiotherapy alone (92–94). Breast carcinoma is usually responsive to radiation but up to 30% of cases may be unresponsive to radiotherapy alone (92,95). Gastrointestinal and renal carcinoma are usually very resistant to radiotherapy.

D. Surgical Treatment of Metastatic Disease

Surgery for metastatic disease continues to change and evolve as ideas and technology change. Not long ago, laminectomy was considered the surgical treatment of choice for patients with neurological compromise produced by epidural metastatic lesions (45,47,96). Although posterior decompression was extensively used for all types of compression, studies began to show that functional results were not significantly improved with laminectomy compared with those produced by radiation therapy alone (4,19,47,97,98). Great strides have been made in tumor surgery with the advent of anterior vertebral body replacement and stabilization (99). Depending on the location of the insulting lesion, both anterior and posterior procedures are used today. In many instances a combination of both approaches is required to achieve the best result.

There are three main goals of surgical treatment of metastatic disease of the spine. These would be the avoidance of neurological injury or treatment of it if it has already developed), the treatment of pain associated with the neoplasm, and the avoidance, or treatment, of spinal deformity due to the neoplasm. Usually a complete cure of the initial neoplasm is not the reason for surgical treatment of a spinal metastasis. The hope is to mobilize the patient by restoring spinal stability, reduce pain to a tolerable level and preserve or improve the neurological status of the patient. Most authors require that the patient to be healthy enough to survive surgery, that he or she will have a survival from the underlying malignancy of at least 6 weeks, and that they not be hopelessly bedridden (12,64,65,100–103). Whereas long-term narcotic usage can often be justified for the symptomatic treatment of metastatic disease, surgical treatment can offer dramatic results. O'Neil reviewed 33 patients with surgical treatment for thoracic and lumbar metastases. Good or excellent pain relief was found in 94% of the patients (104). Kostuik and Errico found good or excellent pain relief in 81% of 71 patients treated with both anterior and posterior approaches for metastatic disease in the cervical, thoracic, or lumbar spine with survival averaging over 11 months (64). Harrington found that 94% of his 77 patients treated by anterior surgery had good or excellent pain relief (50). Therefore, operative treatment for pain relief alone must be considered at times.

When evaluating the effect of surgical treatment on neurological recovery, there appears to be a large difference between anterior vs. posterior treatment. Experimentally Doppman and Girton reported on the results of laminectomies for treatment of anterior epidural masses in an angiographic study of rhesus monkeys. They concluded that an epidural mass of more than 4 mm could not be adequately decompressed by posterior laminectomy alone (105). Several reports have shows that posterior decompression alone has a very low rate of neurological improvement. Livingston and Perrin (18) reviewed 100 laminectomies for neurological deficits in metastatic disease, with only 40% of the patients having satisfactory results in regard to their ability to walk, urinary continence, and survival of more than 6 months. Constans (49) showed only some slight improvement in results when comparing laminectomy vs. radiotherapy alone; 46% of patients treated with laminectomy and radiotherapy had improvement neurologically compared to 39% improvement in patients treated with radiation alone. Others have noted that less than half of those patients treated with radiotherapy and laminectomy have satisfactory results in retaining or regaining neurological function (106). This failure was due to either inadequate decompression of the spinal cord or the resultant destabilization of the spinal column. In a review of several large series (Table 3) comparing posterior decompression to anterior decompression for metastatic disease, Kostuik found the average neurological improvement to be 33% in those treated by posterior decompression versus 78% in those treated by anterior decompression. Only an average of 37% of the patients had a satisfactory outcome in those cases treated posteriorly vs. an 80% satisfactory outcome in those treated anteriorly (8).

1. Surgical Approaches and Tumor Location

In general the location of the neoplasm within the vertebral body or spinal canal will determine the symptoms and signs produced and in part dictate the surgical approach. The choice is determined by the extent of involvement of the spine, the presence of skip lesions, and the degree of epidural tumor. A close review of the preoperative testing including x-rays, CT/myelogram, or MRI will be necessary to plan the best approach. Almost every area of the spinal canal can be approached from either a posterior, anterior, or posterior-

Table 3 Maintenance and Recovery of Neurological Function in Patients Treated Surgically (Anterior vs. Posterior Decompression) for Cord Compression Due to Metastatic or Primary Spinal Tumor

Anterior decompression

Reference	Number of patients		% Improvement		% Satisfactory outcome
Sundaresan et al. (107)	160		80		78
Siegal and Siegal (108)	75		80		80
Fidler (63)	17		73		78
Harrington (50)	77		84		73
Kostuik (64)	70		73		84
Manabe et al. (65)	28		82		89
Total Patients	427	Average	78	Average	80

Posterior decompression

Reference	Number of patients		% Improvement		% Satisfactory outcome
Wright (109)	86		35		33
White et al. (96)	226		38		37
Hall and Mackay (45)	123		30		29
Gilbert et al. (47)	65		45		46
Nather and Bose (13)	42		13		29
Siegal et al. (56)	25		39		39
Sherman and Waddell (44)	149		27		48
Kostuik et al. (64)	30		36		37
Total Patients	746	Average	33	Average	37

Source: Ref. 8.

lateral or anterior-lateral approach. The addition of some form of spinal stabilization after any decompression is usually possible from any of the approaches chosen and will usually improve pain relief and avoid neurological deterioration from progressive instability. Whether this stabilization is provided by instrumentation and bone graft or with instrumentation and methyl-methacrylate is debated by different authors. In general if survival is anticipated to be less than 1 year methylmethacrylate is used and if it is more than 1 to 2 years, some form of bone grafting may be used.

A laminectomy alone should be restricted in rare cases where the site of compression is strictly posterior to the spinal cord (63). In the thoracic cord area, the surgical manipulation necessary to reach anterior tumor tissue from a posterior approach and the narrowness of the thoracic spinal canal can pose an increased risk for neurologic deficit (110).

Anterior decompression is usually restricted to patients with disease limited to one or two adjacent segments or with significant kyphosis in conjunction with vertebral body destruction. Skip lesions with single-level destruction at separate locations can be treated anteriorly but usually multiple-level disease is best treated by a posterior approach (8). If the metastatic disease is at more than two adjacent levels and is essentially posterior or where there is extensive epidural spread, the decompression can be carried out by a posterior-lateral approach. Occasionally in the thoracic spine one or two segmental nerve roots may be sacrificed to provide access for anterior tumor removal, and then stabilization can be achieved by posterior segmental instrumentation.

2. Anterior Surgery

Anterior surgery offers the ability to provide wide spinal cord decompression under direct visualization. Kyphotic deformity can be directly addressed and reconstructed. Johnson wrote about the effectiveness of anterior decompression for a wide range of conditions, including tumors, and found that neurological improvement was especially dramatic in cases involving metastatic disease and that early intervention had the best outcome with respect to neurological recovery (111). Many authors have reported favorable results from anterior surgery for metastatic disease of the spine (10,48,63,99,111–113). Patients who have undergone radiation therapy are at a lesser risk of having problems with wound healing and skin slough with anterior procedures as compared to posterior surgery (5, 12).

Vertebral replacement with methylmethacrylate is advantageous in patients with a limited prognosis or who may require radiation treatment after surgery (Fig. 19). Replacing the vertebral body with a large bone graft requires bracing for 2 to 4 months while the graft is incorporating. Corpectomy, especially of more than one level, requires a large graft and this can add significantly to the morbidity of a patient whose general condition may be frail to begin with. Patients with metastatic cancer often have osteopenic bone that has limited compressive strength. The risk of graft collapse may also increase with the use of postoperative irradiation, because therapeutic doses that will destroy tumor may also cause bone necrosis or delay healing (114). Methylmethacrylate is advantageous in that it offers immediate stability to compressive loads and can withstand radiation therapy without loss of strength or risk of dislodging. Methylmethacrylate is strongest in compression but weakest in tension; therefore, it is usually not as well indicated in posterior surgery. It functions best in an area,

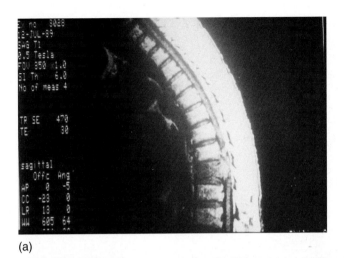

(a)

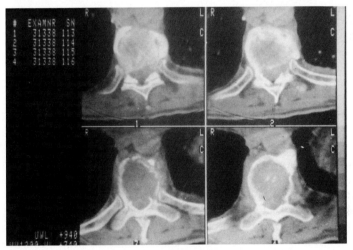

(b)

Figure 19   (a) A 49-year-old male presented with metastatic melanoma and paraparesis with a lesion of T7. Sagittal MRI shows a large anterior epidural tumor mass with replacement of the T7 vertebral body with tumor. (b) A CT scan after myelogram shows almost total replacement of vertebral body with erosion of posterior vertebral body and complete blockage. (c) Lateral postoperative radiograph showing replacement of T7 vertebra with methylmethacrylate in a Silastic tube without instrumentation.

(*Fig. continues*)

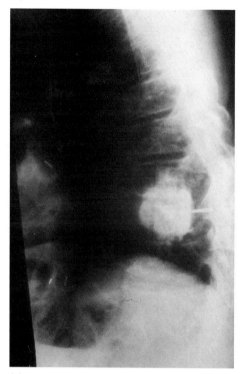

(c)

Figure 19 Continued

such as anterior vertebral body, where it will see compressive loads and function as a spacer (115). Cement is usually combined with some form of internal fixation that can be immediately stable and obviate the need for postoperative bracing. Lesions affecting one or two vertebrae can usually be treated without posterior supplemental fixation. More widespread involvement will usually require that an additional posterior stabilization be carried out (10,112). The use of cement alone without some form of bone grafting should also be avoided when the primary tumor is a type that may have a long survival, such as a lymphoma or some estrogen-sensitive breast carcinomas. In these cases, fusion should be attempted by using autogenous bone graft, because if a solid arthrodesis is not obtained, it may be only a matter of time before the construct fails (116).

3. Anterior Thoracic or Lumbar Techniques

The thoracic spine is prone to neurological injury resulting from what may be considered only a modest-sized lesion. For patients with thoracic disease a direct thoracotomy or using a retropleural technique can expose the diseased area and provide enough room for stabilization A double lumen endotracheal tube should be used to allow for selective lung deflation if necessary. The patient is usually placed in a right lateral decubitus position; the left side is chosen because the aorta is easier to mobilize rather than the more fragile vena cava. In the upper thoracic spine, the right side can be chosen with the azygous vein and superior vena cava being mobilized (117). In order to adequately expose the area and avoid working upward, it is usually best to begin the incision one or two ribs proximal to the most cranial vertebrae exposed.

For the T11 to L1 area, a thoracolumbar approach is employed. The diaphragm is taken down for exposure and this can be extended into the chest or distally into the abdomen. Below L2, a retroperitoneal approach, without exposing above the diaphragm, can be achieved using a left-sided approach (117).

Once the exposure has been performed a vertebrectomy can proceed from the anterolateral approach, with the anterior shell of the vertebrae being left if it is not involved with tumor. Different surgeons have advocated several techniques for achieving internal fixation after anterior vertebrectomy. Sundaresan has written of using two or more Steinmann pins imbedded in the adjacent superior and inferior vertebral bodies before placing the methylmethacrylate into the void (Fig. 20). These Steinmann pins enhance the bending resistance of the construct (57). Siegel has advocated placing Harrington distraction rods and, recently, sacral hooks with threaded rods for anterior purchase (56). Harrington has used Knodt rods, placed anteriorly in distraction, for the same purpuse (12, 99) (Fig. 21). In addition, Harrington has used Edwards hooks into the vertebral bodies anteriorly. Kostuik has used a modification of the Harrington instrumentation with Harrington-Kostuik screws placed in the vertebral bodies (118). Chang and Errico reported good results from a technique of using a Silastic tube filled with methylmethacrylate supplemented by anterior Harrington-Kostuik instrumentation. (119,120) (Figs. 22 & 23).

As minimally invasive surgery is becoming more prevalent, thorascopic anterior spinal procedures are beginning to carve a niche in tumor surgery. Regan et al. reported favorable results with thoracoscopic anterior vertebrectomy and stabilization (121). Although investigational at present, these techniques offer the potential benefits of anterior spinal surgery with reduced operative morbidity to those patients who may be quite ill to begin with.

Another new technique has involved the use of hollow metal cages that are placed between the vertebral bodies and can be filled either with morsalized autogenous bone graft or methylmethacrylate to reconstruct a vertebral body defect.

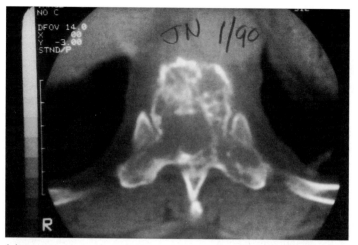

(a)

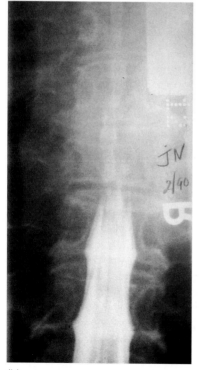

(b)

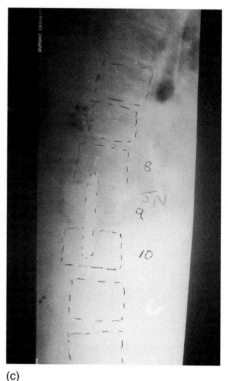

(c)

Figure 20 (a) A 62-year-old male with metastatic lung carcinoma (same patient as Figure 6). A CT scan shows destruction of vertebral body and transverse processes of T9. (b) Anteroposterior myelogram shows almost complete block of dye at T9. (c) Lateral postoperative radiograph after placement of Steinmann pin from T8-T10 with addition of methylmethacrylate.

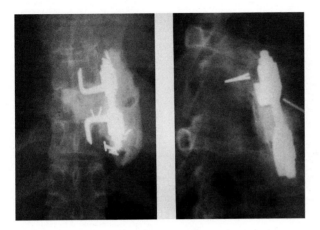

Figure 21 Example of reversed Edwards hooks used in distraction with methyl-methacrylate for a thoracic metastasis. (From Ref. 8.)

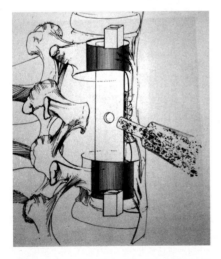

Figure 22 Technique using a soft Silastic tube that is placed in the vertebrec-tomy defect and into the intact proximal and distal vertebrae partially through the end plates. The Harrington-Kostuik screws have been placed into the verte-brae proximally and distally prior to filling the Silastic tube with methylmethacry-late. The liquid cement is placed into a Toomey syringe and injected into the Silastic tube through a small opening made laterally in the tube. This pressurizes the cement and also injects it into the vertebrae above and below for added support. The dura is covered with Gelfoam during the cement injection and, once hardened, the connecting rod is connected to the hooks. (From Ref. 135.).

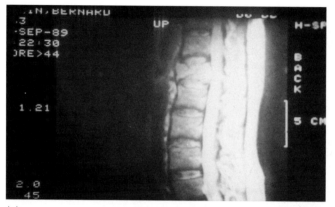

(a)

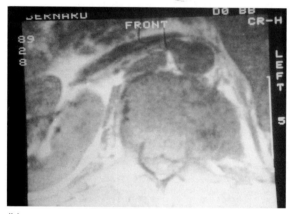

(b)

Figure 23 Example of the technique using a Silastic tube and anterior instrumentation. (a) Sagittal T2 MRI of a 62-year-old male with metastatic lung carcinoma and an L1 metastasis. (b) Axial MRI showing a large amount of tumor in the anterior epidural space with a pathological fracture of the posterior vertebral body. (c) Postoperative anteroposterior film after vertebrectomy and replacement with a Silastic tube with methylmethacrylate and anterior instrumentation. (d) Postoperative lateral view.

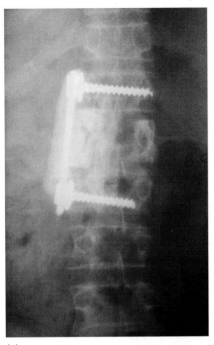

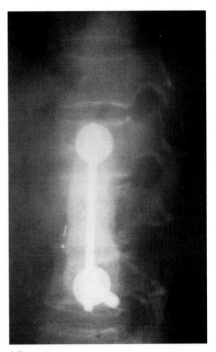

(c)   (d)

4. Posterior Surgery and Techniques

Although performed much less frequently, laminectomy still has a role in treating metastatic disease to the spine. Tumors that are primarily causing posterior compression should be decompressed via laminectomy. The lumbar spine offers more leeway toward posterior surgery than the thoracic or cervical spine, because distal to the termination of the spinal cord, the dura with the lumbar nerve roots can be retracted more vigorously. In the event that laminectomy is performed, it should have posterior fusion and stabilization included. Posterior decompression and stabilization are also useful for treatment of multiple levels of disease that may span from the cervical to the sacral area (Fig. 24), or to supplement anterior surgery when all three spinal columns have been invaded (Fig. 25). If more than two levels are decompressed from the anterior approach, then supplimental posterior stabilization should be considered. In the lower lumbar spine below L3, anterior stabilization is difficult to achieve and tumors in this area may be best treated with anterior excision and posterior fusion as a supplement (50). If radiotherapy is to be considered postoperatively after posterior stabilization, it should be delayed at least 2 weeks to allow for wound

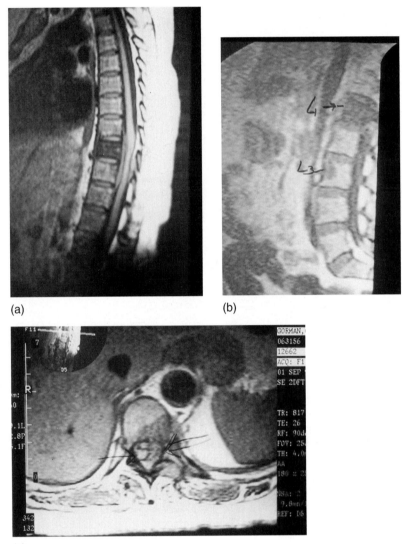

(a)   (b)

(c)

Figure 24 A 59-year-old female presented with back pain and paraparesis with a lesion of T9 that, on biopsy, was an adenocarcinoma from unknown origin. (a) Sagittal MRI shows a lesion of T9 without collapse but with epidural spread from T8 to T11. (b) Sagittal MRI of lumbar area shows involvement of L1 and also L3. (c) Axial MRI shows large left-sided epidural tumor mass. (d) and (e) Due to multiple tumor sites, the patient was treated with laminectomy from T8 to T11 and posterior fusion using Cotrel-Dubousset instrumentation from T4 to L3. Supplementary fixation was provided by intraspinous process wiring and wires placed through the foramen and transverse processes at the laminectomy sites.

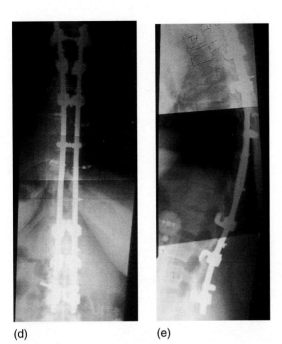

(d)　　　　　　　　(e)

healing. Additional techniques helpful in proving wound coverage in a less than adequate posterior area include meticulous muscle closure and possibly the use of soft tissue and skin expanders popularized by plastic surgeons (122,123). Because patients with metastatic disease often have weakened osteopenic bone, multiple levels of fixation are needed to reduce the risk of pullout (101). The thoracic and lumbar spine is amenable to traditional sublaminar wiring or current rod-hook constructs. Luque sublaminar wires may provide better fixation in soft bone than the traditional Harrington system (10,124) but have the added risk for sublaminar wire placement. Rod-hook constructs can also be supplemented by additional fixation points using spinous process wires and with wires passed around the transverse processes or through the neural foramen at operated segments (101) (Fig. 26). Posterior instrumentation in the thoracic spine should span three levels above and below the operated levels (5,20). This will further enhance the implant's hold but also can safeguard against further disease spread to adjacent levels.

Some authors advocate adding methylmethacrylate to the hardware posteriorly to increase fixation (Fig. 27) (48,112,116,125,126). This is believed to help mobilize the patient sooner without the need for postoperative bracing but has not been universally accepted.

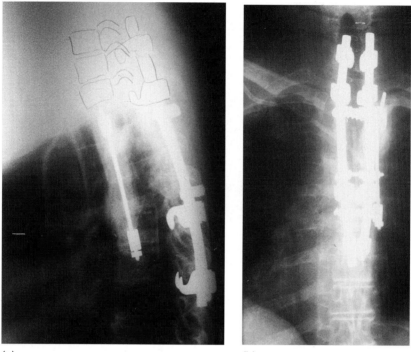

(a)   (b)

Figure 25 Example of a 50-year-old female with metastatic breast carcinoma
(see Figure 10) with involvement of all three spinal columns and epidural tumor
spread. The patient was treated with anterior vertebrectomy of T3 and T4 and
Harrington-Kostuik instrumentation, along with Silastic tube technique of anterior
reconstruction, the laminectomy posteriorly, and Cotrel-Dubousset instrumentation from C7 to T6. (a) Lateral radiograph. (b) Anteroposterior radiograph.

Costotransversectomy may be useful for masses that are anterolateral to
the thecal sac and may be useful for tumors arising in the spinal canal or for
lesions that can be removed without structurally weakening the vertebral body.
Corpectomy can be done from this approach, but stabilization is difficult due
to limited exposure. Posterior spinal stabilization can be carried out at the same
setting without having to do an anterior/posterior exposure, possibly lessening
the morbidity and surgical time required (127).

5. Cervical Techniques

Anterior surgery of the cervical spine has certain advantages over thoracic and
lumbar surgery. A general or thoracic surgeon is not needed for the approach.

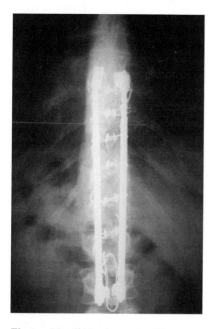

Figure 26 If Harrington rods are to be used posteriorly, they should be supplemented by some form of intraspinous or sublaminar fixation. This case was managed with Drummond intraspinous process wires.

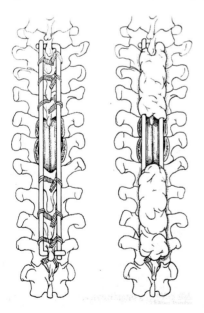

Figure 27 Example of technique described by Harrington using either Luque rods or Harrington rods posteriorly, with sublaminar wires above and below a laminectomy, and then reinforcing them with methylmethacrylate. (From Ref. 125.)

Postoperatively, a chest tube is not necessary and a prolonged ileus is uncommon. There is usually minimal pain due to the approach as tissue planes are gently spread apart without the need for soft tissue stripping. After cervical fusion, patients can be easily ambulated with either a halo brace or plastic orthosis such as a Philadelphia collar.

Indications for surgery in the subaxial cervical spine are similar to those for the remainder of the spine. In lesions below C3, an anterior approach with decompression and then vertebral body reconstruction with methylmethacrylate is usually advocated, especially if a patient's life expectancy is less than 1 year. If the tumor is limited to the anterior column and to one or two levels then a posterior reinforcement is usually unnecessary. Usually a left longitudinal sternocleidomastoid approach is advocated to decrease the incidence of neurological deficit of the recurrent laryngeal nerve but this can be at the discretion and training of the surgeon. Once decompression is complete, some form of stabilization is performed. Depending on the tumor virulence and the patient's long-term prognosis, the corpectomy site is filled with either methylmethacrylate, bone, or a combination of both (48).

A recent technique that can also be considered is the use of an anterior cervical plate in addition to an acrylic vertebral reconstruction. Six patients with cervical metastases treated in this way were presented by Atanasiu et al. (128), and apparently good fixation was reported (Fig. 28). If disease is more extensive or if there is also posterior involvement, then a posterior reinforcement is necessary (Fig. 29). When performing the anterior reconstruction, it is necessary to assess the quality of the vertebral bodies adjacent to the ones being removed. If there is even a small amount of tumor in these bodies at the time of surgery, the risk of recurrence should be considered. Because tumor recurrence often involves the vertebrae above and below the site of a previous resection, it is recommended that if a posterior cervical fusion is performed, it should be done two levels above and below the area of resection (129).

If the disease is primarily posterior, then a posterior approach with posterior stabilization using some form of metal instrumentation can be done. Techniques for posterior stabilization include using a Luque rectangle with either sublaminar or intraspinous process wiring or possibly a posterior lateral mass plating technique. Lesions at the cervicothoracic junction may need to be treated with a segmental posterior spinal system that can provide hooks for the thoracic spine and wires for the cervical spine (Fig. 30).

Lesions at the cervicothoracic junction may be particularly difficult to expose anteriorly. A modified anterior approach that involves splitting the proximal sternum and removing the medial left clavicle, using it for a possible bone graft, has been described. This permits exposure to the T4 area distally (130). Once this area has been exposed, reconstruction can be done using either ante-

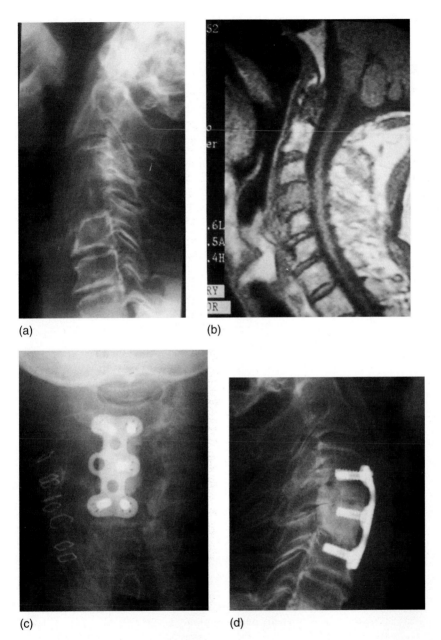

(a)　　　　　　　　　　(b)

(c)　　　　　　　　　　(d)

Figure 28　A 70-year-old male presented with neck pain 4 months after having a metastatic adenocarcinoma of unknown origin of his femur treated. (a) Lateral radiograph shows almost complete replacement of the C4 vertebrae with an early collapse pattern. (b) Sagittal MRI shows early epidural compression. (c) and (d) Anteroposterior and lateral radiographs after vertebral replacement with methylmethacrylate and anterior plating with AO locking plate from C3 to C5.

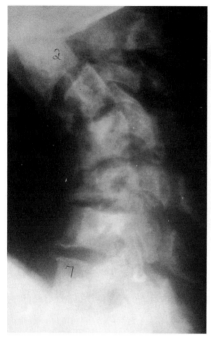

(a)

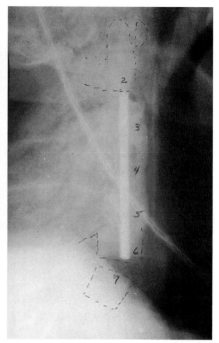

(b)

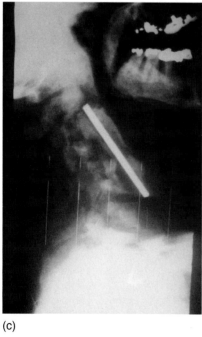

(c)

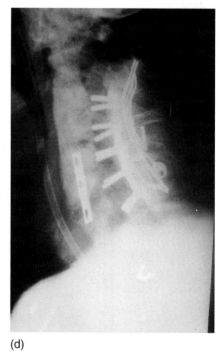

(d)

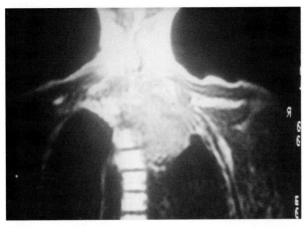

(a)

Figure 30 A 62-year-old male presented with a large right lung "pancoast tumor" with paraparesis secondary to thoracic and lower cervical vertebral body involvement. (a) Coronal MRI showing large right lung tumor. (b) Sagittal MRI showing involvement of lateral aspect of three vertebrae. (c) Axial MRI showing destruction of lateral vertebrae. (d) The patient was treated with posterior laminectomy from C6 to T2 with posterior fusion using Luque rods and a combination of sublaminar and intraspinous process wiring. Anteroposterior radiograph postoperatively. (e) Lateral radiograph postoperatively.

(*Figure 30 continues*)

rior cervical plates, or small Kirshner wires, or larger rods such as Knodt rods reinforced with methylmethacrylate (128).

The upper cervical spine, however, should be considered separately. Tumor that has infiltrated C1 or C2 carries the risk of sudden death and increased instability due to respiratory depression. Lesions in that location should be considered for prophylactic posterior stabilization. Although transoral decompres-

Figure 29 A 72-year-old male with metastatic prostate carcinoma presented with several weeks of neck pain and a fixed kyphotic deformity of his neck. (a) Lateral radiograph shows a kyphosis secondary to extensive disease with partial collapse of C3, C4, and C5. (b) The patient was initially treated with anterior vertebral reconstruction using cement and a Steinmann pin from C2 to C6. (c) One week postoperatively, he suffered graft dislodgment. (d) He was revised with repeat anterior cement replacement and posterior fusion from C2 to C6 with posterior plates, wires, and cement.

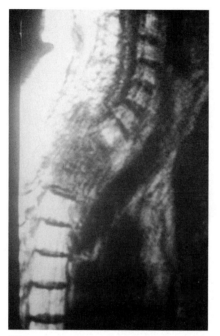

(b)

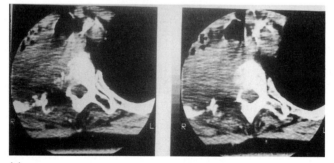

(c)

Figure 30 Continued

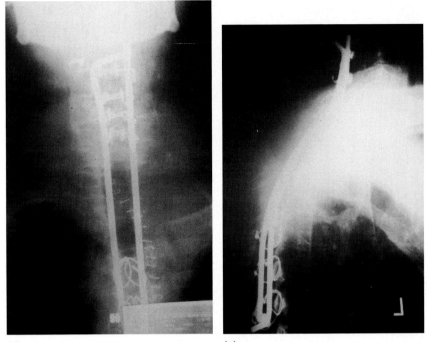

(d)   (e)

sion is the most direct route to lesions about the dens, this approach is not without considerable risk (131). In lesions above C3, a posterior approach is usually advocated but if the dens is preserved and the body of C2 is destroyed, an anterior approach can be used, fixing the dens to C3 or C4 with metal and methylmethacrylate (132). If the dens is destroyed, a posterior stabilization from C1 or the occiput to distal at C3 or C4 is necessary (Fig. 31).

Results from treatment of cervical lesions have been good. Fielding reported on 20 cases of cervical tumors treated with anterior vertebrectomy and bone grafting, with 13 requiring additional posterior fusion for stability augmentation. There were no graft failures; there was good resolution of neurological symptoms and pain with the quality of life and longevity all improved (129). These good results for similar treatment were also found by other authors (64,133,134). Fidler reported on 11 patients with upper cervical metastases treated with posterior decompression and stabilization that provided good to excellent pain relief in all patients; however, one patient still developed vertebral collapse due to severe anterior vertebral body destruction (63).

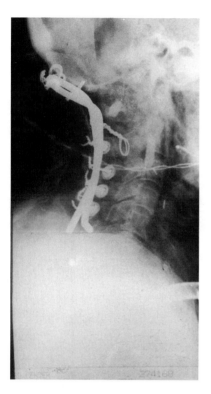

Figure 31 Example of lateral radiograph after fusion from occiput to C5 using Luque rectangle and Drummond intraspinous process wires and cranial wiring to occiput.

IV. SPECIAL CONSIDERATIONS

A. Renal Carcinoma

Renal carcinoma can be especially difficult to treat for several reasons. Frequently it presents with osseous metastases at the time of first diagnosis, which can demonstrate a highly variable course with respect to long-term survival (135,136). In addition it is notoriously radioresistant and unresponsive to chemotherapy. Renal cell carcinoma is also a very vascular tumor when metastatic to a skeletal area and a significant bleeding may be encountered. Angiography is usually recommended before operative treatment to help control this bleeding. Whereas this may only be necessary in a small number of patients, it may avoid a situation in which bleeding is severe enough to cause premature abandonment of surgical treatment (8) (Fig. 32).

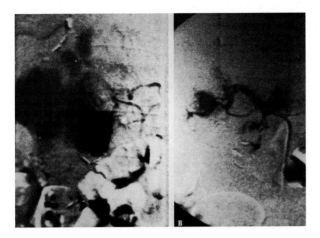

Figure 32 Example of a lateral digital subtraction angiogram of vertebral metastasis of renal carcinoma treated with preoperative embolization. Left-side film is preembolization; right-side film is postembolization. (From Ref. 120.)

King and Kostuik (137) presented 33 patients with renal cell metastatic to the spine that was treated surgically. Fifty percent of the patients had local recurrence of the tumor after decompression but all were helped by repeat decompression. Six patients needed more than two decompressions because of recurrent disease. Recurrence was more frequent in patients with more posterior than anterior involvement. Sundaresan (138) reported on 43 patients with renal cell carcinoma, 32 treated with anterior resection for cord compression and 11 treated with radiation only. The surgical group had a mean survival rate of 13 months compared to only 3 months for the radiation-treated group. The patients treated with complete resection of the tumor anteriorly had a 37% survival at 2 years, whereas none of the radiation-treated group survived 2 years. Neurological improvement was seen in 70% of the surgically treated patients compared to 45% of the radiated patients.

B. Tumors in Children

Metastatic spinal tumors can occur in children even though they are less common than primary bone tumors. The concern over treatment of the actual tumor is compounded by concern over management of the spinal deformity that may result from treatment. The usual metastatic tumors of adulthood are absent, but metastatic lesions or lesions from contiguous invasion can occur from neuroblastoma, embryonal carcinoma, or various sarcomas (9). In Tachdjian's series (139), which excluded intramedullary spinal cord tumors, 37% of the tumors found were malignant, with neuroblastoma occurring in 20% of the cases. Fraser (140) reviewed 40 pediatric spinal tumors and found that 30% were metastatic neuroblastomas.

Leukemia can also involve the vertebrae and cause potential treatment problems. In 6% of patients with pediatric leukemias, back pain and vertebral collapse are the initial findings at time of presentation. Up to 10% of patients with leukemia during the course of their disease sustain a pathological vertebral fracture (9). Radionucleotide bone scans are notoriously unreliable in diagnosing vertebral body involvement with leukemia. Many times they will show no uptake in an area of obvious bony destruction (141).

V. COMPLICATIONS

Unfortunately in any spinal disorder that requires operative treatment, there are instances in which complications may occur. These may be minor and involve medical problems such as wound infections, delayed healing of incisions, or pulmonary and gastrointestinal complications, or they may be major losses of fixation or neurological deterioration. As opposed to patients with nonpathological fractures whose spinal instability is assumed to lessen as their fracture heals, many patients with instability due to metastatic disease may never develop more spinal stability than they have at the termination of their operative treatment. This may be especially true for the patient who has had replacement of parts of the vertebrae by methylmethacrylate or who has had irradiation or chemotherapy as part of the original malignancy.

A number of studies have implicated iatrogenic instability and deformity as a reason for lack of neurological improvement and for occasional progression of neurological dysfunction after surgical treatment. Prevention of postoperative kyphosis and instability is crucial to maintenance of neurological improvement. Instability may result from inadequate reconstruction or stabilization at the time of the initial surgery or from late failure of fixation due to progressive disease or implant failure (8) (Fig. 33).

In Harrington's series (103) of 77 patients treated with posterior stabilization with methylmethacrylate, 5 suffered loss of fixation and required restabilization. Six patients developed spinal instability due to metastatic disease at other levels of the spine. In 100 patients treated by Kostuik (64), there were 3 cases of instrumentation failure, 1 with methylmethacrylate in the cervical spine, and 2 treated with Harrington instrumentation in the thoracic spine with methylmethacrylate but without sublaminar wires. All three cases required secondary surgeries. Kostuik had 75 patients treated with anterior constructs using methylmethacrylate-reinforced metal rods passed into the vertebral bodies proximal and distal to the resected level with only 1 failure, and with some constructs lasting as long as 4 years.

There appears to be a higher complication rate if the methylmethacrylate is used posteriorly for stabilization. McAfee (142) reported on 24 complications, with only 5 occurring after anterior stabilization and 19 occurring after methylmethacrylate was used posteriorly. Of these 19 patients, 15 suffered loss of fixation and a large number developed kyphosis. Six developed deep infections and three suffered associated significant neurological deterioration.

Most people agree that methylmethacrylate can last a very long time, but most feel that added bone graft should be used in cases with an anticipated survival of more than 1 year.

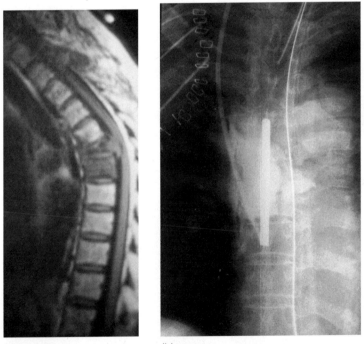

(a)   (b)

Figure 33 Example of failure of instrumentation due to inadequate fixation and poor bone quality. (a) Sagittal MRI of a 60-year-old female with metastaic breast carcinoma of T6 and T7. (b) The patient was treated with anterior reconstruction from T5 to T8 with Steinmann pin and methylmethacrylate. (c) Ten days postoperatively, she started to show early graft dislodgement superiorly. (d) She was treated with posterior short fusion two levels above and below the levels of anterior fusion and was noted to be very osteopenic. (e) and (f) Lateral and anteroposterior radiographs 4 months later showing dislodgement of inferior hooks and further lateral dislodgement of anterior graft. Patient and family refused further revision. This might have been avoided by performing longer posterior fusion along with multiple fixation points.

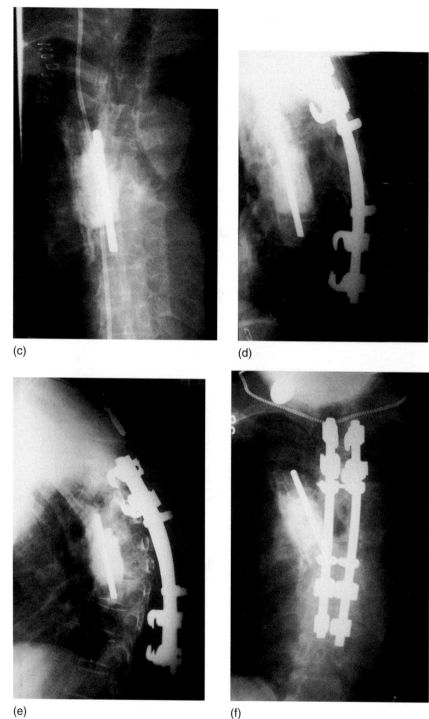

(c)

(d)

(e)

(f)

Figure 33 Continued

VI. SUMMARY

The treatment of patients with metastatic lesions involving the spinal column has advanced greatly in the last 20 years. With the advent of more sophisticated and quicker diagnosis and with refinements in the treatment available, the dismal prognosis that once was common has been replaced by the ability to continue a patient as a neurologically intact, active, and hopefully relatively pain-free individual who may still remain involved in society and family. For this to occur, it takes a concentrated effort via a team approach, with the spinal surgeon having a vital but not isolated part in the treatment plan. As refinements occur in the treatment plans, hopefully we will see the complication rate of these difficult spinal problems decrease, improvement in the life expectancy of these patients, and more definitive guidelines for their treatment.

REFERENCES

1. Dahlin DC. Bone Tumors: General Aspects and Data on 6,221 Cases. 3rd ed. Springfield: Charles C. Thomas, 1978.
2. American Cancer Society. Cancer Facts and Figures. New York: ACS, 1982.
3. Jaffee WL. Tumors and Tumorous Conditions of Bones and Joints. Philadelphia: Lea & Febiger, 1958.
4. Black P. Spinal metastases: Current status and recommended guidelines for management. Neurosurgery 1979; 5:726–746.
5. Harrington KD. Metastatic disease of the spine. In: Harrington, KD, ed. Orthopaedic Management of Metastatic Bone Disease. St. Louis: CV Mosby Co, 1988; 309–393.
6. Krishnamurthy GT, Tubis M, Hiss J, Blahd WH. Distribution pattern of metastatic bone disease. A need for total body skeletal image. JAMA 1977; 237:2504.
7. Schaberg JC, Gainor BJ. A profile of metastatic carcinoma of the spine. Spine 1985; 10:19.
8. Kostuik JP, Weinstein JN. Differential diagnosis and surgical treatment of metastatic spine tumors. In: Frymoyer JW, ed. The Adult Spine: Principles and Practice. New York: Raven Press, 1991; 861–888.
9. Weinstein JN, McLain RF. Tumors of the spine. In: Rothman RH, ed. The Spine. Philadelphia: WB Saunders Co, 1992: 1279–1318.
10. Dewald RL, Bridwell KH, Prodromas C, Rodts MF. Reconstructive spinal surgery as palliation for metastatic malignancies of the spine. Spine 1985; 10:21–26.
11. Drury AB, Palmer PH, Highman WH. Carcinomatous metastasis to the vertebral bodies. J Clin Pathol. 1964; 17:448–457.
12. Harrington KD. Current Concepts Review. Metastatic Disease of the Spine. J Bone Joint Surg 1986; 68A:1110–1115.
13. Nather A, Bose K. The results of decompression of cord or cauda equina compression from metastatic extradural tumors. Clin Orthop 1982; 169:103–108.

14. Perrin RG, McBroom RJ. Anterior versus posterior decompression for symptomatic spinal metastasis. Can J Neurol Sci 1987; 14:75.

15. Brihaye J, Ectors P, Lemort M, Van Houtte P. The management of spinal epidural metastases. Adv Tech Stand Neurosurg 1988; 16:121.

16. Viadana E. Autopsy study of metastatic sites of breast cancer. Cancer Res. 1973; 33:179–181.

17. Alexander E, Davis CH, Field CH. Metastatic lesion of the vertebral column causing cord compression. Neurology 1956; 6:103.

18. Livingston KE, Perrin RG. The neurosurgical management of spinal metastases causing cord and cauda equina compression. J Neurosurg 1978; 49:839.

19. Nicholls PJ, Jarecky TW. The value of posterior decompression by laminectomy for malignant tumors of the spine. Clin. Orthop. 1985; 201:210–213.

20. Nottebaert M, Von Hochstetter AR, Exner GU, Schreiber A. Metastatic carcinoma of the spine: A study of 92 cases. Internat Orthop 1987; 11:345.

21. Roy-Camille R, Saillant G, Lapresle PH. Fixation of spinal metastases using plates and pedicular screws. Rev Chir Orthop 1985; 71:483.

22. Zevallos M, Chan PYM, Munoz L. Epidural spinal cord compression from metastatic tumor. Int J Radiat Oncol Biol Phys 1987; 13:875.

23. Engell HC. Cancer cells in the circulating blood. Acta Chir Scand(Suppl) 1955; 201:1.

24. Nicholson G. Cancer metastases Sci Am 1979; 240:66.

25. Roos E, Dingemans KD. Mechanisms of metastasis. Biochem Biophys Acta 1979; 560:135.

26. Stoll BA. Natural history, prognosis, and staging of bone metastases. In Stoll BA, Parbhoo S. eds. Bone Metastases: Monitoring and Treatment. New York, Raven Press, 1983; 1–20.

27. Batson OV. The role of the vertebral veins in metastatic processes. Ann Intern Med. 1942; 16:38–45.

28. Bullough PG, Vigorita VJ. Atlas of Orthopaedic Pathology with Clinical and Radiographic Correlations. New York; Gower Medical Publishing Ltd, 1984.

29. Galasko CSB. The development of skeletal metastases. In: Weiss L., Gilbert HA, eds., Bone Metastases. Boston: GK Hall Medical Publishers, 1981.

30. Powles TJ. Breast cancer osteolysis, bone metastasis, and the antiosteolytic effect of aspirin. Lancet, 1976; 1:608–610.

31. Braunstein EM, Kuhns LR. Computed tomographic demonstration of spinal metastases. Spine 1983; 8:912.

32. Asdorian PL, Weidenbaum M, Hammerberg KW, Dewald RL. The pattern of vertebral involvement in metastatic vertebral breast cancer. Clin Orthop 1990; 250:164.

33. Willis RA. The spread of tumors in the human body. 3rd ed. London: Butterworths, 1973.

34. Fischer B. Fisher ER, Feduska N. Trauma and the localization of tumor cells. Cancer 1967; 20:23.

35. Vernon-Roberts B, Pirie CJ. Healing trabecula microfractures in the bodies of the lumbar spine. Ann Rheum Dis 1973; 32:406.

36. Dommisse GF. The blood supply of the spinal cord: A critical vascular zone in spinal surgery. J. Bone Joint Surg 1974; 56B:225.

37. Crook HW, Yoshizawa H. The blood supply of the vertebral column and spinal cord in man. New York: Wein, Springer, 1977.

38. Louis R. Surgery of the spine. Surgical anatomy and operative approaches. Berlin: Springer-Verlag, 1983.

39. Bullough PG, Boachie-Adjei O. Atlas of Spinal Diseases. New York: Gower Medical Publishing, 1988.

40. Asdorian PL, Mardjetko S, Rauschning W, Jonsson J, Hammerberg K, Dewald R. An evaluation of spinal deformity in metastatic breast cancer. J Spinal Disord 1990; 3:119.

41. Pittaluga S, Soffer D, Siegel T, Siegel T. Massive hemorrhagic necrosis of the spinal cord in metastatic cord compression. Clin Neuropathol 1983; 2:114.

42. Barron KD, Hirano A, Araki S, Terry RD. Experiences with metastatic neoplasms involving the spinal cord. Neurology 1959; 9:91.

43. Asdorian PL. Metastatic disease of the spine. In: Bridwell KH, Dewald RL, eds. The textbook of Spinal Surgery. Philadelphia: JB Lippincott, 1991.

44. Sherman RMP, Waddell JP. Laminectomy for metastatic epidural cord tumors. Clin Orthop 1986; 207:55–63.

45. Hall AJ, MacKay NNS. The results of laminectomy for compression of the cord or cauda equina by extradural malignant tumor. J Bone Joint Surg 1973; 55B:497–505.

46. Arseni CN, Simionescu MD, Horwath L. Tumors of the spine. A follow up study of 350 patients with neurosurgical considerations. Acta Psychiatr Scand 1959; 34:398.

47. Gilbert RW, Kim JH, Posner JB. Epidural spinal cord compression from metastatic tumor: Diagnosis and treatment. Ann Neurol 1978; 3:40–51.

48. Boland PJ, Lane JM, Sundaresan N. Metastatic disease of the spine. Clin Orthop 1982; 169:95–102.

49. Constans JP, Divitiis E, Donzelli R, et al. Spinal metastases with neurologic manifestations: A review of 600 cases. J Neurosurg 1983; 59:111–118.

50. Harrington KD. Anterior decompression and stabilization of the spine as a treatment for vertebral collapse and spinal cord compression from metastatic malignancy. Clin Orthop 1988; 233:177–197.

51. Liaw CC, Leung W, Ng KT, et al. Malignant lesions causing spinal compression: Review of 139 cases. J Formosan Med Assoc 1988; 87:310.

52. Ono K, Tada K. Metal prosthesis of the cervical vertebrae. J Neurosurg 1975; 42:562.

53. Phillips E, Levine AM. Metastatic lesions of the upper cervical spine. Spine 1989; 14:1071.

54. Shaw B, Mansfield FL, Borges L. One stage posterolateral decompression and stabilization for primary and metastatic vertebral tumors in the thoracic and lumbar spine. J Neurosurg 1989; 70:405.

55. Sherk HH. Lesions of the atlas and axis. Clin Orthop 1975; 109:33.

56. Siegel T, Tiqva P, Siegel T. Vertebral body resection for epidural compression by malignant tumors. J. Bone Joint Surg 1985; 67A:375–382.

57. Sundaresan N, Galicich JH, Lane JM, et al. Treatment of neoplastic epidural cord compression by vertebral body resection and stabilization. J Neurosurg 1985; 63:676–684.

58. Sundaresan N, Galicich JH, Lane JM, Greenberg HS. Treatment of odontoid frac-
     tures in cancer patients. J. Neurosurg 1981; 54:187.
59. Galasko CSB. The role of the orthopaedic surgeon in the treatment of bone pain.
     Cancer Surv 1988; 7:103.
60. Shives TC, Dahlin DC, Sim FH, et al. Osteosarcoma of the spine. J Bone Joint
     Surg. 1986; 68A:660–668.
61. Sim FH, Dahlin DC, Stauffer RN, Laws ER. Primary bone tumors simulating lum-
     bar disc syndrome. Spine 1977; 2:65–74.
62. Swanson DA, Orovan WL, Johnson DE, Giacco G. Osseos metastases secondary
     to renal cell carcinoma. Urology 1981; 18:556.
63. Fidler MW. Anterior decompression and stabilization of metastatic spinal fractures.
     J Bone Joint Surg. 1986; 68B:83–90.
64. Kostuik JP, Errico TJ, Gleason TF, Errico CC. Spinal stabilization of vertebral
     column tumors. Spine 1988; 13:250–256.
65. Manabe S, Tateisni A, Abe M, Ohno T. Surgical treatment of metastatic tumors of
     the spine. Spine 1989; 14:41–47.
66. Edelstyn GA, Gillespie PJ, Grebell ES. The radiologic demonstration of osseos
     metastases experimental observations. Clin. Radiol. 1967; 18:158–164.
67. Lodewick GS. Determining growth rates of focal lesions of bone from radiographs.
     Radiology 1980; 134:577–583.
68. Mullan J, Evans JP. Neoplastic disease of the spinal extradural space: A review of
     50 cases. Arch Surg 1957; 74:900.
69. Spjut HJ, Dorfman HD, Fechner RE, Ackerman LV. Tumors and Cartilage. Wash-
     ington DC: Armed Forces Institute of Pathology, 1971.
70. Galasko CSB. Skeletal metastases. Clin Orthop 1986; 210:18.
71. Joo KG, Parthasaranthy KL, Bakshi SP, Posner D. Bone scintigrams: Their clinical
     usefulness in patients with breast carcinoma. Oncology 1979; 36:94.
72. Roberts JG, Gravalle IH, Baum M. Evaluation of radiography and isotope scintig-
     raphy for detecting skeletal metastases in breast cancer. Lancet 1976; 1:237.
73. Galasko CSB. Mechanisms of bone destruction in the development of skeletal me-
     tastases. Nature 1976; 263:507.
74. Galasko CB. The pathologic basis for skeletal scintigraphy. J Bone Joint Surg 57
     1975; B:353.
75. Milch A, Changus GW. Response of bone to tumor invasion. Cancer 1956; 9:340–
     351.
76. Corcoran RJ, Thrall JH, Kyle RW, et al. Solitary abnormalities in bone scans of
     patients with extraosseos malignancies. Radiology 1976; 121:663–667.
77. Citrin DL, Bessent RG, Greig WR. A comparison of sensitivity and accuracy of
     the 99m Tc phosphate bone scan and skeletal radiograph in the diagnosis of bone
     metastases. Clin Radiol. 1977; 28:107–111.
78. Waxman AD. Bone scans are of sufficient accuracy and sensitivity to be part of
     the routine work up prior to definitive surgical treatment of cancer. In: Van Scoy-
     Mosher MB, ed. Medical Oncology-Current Controversies in Cancer Treatment.
     Boston: GK Hall Medical Publishers, 1981; 69–76.
79. Weinstein JN, McLain RF. Primary tumors of the spine. Spine 1987; 12:843–851.

80. Weinstein JN. Surgical approaches to spine tumors. Orthopaedics 1989; 12:843–851.

81. Rodichok LD, Harper GR, Ruckdeschel JC, et al. Early diagnosis of spinal epidural metastases. Am J Med 1981; 70:1181.

82. Rodichok LD, Ruckdeschel JC, Harper GR, et al. Early detection and treatment of spinal epidural metastases. The role of myelography Ann Neurol 1986; 20:696.

83. Hollis PH, Malis LI, Zappulla RA. Neurologic deterioration after lumbar puncture below complete spinal subarachnoid block. J Neurosurg 1986; 64:253.

84. Godersky JC, Smoker WRK, Knutzon R. Use of magnetic resonance imaging in the evaluation of metastatic spinal disease. Neurosurgery 1987; 21:676.

85. Smoker WRK, Godersky JC, Knutzon RK, et al. The role of MR imaging in evaluating metastatic spinal disease. AJR 1987; 149:1241.

86. Hewes RC, Vigorita VJ, Freiberger RH. Percutaneus bone biopsy: The importance of aspirated osseous blood. Radiology 1983; 148:69.

87. Tehtanzadeh J, Freiberger RH, Ghelman B. Closed skeletal needle biopsy: Review of 120 cases. AJR 1983; 140:113.

88. Mink J. Percutaneus bone biopsy in the patient with known or suspected osseous metastases. Radiology 1986; 161:191.

89. Murphy WA, Destouet JM, Gilula LA. Percutaneus skeletal biopsy 1981: A procedure for radiologists—results, review and recommendations. Radiology 1981; 139:545.

90. Abitbol JJ, Botte MJ, Garfin SR, Akeson WH. The treatment of multiple myeloma of the cervical spine with a halo vest. J Spinal Disord 1989; 2:4:263–267.

91. Danzig LA, Resnick D, Akeson WH. The treatment of cervical spine metastasis from the prostate with a halo cast. Spine 1980; 5:395–398.

92. Tomita T, Galicich JH, Sundaresan N. Radiation therapy for spinal epidural metastases with complete block. Acta Radiol Oncol 1983; 22:135–143.

93. Bruckman JE, Bloomer WD. Management of spinal cord compression Semin Oncol 1978; 5:135–140.

94. Millburn L, Hibbs GC, Hendrickson FR. Treatment of spinal cord compression from metastatic carcinoma. Cancer 1968; 21:447–452.

95. Greenberg HS, Kim JN, Posner JB. Epidural spinal cord compression from metastatic tumor. Ann Neurol 1980; 8:361–366.

96. White WA, Patterson RH, Bergland RM. Role of surgery in the treatment of spinal cord compression by metastatic neoplasm. Cancer 1971; 27:3:558–561.

97. Barcena A, Lobato RD, Rivas JJ, et al. Spinal metastatic disease: Analysis of factors determining functional prognosis and the choice of treatment. Neurosurgery 1984; 15:820–827.

98. Young RF, Post EM, King GA. Treatment of spinal epidural metastases randomized prospective comparison of laminectomy and radiotherapy. J. Neurosurg 1980; 53:741–748.

99. Harrington KD. The use of methylmethacrylate for vertebral body replacement and anterior stabilization of pathologic fracture-dislocations of the spine due to metastatic disease. J Bone Joint Surg 1981; 63A:36–46.

100. Dolin MG. Acute massive dural compression secondary to methylmethacrylate replacement of a tumorous lumbar vertebral body. Spine 1989; 14:108–110.

101. Flatley TJ, Anderson MH, Anast GT. Spinal instability due to malignant disease. J Bone Joint Surg 1984; 66A:47–52.

102. Fraser RD, Paterson DC, Simpson DA. Orthopaedic aspects of spinal tumors in children. J Bone Joint Surg 1984; 59B:143–151.

103. Harrington KD, Sim FH, Enis JE, et al. Methylmethacrylate as an adjunct in internal fixation of pathologic fractures. J Bone Joint Surg 1976; 58A:1047–1055.

104. O'Neil J, Gardner V, Armstrong G. Treatment of tumors of the thoracic and lumbar spinal column. Clin. Orthop 1988; 227:103–112.

105. Doppman JL, Girton M. Angiographic study of the effect of laminectomy in the presence of acute anterior epidural masses. J Neurosurg 1976; 45:195–202.

106. Shaw MDM, Rose JE, Paterson A. Metastatic extradural malignancy of the spine. Acta Neurochir 1980; 52:113–120.

107. Sundaresan N, Scher H, DiGiacinto GV, et al. Surgical treatment of spinal cord compression in kidney cancer. J Clin Oncol 1986; 4:1851–1856.

108. Siegel T, Siegel T. Surgical decompression of anterior and posterior malignant epidural tumors compressing the spinal cord: A prospective study. Neurosurgery 1985; 17:424–432.

109. Wright RL. Malignant tumors in the spinal extradural space. Results of surgical treatment. Ann Surg 1963; 157(2):227–231.

110. Martin NS, Williamson J. The role of surgery in the treatment of malignant tumours of the spine. J Bone Joint Surg 1970; 52B:227–237.

111. Johnson JR, Leatherman KD, Holt RT. Anterior decompression of the spinal cord for neurologic deficit. Spine 1983; 8:396–405.

112. Kostuik JP. Anterior spinal cord decompression for lesions of the thoracic and lumbar spine; technique, new methods of internal fixation and results. Spine 1983; 8:512–531.

113. Siegel T, Siegel T. Current considerations in the management of neoplastic spinal cord compression. Spine 1989; 14:223–228.

114. Arpin H. Metastatic tumors of the spine. Spine: State of the Art reviews 1987; 2:301–311.

115. White AA III, Panjabi MM. Surgical constructs employing methylmethacrylate. In Clinical Biomechanics of the spine. Philadelphia, JB Lippincott Co, 1978; 423–431.

116. Clark CR, Keggi KJ, Panjabi MM. Methylmethacrylate stabilization of the cervical spine. J Bone Joint Surg 1984; 66A:40–46.

117. Bradford DS. Techniques of surgery. In: Moes Textbook of Scoliosis and other Spinal Deformities, 2nd ed. Philadelphia, WB Saunders Co, 1987; 135–189.

118. Kostuik JP. Anterior Kostuik-Harrington distraction systems. Orthopaedics 1988; 11:10:1379–1391.

119. Chang MK, Errico TJ, Cooper PR, Crawford B. A new technique for anterior spinal reconstruction for neoplastic disease. Abstract. NASS meeting, San Diego 1993.

120. Errico TJ, Kostuik JP. Diagnosis and treatment of pathologic spinal fractures secondary to metastatic disease. In: Spinal Trauma. Errico TJ, Bauer RD, Waugh T, eds. Philadelphia: JB Lippincott Co, 1991.

121. Regan JJ, Mack MJ, Picetti GD III, et al. A comparison of video-assisted thoracoscopy (VAT) to open thoracotomy in thoracic spinal surgery. Abstract. NASS meeting, San Diego, 1993.

122. Zide BM, Wisoff JH, Epstein FJ. Closure of extensive and complicated laminectomy wounds. J Neurosurg 1987; 67:59–64.

123. Paonessa KJ, Zide B, Errico T, Engler GL. Using tissue expanders in spinal surgery for deficient soft tissue or postirradiation cases. Spine 1991; 16S:324–327.

124. Cybulski GR, Von Roenn KA, D'Angelo CM, Dewald RL. Luque rod stabilization for metastatic disease of the spine. Surg Neurol 1987; 28:277–283.

125. Harrington KD. Metastatic Tumors of the spine: Diagnosis and treatment. J Amer Acad Orthop Surg 1993; 1:76–86.

126. Errico TJ, Kostuik JP. Diagnosis and treatment of metastatic disease of the spinal column: A review. Contemp Orthop 1986; 13:15–26.

127. Overby MC, Rothman AS. Anterolateral decompression for metastatic epidural spinal cord tumors. J Neurosurg 1985; 62:344–348.

128. Atanasiu JP, Badatcheff F, Pidhorz L. Metastatic lesions of the cervical spine: A retrospective analysis of 20 cases. Spine 1993; 18:1279–1284.

129. Fielding JW, Pyle RN, Fietti VG. Anterior cervical vertebral body resection and bone grafting for benign and malignant tumors. J Bone Joint Surg 1979; 61A:251–253.

130. Kurz LT, Pursel SE, Herkowitz HN. Modified anterior approach to the cervicothoracic junction. Spine 16(Suppl): 1991; 542–547.

131. Fang HSY, Ong GB. Direct anterior approach to the upper cervical spine. J Bone Joint Surg 1962; 44A:1588.

132. McAfee PC, Bohlman HH, Riley LH Jr, et al. The anterior retropharyngeal approach to the upper part of the cervical spine. J Bone Joint Surg 1987; 69A:1371.

133. Bohlman HH, Sachs BL, Carter JR, et al. Primary neoplasms of the cervical spine. J Bone Joint Surg 1986; 68A:483–494.

134. Verbiest H. From anterior to lateral operations on the cervical spine. Neurosurg. Rev. 1978; 47:1–2.

135. Saitoh H, Hida M. Metastatic processes and a potential indication of treatment for metastatic lesions of renal adenocarcinoma. J Urol 1982; 128:916–918.

136. Skinner DG, Colvin RB. Diagnosis and management of renal cell carcinoma. Cancer 1971; 28:1165–1177.

137. King GJ, Kostuik JP, McBroom RJ, Richardson W. Surgical management of metastatic renal carcinoma of the spine. Spine 1991; 16:265–271.

138. Sundaresan N, Scher H, Digiacinto GV, et al. Surgical treatment of spinal cord compression in kidney cancer. J Clin Oncol 1986; 4:1851–1856.

139. Tachdjian MO, Matson DD. Orthopaedic aspects of intraspinal tumors in infants and children. J Bone Joint Surg 1965; 47A:223–248.

140. Fraser RD, Paterson DC, Simpson DA. Orthopaedic aspects of spinal tumors in children. J Bone Joint Surg. 1977; 59B:143–151.

141. Clausen N, Goetze H, Pedersen A, et al. Skeletal scintigraphy and radiography at
      onset of acute lymphocytic leukemia in children. Med Pediatr Oncol 1983;
      11:291–296.
142. McAfee PC, Bohlman HH, Ducker T, Eismont FJ. Failure of stabilization of the
      spine with methylmethacrylate. J Bone Joint Surg 1986; 68A:1145–1157.

16

Spinal Features of Multiple Sclerosis

Clive Paul Hawkins
Keele Postgraduate Medical School and Royal Infirmary, Stoke-on-Trent, England

Multiple sclerosis (MS) is a disease of the central nervous system with particular involvement of the spinal cord, optic nerve, and brainstem. Prevalence in Britain approaches 80–100 cases per 100,000 population. The definitive clinical and pathological description of the disease was established by Charcot (Histologie de la Sclerose en Plaques). It usually follows a relapsing and remitting course, with progression of disability in time leading to spastic weakness, visual loss, and ataxia (1). The hallmarks of the condition include demyelination, inflammatory change, and gliosis (2–5) resulting in a multifocal disorder of white matter. At the present time there is no proven effective treatment to ameliorate progression of the condition in the long term, but a course of high-dose intravenous methylprednisolone shortens the duration of symptoms and clinical signs during relapse (6).

There is evidence for both genetic and environmental factors in the etiology of the disease (1). Support for the former comes from family studies. The risk of developing MS in a monozygotic twin, whose twin is affected, is as high as 30%, whereas for a dizygotic twin, the risk may be as low as that for other family members—between 0.6% and 2.5% (7). There is an association between MS and certain HLA groups, particularly DR2, DR4 and DQw1 (8, 9). Evidence for an environmental factor is suggested from migration studies: children migrating from a region of high risk to a low-risk area have a lower incidence of the disease than migrating adults (10). Further support comes from a possible "epidemic" of MS in the Faeroe Islands between 1943 and 1960 attributed to the influx of British troops during the Second World War (11).

There are several lines of evidence to suggest that MS is an immune-mediated condition, either resulting from an abnormality of systemic immunity (12, 13) or a more localized central nervous system disorder (14, 15). The nature of the immune antigen(s) is uncertain, and it is noticeable that a somewhat clinically similar condition involving the spinal cord and optic nerves (previously known as tropical spastic paraparesis or Jamaican myelopathy) is associated with slow virus infection (HTLV1) (16, 17). Animal models of demyelination may occur as a result of viral infection, in which the chronic phase of demyelination is mediated by activated immune cells (18). There are also important similarities in the morphological and pathogenetic characteristics between MS and a model of autoimmune-mediated demyelination, experimental allergic encephalomyelitis (EAE) (19, 20). In both conditions there is inflammatory demyelination and blood-brain barrier (BBB) breakdown with, in the chronic form of EAE, a relapsing and remitting course. Genetic restriction operates in both and there may be similar immune mechanisms: EAE is T lymphocyte-mediated and changes in peripheral blood lymphocyte subsets are seen in MS (1, 13). There is evidence for abnormal antibody production in EAE lesions, and oligoclonal IgG bands are a frequent finding in the cerebrospinal fluid in MS (20, 21). Breach of the BBB in both conditions allows access of immune cells to the normally forbidden ground of the central nervous system (22), with the potential for antigen presentation by locally resident cells.

Blood-brain barrier breakdown in multiple sclerosis was first observed by Broman when leakage of Trypan blue occurred into active plaques, and less so into chronic ones, after supravital injection (23). Other evidence for a central role of vascular changes in the evolution of the MS plaque came from Dawson (3), who described finger-like projections of plaque along draining venules and veins and from Fog (24), who established that virtually all lesions in the cerebral hemispheres are perivenular in distribution. More recently, Allen has found changes of perivascular inflammation affecting the normal-appearing white matter of patients with mild or spinal MS (4). The question of ensuing vascular damage in MS has been recently addressed, and evidence for past BBB breakdown was observed in many vessels in and around plaques—the presence of hemosiderin deposition indicating past extravasation of red blood cells (Adams et al., 5). Adams et al. indeed considered MS as a form of central nervous system venulitis or vasculitis. The most convincing evidence that inflammation in MS can occur in the absence of myelin breakdown products, and that demyelination is not a necessary precursor of it, comes from the observation that retinal periphlebitis with leakage of injected fluorescein is a frequent finding in patients with optic neuritis (25), which is often the presenting feature of MS. The fact that such retinal changes occur in a region free of myelin and its breakdown products raises the question whether vascular changes are a very early, perhaps primary event in the development of the new lesion.

With computed tomographic (CT) scanning and magnetic resonance imaging (MRI), it has been possible to visualize the MS lesion in vivo for the first time. Breakdown of the BBB can be assessed using iodine-contrast media with CT scanning (26) and vascular changes observed by MRI using the contrast agent, gadolinium-DTPA (Gd-DTPA). Gadolinium enhancement is seen in patients with active disease (27–29). In serial studies, when patients are rescanned 1 month apart, two-thirds of the previously Gd-enhancing lesions cease to enhance (29); thus, Gd enhancement appears to be of relatively short duration. Similarly, in chronic relapsing EAE, Gd enhancement in the spinal cord is short-lived, and histological studies show that areas of enhancement correspond to BBB breakdown and accompanying inflammatory change within the spinal cord (30, 31). Thus MS is a demyelinating disease in which inflammation is known to occur.

A minority of patients, up to 30%, have benign MS and are minimally disabled 10 years or more after diagnosis. Usually, an initial relapsing and remitting course is followed—in up to 60% of patients—by the development of progressive disability, secondary progressive disease (2°P). In a small group, up to 10%, the condition is progressive from onset (usually of spinal-type, progressive spastic paraparesis) without clinical relapses or remissions—primary progressive disease (1°P). There is evidence for immunogenetic differences between the two types of MS (32). Magnetic resonance imaging has demonstrated differences in the pattern and extent of abnormality seen in the cerebrum between the two groups (33). In a serial study with Gd-enhanced MRI (34, 35), 24 patients (12 with 1°P and 12 with 2°P disease) were scanned during a 6-month period. In the 2°P group, 109 new lesions were seen during the study period, and 87% of these showed enhancement. By contrast, in the 1°P patients only 20 new lesions were seen and only one of these enhanced. There was no difference in the degree of clinical deterioration between the two groups during the study. These findings suggest that there may be a less significant inflammatory component in the evolution of new lesions in patients with 1°P MS when compared to those with 2°P disease.

I. CLINICAL FEATURES

Spinal symptoms or signs are almost invariably present in the course of MS and, in up to 60% of patients, are the presenting feature of the disease. Usually spinal symptoms are relapsing and remitting, with an average relapse rate once every 2 years; with progression of the condition, spinal symptoms become persistent and clinical signs develop with ensuing neurological disability. The cervical and thoracic cords are particularly involved, and the lumbosacral cord is occasionally affected. As might be expected from the evolution of BBB changes accompanying inflammatory demyelination (shown by Gd-enhanced MRI), spinal symptoms, and clinical signs develop subacutely over a period of days to a few weeks, to reach a plateau, usually for a matter of weeks before gradual recovery. Sometimes, as in primary progressive disease, spinal symptoms and signs are progressive from onset without an initial relapsing and remitting phase, and they may or may not be accompanied by clinically apparent involvement of one or both optic nerves or brainstem. In contrast, recurrent episodes of spinal cord inflammation (myelitis) may be the only manifestation of the disease, and on occasion, such episodes might be stereotyped, mimicking a structural lesion. Usually, episodes of myelitis due to MS result in partial cord disturbance (incomplete transverse myelitis), often confined to sensory disturbance.

Commonly, spinal disease is accompanied by urinary tract symptoms, usually of frequency and urgency of micturition and occasionally urinary incontinence. Urinary retention is rare in the early stages of the condition and almost never the presentation of MS. Usually, deep tendon reflexes are exaggerated in the lower limbs and often in the upper limbs, although on occasion, one or more reflexes are found to be depressed or absent, particularly in the upper limbs, probably as a result of dorsal root or dorsal column involvement in the cervical cord. Spinal symptoms are often induced or aggravated by minor increases in body heat. Temperature sensitivity was originally described by Uhthoff in patients who suffered temporary visual disturbance in association with hot baths or exercise. Its effect is generally short-lived, lasting a matter of minutes, and is most likely the result of temporary conduction block in demyelinated nerve fibers.

Neurological examination of a patient with MS in the later stages of the disease will reveal particularly a loss of vibration sense and often joint position sense in the lower limbs with spinothalamic disturbance and spastic paraparesis or paraplegia. The latter is due in part to axonal loss accompanying demyelination. The measured transverse area of the cervical cord on MRI corresponds to the degree of neurological disability expected from spinal cord involvement (36).

A. Cervical Cord

Inflammatory disease in the cervical cord often leads to sensory symptoms in the lower limbs in ascending fashion, but not always ascending to cervical sensory level. Weakness of the lower limbs or a feeling of heaviness is a common accompaniment. When dorsal columns are affected, the phenomenon of deafferentation may develop and joint position sense might be lost in one upper limb, leading to the useless hand of Oppenheimer, or in milder cases, pseudo-athetosis. More commonly, dorsal column inflammation will lead to positive symptoms (tingling, pins and needles, or a feeling of tightness and constriction). At other times, in up to 40% of patients, such involvement results in Lhermitte's sign, when flexion of the neck leading to stretching and stimulation of inflamed or demyelinated dorsal column tracts results in sudden sensations of electric shock or painful tingling down the spine, affecting upper and lower limbs, usually on both sides but sometimes only on one side. Lhermitte's sign commonly lasts a matter of days or weeks only, but on occasion may be persistent due to established demyelination. With progression of the disease, spastic paraparesis usually develops to a greater or lesser extent and may be the only feature of MS developing in middle age or later in life, progressing slowly to spastic paraplegia.

B. Thoracic and Lumbar Cord

Often, disease in the thoracic cord is accompanied by girdle pain due to dorsal root involvement, with sensory disturbance in ascending fashion to the thoracic level. Symptoms and signs may conform to a Brown-Séquard syndrome or almost such a syndrome (of hemisection of the cord), resulting in proprioceptive loss (loss of vibration and joint position sense and of light touch), pyramidal tract deficit (weakness of hip and knee flexion and ankle dorsiflexion and eversion, with enhanced knee and ankle reflexes and an extensor plantar response) ipsilaterally, and contralateral spinothalamic loss (loss of pinprick and temperature sensation).

On occasion, disease in the lumbosacral cord results in a "conus" syndrome—a pattern of weakness and sensory loss in the lower limbs consistent with lumbosacral radiculopathy but with signs of pyramidal tract involvement (for example, extensor plantar responses). Urinary tract symptoms are a common accompaniment, usually of frequency, urgency, and incontinence, but sometimes urinary retention as well.

II. DIFFERENTIAL DIAGNOSIS

Postviral syndromes, including acute disseminated encephalomyelitis (ADEM), may lead to spinal inflammatory demyelination identical to that seen in MS, although recurrence of symptoms is unusual in the former conditions and expected in MS. A complete transverse myelitis with paraplegia and distinct sensory level is usually of postviral type and occurs infrequently in the presentation of MS. Limited forms of ADEM occur with clinical manifestations almost entirely confined to the spinal cord, although characteristic and rather symmetrical lesions may often be seen on brain MRI; cerebellar lesions are particularly suggestive [37]. The occurrence of mental changes, or accompanying bilateral rather than unilateral optic neuritis, and a particularly high cerebrospinal fluid (CSF) cell count or protein content, favor a diagnosis of ADEM (or other post-viral causes) rather than MS.

Several immune-mediated conditions can result in spinal cord disturbance of the type seen in MS. Systemic lupus erythematosis (SLE), sarcoidosis, and Behçet's disease may lead to variable sensory symptoms, a sensory level and spastic paraparesis, although a raised CSF protein content or persistent CSF pleocytosis should raise suspicion of these disorders and cast doubt on a diagnosis of MS.

Infection with HTLV-1 (formerly known as tropical spastic paraparesis or Jamaican myelopathy) almost exclusively affects the West Indian population in Britain. It is also common in the Japanese. The clinical presentation may be similar to MS, leading to difficulty in diagnosis in the descendants of West Indian immigrants. The usual clinical presentation is of a slowly progressive spastic paraparesis with subclinical optic nerve involvement, but also radicular symptoms and often myositis. Syndromes of myelitis and myelopathy (often vacuolar myelopathy) can also be seen after HIV infection, although additional features of the condition will usually be present.

Devic's disease (neuromyelitis optica), with rapid progression of bilateral optic neuropathy and spastic paraplegia, is probably in many cases a variant of MS, but a more florid and necrotizing form. However, such a presentation can be due to SLE, Behçet's disease and ADEM.

Hereditary spastic paraparesis or paraplegia (HSP) is usually inherited in an autosomal dominant form. In the absence of a documented family history, the condition may be mistaken for MS. However, a cardinal feature of HSP is a degree of spasticity in the lower limbs out of proportion to weakness. Indeed, often the only clinical finding is marked spasticity with minimal or no detectable weakness. Sensation is generally preserved and additional features, including pigmentary retinopathy, choreoathetosis, or mental changes may help to differentiate the condition.

Lastly, it is to be remembered that structural lesions in the spinal cord can lead to clinical symptoms and signs indistinguishable from MS. Particularly, arteriovenous malformations (AVM) are often overlooked. Back pain and sensory or motor symptoms related to exercise are typical features. A spinal bruit may be evident. Cervical or thoracic disc protrusion and thoracic meningioma (particularly common in women) may lead to disabling root and girdle pain and progressive paraplegia.

III. INVESTIGATION

The investigation of choice in a patient presenting with spinal symptoms and signs of the type seen in MS is spinal MRI. Inflammatory and demyelinating plaques may be visualized in the spinal cord, and multiple lesions are highly suggestive of MS. Active plaques can be seen to enhance after Gd-DTPA injection, indicating BBB breakdown and inflammation (30, 38) (Fig. 1). Spinal MRI serves to exclude cord compression and, in general, is useful in detecting an AVM. Myelography is no longer justified in the routine investigation of MS with the advent of MRI. Sometimes myelography can be useful in suggesting the presence of an AVM when such is suspected on clinical grounds and the MRI is normal.

A brain MRI is abnormal in 99% of patients with definite MS (39). The characteristic appearance is of multiple lesions in the periventricular and subcortical white matter. In patients presenting with spinal disease of the type seen in MS, brain MRI will reveal periventricular lesions of variable extent in 60–70% of cases. When a cohort of patients is followed up for a period of 5 years, between 60% and 70% of those with an abnormal MR brain scan at presentation will develop clinically definite MS, compared to less than 10% of those with a normal brain MRI at presentation (40). Thus, MRI is not only valuable in confirming a diagnosis of MS, but it is also a useful prognostic indicator. Internationally agreed Poser criteria require two episodes of inflammatory demyelination affecting different parts of the central nervous system, separated by 1 month to establish a diagnosis of MS (41); two episodes of incomplete transverse myelitis, despite involving different regions of the spinal cord, are not sufficient to make such a diagnosis. However MRI can now be used to show involvement of the cerebrum (or optic nerves) and may serve as a means of laboratory supported diagnosis (Fig. 2).

Evoked potentials continue to be valuable in diagnosis. Particularly, delayed visual evoked potentials can contribute to a laboratory-supported diagnosis. Delayed somato-sensory evoked potentials may be useful in the differential diagnosis of patients presenting with lower limb weakness in the absence of sensory symptoms or convincing sensory signs (for example, in excluding HSP). Auditory evoked potentials are of limited value, although when abnormal, they provide additional support for dissemination of the condition.

The CSF examination remains an important investigation to exclude conditions that resemble MS. In particular, a high inflammatory cell count (greater than 50/cu mm) or raised protein content, when sustained, should raise suspicion of an alternative immune-mediated condition (SLE, sarcoid, Behçet's or ADEM). The presence of oligoclonal IgG bands may confirm a diagnosis of

MS in the absence of known immune-mediated disease, particularly when bands are persistent (oligoclonal IgG bands in ADEM tend to be transitory).

IV. MANAGEMENT

Treatment of an acute relapse of spinal MS, which is disabling due to weakness or sensory ataxia, with high-dose intravenous methylprednisolone (0.5 g daily for 5 days or 1 g daily for 3 days) reduces the duration of symptoms and clinical signs, although this has no long-term effect on the disease (8). In general, sensory disturbance responds less well, and a course of steroids is not routinely advised for mild sensory relapse. High-dose steroids administered in this way appear to diminish the extent of BBB breakdown associated with in-

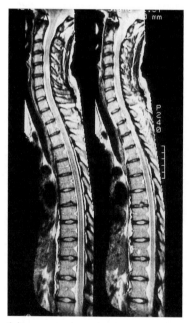

(a)

Figure 1 Spinal cord MRI from a patient with secondary progressive disease. (a) T2-weighted image (SE2500/100) showing a large, high-signal lesion at C4-5 and smaller lesions at T2 and T8. (b) T1-weighted image (SE500/20) before injection of gadolinium-DTPA. (c) Postgadolinium image (SE500/20) showing enhancement of the lateral cord at C4-5 corresponding to the large lesion seen on the T2-weighted image in (a). (With kind permission of Dr. D. Kidd, Institute of Neurology, Queen Square, London, England.)

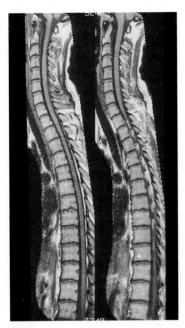

(b)

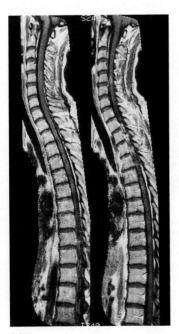

(c)

flammatory change, although temporarily so (Gd enhancement on MRI is suppressed, but has returned to its previous intensity by the end of 1 week (42)). Most immunosuppressive treatments have been relatively ineffective in reducing disease activity in controlled trials (including azathioprine, cyclosporine, cyclophosphamide, and plasma exchange). However a cytokine, beta-interferon, has recently been shown to reduce the relapse rate in relapsing and remitting patients, although modestly so—by 30%—and reduce lesion load apparent on MRI (43). The medication needs to be given three times per week by subcutaneous injection. This frequently induces a local inflammatory reaction at the injection site and flu-like symptoms helped by paracetamol. A large multicenter international study is underway to determine whether a higher dose of beta-interferon, if tolerated, will reduce the frequency of relapse further, and whether

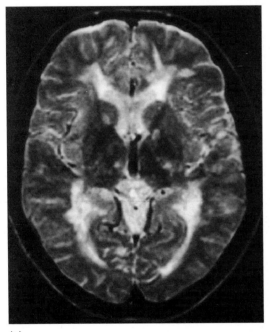

(a)

Figure 2 Brain MRI from a patient with relapsing-remitting disease. (a) T2-weighted image (SE2000/80) showing multiple and confluent periventricular and subcortical lesions. (b) FLAIR (fluid-attenuated inversion recovery), T2-weighted IR3000/1200/150, allows improved detection of cortical lesions and those at the gray-white matter border. (c) Postgadolinium study (SE1000/40) demonstrates enhancement of subcortical white matter lesions. (With kind permission of Dr. M. Boggild, Department of Neurology, North Staffordshire Royal Infirmary, Stoke-on-Trent, England.)

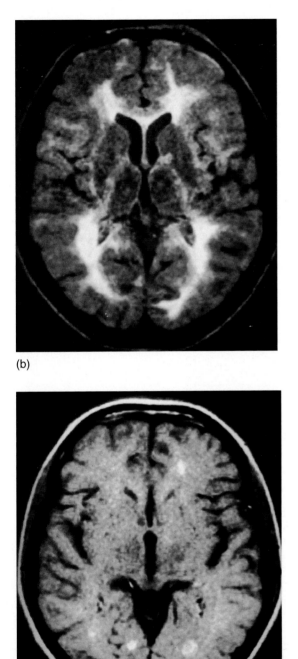

(b)

(c)

such treatment, as might be expected, will slow the progression of neurological disability in secondary progressive disease.

Meanwhile, management should be directed toward alleviating bladder symptoms and spasticity. Urinary frequency and urgency can be suppressed by oxybutinin. Sometimes, in resistant cases, bladder denervation may be necessary. When bladder emptying is a problem, intermittent self-catheterization should be encouraged. For spasticity, both baclofen and dantrolene are effective in increasing doses. In resistant cases and when the patient is bedbound as a result of spasticity, intermittent or continuous infusion of intrathecal baclofen may be considered (44). Whether such therapy is helpful in ambulant patients is uncertain. Attention to the psychological needs of the patient may require the assistance of an experienced clinical neuropsychologist with a special interest in the condition. It should be emphasized that the role of a dedicated neurorehabilitation unit with particular facilities for MS patients and for spinal disabilities cannot be underestimated. In the late stages of the disease, such a unit can mean the continuity of a lifestyle at home in a setting familiar to relatives and friends. Without such support, a gradual withdrawal of the individual ensues, and with it, his or her self-esteem.

REFERENCES

1. McDonald WI, Silberberg DH. Multiple sclerosis. London/Boston/Durban/Singapore/Sydney/Toronto/Wellington: Butterworths, 1986.
2. Charcot J-M. Histologie de la sclerose en plaques. Gazette Hospital, Paris 1868; 41:554–555;557–558;566.
3. Dawson JW. The histology of disseminated sclerosis. Transactions of the Royal Society of Edinburgh 1916; 50:517–740.
4. Allen IV. Demyelinating diseases. In: ADAMS JH, Corsellis Jan, Duchen LW, eds. Greenfield's Neuropathology, 4th ed. London: Edward Arnold, 1984:338–384.
5. Adams CWM, Poston RN, Buk SJ, Sidhu YS, Vipond H. Inflammatory vasculitis in multiple sclerosis. J Neurol Sci 1985; 69:269–283.
6. Compston A. Methylprednisolone and multiple sclerosis. Arch Neurol 1988; 45:669.
7. Ebers GC, Bulman DE, Sadnovik AD, et al. A population-based study of multiple sclerosis in twins. N Engl J Med 1988; 315:1638–1642.
8. Compston A. Genetic factors in the aetiology of multiple sclerosis. In: Mcdonald WI, Silberberg WH, eds. Multiple Sclerosis. London: Butterworths, 1986:56–73.
9. Francis DA, Batchelor JR, McDonald WI, et al. Multiple sclerosis in north-east Scotland. An association with HLA-DWQ1. Brain 1987; 110:181–196.
10. Dean G, Kurtzke JF. On the risk of multiple sclerosis according to age at immigration to South Africa. Br Med J 1971; 3:725–729.
11. Kurtzke JF, Beebe GW, Norman JE. Epidemiology of multiple sclerosis in United States veterans. III. Migration and the risk of MS. Neurology 1985; 35:672–678.

12. Hafler DA, Weiner HL. MS: a CNS and systemic autoimmune disease. Immunology Today 1989; 10:104–107.
13. Waksman BH. Multiple sclerosis. Current Opinions in Immunology 1989; 1:733–739.
14. Esiri MM. Multiple sclerosis: a qualitative and quantitative study of immunoglobulin containing cells in the central nervous system. Neuropathol Appl Neurobiol 1988; 6:9–21.
15. Calder V, Owen S, Watson C, Feldmann M, Davison A. MS: a localised immune disease of the central nervous system. Immunology Today 1989; 10:99–103.
16. Gessain A, Vernant JC, Maurs I et al. Antibodies to Human T-Lymphotropic Virus type-I in patients with tropical spastic paraparesis. Lancet 1985; 11:407–409.
17. Cruickshank JK, Richardson JH, Morgan OC et al. Screening for prolonged incubation of HTLV-I infection in British and Jamaican relatives of British patients with tropical spastic paraparesis. Br Med J 1990; 300:300–304.
18. Watanabe R, Wege H, Ter Meulen V. Comparative analysis of corona virus JHM-induced demyelinating encephalomyelitis in Lewis and Brown Norway rats. Laboratory Investigations 1987; 37:375–384.
19. Wisniewski HM, Keith AB. Chronic relapsing experimental allergic encephalomyelitis. An experimental model of multiple sclerosis. Ann Neurol 1977; 1:144–148.
20. Lassmann Hans. Comparative Neuropathology of Chronic Experimental Allergic Encephalomyelitis and Multiple Sclerosis. Berlin/Heidelberg/New York/Tokyo: Springer-Verlag, 1983.
21. Lisak RP. Immunological abnormalities. In: McDonald WI, Silberberg DH, eds. Multiple Sclerosis. London: Butterworths, 1986:74–98.
22. Wekerle H, Linington C, Lassmann H, Meyermann R. Cellular immune reactivity within the CNS. Trends in Neurosciences 1989;9:271–277.
23. Broman T. The permeability of the cerebrospinal vessels in normal and pathological conditions. Copenhagen: Munksgaard, 1949.
24. Fog T. The topography of plaques in multiple sclerosis. Acta Neurol Scand 1965; 41(Suppl 15):7–16.
25. Lightman S, McDonald WI, Bird AC, et al. Retinal venous sheathing in optic neuritis: Its significance for the pathogenesis of multiple sclerosis. Brain 1987; 110:405–414.
26. Harding AE, Radue EW, Whiteley AM. Contrast-enhanced lesions on computerised tomography in multiple sclerosis. J Neurol Neurosurg Psychiatry 1978; 41:754–758.
27. Grossman RI, Gonzalez-Scarano F, Atlas SW, Galetta S, Silberberg DH. Multiple sclerosis: Gadolinium enhancement in MR imaging. Radiology 1986; 161:721–725.
28. Kappos L, Stadt D, Roharbach E, Keil W. Gadolinium-DTPA enhanced magnetic resonance imaging in the evaluation of different disease courses and disease activity in MS. Neurology 1988; 38(Suppl 1):255.
29. Miller DH, Rudge P, Johnson G, et al. Serial Gadolinium enhanced magnetic resonance imaging in multiple sclerosis. Brain 1988; 111:927–939.

30. Hawkins CP, Munro PMG, Mackenzie F, et al. Duration and selectivity of blood-brain barrier breakdown in chronic relapsing experimental allergic encephalomyelitis by gadolinium-DTPA and protein markers. Brain 1990; 113:365–378.

31. Hawkins CP, MacKenzie F, Tofts PS, du Boulay EPGH, McDonald WI. Patterns of blood-brain barrier breakdown in inflammatory demyelination. Brain 1991; 114:801–810.

32. Olerup O, Hillert J, Fredrikson S, et al. Primarily chronic progressive and relapsing/remitting multiple sclerosis: Two immunogenetically distinct disease entities. Proc Natl Acad Sci USA 1989; 86:7113–7117.

33. Thompson AJ, Kermode AG, MacManus DG, et al. Patterns of disease activity in multiple sclerosis: Clinical and magnetic resonance imaging study. Br Med J 1990; 300:631–634.

34. Hawkins CP, Thompson AJ, Kermode AG, et al. Gadolinium-enhancement of new MRI lesions in progressive multiple sclerosis: Its significance and predictive value. Proceedings of XIV Symposium Neuroradiologicum (London), 1990:65.

35. Thompson AJ, Kermode AG, Wicks D, et al. Major differences in the dynamics of primary and secondary progressive multiple sclerosis. Ann Neurol 1991; 29:53–62.

36. Thorpe JW, Kidd D, MacManus DG, Barker GJ, Miller DH, McDonald WI. Planimetric analysis of spinal cord atrophy using MRI. Proc Soc Magnetic Resonance in Medicine (Berlin) 1992; 1:1607.

37. Kesselring J, Miller DH, Robb SA, et al. Acute disseminated encephalomyelitis: MRI findings and the distinction from multiple sclerosis. Brain 1990; 113:291–302.

38. Katz J, Tauberger J, Raine C, McFarlin D, McFarland H. Gadolinium-enhancing lesion on magnetic resonance imaging: Neuropathological findings. Ann Neurol 1990; 28:243.

39. Ormerod IEC, Miller DH, McDonald WI, et al. The role of NMR imaging in the assessment of multiple sclerosis and isolated neurological lesions. Brain 1987; 110:1579–1616.

40. Morrissey SP, Miller DH, Kendall BE, et al. The significance of brain magnetic resonance imaging abnormalities at presentation with clinically isolated syndromes suggestive of multiple sclerosis. Brain 1993; 116:135–146.

41. Poser CM, Paty DW, Scheinberg L, et al. New diagnostic criteria for multiple sclerosis: Guidelines for research protocols. Ann Neurol 1983; 13:227–231.

42. Miller DH, Morrissey SP, Thompson AJ, et al. The influence of intravenous methylprednisolone on gadolinium-enhancement of multiple sclerosis lesions. Proc Soc Magnetic Resonance in Medicine (San Francsico) 1991; 1:6.

43. The IFNB Multiple Sclerosis Study Group. Interferon beta-1b is effective in relapsing-remitting multiple sclerosis. 1. Clinical results of a multicenter, randomised double-blind, placebo-controlled trial. Neurology 1993; 43:655–661.

44. Coffey RJ, Cahill D, Steers W, et al. Intrathecal baclofen for intractable spasticity of spinal origin: Results of a long-term multicenter study. J Neurosurg 1993; 78:226–232.

17

Motor Neuron Disease (Amyotrophic Lateral Sclerosis)

Catherine M. Lloyd and P. Nigel Leigh
Institute of Psychiatry, London, England

I. INTRODUCTION

Motor neuron disease (MND) is a progressive neurodegenerative disorder involving mainly the corticospinal tracts and lower motor neurons of the brainstem and spinal cord. The cause of MND is unknown, with the exception of rare familial forms of the disease, in which specific mutations have been identified. Neurologists use the term MND to refer to a characteristic clinical syndrome, but there are many other motor neuron disorders, most of them very rare. Typical MND is not a common disease, and the general practitioner with an average list might be expected to see only one new case in about 20 years.

The identification of mutations in the Cu/Zn superoxide dismutase (SOD) gene in 10–20% of families with autosomal dominant familial MND has opened up new possibilities for understanding pathogenesis in the sporadic form of the disease, and has important implications for treatment. Likewise, the increasing but still circumstantial evidence for the involvement of excitotoxicity in the pathogenesis of the disease has led to new therapeutic initiatives, with indications that glutamate antagonist drugs may slow the progression of the disease.

In this chapter we review the natural history, pathogenesis, pathology, diagnosis, and management of MND and other motor neuron disorders. Charcot and Joffroy in 1869 (1) first clearly described what we now refer to as MND, and used the term amyotrophic lateral sclerosis (ALS) to denote the association of progressive muscle wasting with degeneration of the lateral corticospinal tracts in the spinal cord. In current usage, ALS is often used to denote all variants of MND, including typical (Charcot) ALS with widespread upper and lower motor neuron signs; progressive bulbar palsy (PBP), which presents with bulbar symptoms but almost always progresses to involve the limbs as in typical ALS; and progressive muscular atrophy (PMA), in which only lower motor neuron signs are evident.

II. EPIDEMIOLOGY AND NATURAL HISTORY

Motor neuron disease is a syndrome of upper and lower motor neuron degeneration, reflecting a variety of molecular abnormalities. Neurologists often comment on the remarkable homogeneity of typical MND, and in 90% of cases, diagnosis in the clinic is straightforward. Diagnosis is based on the characteristic combination of upper and lower motor neuron signs in the same region of the body, and this feature has been incorporated in the diagnostic criteria developed by a working party of the World Federation of Neurology in 1990—the El Escorial criteria (Table 1). The criteria can be supported by investigations such as the electromyograph (EMG), and although these are desirable, they are not essential for classification.

The incidence of MND varies between 1 and 2 per 100,000 in most studies (2,3), and the prevalence is 4–6 per 100,000. The exception to this is the focus of high prevalence in the western Pacific, including the island of Guam, the Kii peninsula of Japan, and remote parts of New Guinea. In Guam, the incidence of MND at one stage was nearly 100 times that in most parts of the world, but the incidence seems to have fallen from around 87 per 100,000 in 1962 to around 5 per 100,000 in 1985 (4). There have been suggestions that the incidence of MND in the northern hemisphere (where it has been most intensively studied) has been rising, although it is still debated whether this is a real phenomenon. Mortality for MND closely approximates incidence and may differ in various ethnic groups. For example, mortality may be lower among Asian immigrants to England compared with the general population.

Specific risk factors include increasing age and male sex. The peak incidence is between 60 and 70 years, ranging from teens to the tenth decade, although very young and old cases are extremely rare. Three men are affected for every two women, although in the very elderly the ratio approaches one (5,6). Many other risk factors have at times been implicated but have not stood the test of rigorous analysis. As in some other neurodegenerative conditions, there is a weak association between previous trauma and MND, but even this is of doubtful validity.

Table 1 El Escorial Criteria

The diagnosis of ALS requires the presence of:
1. LMN signs (may include EMG signs in clinically normal muscles)
2. UMN signs
3. Progression of the disorder

Subclassification of diagnostic criteria:

Definite ALS—UMN and LMN signs in three regions

Probable ALS—UMN and LMN signs in two regions, with UMN signs rostral to LMN

Possible ALS—UMN and LMN signs in one region, or UMN signs in two or three regions

Suspected ALS—LMN signs in two or three regions

Regions are defined as brainstem, brachial, thorax and trunk, and crural.

The diagnosis of ALS is supported by the following features:
1. Fasciculation in one or more regions
2. Neurogenic change in EMG studies
3. Normal motor and sensory nerve conduction
4. Absence of motor conduction block

The diagnosis of ALS requires the absence of the following clinical features:
1. Sensory signs
2. Sphincter disturbances
3. Visual disturbances
4. Autonomic dysfunction
5. Parkinson's disease
6. Alzheimer-type dementia
7. Certain "mimic" syndromes, e.g., lymphoma, acute infections, postradiation.

Abbreviations: LMN, lower motor neuron; UMN, upper motor neuron.

A. Pathology

In the MND spinal cord, the characteristic and diagnostic finding is the loss of the large anterior motor neurons (α and γ motor neurons) in the anterior horns. The extent of this loss varies from case to case and ranges from complete (where it is impossible to find a surviving motor neuron) to mild, if the patient dies from rapidly progressive ventilatory failure before the limbs are severely affected. In such cases, it is possible to see the early phases of motor neuron degeneration, comprising accumulations of neurofilamentous material within neuronal perikarya and large proximal axonal swellings (spheroids) also composed of accumulations of highly phosphorylated neurofilaments (7). True chromatolysis is very rare in MND, but neurons that contain neurofilamentous accumulations appear achromasic and swollen. In about 70% of cases, small eosinophilic intracytoplasmic inclusions known as Bunina bodies can be identified, and in about 20% of cases, surviving motor neurons contain Lewy body-like inclusions (8–10). The most common pathological picture in the cervical and lumbar expansions of the spinal cord is marked depletion (more than 70% loss) of anterior horn motor neurons, with severe shrinkage of surviving motor neurons.

Although the molecular composition of Bunina bodies is unknown, antibodies against ubiquitin, a protein involved in the nonlysosomal degradation of abnormal or short-lived proteins, detect characteristic intracytoplasmic inclusions that take the form of rounded or irregular masses or "skeins" (10–12). These ubiquinated inclusions are not labeled by antibodies against cytoskeletal proteins, and thus differ from neurofibrillary tangles in Alzheimer's disease and Lewy bodies in Parkinson's disease, which react not only with ubiquitin antibodies but also with antibodies against neurofilaments, microtubule-associated protein, and other cellular proteins. Although ubiquitin-immunoreactive inclusions in lower motor neurons (including lower motor neuron nuclei of the brainstem) are characteristic for MND, they are not found in all cases that otherwise satisfy the usual pathological criteria.

Aside from degeneration of lower motor neurons, typical MND cases show degeneration of the lateral corticospinal tracts, and degeneration of the corticospinal tracts can be traced upward through the brainstem to the internal capsules and centrum semiovale.

We now recognize that the selective vulnerability of upper and lower motor neurons in MND is a relative phenomenon, and that most patients show involvement of the column of Clarke (13), with degeneration of the spinocerebellar tracts, and that some patients have degeneration of the frontal and temporal neocortex. Patients in whom frontotemporal degeneration is prominent often present with a frontal-type dementia (14,15). In Japan a number of patients have been maintained alive with assisted ventilation for many years, and neuropathological examination has shown extensive degeneration of subcortical structures, including the substantia nigra, as well as the posterior columns of the spinal cord. In typical MND, posterior column involvement is minimal. In addition to the evidence from pathology, recent positron emission tomography (PET) scan studies show distinctive abnormalities of brain function involving the parahippocampal gyrus, the anterior thalamus, and the medial frontal areas (16,17).

In the western Pacific form of MND, which is associated with parkinsonism and dementia (see below), the pathology of motor neuron degeneration is essentially the same as in sporadic MND elsewhere in the world, but in addition the brain contains many neurofibrillary tangles (18).

In summary, the pathological hallmarks of motor neuron disease are degeneration of the corticospinal tracts, degeneration and loss of spinal cord anterior horn motor neurons, and the presence within surviving motor neurons of characteristic inclusions, including Bunina bodies and ubiquitin-immunoreactive dense bodies and skeins. The full range of neuronal vulnerability in extramotor cortex has still to be defined but probably varies considerably from case to case.

B. Clinical Features

Motor neuron disease is a disorder with an insidious onset. Common early symptoms include cramps, tripping due to foot drop, difficulty opening bottle tops because of weakness of one hand, slurring of speech (in the bulbar form of the disease), and rarely (less than 1% of patients), shortness of breath. It is rare for patients to notice fasciculations; these are usually pointed out to them by a doctor or a member of the family. Wasting is usually noticed after weakness, but sometimes can be the first symptom. Two-thirds of patients with MND present with weakness in the limbs, and about one-third present with bulbar symptoms (2,19). Only about 5% of patients have widespread disease involving both bulbar musculature and limbs from the outset. When the onset is in the limbs, weakness usually begins distally and is asymmetrical. The legs are more commonly affected before the arms (2,9). Less commonly, the onset of weakness may be proximal, either in the upper or lower limbs. A distinct subgroup of patients presents with progressive upper limb weakness that may begin proximally or distally, and lead to flail arms, severe weakness persisting in the arms, sometimes for many months or even years before lower limb and bulbar involvement becomes obvious. Muscle cramps after stretching or exercise are common and may precede weakness or wasting by many months. The rare patients who present with dyspnea have diaphragmatic weakness and occasionally present to neurologists, having been admitted to intensive care units with ventilatory failure of unknown cause.

Upper motor neuron involvement results in spasticity, exaggerated deep tendon reflexes and, in about 60% of patients, a positive Babinski sign. A brisk jaw jerk, brisk facial reflexes, and a snout response are common in the bulbar form of the disease, in which the predominant features are those of pseudobulbar palsy. In these cases, emotional lability is common. A combination of lower motor neuron signs (fasciculations, wasting) with upper motor neuron signs (preserved or exaggerated tendon reflexes in the presence of wasting and weakness, spasticity) in the same region of the body, and observed in several regions simultaneously, is characteristic of the disease. Nevertheless, initial diagnosis should be supported by full investigations, and many would regard a second opinion from an experienced neurologist as desirable.

In patients with limb onset, the bulbar muscles eventually become involved in at least 60–70% of patients. Ultimately the ventilatory muscles fail and death ensues from ventilatory failure, often accompanied by pneumonia. Patients with dysphagia often aspirate, and this may precipitate pneumonia.

Between 10 and 20% of patients have sensory symptoms (20), but objective sensory abnormalities suggest that another diagnosis should be sought, unless a simple explanation can be found (for example, coexisting carpal tunnel compression). Significant disturbance of sphincter function is unusual, but it does occasionally occur in the form of urinary frequency and urgency. If sphincter disturbance is more than minimal, an alternative diagnosis should be sought. The preservation of sphincter function is linked to the relative sparing of Onuf's nucleus in the sacral spinal cord. It is now known that Onuf's nucleus is involved in the disease process, but the degeneration seems to be much slower in this group of motor neurons than in typical somatic motor neurons. Other parts of the neuromuscular system that are spared include the ocular muscles and the autonomic nervous system. Just as with Onuf's nucleus, this sparing is relative, and abnormalities of eye movement and autonomic function have been documented, although they are seldom clinically significant (21,22).

Familial and sporadic forms of MND are usually clinically indistinguishable, but within kindreds with typical autosomal dominant familial MND, some individuals may present with only lower motor neuron signs, and some with typical MND of Charcot type (ALS) (23). About 10% of patients with sporadic MND have only lower motor neuron signs and may therefore be classified as suffering from PMA. Where the progression is slow, with survival of more than 5 years, differentiation between a lower motor neuron form of ALS and some of the late-onset forms of spinal muscular atrophy (SMA) can be well nigh impossible. In this context it is particularly important to remember Kennedy's disease (see below).

Overall, the prognosis of MND is poor, the median survival for all cases being around 3 to 5 years, but just over 2 years for patients with bulbar onset. Bulbar onset is more common in elderly women, accounting for the worse prognosis in this particular group. In a recent study of more than 700 cases, Norris, et al. found an average survival of just over 3 years, with a range of 5 months to 33 years (3). A group of young-onset patients with a more benign course was identified and in our experience, these are often patients with predominantly upper motor neuron signs. There is little doubt that patients with MND, particularly where the onset is early, may enter a long period of stability and survive for many years, as witnessed in the physicist Stephen Hawkings. There are also a number of instances of apparent recovery from MND (24,25), although in the large study of Norris, et al. (3), no such case was identified. If spontaneous recovery occurs, it must be very rare indeed (Table 2).

Table 2 Summary of Clinical Characteristics

	ALS	PLS	PMA	Kennedy's syndrome	Motor neuropathies
Age of onset (average)	60–70 yrs	30–50 yrs	50–70 yrs	20–70 yrs	<45 yrs
Site of onset	Bulbar/arms/legs	Usually legs	Proximal	Proximal	Arms asymmetrical
Sex	M>F (3:2)	M=F	M>F	Males only	Usually male
Wasting	Yes	No	Yes	Yes	Yes
Fasciculations	Yes	No	Yes	Yes	Yes
Reflexes	Brisk	Brisk	Reduced/Absent	Reduced/Absent	Reduced/Absent
Babinski reflex	Extensor in 60%	Extensor	Flexor or equivocal	Flexor	Flexor
Inheritance	5–10% AD Majority sporadic	Sporadic	Sporadic	Sex-linked recessive	Sporadic
Endocrine abnormalities	None	None	None	Gynecomastia Infertility Diabetes mellitus	None
IgM Anti-GM$_1$ antibodies	10–20% (same as normals)	10–20%	10–20%	10–20%	60–80%
Motor conduction block on EMG	No	No	No	No	Yes
Prognosis	3–5 yrs (less in bulbar onset)	15–18 yrs	5–10 yrs	Near-normal life expectancy	May respond to immunosuppression

Abbreviation: AD, autosomal dominant.

III. PRIMARY LATERAL SCLEROSIS

Primary lateral sclerosis (PLS) is a form of MND, with the disease confined to the upper motor neuron. It is much rarer then classical MND, with studies from North America suggesting an incidence of 4% (3), although in the authors' experience it accounts for an even smaller percentage of patients seen.

Primary lateral sclerosis presents insidiously in the fourth to sixth decades, men and women being equally affected. Presentation is usually with a spastic paraparesis or more occasionally, a spastic dysarthria. It progresses to result in a spastic quadriparesis with minimal associated weakness, pathological hyper-reflexia with an extensor plantar response and clonus, a spastic dysarthria, dysphagia, and emotional lability. There is no evidence of muscular atrophy or fasciculations. Primary lateral sclerosis is much more benign than ALS, with a life expectancy of 15 to 18 years (3,26), compared with 2 to 5 years for classical MND.

The EMG is normal early in the disease, with only patchy mild denervation occurring later (27). There is no evidence of anterior horn cell involvement histologically. The differential diagnosis includes hereditary spastic paraplegia, multiple sclerosis affecting the spinal cord, adrenomyeloneuropathy, HTLV-1 infection, and a structural lesion of the cervical spinal cord or the foramen magnum.

A. Motor Neuron Disease–Dementia

About 2% of patients with MND develop dementia, which is usually of frontal lobe type (28). Although many such patients present with behavioral abnormalities and changes in character, progressive memory impairment may be the initial feature, and some patients develop frankly psychotic behavior. The relationship between the more subtle cognitive changes suggestive of frontal lobe dysfunction that can be detected in many patients with MND (29) and the MND-dementia syndrome is uncertain, because the pathological basis for these cognitive changes in nondemented patients is unknown. The great majority of patients with cognitive impairments only detectable on formal neuropsychological testing do not progress to clinically significant dementia. It is still not clear, however, whether such cognitive changes have any significant impact upon quality of life for patients and carers; our impression is that they quite frequently do.

The pathological changes in the MND-dementia syndrome are characteristic, although not specific. Typically, there is frontal and temporal atrophy, which may be very marked. At a microscopic level, there is usually striking neuronal loss in the more superficial cortical layers of the frontotemporal neocortex, with marked cortical and subcortical gliosis. Immunocytochemistry with antibodies against ubiquitin frequently reveals intraneuronal ubiquitin-immunoreactive inclusion bodies in surviving neurons of layers 2 and 3 of the frontotemporal neocortex, together with round or oval intraneuronal inclusions in the granule cells of the hippocampal dentate gyrus (15). These ubiquitin-immunoreactive inclusions differ from those of typical Pick's disease in that they are not labeled by antibodies directed against microtubule-associated protein tau or against neurofilament proteins, nor are they revealed by silver stains. They thus have the same molecular pathological features as the ubiquitin-immunoreactive inclusions found in lower motor neurons of the brainstem and spinal cord. A further feature differentiating the MND-dementia syndrome from typical Pick's disease is the absence of ballooned neurons in cortical and subcortical areas.

About 40% of patients with the MND-dementia syndrome have a family history of dementia or MND in a first degree relative. One family has been described in which dementia of frontal lobe type occurred in several generations and MND with and without dementia in only one generation (30).

The prognosis in MND-dementia syndrome is poor, patients seldom surviving more than 3 years from the onset.

B. Guam

The island of Guam in the western Pacific ocean, inhabited by Chamorro Indians, has been known to have a very high incidence of ALS since 1945 when a naval pathologist from the United States reported the deaths of seven Chamorro natives in 1 month from ALS (31). The disease, however, has been recognized on the island since the last century. In 1954 the incidence was reported as being fifty to one hundred times the incidence in the rest of the world (32,33), with a tendency for the disease to aggregate in families. In more recent years, the incidence has been falling and is now approaching that found in the rest of the world.

Clinically the Guam ALS differs from sporadic ALS seen in the rest of the world only in its association with parkinsonism and dementia. Parkinsonism and dementia also occur independently of ALS. The syndrome was termed the ALS-parkinsonism-dementia complex (ALS/PDC) of Guam. About 20% of the patients with PDC have clinical evidence of ALS (34).

Initially it was thought that there was a genetic etiology to the ALS/PDC of Guam. There is, however, no increase in the incidence of the ALS/PDC in the offspring of children with both parents affected, compared with those with only one or neither parent affected. Nor is there an increased incidence in Chamorros with the same genetic background living on Saipan, an island 80 miles north of Guam. In addition in the mid-1970s, there was a small outbreak among Filipino immigrants, who had lived on the island for 20 years (35).

The cause of the ALS/PDC remains obscure. One theory is that the Guam population is exposed to a toxin as a result of the ingestion of flour from the cycad seed of the false sago palm tree, *Cycas circinalis*. This contains an excitatory neurotoxin, β-methylamino-1-alanine (BMAA), as well as cycasin, also a potential neurotoxin. The seeds are used to make a flour and also as a traditional medicine. The raw cycad seed is highly toxic, producing severe hepatic necrosis and death; hence the seeds are soaked in water for several days prior to being used as a flour. During World War II, when the islands were invaded by the Japanese, the Chamorros depended heavily on the cycad flour, but since 1945 have eaten far more wheat flour, which could account for the fall in incidence (36). In 1987 it was reported by Spencer (37) that monkeys fed extremely high doses of BMAA developed anterior horn cell and pyramidal tract dysfunction. However, humans would have to consume about 70 kg of the flour daily to reach doses of BMAA equivalent to those fed to the monkeys. The case for the cycad seed, and for BMAA being involved in the pathogenesis, remains unproven. The role of cycasin likewise remains uncertain.

Soil on Guam has been found to have up to 42 times the amount of aluminum found on geologically similar islands that do not have the high incidence of ALS/PDC. The neurofibrillary tangles of the patients on Guam have been found to have up to 10 times the quantity of aluminum found in other Alzheimer disease patients, and more than 100 times that found in normal controls. Nevertheless, there is no consensus that aluminum or other trace metals are the trigger for ALS/PDC.

C. Motor Neuropathies

Multifocal motor neuropathy (MMN) is a syndrome of asymmetrical lower motor neuron weakness that begins distally in the arms and spreads slowly. It is more frequent in men and tends to occur in those less than 45 years of age.

Elecrophysiological studies of the motor nerves show multifocal conduction block, although this may have to be looked for carefully, with multiple nerves being sampled. Sensory conduction is normal. High levels of serum antibodies to GM_1 and GD_{1b} gangliosides have been found in 60–80% of patients (38). Patients with MMN have responded to treatment with cyclophosphamide, both clinically and with falls in antibody levels, having previously failed to respond to high-dose prednisolone; indeed, steroids may be deleterious. Some patients may respond to plasmapheresis (39–41). Other patients with MMN have been treated with human immune globulin (HIG), with an encouraging clinical response (41,42).

The role of anti-GM_1 ganglioside antibodies in typical MND remains controversial. It was initially suggested that they were a frequent finding, occurring in 50–60% of patients (38,43). More recent studies have shown them to occur in only 10–20% of patients, a prevalence similar to many disease controls (44,45). In our experience, they are not significantly raised in typical MND (ALS).

D. Familial MND

Familial MND (FMND) has been recognized since the middle of the last century. It accounts for 5–10% of cases of MND (46). In the majority of these patients the inheritance is of autosomal dominant type, although rare autosomal recessive forms have been described in consanguineous kindreds in North Africa (47). Most studies have shown that penetrance is high, particularly within early-onset families with autosomal dominant inheritance (48,49), although a study from Australia found that in some families the penetrance was low and proposed that because of this, the incidence of FMND is underestimated (50).

The histological findings in FMND are similar to those of sporadic MND, with marked anterior horn cell loss, and corticospinal tract degeneration. Initial suggestions that involvement of the posterior columns, the spinocerebellar tracts, and the columns of Clarke were characteristic of FMND were inaccurate in as much as these pathways are also involved in sporadic MND (51–54).

Both dementia (of the frontal lobe type) and extrapyramidal signs are said to be more common in patients with familial MND (29,55).

In 1991, the MND gene was mapped to chromosome 21 by the collaboration of three laboratories in North America with access to 300 families (56). In 1993 the same laboratories showed mutations of the gene encoding for Cu,Zn superoxide dismutase (Cu,Zn SOD) (57), and this has since been confirmed by other centers. These point mutations are found in 10–20% of the families with autosomal-dominant FMND and have been detected in apparently sporadic cases. Cu,Zn SOD removes potentially harmful superoxide free radicals, but it is not clear why motor nerves should be selectively damaged given that Cu/Zn SOD is widely expressed.

E. Kennedy's Syndrome

Kennedy's syndrome or bulbospinal muscular atrophy is inherited as a sex-linked recessive disorder (58,59). Men present in their third to fifth decades with a proximal muscular weakness resulting in a lordotic gait, although cramps may have preceded the weakness by several years. Weakness is associated with wasting and fasciculations and spreads to affect the more distal musculature. The arms are more prominently affected than the legs. The deep tendon reflexes are reduced or absent. Facial weakness is prominent, with associated fasciculations of the chin. These are often present at rest but are much more marked when the patient is asked to whistle or blow. In addition there is a mild dysarthria, a wasted and fasciculating tongue, and a degree of dysphagia, although this is rarely severe enough to interfere with nutrition. Sensation is normal. A fine essential tremor is frequently present.

Kennedy's syndrome has a more indolent course than classical MND, and patients are often ambulant until just before death. Life expectancy is usually little shortened and may be normal.

In addition to the neurological findings, several endocrine features have been reported. These can precede the neurological symptoms by many years. Gynecomastia and reduced fertility occur in more than 50% of patients and may be associated with testicular atrophy. Hormonal studies generally suggest primary testicular failure (59). Maturity-onset diabetes is also recognized.

Kennedy's syndrome is due to an expansion of a CAG repeat in the coding region of the androgen receptor gene (60). This trinucleotide repeat codes for a polyglutamine tract. Most people have between 20 and 29 repeats, but patients with the mutation have more than 40. This allows for genetic counseling, enabling female carriers to make fully informed choices prior to pregnancy (see Table 2).

F. Juvenile-Onset ALS

In Europe and North America, there have been a few recorded cases of classical ALS occurring before the age of 20 years. In one center in the United States, this accounted for only three out of a thousand patients seen (28). In Tunisia, Ben Hamida (47) has studied more than 50 patients. Juvenile ALS is usually familial, with autosomal recessive inheritance, and the high incidence in Tunisia is probably because of consanguineous marriages. Linkage has recently been made to chromosome 2q33-q35 (61).

G. Konzo

Konzo is a rare form of MND found in remote rural areas of Mozambique, Tanzania, and Zaire. It is caused by the combined effect of a high cyanide and low sulphur intake from the exclusive consumption of insufficiently processed bitter cassava roots, which occurs in time of drought, when up to two-thirds of the inhabitants of a single village may be affected. Konzo presents with the sudden onset of a symmetrical, spastic paraparesis developing over a few days. It is nonprogressive, and some improvement may occur during the ensuing months. The arms are affected less frequently. Only the upper motor neuron is involved generally with no sensory or autonomic changes, although an optic neuropathy has been described (62,63).

H. Neurolathyrism

Neurolathyrism is a form of MND predominantly affecting the upper motor neuron. It is found in Africa and Asia, where the prevalence rate is up to 2.5% (64). The symptoms are usually confined to the legs, resulting in a spastic paraparesis, although upper limbs may be affected. The weakness is usually minimal, but walking is impaired due to severe spasticity, with associated clonus, hyperreflexia, and extensor plantars. Patients also complain of altered sensation, although no abnormalities are detected on clinical examination. Other symptoms involve the urinary tract, the bowel, and sexual function (65). Lathyrism tends to be nonprogressive.

Lathyrism is caused by excessive consumption of the chickling pea, *lathyrus sativus*, which contains β-N-oxalyl-L-α,β-diaminopropionic acid (β-OADP) also known as β-N-oxalylamino-L-alanine (BOAA). This is a potent neuroexcitatory aminoacid and is thought to be the toxic constituent. β-OADP is a glutamate agonist and fed to primates in large quantities, can induce corticospinal dysfunction (65).

I. MND with Lymphoma

The syndrome of MND in association with a lymphoma, both Hodgkin's disease and non-Hodgkin's lymphoma, has been recognized for a long time, although it is very rare. The majority of patients have both upper and lower motor neuron signs, resulting in an ALS-like syndrome, and this has been confirmed histologically, with postmortems revealing corticospinal tract involvement. Approximately 50% of patients studied have an associated paraprotein. Very occasionally, the neurological symptoms will respond to treatment of the lymphoma (66).

J. Spinal Muscular Atrophy

The spinal muscular atrophies (SMAs) are a group of genetically inherited diseases affecting the lower motor neuron most commonly found in infancy or early childhood. They were originally described in infants at the end of the last century, but other forms have since been described, including rare forms seen in adults.

Children present with reduced spontaneous movements and muscular weakness. Proximal musculature is most severely affected, with any remaining movement being in the small muscles of the hands and feet. Atrophy occurs but can be difficult to see because of subcutaneous fat in children. There is severe hypotonia, and marked reduction or absence of the deep tendon reflexes. The condition spreads to affect the bulbar musculature with atrophy and fasciculations of the tongue. Death occurs from respiratory failure often complicated by a chest infection. As with most forms of MND, there is no sensory impairment, sphincter involvement, or intellectual impairment.

Type I SMA, or Werdnig-Hoffmann disease, accounts for about 25% of childhood forms. Infants who present at birth with severe hypotonia rarely survive their first year. Those children presenting in the postnatal period tend to progress more slowly, but still rarely survive past 3 years.

Type II SMA accounts for 50% of cases (67) and has a more benign course. Children develop normally for the first 6 months of life and then show motor retardation, usually with failure to stand or walk unaided. The weakness is usually symmetrical. Bulbar symptoms occur with wasting and fasciculation of the tongue. A tremor affecting the arms is typical. The weakness is usually nonprogressive, and prognosis depends on the onset of respiratory failure, either due to weakness of the intercostal muscles or restrictive lung disease secondary to the development of a scoliosis. The median age at death in this group is 10 years, but some survive into adult life (68).

Wohlfart-Kugelberg-Welander disease, or type III SMA, presents later and runs a much slower progressive course, with patients surviving on average 35 years from diagnosis. Children present, at an average age of 9 years, with difficulty in walking, running, or jumping. Proximal muscles are affected first, and the arms may be unaffected for several years. Atrophy, fasciculations, and absence of tendon reflexes are characteristic. Cranial nerves are not involved other than those supplying the sternomastoids and the tongue. Patients are often mistakenly thought to have a muscular dystrophy. There are no signs of corticospinal tract involvement.

These spinal muscular atrophies may not represent distinct disease entities, as all forms have been described within the same families. The gene locus for Werdnig-Hoffmann and Wohlfart-Kugelberg-Welander disease has been mapped to the long arm of chromosome 5q12-14 (69,70), and it is interesting that this is in close proximity to the gene for hexosaminidase A, mutations of which cause Tay-Sachs disease. They are usually inherited as autosomal recessive, but autosomal-dominant cases have also been described. The hexosaminidase A gene has been excluded, however, as a candidate gene for SMA types I–III (see Table 3), and recently mutations have been identified in two genes at the 5q 12–14 locus. These are the survival motor neuron (SMN) and neuronal apoptosis inhibitory protein genes.

K. Hexosaminidase Deficiency

Hexosaminidase deficiency is most commonly seen in infants as Tay-Sachs disease. Rarely, it presents in the second or third decade with a syndrome comprising progressive muscle wasting and weakness associated with fasciculations due to lower motor neuron involvement, with signs of pyramidal tract and cere-

Table 3 Spinal Muscular Atrophies

Type	Also known as	Age at onset	Age at death	Inheritance/ chromosome
I	Werdnig-Hoffman acute infantile Amyotonia congenita	In utero, at birth, or early postnatal	If present at birth, by 1 year; otherwise by 3 years	AR 5q12–14
II	Intermediate SMA	6–12 months	10 years (mean)	AR 5q12–14
III	Wohlfart-Kugelberg-Wellander Mild SMA	9 years (range 2–18 years)	Mid-30s	AR 5q12–14
IV		Teens; adults	Adult	AR 5q12–14
V		Adult	Adult	AD

Abbreviations: AR, autosomal recessive; AD, autosomal dominant.

bellar involvement. Patients may present with neuropsychiatric syndromes including psychosis (71,72).

L. Pathogenesis: Summary of Current Hypotheses

Although the evidence for excitotoxicity in MND is largely circumstantial (73), the finding of mutations in the gene coding for Cu/Zn SOD strongly supports the notion that free-radical damage is an important mechanism for selective neuronal damage in MND. It must be remembered, however, that patients with these mutations represent a small minority of all patients with MND and only 20% of patients with familial MND. The evidence for free-radical damage in sporadic MND is weak, although Bowling (74) found evidence of protein carbonyl formation in postmortem tissue from such patients. This is thought to be a marker of free-radical damage.

Despite many years of epidemiological study, it has not been possible to identify with constancy any specific environmental toxin that might cause MND. Unlike Parkinson's disease, MND patients do not show an increased prevalence of null mutations for the cytochrome P450 debrisoquine hydroxylase (CYP-2D6 gene), although it has been claimed that they have a defect in sulphur metabolism (75).

Abnormalities of neurofilament function have long been implicated on the basis of neuropathological studies, and recently, mutations have been described in the gene coding for the neurofilament heavy chain subunit (NFH), although these mutations were found in sporadic rather than familial cases. Disruption of neurofilament production and assembly using transgenic models leads to accumulation of neurofilaments in motor neurons and motor neuron death (7).

At present it seems likely that MND represents a syndrome resulting from several molecular causes. The challenge is to find the precise mechanisms of selective neuronal death and to understand how on the one hand, mutations of Cu/Zn SOD, and on the other, abnormalities of neurofilament function, can lead to the same or very similar clinical syndrome.

IV. THE EL ESCORIAL CRITERIA FOR DIAGNOSING MND

After a conference of the World Federation of Neurology at El Escorial in Spain in 1990, a consensus was reached on a set of criteria for diagnosing and classifying MND. They take into account the difficulties associated with early diagnosis and utilize the varying distribution of upper and lower motor neuron signs, including EMG findings. Positive features that help in the diagnosis are included and features that should be absent are also listed (76) (Table 1).

A. Investigations

There is no specific diagnostic test for MND, and many of the following tests are performed to exclude an alternative and a possibly treatable condition.

The EMG and nerve conduction studies, which ideally should be performed in all patients in whom the diagnosis is suspected, can give positive evidence of anterior horn cell disease but are not specific for MND. The diagnostic criteria for MND, which were suggested by Lambert (77) and are still widely used are as follows:

1. Fibrillation and fasciculations should be present in the muscles of the upper and lower extremities, or in the extremities and the head.
2. Reduction in number and increase in amplitude and duration of motor unit action potentials.
3. Normal electrical excitability of remaining motor nerves fibers and motor fiber conduction velocity, within the normal range of relatively unaffected muscles and not less then 70% of the average normal value, according to age, in nerves of more severely affected muscles.
4. Normal excitability and conduction velocity of sensory nerve fibers even in severely affected extremities.

The above findings will differentiate MND from myopathies, local spinal cord lesions, and upper motor neuron lesions, but not from other causes of anterior horn cell disease, such as poliomyelitis. It is important to examine more than a single nerve. Useful information in support of the diagnosis may be gained by showing evidence of denervation in an area that also has upper motor neuron signs.

In a recent review, it was noted that just under half the patients did not fit Lambert's criteria at presentation, which was frequently due to the absence of fibrillation potentials, and if this is the case, the tests should be repeated after several weeks (78). It is also necessary to exclude multifocal conduction block, such as is found in MMN, which may mimic the lower motor neuron form of MND, and may be treatable with immunosupression. Conduction block is not by itself diagnostic of MMN, particularly if it is only present at common sites of nerve compression, and therefore should be looked for at other sites. In conduction block, there should be a greater than 50% reduction in the compound muscle action potential amplitude and the negative peak area after proximal vs. distal nerve stimulation, with less than 15% change in the duration of the negative peak. A reduction in sural nerve action potential does not exclude a diagnosis of MND. If low amplitude of compound action potentials and a decremental response to repetitive nerve stimulation are present, it may suggest rapid progression.

Transcutaneous cortical and spinal stimulation has shown marked reductions in central motor conduction in MND and may be evidence of subclinical involvement in patients (79). In patients with signs only below the level of the craniocervical junction and particularly in patients with only lower motor neuron signs. It may be necessary to image the spinal cord to exclude a compressive lesion, such as cervical spondylosis, a spinal cord tumor, or syringomyelia. Demyelinating plaques due to multiple sclerosis may be seen in patients with only upper motor neuron signs. In MND, magnetic resonance imaging (MRI) of the spinal cord is likely to be normal, although the cord may be thinned especially in the cervical region. Magnetic resonance imaging scans of the brain may show high intensity lesions in the motor cortex, internal capsule, and brainstem, although this may not always reflect degeneration of the corticospinal tracts, because this appearance is seen in some normal individuals with different pulse sequences. In addition, atrophy may be seen, particularly in the frontotemporal region in patients with MND and dementia. An MRI scan of the brain should be carried out in cases of MND with atypical features, for example, if only upper motor neuron signs are present, or if rare conditions such as adrenoleukodystrophy are suspected.

In atypical cases, a muscle biopsy should be considered. In MND, the muscles show typical denervation atrophy of different ages.

Other investigations that may be indicated are listed in Table 4.

Table 4 Investigations

Investigation	Reason	Comments
CPK	Often raised	No specific diagnostic purpose. Low levels indicate poor prognosis.
TSH, T_3, and T_4	Exclude thyrotoxicosis	Very rarely causes a syndrome of fasciculations, weakness, and hyperreflexia.
Ca^{2+} and parathyroid hormone	Exclude hyperparathyroidism	
Chest x-ray	Exclude carcinoma of lung	MND has been reported as a paraneoplastic condition in association with lung cancer.
Plasma protein electrophoresis	Detect a paraprotein	May be associated with a lymphoma.
Hexosamindase A and B	Exclude Tay-Sachs and Sandhoffs diseases	May rarely present in adults.
Anti-GM_1 ganglioside antibodies	Positive in motor neuropathies	Present in 10–20% of normal population. Need high levels to diagnose multifocal motor neuropathy.
HTLV-1	Exclude tropical spastic paraparesis	May mimic PLS.
Serum and urine lead	Exclude lead toxicity	Excess lead may cause a motor neuropathy, which is usually clinically distinct from MND.
Androgen receptor gene mutation	Diagnose Kennedy's syndrome	
VDRL/TPHA	Exclude syphilis	
Long-chain fatty acids	Raised in adrenoleukodystrophy	Combination of Addison's disease, degeneration of motor cortex and spinal cord, with a pseudobulbar palsy and cortical blindness, occurring in males. Occasional presentation in adults described.

B. Treatment

No treatment exists to reverse or halt the progression of MND, and therefore much of the management of these patients is supportive and involves the treatment of specific symptoms. In the ideal situation, there is a neurocare team to care for the MND patient. The team consists of various professionals who have skills to offer the disabled and terminally ill patient. The team members will vary according to local needs and resources but usually includes a consultant neurologist, a speech therapist, a physiotherapist, an occupational therapist, and a social worker. In addition there may be a representative from the local hospice, a general practitioner, and the local Motor Neurone Disease Association Regional Care Adviser. Each patient is allocated a key worker, who is the patient's first line of contact for assistance, and who would then be able involve other members of the team as the individual's needs change. For example a patient presenting with a dysarthria may have as his key worker the speech therapist. If the patient then develops difficulty walking, the speech therapist would be able to liaise with colleagues on the team so the physiotherapist and the occupational therapists could offer their expertise with minimal delay. The team aims to anticipate needs, allowing appropriate equipment and adaptations to be provided prior to a crisis. Patients are often reluctant to accept such advice in advance, and this issue needs delicate handling to avoid causing distress to the patient and carers.

Excess salivation is one of the most distressing symptoms for MND patients. It is often difficult, using anticholinergic drugs, to reach a satisfactory balance between drying up secretions and leaving an unpleasantly dry mouth, making it even more difficult for a dysphagic patient to swallow food. Benzhexol has been shown to reduce secretions by 85%, benztropine by 65–70%, and atropine sulphate by 50%. Hyoscine patches, licensed for use in motion sickness, reduce secretions by 30% when one patch is used and up to 60% when two patches are used. Antidepressant drugs such as amitriptyline and dothiepin may also have a role in treating sialorrhea, in addition to their beneficial role in improving mood and sleep. Referral to an oral surgeon can be considered for an intraoral prosthesis, to aid in approximating the lips and creating an oral seal. In addition, radiotherapy to the parotid glands can be considered in refractory cases. Oral suction units should be provided when excess secretions remain a problem.

Initial symptoms of dysphagia should prompt referral to a speech therapist for an assessment of swallowing and may involve videofluoroscopy. The therapist will be able to advise on techniques to improve swallowing such as posture and lip closure. Sucking an ice cube prior to eating can improve deglutination. Advice can be given on the ideal consistency of food for a particular patient, including proprietary thickeners containing modified maize starch. Advice from a dietician at this stage may often be beneficial.

At a later stage, when adequate nutrition is not being maintained or when the patient is aspirating food, a gastrostomy should be offered to the patient. Ideally this is discussed well in advance and performed before significant weight loss occurs. The most frequently performed procedure is a percutaneous endoscopic gastrostomy (PEG), when a small-bore tube is inserted under local anesthetic and endoscopic control into the stomach. Some centers perform gastrostomies under radiological control or via a minilaparotomy. In addition to the gastroenterologist, a dietician should be involved before the procedure being performed. Proprietary feeds can then be infused via a pump directly into the stomach. Some patients find this most convenient at night. Complications include diarrhea, which often resolves on slowing down the speed of the feed, and reflux, which responds to antacids. The rate of sepsis is low. There is a risk of aspiration pneumonia at the time of the procedure and gastric perforation. Providing the risk of aspiration is not great, patients can continue to eat and drink if they so wish.

Dysarthria is the presenting complaint in about one-third of patients and also affects up to 70% of patients with limb onset at a later stage. Speech therapists have an important role initially in encouraging techniques to make the best use of remaining functions. At a later stage, they will be able to advise on communication aids such as lightwriters, the SAMM communicator (onto which the patient's own voice can be recorded at an early stage in the disease), or more sophisticated computer aids, such as the Possum Communicator.

Constipation is a frequent complaint in patients, due to a combination of factors including reduced fluid intake, poor diet, reduced mobility, and weakening of the abdominal and pelvic floor muscles. In addition to encouraging patients to drink plenty of fluids, drugs such as co-danthramer, lactulose, and isphagula husk can be prescribed. As the disease progresses, suppositories and enemas may be required.

Spasticity can cause both discomfort and pain, in addition to hindering walking. Baclofen, dantrolene, and diazepam can all be tried. Cramp, another troubling symptom, often responds well to quinine or magnesium salts.

The majority of patients with MND die of respiratory failure, often complicated by aspiration pneumonia. Chest infections should be treated promptly with antibiotics, rehydration, and chest physiotherapy. In the later stage of the disease, careful thought and discussion with the patient and caregivers should occur prior to commencing aggressive treatment of pneumonia, if this will prolong a life that has become a burden to the patient. Many patients will have made their preferences known in advance, and there is an increasing trend toward make a "living will."

Diaphragmatic weakness occurs frequently, with dyspnea on minimal exertion and orthopnea, progressing to disturbed sleep, daytime somnolence, morning headache, and ankle edema. Paradoxical movement of the abdomen is observed on inspiration when supine. Vital capacity is usually 50% of the predicted normal on standing, falling by half again in the supine position.

Symptomatic relief of dyspnea can be achieved with diazepam, or more effectively by oral or subcutaneous morphine.

The question of whether more invasive forms of ventilation should be used is not easy. In the United Kingdom only in exceptional circumstances would a patient with MND have a tracheotomy performed and intermittent positive pressure ventilation (IPPV) instigated. In North America and other parts of Europe, the practice is more common. In the United States, about 10% of MND patients are offered and accept home ventilation, usually by IPPV. The cost is on average $150,000 (£ 100,000) per year. In a study from northern Illinois, 90% of patients receiving IPPV said they were glad they had chosen the option and would do so again, although families of the patients reported major burdens and only 50% said they would choose it for themselves (80).

In the United Kingdom, other forms of ventilatory support are more commonly tried. Considerable relief from the symptoms of diaphragmatic weakness can be achieved by negative pressure ventilation with a cuirass. These are initially used mainly at night, but as the condition progresses, patients tend to use them for an increasing number of hours. Negative pressure ventilation increases the risk of aspiration of secretions. Other patients have been treated by nasal continuous positive airway pressure (CPAP), often just at night, although patients frequently find it difficult to tolerate the mask, especially if they are troubled by excessive secretions. A rocking bed can be effective in relieving the symptoms of diaphragmatic weakness in the later stages (81).

The role of respiratory support in patients with MND presents complicated medical and ethical problems, and careful thought and discussion with patients and caregivers should be entered into before embarking on a particular form of management.

C. Clinical Trials

There is no treatment that has been shown conclusively to slow or halt the progression of MND, let alone restore lost motor neurons. At best all we can currently offer patients is a place in a double-blind, randomized, placebo-controlled trial of one of the new therapeutic agents being tested in MND. Entry into these trials is strictly controlled, and usually only patients with definite or probable MND according to the El Escorial research criteria are included. The major trials currently underway are:

1. Riluzole

This is a glutamate release inhibitor, known to inactivate the neuronal Na^+ channel and so decrease neuronal excitability. It may also have postsynaptic glutamate receptor blocking actions. It was originally tried in MND because of the evidence for raised cerebrospinal fluid (CSF) levels of glutamate and reduced tissue levels. In the original study by Bensimon, et al. (82) carried out in 155 patients, survival was significantly prolonged in the treated group as compared with the control group. The effect was most marked in the bulbar-onset patients.

As discussed above, glutamate toxicity has been implicated in the neuronal damage associated with ALS. Riluzole has been shown to have neuroprotective activity, possibly by presynaptic inhibition of glutamate release. An earlier trial, (randomized, double-blind, placebo-controlled) had shown that in 155 patients, riluzole (100 mg per day) appeared to retard disease progression (82). The next stage was to conduct a multicenter trial under similar trial conditions, only this time looking at doses of 50 mg, 100 mg or 200 mg daily. The effects of the drug were compared in terms of time since diagnosis (12 and 18 months) and clinical presentation (bulbar vs. limb onset) (83).

Overall, 959 patients with clinically probable or definite ALS of fewer than 5 years' duration were randomly assigned to treatment with placebo or one of the above doses daily. Randomization was stratified by center and site of disease onset. The primary outcome was survival without tracheostomy. Secondary outcomes were rates of change in functional measures (muscle strength, functional status, respiratory function, patient's assessment of fasciculation, cramps, stiffness, and tiredness).

At the end of the study (median, 18 months), 122 (50.4%) placebo-treated patients and 134 (56.8) of those who had received 100 mg per day of riluzole were alive without tracheostomy. In those who had received 50 mg or 200 mg per day of riluzole, 55.3% and 57.8%, respectively, were alive without tracheostomy. There was a significant inverse dose response in risk of death. No functional scale discriminated between the treatment groups. The most common adverse reactions were asthenia, dizziness, GO disorders, and increases in liver enzymes. These were most common in the higher doses.

Thus the use of riluzole was associated with enhanced survival: the risk of death or survival with tracheostomy at 18 months was 35% lower on 100 mg of the drug than with placebo in patients with both bulbar and limb onset. Of course it is not possible to know whether this small prolongation of life is reflected in positive or negative changes in the quality of life. Our experience as clinicians, however, does suggest that psychological well being is enhanced by the availability of a drug that is safe and well tolerated and that has a proven effect on the disease. Riluzole is effective and represents the first step in the development of treatments for ALS.

2.   Ciliary Neurotrophic Factor

Neurotrophic factors are required for the survival of neurons in development. Ciliary neurotrophic factor (CNTF) was originally shown to prevent the death of facial motor neurons in rats after axotomy by Sendter, et al. in 1990 (84). In 1992, the same laboratory reported work showing that CNTF prolonged survival and greatly improved function in the progressive motor neuronopathy mouse, a model for human spinal MND (85). Trials are currently being carried out in North America of subcutaneous CNTF in ALS. Doubts have been raised as to whether CNTF given subcutaneously can cross the blood-brain barrier.

3. Insulin-Like Growth Factor

Insulin-like growth factor-1 (IGF-1) has been shown to enhance motor neuron sprouting and to increase muscle end-plate size in rats. Multicenter trials in MND are underway in North America and Europe.

4. Brain-Derived Neurotrophic Factor

Brain-derived neurotrophic factor (BDNF) has been shown to enhance the survival of motor neurons after axotomy and rescue motor neurons from death in mice. The first human trials are underway in North America.

5. N-Acetylcysteine

N-Acetylcysteine (NAC) is a free radical scavenger, widely used in the treatment of paracetamol overdose. It is a precursor of glutathione, which plays a major part in the body's intracellular oxidant defense mechanisms. Preliminary reports of a double-blind, placebo-controlled trial showed a significant improvement in the survival of the treated group of patients with spinal-onset MND (86).

In addition to the trials mentioned above, many other forms of treatment have been tried in MND. Although, apart from in a few specific situations, i.e., those patients with monoclonal paraproteinemia, lymphoma, or high titers of antibodies to GM_1 ganglioside, there is no evidence that MND is an autoimmune disease. Many treatments aimed at the immune system have been tried without success. These include high-dose steroids (87), plasmapheresis (88) azathioprine, cyclophosphamide (89), cyclosporine (90), and total lymphoid irradiation (91).

Other glutamate antagonists have been tried in addition to riluzole, but neither lamotrogine or dextrometrophan (92) had any effect. In a small pilot study, Plaitakis (93) treated patients with branched-chain amino acids and showed muscle strength and function was maintained, but this was not confirmed in the much larger European study. Selegiline, a monoamine oxidase B inhibitor, which possibly slows down the progression of Parkinson's disease, has no effect on MND (94). Miscellaneous agents including thyrotrophin-releasing hormone (95), L-dopa, amantidine, guanadine, naloxone, bovine ganglioside, testosterone, and pancreatic extracts have all been tried without success.

After the finding of a SOD1 mutation in some families with MND, many neurologists recommend that patients should try vitamin E, 1 g daily, in view of its role as a free radical scavenger, although there is no direct evidence to support its use or that of vitamin C.

V. CONCLUSIONS

The motor neuron disorders are a large group of disorders of varying etiology. One hundred twenty-five years after the classic description of MND (ALS) by Charcot and Joffroy, we know the cause of one type of familial MND, but we do not yet know how mutations of the Cu/Zn SOD gene lead to late-onset, progressive, and selective neuronal death, nor whether damage by free radicals holds the key to understanding motor neuron death in the sporadic form of the disease and in other familial forms in which Cu/Zn SOD gene mutations have been excluded. We also do not yet understand why mutation of the androgen receptor leads to selective degeneration of lower motor neurons in Kennedy's disease.

Nevertheless, these advances provide new opportunities for research into pathogenesis, and it is likely that mutations causing SMA will soon be identified, providing another insight into the molecular mechanisms leading to motor neuron death.

The role of excitotoxicity in MND remains speculative, but a combination of vulnerability to excitotoxicity and free radical damage might account for the selective loss of motor neurons, and the excitotoxin and free radical hypothesis provides new therapeutic opportunities currently being tested in large and well-defined clinical trials.

The management of MND is demanding and requires a positive approach from all concerned, preferably through a team of professionals with experience of the disease. At various stages, specialist advice in rheumatology and rehabilitation, orthopedics, ENT, respiratory medicine, gastroenterology, and psychiatry may be required, and the neurologist often acts as a coordinator for these inputs, although coordination of care is often best achieved by a key worker based in the community. Indeed the support of the therapists, district nurses, general practitioners, and hospice teams is usually of greater importance than that of the hospital specialists, including the neurologists. Nevertheless, the neurologist should wherever possible take an active role in supporting the patient and caregivers, keeping them (and the care team) informed of research progress and advising on symptomatic relief. The rapidly changing needs of individuals with MND provide a major challenge for all concerned with their care.

REFERENCES

1. Charcot JM, Joffroy A. Deux cas d'atrophie musculaire progressive avec lésions de la substance grise et des faisceaux antérolatéraux de la moëlle épinière. Arch Physiol Norm Pathol 1869; 2:354–367, 629–649, 744–760.
2. Juergens SM, Kurland LT, Haruo Okazaki PH, Mulder DW. ALS in Rochester, Minnesota. Neurology 1980; 30:463–470.
3. Norris F, Shepherd R, Denys E, Onset, natural history and outcome in idiopathic adult motor neuron disease. J Neurol Sci 1993; 118:48–55.
4. Gurruto RM, Yanagihara R, Gajdusek DC. Disappearance of high incidence amyotrophic lateral sclerosis and parkinsonism dementia on Guam. Neurology 1985; 35:193–198.
5. Chancellor AM, Warlow CP. Adult onset motor neuron disease: Worldwide mortality, incidence and distribution since 1950. J Neurol Neurosurg Psychiatry 1993; 55:1106–1115.
6. Dean G, Quigley M, Goldacre M. Motor neuron disease in defined English population: Estimates of incidence and mortality. J Neurol Neurosurg Psychiatry 1994; 57:430–434.
7. Matsumoto S, Hirano A, Goto S. Spinal cord neurofibrillary tangles of Guamanian amyotrophic lateral sclerosis and parkinsonism-dementia complex. Neurology 1990; 40:975–979.
8. Bunina TL. On intracellular inclusions in familial amyotrophic lateral sclerosis. Zhurnal Nevropathol Psikhiatri Iimeni SS Korsaakova. 1962; 62:1293–1299.
9. Chou SM. Pathognomy of intaneuronal inclusions in ALS. In: Tsubaki T, Toyokura Y, eds. Amyotrophic Lateral Sclerosis. Tokyo. Tokyo University Press; Baltimore: University Park Press, 1979; 744–760.
10. Leigh PN, Whitwell H, Garofalo O. Ubiquitin-immunoreactive intraneuronal inclusions in amyotrophic lateral sclerosis: morphology, distribution, and specificity. Brain 1991; 114:755–788.
11. Leigh PN, Anderton BH, Dodson A, Gallo J-M, Swash M, Power DM. Ubiquitin deposits in anterior horn cells in motor neuron disease. Neurosci Lett 1988; 93:197–203.
12. Lowe J, Lennox G, Jefferson D, A filamentous inclusion body within anterior horn neurons in motor neuron disease defined by immunocytochemical localization of ubiquitin-protein conjugates. Neurosci Lett 1988; 94:203–210.
13. Williams C, Kozlowski MA, Hinton DR, Miller CA. Degeneration of spinocerebellar neurons in amyotrophic lateral sclerosis with dementia. Ann Neurol 1990; 27:269–274.
14. Neary D. Snowdon JS, Northern B, Goulding PJ, MacDermott N. Frontal lobe dementia and motor neuron disease. J Neurol Neurosurg Psychiatry 1990; 53:23–32.
15. Wightman G, Anderson VER, Martin J, Hippocampal and neocortical ubiquitin-immunoreactive inclusions in amyotrophic lateral sclerosis with dementia. Neurosci Lett 1992; 139:269–264.

16. Kew JJM, Leigh PN, Playford ED. Cortical function in amyotrophic lateral sclerosis. A positron emission tomography study. Brain 1993; 116:655–680.

17. Kew JJM, Goldstein LH, Leigh PN, The relationship between abnormalities of cognitive function and cerebral activation in amyotrophic lateral sclerosis: A neuropsychological and positron emission tomography study. Brain 1994; 116:1399–1424.

18. Hirano A, Malamud N, Kurland LT. Parkinsonism-dementia complex, an endemic disease on the island of Guam. II. Pathological features. Brain 1961; 84:662–679.

19. Jokelainen M. Amyotrophic lateral sclerosis in Finland. Acta Neurol Scand 1977; 56:194–204.

20. Hamida MB, Letaief F, Hentati F, Hamida CB. Morphometric study of the sensory nerve in classical (or Charcot disease) and juvenile amyotrophic lateral sclerosis. J Neurol Sci 1987; 78:313–329.

21. Nogues MA, Stalberg EV. Automatic analysis of heart rate variation. II. Findings in patients attending an EMG laboratory. Muscle Nerve 1989; 12:1001–1008.

22. Kihira I, Yoshida S, Uebayashi Y, Yase Y, Yoshimasu F. Involvement of Onuf's nucleus in ALS. Demonstration of intraneuronal inclusions and Bunina bodies. J Neurol Sci 1991; 104:119–128.

23. Veltema AN, Roos RAC, Bruyn GW. Autosomal dominant adult amyotrophic lateral sclerosis. J Neur Sci 1990; 97:93–115.

24. Tucker T, Layzer RB, Miller RG, Chad D. Subacute, reversible motor neuron disease. Neurology 1991; 41:1541–1544.

25. Tsai C, Ho H, Yen D, Reversible motor neuron disease. Eur Neurol 1993; 33:387–389.

26. Pringle CE, Hudson AJ, Munoz DG, Kiernan JA, Brown WF, Ebers GC. Primary lateral sclerosis. Clinical features, neuropathology and diagnostic criteria. Brain 1992; 115:495–520.

27. Rowland LP, Natural history and clinical features of amyotrophic lateral sclerosis and related motor neuron diseases. In: Calne DB, ed. Neurodegenerative diseases. WB Saunders Co., 1994; 507–521.

28. Kew J and Leigh PN. Dementia with motor neuron disease. In: (Rosor MN, ed.) Unusual Dementias. Vol 1 (3). Baillière's Clinical Neurology. London: Baillière Tindall,

29. Kew JJM, Leigh PN, Playford ED, Cortical function in amyotrophic lateral sclerosis: a positron emission tomographic study. Brain 1993; 116:655–680.

30. Gunnarsson L-G, Dahlbom K, Strandman E. Motor neuron disease and dementia reported among 13 members of a single family. Acta Neurol Scand 1991; 84:429–433.

31. Zimmerman HM. Monthly report to the Medical Officer in Command. US Navy medical research. Unit No. 2, June 1, 1945.

32. Kurland LT, Mulder DW. Epidemiologic investigations of amyotrophic lateral sclerosis. 1. Preliminary reports on geographic distribution, with special reference to the Marina Islands, including pathologic observations. Neurology 1954; 4:335–378, 438–448.

33. Mulder DW, Kurland LT. Amyotrophic lateral sclerosis in Micronesia. Proc Staff Meet Mayo Clin 1954; 29:666–670.

34. Hirano A, Kurland LT, Krooth RS, Lessel S. Parkinsonism-dementia complex, an endemic disease on the island of Guam. I. Clinical features. Brain 1961; 84:642–661.

35. Garruto RM, Gajdusek DC, Chen K-M. Amyotrophic lateral sclerosis among Chamorro migrants from Guam. Ann Neurol 1980; 8:612–618.

36. Kurland LT. An appraisal of the neurotoxicity of cycad and the aetiology of amyotrophic lateral sclerosis on Guam. Fed Proc 1972; 31:1540–1542.

37. Spencer PS, Nunn PB, Hugon J, Linkage of Guam amyotrophic lateral sclerosis-parkinsonism-dementia to a plant excitant neurotoxin. Science 1987; 237:517–522.

38. Pestronk A, Chaudhary V, Feldman. Lower motor neuron syndromes defined by patterns of weakness, nerve conduction abnormalities, and high titres of antiglycolipid antibodies. Ann Neurol 1990; 27:316–326.

39. Pestronk A, Cornblath DR, Ilyas AA. A treatable multifocal motor neuropathy with antibodies to GM1 ganglioside. Ann Neurol 1988; 24:73–78.

40. Krarup C, Stewart JD, Sumner AJ, A syndrome of asymmetrical limb weakness and motor conduction block. Neurology 1990; 40:118–127.

41. Donaghy M, Mills KR, Boniface SJ, Pure motor demyelinating neuropathy: Deterioration after steroid treatment and improvement with intravenous immunoglobulin. J Neurol Neurosurg Psychiatry 1994; 57:778–783.

42. Chaudhry V, Corse AM, Cornplath DR. Multifocal motor neuropathy: Response to human immune globulin. Ann Neurol 1993; 33:237–242.

43. Shy ME, Evans VA, Dublin FD. Antibodies to GM1 and GD1b in patients with motor neuron disease without plasma cell dyscrasia. Ann Neurol 1989; 25:511–513.

44. Latov N, Hays AP, Donofrio, Monoclonal IgM with unique reactivity to gangliosides GM1b and lacto-N-tetraose in two patients with motor neuron disease. Neurology 1988; 38:763–768.

45. Salazas-Grueso EF, Routbort MJ, Martin, Polyclonal IgM anti-GM1 ganglioside antibody in patients with motor neuron disease and variants. Ann Neurol 1990; 27:558–563.

46. Kurland LT, Mulder DW. Epidemiological investigations of amyotrophic lateral sclerosis. 2. Familial aggregations indicative of dominant inheritance, parts I and II. Neurology 1955; 5:182–196. 249–268.

47. Ben Hamida M, Hentati F, BeHamida C. Hereditory motor system diseases (chronic juvenile amyotrophic lateral sclerosis). Brain 1990; 113:347–363.

48. Emery A, Holloway S. Familial motor neuron disease. In: Rowland LP, ed. Human Motor Neuron Diseases. New York: Raven Press, 139–147.

49. Siddique T, Periacak-Vance MA, Brook BR, Linkage analysis in familial amyotrophic lateral sclerosis. Neurology 1989:919–926.

50. Williams DB, Floate DA, Leicester J. Familial motor neuron disease: Differing penetrance in large pedigrees. J Neurol Sci 1988; 86:215–230.

51. Engel WK, Kurland LT, Latzo I. An inherited disease similar to amyotrophic lateral sclerosis with a pattern of posterior column involvement: An intermediate form? Brain 1959; 82:203–303.

52. Hirano A, Kurland LT, Sayre GP. Familial amyotrophic lateral sclerosis. Arch Neurol 1967; 16:232–243.

53. Swash M, Scholtz CL, Vowles G, Selective and asymmetric vulnerability of corti-cospinal and spinocerbellar tracts in motor neuron disease. J Neurol Neurosurg Psychiatry 1988; 51:785–789.
54. Williams C, Kozlowski MA, Hinton DR, Degeneration of spinocerebellar neurons in amyotrophic lateral sclerosis. Ann Neurol 1990; 27:215–225.
55. Hudson AJ. Amyotrophic lateral sclerosis and its association with dementia, par-kinsonism and other neurological disorders: A review. Brain 1981; 104:217–253.
56. Siddique T, Figlewicz DA, Pericak-Vance MA, Linkage of a gene causing familial amyotrophic lateral sclerosis to chromosome 21 and evidence of genetic-locus het-erogeneity. New Engl J Med 1991; 324:1381–1384.
57. Rosen DR, Siddique T, Patterson D, Mutations in Cu/Zn superoxide dismutase gene are associated with familial amyotrophic lateral sclerosis. Nature 1993; 362:59–62.
58. Kennedy W, Alter M, Sung K. Progressive proximal spinal and muscular atrophy of late onset: A sex linked recessive trait. Neurology 1968; 18:671–680.
59. Harding AE, Thomas PK, Barrister M, Bradbury PG, Morgan-Hughes JA, Pons-ford JR. X-linked recessive bulbospinal neuronopathy: A report of ten cases. J Neurol Neurosurg Psychiatry 1982; 45:1012–1019.
60. La Spada AR, Wilson EM, Lubahn EB, Androgen receptor gene mutations in X-linked spinal and bulbar muscular atrophy. Nature 1991; 352:77–79.
61. Hentai A, Bejaoui K, Periack-Vance M A, Linkage of recessive familial amyotro-phic lateral sclerosis to chromosome 2q33-q35. Nature Genetics 1994; 7:425–428.
62. Tylleskär T, Banea M, Bikangi N, Cooke R, Poulter NH, Rosling H. Cassava cy-anogens and konzo, an upper motor neuron disease found in Africa. Lancet 1992; 339:208–211.
63. Tylleskär T, Howlett WP, Rwiza HT, Konzo: A distinct disease entity with selective upper motor neuron damage. J Neurol Neurosurg Psychiatry 1993; 56:638–643.
64. Gebre-Ab T, Wolde Gabriel Z, Maffi M, Ahmed Z, Ayele T, Fanta H. Neurolathyr-ism. A report and a review of an epidemic. Ethiop Med J 1978; 16:1–11.
65. Spencer PS, Roy D, Ludolph A, Hugon J, Dwived MP, Schaumberg HH, Lathyr-ism: Evidence for the role of the neuroexcitatory aminoacid BOAA. Lancet 1986; ii:1066–1067.
66. Younger DS, Rowland LP, Latov N, Lymphoma, motor neuron disease and amyo-trophic lateral sclerosis. Ann Neurol 1991; 29:78–86.
67. Brandt S. Course and symptoms of progressive infantile muscular atrophy. A fol-low-up study of one hundred and twelve cases in Denmark. Arch Neuro Psych 1950; 63:218–228.
68. Pearn J. Classification of spinal muscular atrophies. Lancet 1980; i:919–922.
69. Brzustowicz LM, Lehner T, Castilla LH, Genetic mapping of chronic childhood onset spinal muscular atrophy to chromosome 5q11.2-13.3. Nature 1990; 334:540–541.
70. Melki J, Abdelhak S, Sheth P, Gene for chronic proximal spinal muscular atrophies maps to chromosome 5q. Nature 1990; 334:767–768.
71. Johnson WG. The clinical spectrum of hexosaminadase deficiency diseases. Neu-rology 1981; 31:1453–1456.
72. Johnson WG. Hexosaminadase deficiency: A cause of recessively inherited motor

neuron diseases. In: Rowland LP, ed. Human Motor Neuron Diseases. New York: Raven Press, 1982; 159–164.

73. Zeman S, Lloyd C, Meldrum B, Leigh PN. Excitatory amino acids, free radicals, and the pathogenesis of motor neuron disease. Neuropathol and Appl Neurobiol 1994; 20:219–231.

74. Bowling AC, Schulz JB, Brown Jr RH, Flint Beal M. Superoxide dismutase activity in familial and sporadic amyotrophic lateral sclerosis. J Neurochem 1993; 61:2322–2325.

75. Heafield MT, Fearn S, Steventon, Plasma cysteine and sulphate levels in patients with motor neuron, Parkinson's and Alzheimer's disease. Neurosci Lett 1990; 110:216–220.

76. Swash M, Leigh PN. Workshop report. Criteria for diagnosis of familial amyotrophic lateral sclerosis. Neuromuscular Disorders 1990; 2(1):7–9.

77. Lambert EH, Mulder DW, Electromyographic studies in amyotrophic lateral sclerosis. Mayo Clinic Proc 1957; 32:441–446.

78. Behnia M, Kelly JJ. Role of electromyography in amyotrophic lateral sclerosis. Muscle Nerve 1991; 14:1236–1241.

79. Ingram DA, Swash M. Central motor conduction is abnormal in motor neuron disease. J Neurol Neurosurg Psychiatry 1987; 50:159–166.

80. Moss MD, Cassey MSOT, Stocking CB, Roos MD, Brooks MD. Siegler MD. Home ventilation for amyotrophic lateral sclerosis patients: Outcomes, costs, and patient, family, and physician attitudes. Neurology 1993; 43:438–443.

81. Howard RS, Wiles CM, Loh L. Respiratory complications and their management in motor neuron disease. Brain 1989; 112:1155–1170.

82. Bensimon G, Lacomblez L, Meininger V, ALS/Riluzole Study Group. A controlled trial of riluzole in amyotrophic lateral sclerosis. New Engl J Med 1994; 330:585–591.

83. Lacomblez L, Bensimon G, Leigh PN, Guillet P, Meininger V. Dose-ranging study of riluzole in amyotrophic lateral sclerosis. Lancet 1996; 347:1425–1431.

84. Sendtner M, Kreutzberg GW, Thoenen H. Ciliary neurotrophic factor prevents the degeneration of motor neurons after axotomy. Nature 1990; 1990:345:440–441.

85. Sendtner M, Schmälbruch H, Stöckli KA, Ciliary neurotrophic factor prevents the degeneration of motor neurons in mouse mutant progressive motor neuropathy. Nature 1993; 358:502–504.

86. Louwerse ES, Weverling GJ, Tijssen J-GP, Meyjes FEP, de Jong JMPV. The efficacy of N-acetylcysteine in amyotrophic lateral sclerosis. Abstract, 4th International Symposium on ALS/MND. Neuroprotection and Clinical Trials, Paris, 1993.

87. Bauman J, Results of treatment of certain diseases of the central nervous system with ACTH and corticosteroids. Acta Neurol Scand 1965; 41(suppl13):453–461.

88. Kelemen J, Hedlund W, Orlin JB, Berkman EM, Plasmapheresis with immunosuppression in amyotrophic lateral sclerosis. Arch Neurol 1983; 40:752–753.

89. Brown RH, Hauser SL, Harrington H, Weiner HL. Failure of immunosuppression with a 10- to 14-day course of high-dose intravenous cyclophosphamide to alter the progression of amyotrophic lateral sclerosis. Arch Neurol 1986; 43:383–384.

90. Appel SH, Stewart SS, Appel V. A double-blind study of the effectivness of cyclosporine in amyotrophic lateral sclerosis. Arch Neurol 1988; 45:381–386.

91. Drachmam DB, Chaudhry V, Cornblath D. Trial of immunosuppression in amyo-
    trophic lateral sclerosis using total lymphoid irradiation. Ann Neurol 1994; 35:142–
    150.
92. Goldberg MP, Pham P-C, Choi DW. Dextrorphan and dextrometrophan attenuate
    hypoxic injury in neuronal culture. Neurosci Lett 1987; 80:11–15.
93. Plaitakis A, Smith J, Mandeli J, Yahr MD. Pilot trial of branched-chain aminoacids
    in amyotrophic lateral sclerosis. Lancet 1988; 1:1015–94.93.
94. Mitchell JD, Houghton E, Kilshaw J. Free radicals, sporadic motor neuron disease
    and selegeline. Abstract. 4th International Symposium on ALS/MND. Neuroprotec-
    tion and Clinical Trials, Paris, 1993.
95. Brooks BR. A summary of the current position of TRH in ALS therapy. Ann NY
    Acad Sci 1989; 553:431–461.

18

Rheumatological Aspects of Spinal Disease

Cyrus Cooper and Michael I. D. Cawley

Southampton General Hospital, Southampton, Hampshire, England

I. INTRODUCTION

Rheumatology is primarily concerned with diseases of the musculoskeletal system, of which the spine is an important component. The intimate relationship of the spinal cord to the vertebral column and related soft tissue structures means that there may be a close relationship between lesions of the spinal cord and the nonneurological tissues of the spine. In this chapter we will consider diseases involving the vertebrae; intervertebral discs; intervertebral and sacroiliac synovial joints; and the muscles, ligaments, and other connective tissue structures associated with these organs. The chapter will emphasize inflammatory diseases involving the spine; other spinal skeletal diseases will be mentioned in brief.

II. DIAGNOSTIC AND THERAPEUTIC APPROACH

The following are important in the history and examination of spinal disease:

Analysis of pain patterns, especially referred pain.
Is the condition local or diffuse? If local, which segments are involved?
Are specific physical signs of bone, joint, or disc lesions present?

Are there psychosomatic or social issues influencing the patient's symptoms?

III. PRIMARY INFLAMMATORY DISORDERS

A. Ankylosing Spondylitis and Related Spondyloarthropathies

Ankylosing spondylitis (AS) is the most common primary inflammatory disorder of the spine in the western world. It is a chronic inflammatory disease that predominantly affects the axial skeleton. It is the prototype of a group of diseases, the spondyloarthropathies, that are interrelated clinically, pathologically, and genetically. This group of diseases includes conditions in which musculoskeletal inflammation coexists with disease in other organ systems, such as the skin and the gastrointestinal tract (Table 1). These other spondyloarthropathies will be mentioned further, where the spinal manifestations differ from AS with which this section is mainly concerned.

Ankylosing spondylosis was first described in 1691, although paleopathologists have reported the occurrence of ankylosing spinal disease in skeletal remains from as early as the third millenium, B.C. However, the clearest descriptions of patients with AS were only made toward the end of the last century when Strumpell in Berlin, Marie in Paris, and von Bechterew in St. Petersburg almost simultaneously described subjects with anterior syndesmophytes, sacroiliitis, peripheral arthritis, and a cluster of extraskeletal manifestations. This disorder was known as spondylitis deformans in Continental Europe and rheumatoid spondylitis in the United States for several decades before the designation AS was given in 1961 and diagnostic criteria were established. Three sets of such diagnostic criteria have been proposed (Table 2). Central to each of these is the presence of radiographically determined sacroiliitis using a grading system dependent upon standard radiographs, together with various symptoms and signs of spinal inflammation. They include back pain, limitation of lumbar

Table 1 The Spondyloarthropathies

Classic ankylosing spondylitis
Sacroiliitis
Reiter's syndrome
Reactive arthritis (enteric or genito-urinary)
Psoriatic arthritis and spondylitis
Enteropathic arthritis and spondylitis (ulcerative colitis or Crohn's disease)
Juvenile chronic arthritis—some cases
Undifferentiated spondyloarthritis

Table 2 Diagnostic Criteria for Ankylosing Spondylitis (Modified New York Criteria, 1984)

1. Low back pain, 3 months' duration, improved by exercise and not limited by rest
2. Limitation of motion of the lumbar spine in sagittal and frontal planes
3. Chest expansion decreased relative to normal values for age and sex
4. Bilateral sacroiliitis, grade 2–4
5. Unilateral sacroiliitis, grade 3–4

Definite AS = unilateral sacroiliitis grade 3–4 or bilateral sacroiliitis grade 2–4 + one of three clinical criteria.

spine movement, and limitation of chest expansion. Recent advances in our understanding of the etiopathogenesis and optimal management of AS relate to the discovery of the association with HLA-B27. We have experienced improvement in our understanding of the genetics of this and other disorders, as well as of the underlying pathology and its differences from other forms of inflammatory joint disease.

B. Epidemiology of Ankylosing Spondylitis and Spondyloarthropathies

Early studies of the frequency of AS in western populations gave estimates of between 0.8 and 1.8 per thousand population. The striking similarity between the results of these studies and those based upon more detailed prevalence estimates using improved case ascertainment and diagnostic criteria suggests that the overall prevalence of AS in Caucasian populations is of the order of 15 cases per 10,000 population. The frequency of AS in non-Caucasian populations is variable. Estimates from the south and west of Africa have suggested very low prevalence rates, whereas the disorder has its highest frequency among Haida Indians, native inhabitants of Northern Canada, of whom 4–6% have AS. Although initially thought to be a disorder almost exclusively of men, with early male-to-female ratios estimated at 20:1, more recent population surveys suggest that AS occurs fairly frequently among women but is less serious. Current estimates of the sex ratio suggest this to be closer to 3:1.

Only one well-performed incidence study of AS has been done, based on the record linkage system of the Rochester Epidemiology Project in the United States. The overall age and sex-adjusted incidence rate for the disorder was 7.3 per 100,000 person years between 1935 and 1989. The age-adjusted incidence ratio in men was four times greater than in women, and age-adjusted incidence rates in both sexes appeared to decline between the periods 1935 to 1949 and 1980 to 1989. The median ages at symptom onset and at diagnosis remained constant during the 55-year period of the study, with the highest age-specific incidence rate occurring in men and women aged 25 and 34 years.

The prevalence of the other defined spondyloarthropathies is approximately as follows:

Psoriatic arthritis, of which less than 10% have spondylitis
Reiter's syndrome
Enteropathic spondyloarthritis associated with ulcerative colitis or Crohn's disease

1. Clinical Features

One of the hallmarks of the spondyloarthropathies is sacroiliac joint inflammation (sacroiliitis), which may be clinically silent. Other joints in the spine characteristically affected include discovertebral, apophyseal, costovertebral, and costotransverse joints. Paravertebral ligamentous structures are commonly involved, and a striking feature of the disease is the high frequency of inflammation at entheses (the sites where connective tissue, especially tendon or ligament, is inserted into bone). This enthesitis frequently results in pain and stiffness and ultimately may lead to bony ankylosis and the appearance of patients with late disease who have kyphotic fused thoracolumbar spines. Clinical features of AS can be characterized as skeletal and extraskeletal.

Skeletal Features

The common and characteristic initial symptom is chronic low back pain of insidious onset. The inflammatory back pain due to AS has special features that differentiate it from much more common noninflammatory causes of back pain including: (1) onset of back pain before the age of 40 years (2) insiduous onset (3) persistence for at least 3 months (4) association with morning stiffness and (5) improvement with exercise. The back pain associated with AS is usually dull, poorly localized, and felt deep in the lumbar and sacroiliac region and buttocks. A more prominent early symptom may be stiffness in the back that is worse in the morning and tends to be eased by moving about or a hot shower. The patient may be awakened in the early hours of the morning by stiffness and pain in the spine. Back complaints are the primary manifestation in about three-quarters of all patients. In the remainder constitutional symptoms, peripheral arthritis, or extraskeletal features may occur before back pain. Involvement of the cervical, thoracic, or lumbar spine contributes to axial pain, and enthesitis may cause pain and tenderness at sternocostal junctions, spinous processes, iliac crests, greater trochanters, and inferior or posterior heels, as well as less commonly at other bony sites. Pain and tenderness arising from the thoracolumbar junction is a common finding.

Peripheral arthritis occurs in about half of patients with AS. The major peripheral joints involved are the hips and shoulders, which are affected at some stage of the disease in one-third of patients. Hip disease is usually bilateral, insidious in onset, and potentially more crippling than involvement of any other limb joint. Flexion contractures of the hip are common in most AS patients with late stage disease. Involvement of other large limb joints such as the knee is also common, but involvement of the smaller peripheral joints of the extremities is much less frequent in primary AS as compared with the spondylitis associated with psoriatic arthropathy, Reiter's disease, or inflammatory bowel disease, in which small joint peripheral arthritis is more common.

A careful physical examination of the spine, sacroiliac, and peripheral joints is crucial to early diagnosis of AS. There is often limitation of lumbar spine movement. This is characteristically symmetrical and involves all planes of movement. Patients with restricted lumbar mobility may still be able to touch the floor with fingertips while keeping the knees extended if hip movement is retained. Lumbar flexion can be measured by the Schober test or modified Schober test. With the patient erect, a mark is placed on the skin overlying the fifth lumbar spinal process and another 10 cm above this. In the modified Schober test, an additional mark is made 5 cm below the fifth lumbar spine. The patient is asked to flex forward maximally without flexing the knees. In normal healthy individuals, the distance between the two marks on the skin should increase by at least 5 cm. Diminished lumbar spine mobility is indicated by a failure to do so. Sacroiliac joint pain due to active sacroiliitis may be elicited by pressure over the anterior superior spine, by compressing the two iliac bones toward each other, or by pressing the flexed knee toward the contralateral shoulder.

Involvement of costovertebral and costrotransverse joints results in a restriction of respiratory movement and therefore in the later stages of the disease, patients with AS may breathe mainly by using the diaphragm. Chest expansion, although age and sex dependent, is usually at least 5 cm in healthy individuals. Limited chest expansion is a frequent finding in established or advanced AS, although not in early disease. It is measured in the fourth intercostal space on maximal inspiration after forced maximal expiration. The presence of enthesopathy over the ischial tuberosities, greater trochanters, costochondral or manubriosternal junctions and calcanei, should be ascertained by local digital pressure. The entire spine becomes increasingly stiff after many years of disease progression, and the patient loses normal posture because of flattening of the lumbar lordosis and the development of an increased thoracic kyphosis. At this stage of disease, the pain from spinal involvement often diminishes and there is less early-morning stiffness. Spinal ankylosis develops at a variable rate and pattern. Occasionally the disease may be confined to one part of the spine throughout life. Often there is diffuse involvement, and the cervical spine may become markedly restricted in established disease, with the consequence of severe disability and a risk of fracture. Typical deformities may, however, usually evolve only after 10 or more years of the disease. In extreme cases, the entire spine may be fused in a flexed position and the field of vision may become progressively limited because of the kyphosis. A convenient means of assessing kyphosis is by standing the patient with heels against a wall and measuring the distance from wall to tragus. A full peripheral joint examination should be undertaken and may show asymptomatic restriction of some peripheral joints and tenderness of axial joints, such as the sternoclavicular or acromioclavicular joints.

An important complication of advanced AS is the development of destructive discovertebral lesions between fused areas of the spine. These result in severe local pain and characteristic radiographic features. They are best considered as pseudoarthroses rather than invasive inflammatory lesions.

Extraskeletal Involvement

Acute anterior uveitis is the most common extraskeletal manifestation of AS. It occurs in 25–30% of patients sometime in the course of their disease. An individual episode is almost always unilateral and has a strong tendency to recur. It is of the acute remitting type. Cardiovascular involvement is a relatively rare feature of AS. Aortitis, aortic regurgitation, conduction defects, and pericarditis have all been observed. The risk of significant aortic regurgitation increases with age, duration of AS, and the presence of peripheral arthritis. It has been reported in up to 3.5% of patients with AS of longer than 10 years' duration but is probably less common.

Thoracic spinal disease impairs chest expansion during inspiration. This does not usually result in ventilatory insufficiency unless diaphragmatic movements are also compromised. A slowly progressive upper lobe pulmonary fibrosis is a very rare complication. This is usually bilateral and may cavitate due to secondary *Aspergillus* infection. Patients may complain of cough, increasing dyspnea, and occasional hemoptysis.

Neurological involvement may occur in patients with AS as a consequence of fracture dislocation of the spine, especially the cervical spine, after minimal trauma, or spontaneous atlanto-axial subluxation, which occurs much less frequently than in rheumatoid arthritis. A cauda equina syndrome is a rare complication in which there is scarring and entrapment of the lumbar nerve roots in the exit foramina, somewhat resembling arachnoiditis. Other very rare extraskeletal manifestations include amyloidosis, IgA nephropathy, and an enteropathy that is said to differ from inflammatory bowel disease.

2. Investigations

Imaging

Radiographic evaluation of the spine and sacroiliac joints is the single most useful investigation in confirming the diagnosis. The earliest and most consistent findings are seen in the sacroiliac joints. Sacroiliitis is usually symmetrical and is indicated by blurring of the bony margin on both sides of the sacroiliac joints, followed by erosion and sclerosis of the adjacent bone and eventually by sacroiliac fusion. The early bony erosion can lead to an apparent widening of the sacroiliac joint space, but ultimately there is narrowing and complete bony ankylosis. A posteroanterior (prone) plain radiograph of the pelvis provides the best routine view of the sacroiliac joints, and oblique views can be obtained for further definition if necessary. Computerized tomography and isotope scintigraphy have both been used in an attempt to show sacroiliitis earlier and in more detail, especially when standard radiography is equivocal. However, these techniques are relatively nonspecific and their usefulness is limited. Recently it has been shown that magnetic resonance imaging (MRI) is the most sensitive index of sacroiliac joint inflammation and will probably gain increased application for this purpose.

Inflammatory lesions in the vertebral column affect the superficial layers of the annulus fibrosis at their attachment adjacent to the corners of the vertebral bodies. Bony erosion may be seen at the site of attachment on radiographs. There is also reactive bony sclerosis, which gives the appearance of "squaring" of the anterior vertebrae. These changes are sometimes known as Romanus lesions. These heal by gradual ossification of the superficial layers of the annulus and eventually may lead to bridging between the vertebrae. These fine vertebral bony spurs or bridges are called syndesmophytes. The paraspinal ligaments progressively ossify so that ultimately, there may be complete fusion of the vertebral column in the worst cases, a condition known as "bamboo spine." Radiographic involvement of the periperhal joints is most typical at the hips, where there is symmetrical concentric loss of joint space with irregularity of the subchondral bone and eventually a destructive deformity of the femoral head or, rarely, complete ankylosis of the hip joints. Bony spurs (the peripheral equivalent of syndesmophytes and due to enthesitis) form at the margins of other peripheral joints. In general, the radiographic changes in peripheral joints are nonerosive and nondestructive and tend toward ankylosis.

Other Investigations

A modestly elevated erythrocyte sedimentation rate (ESR) is present in most patients with AS, but the degree of elevation may not correlate with clinical disease activity. The carbon-reactive protein and other acute-phase proteins are also often elevated during active disease. Circulating serum IgA levels may be high in active spondylitis and spondyloarthritis. A mild normocytic normochromic anemia may be found, as may an elevated alkaline phosphatase. The autoantibody profile, including rheumatoid factor, is characteristically negative. Synovial fluid aspirated from inflamed peripheral joints shows nonspecific features of inflammation with increased leukocyte and protein content but no distinctive features to differentiate it from other inflammatory arthropathies. Subtle differences in the synovial lymphocyte infiltrate, as compared with rheumatoid arthritis, have been described. Pulmonary function tests often fail to reveal ventilatory dysfunction, even in advanced disease, but vital capacity and total lung capacity may be diminished.

HLA-B27 Typing

About 95% of patients with AS carry the class I histocompatibility locus antigen HLA-B27. The other spondyloarthropathies are also associated with this genetic marker to a variable extent (Table 3). Class I HLA molecules are expressed on the surface of all nucleated cells. The frequency of HLA-B27 in the general population in Northwest Europe is 6–8%. The role of the HLA-B27 molecule in the pathogenesis of AS and related diseases is not fully understood. One popular hypothesis is that antigenic peptides from certain infecting microorganisms, especially gastrointestinal or genitourinary pathogens, are compatible with the binding groove on the HLA-B27 molecule and are thereby presented to T-helper cells, thus provoking an immune response. However, HLA tissue typing is of limited value as an aid to diagnosis of typical AS, which can usually be recognized on the basis of the history, physical examination, and radiographic findings. However, the predictive value of HLA-B27 can be helpful in some clinical situations, including in patients with inflammatory back pain without radiographic changes, and those with rheumatoid factor-negative peripheral joint inflammation.

Table 3 Frequency of HLA-B27 in Various Diseases

	Approx. % HLA-B27	Controls of HLA-B27
Ankylosing spondylitis	> 95	7
Reiter's syndrome	6	
with sacroiliitis	95	6
Acute anterior uveitis	55	8
CIBD[a] and sacroiliitis	67	6
Juvenile chronic arthritis	25–42	6–10
Enteric reactive arthritis		
yersinia	88	
salmonella	94	14[b]
shigella	85	
Circinale erosive balanitis	88	14[b]

[a]Chronic inflammatory bowel disease.
[b]Finland.

3. Differential Diagnosis

Low back pain is the most frequent musculoskeletal symptom in the general population, and AS is a relatively infrequent, but important, cause of low back pain. It has to be differentiated from the various noninflammatory structural causes of back pain (q.v.) and also from intrinsic bone disease. When peripheral joint inflammation is prominent, AS has to be differentiated from other forms of inflammatory arthritis. Ankylosing spondylitis should be suspected when back pain has inflammatory characteristics, especially in younger patients. A strong family history of back pain, the presence of constitutional symptoms, peripheral arthritis, or characteristic extra-articular lesions such as acute iritis, also suggest AS. In such circumstances, a plain posteroanterior and lateral radiograph of the lumbar spine, including the sacroiliac joints, is helpful. Diagnosis depends on an appropriate association of clinical and radiographic features. However, in early disease, the radiographs may be normal and the diagnosis will be provisional. In these cases HLA-B27 typing will be helpful. The term "preankylosing spondylitis" is sometimes used for radiographically normal patients.

4. Management of Ankylosing Spondylitis

General Measures

The majority of patients with AS have a good prognosis, despite recurrent or chronic discomfort. With early intervention, the disease does not progress to severe and total ankylosis in the majority of patients. Apart from uveitis, systemic involvement is rare and the patient can be reassured of this as part of an overall education program. Contact with other patients through support groups, such as the National Ankylosing Spondylitis Society (NASS) is helpful in these program. Patients should be advised to stop smoking and take regular exercise, especially swimming. In the minority in whom the disease progresses rapidly, patients may need hospitalization for active rehabilitation. Patients should be encouraged to continue working, although job modification may be required. Physical therapy, a regular disciplined program of remedial exercises, is mandatory. The aim is to maintain normal posture and mobility. Long-term morbidity has been improved substantially by active physiotherapy, including hydrotherapy, especially in the early stages. A hot bath or shower in the morning reduces stiffness and, together with appropriate medication, allows the exercise program to be followed. During the day, attention should be given to ergonomic factors including position at work and maintenance of mobility. A long-term active managed approach, which includes physiotherapists and other paramedical staff, provides the best means of achieving these objectives, and often group therapy classes are the most cost-effective way of providing this treatment.

Nonsteroidal Anti-Inflammatory Drug Therapy

Nonsteroidal anti-inflammatory drugs (NSAID) are the core drug treatment for AS and other spondyloarthropathies. There have been few well-controlled studies comparing the efficacy of different anti-inflammatory agents in these diseases. In milder cases, any of the widely used, less potent and better tolerated NSAID can be used. In more severe cases in which more potent anti-inflammatory therapy is necessary, indomethacin is the drug of choice at present. It is more effective to give a slow-acting preparation at night (75–100 mg by capsule or suppository respectively) and if necessary, a further supplement in the morning. If indomethacin fails to control the disease, phenylbutazone, 100 mg two or three times daily may be used; this is probably the most effective anti-inflammatory drug. In the treatment of AS, because statistically significant increased bone marrow toxicity was recorded with this drug years ago, its prescription in the United Kingdom is restricted to hospitals only. If patients go into remission, alternative anti-inflammatory agents should be used.

Other Drugs

Of the disease-modifying antirheumatic drugs used in other inflammatory rheumatic disorders, sulfasalazine is the most promising the treatment of early AS. Trials of this agent in classic AS and psoriatic arthritis have been encouraging, especially with regard to peripheral joint inflammation. In a 6-month randomized, placebo-controlled, double-blind trial, 3 g of sulfasalazine taken daily was shown to result in significant reduction in both clinical and laboratory indices of disease activity. In rheumatological practice, sulfasalazine is given in enteric-coated form. Other disease modifying drugs used in rheumatoid arthritis have not been demonstrated as effective in treating AS. Glucocorticoids are valuable for local intra-articular and periarticular injection treatment, but there is no place for systemic glucocorticoids in the management of AS, except possibly as an occasional intravenous pulse for a rescue procedure from a very severe exacerbation.

Radiotherapy

Radiotherapy was widely used in the middle decades of this century to treat spinal inflammation and was regarded as very effective. However, clear evidence that this therapy was associated with increased mortality, particularly due to hemopoietic malignancy, led to its discontinuation for routine use. There is still an occasional place for radiotherapy for intractable local nonspinal enthesitis, and it may still be considered if all else fails for intractable spinal disease.

Surgery

Vertebral wedge osteotomy is occasionally used to correct advanced spinal kyphosis. More commonly, hip arthroplasty and occasionally arthroplasty of other joints are used to restore mobility to partially ankylosed or eroded joints such as the hip. Unfortunately, there is a tendency for joints to stiffen after surgery in AS, and intensive physiotherapy is necessary. General anesethesia in AS is potentially dangerous if there is fusion or subluxation in the cervical spine.

5. Prognosis

Ankylosing spondylitis is usually a rewarding condition to diagnose and treat. Much can be done to ameliorate symptoms and prevent spinal deformity and ankylosis. The natural history of the untreated disorder remains poorly defined in individual patients. However, in light of clinical experience over several decades, it seems likely that an intensive mobilization program with pharmacological suppression of inflammation can improve the long-term functional prognosis and diminish ankylosis. It must be recognized, however, that there is a wide range of severity of the disease. In some patients, minimal symptoms with limited sacroiliac joint and spinal involvement continue for many decades, whereas in a minority, progressive, widespread disease results in poor functional outcome and even death. Community studies have shown that the majority of patients with AS can continue in gainful employment.

C. Other Spondyloarthropathies

These conditions will be considered insofar as their spinal manifestations differ from classic AS. The group of spondyloarthropathies includes Reiter's disease and other forms of reactive arthritis, psoriatic arthritis in its various clinical forms, the arthropathies associated with inflammatory bowel disease, a proportion of children presenting with juvenile chronic arthritis, and a group of patients with so-called undifferentiated spondyloarthritis, in which associated disease is absent and who usually carry the HLA-B27 antigen.

In all these conditions, spinal and sacroiliac joint inflammation (spondylitis and sacroiliitis) may occur, although these conditions usually present initially with peripheral arthritis. In general, the severity of the spondylitis is not as severe in these conditions as in the classic disease, and the peripheral joint lesions tend to predominate. This may lead to neglect of the spondylitis and failure to receive adequate therapeutic attention. Distinct radiological features have been described, especially in psoriatic arthritis and Reiter's disease, in which the pattern of spinal ankylosis is coarser, and florid thick paravertebral syndesmophytes may occur. Moreover, in these nonclassic forms of AS, sacroiliitis is more likely to be unilateral. The frequency of HLA-B27 in different diseases in this group varies (Table 3). The principles of drug treatment are the same as in AS, but in psoriatic arthritis in particular, there is good evidence that sulphasalazine and especially methotrexate are effective. There is less convincing evidence that gold and azathioprine are effective in treating psoriatic arthritis. However, disease-modifying drugs are more valuable in treating peripheral joint inflammation and overall disease activity than in relation to spinal inflammation. Long-term follow-up studies of patients with reactive arthritis of enteric or genitourinary origin have shown that there is a tendency in the longer term to develop spondylitis, as well as other chronic musculoskeletal lesions.

D. Infectious Spondylitis and Discitis

Direct bacterial infection of the spine is relatively rare in the western world. Infection is usually spread hematologically but may follow surgical and other invasive procedures or trauma. Infection may be due to certain specific organisms, especially tuberculosis and brucellosis, or to a variety of ubiquitous pyogenic organisms. Infection in the spine can result in a space-occupying lesion due to epidural abscess formation which may compromise the spinal cord. Although patients may present with fever and other manifestions of systemic infection, spinal infection is often insiduous in onset and diagnosis may be delayed. Patients will usually experience back pain that may be relatively localized and there may be segmental tenderness. Plain radiographs show bone destruction in affected vertebrae, and other imaging techniques can be used to define the local lesion more accurately. Isotope scintigraphy will show intense uptake at the site of infection, whereas MRI will demonstrate the bone and soft tissue changes in anatomical detail. In septic discitis, the infection appears to start in an intravertebral disc and the disc space may appear widened on radiographs. The endplates of the adjacent vertebral bodies will show evidence of destruction. Septic discitis occurs most commonly as a complication of spinal surgery in adults or spontaneously in children.

1. Tuberculosis

The spine is one of the more common sites of tuberculous infection. It often occurs without any history of tuberculous infection. Patients from areas with a high endemic tuberculosis infection rate and those who are debilitated or immunocompromised are particularly susceptible. However, the infection can arise in otherwise healthy young people who complain of back pain, malaise, weight loss, and low-grade pyrexia. The radiographic appearances are characteristic and include destructive osteolysis with collapse of adjacent vertebrae, often with local abscess formation. In untreated cases, an angular kyphosis may occur due to collapse of one or more vertebral bodies as in classic Pott's disease of the spine. The lower thoracic spine is commonly affected.

2. Brucellosis

In areas where brucellosis is endemic, bone and joint infection are common manifestations, and the spine may be involved in up to 50% of cases, often late in the disease. The lumbar spine is more likely to be involved than other areas, and the infection often involves more than one segment. The onset is insidious, and fever may be absent, but constitutional symptoms and malaise are common. Affected segments may be tender to palpation or percussion. Epidural abscesses may form. Any of the common *Brucella* strains may be responsible including *B. abortus*, *Brucella melitensis*, and *Brucella suis*. Sacroiliitis is also common in brucellosis and tends to occur early in the disease.

3. Diagnosis and Management of Infectious Spondylitis

It is important that diagnosis of infection in the spine is not delayed because of the potentially serious morbidity and even mortality. Blood cultures may be positive but specific diagnosis will often depend on biopsy of the affected bone. It is important that all bone biopsies of the spine are sent for microbiological culture. The principles of treatment of pyogenic spinal infection are prolonged specific antibiotic therapy and sometimes surgery. Where there is marked extensive bony destruction, a spinal brace and possibly delayed surgical spinal fusion may be required. In the case of tuberculous spondylitis, prolonged antituberculous chemotherapy is required until there is no evidence of active infection, as assessed by the patient's clinical condition, negative inflammatory markers such as ESR, and a stable radiological appearance. In the case of brucella spondylitis, prolonged antibiotic therapy is required until all evidence of infection has subsided; this may take several months. Localized septic discitis may fuse spontaneously after appropriate antibiotic treatment.

E. Rheumatoid Disease and Other Autoimmune Connective Tissue Disorders

Although there are synovial joints in the thoracic and lumbar spine, they are not usually involved to a clinically significant degree in rheumatoid arthritis. The main clinical lesions of the thoracolumbar spine in rheumatoid disease are secondary and associated with osteoporosis or occasionally infection.

The cervical spine is particularly vulnerable to the destructive synovitis of rheumatoid disease. This is because the inflammatory granulation tissue attacks the neurocentral joints of the cervical spine, which are not found in the thoracolumbar spine. This erosive arthropathy results in instability of the cervical spine, and subluxation may occur. In addition, there is narrowing of the cervical discs with little, if any, associated bony sclerosis. The destructive changes are best recognized at the atlantoaxial level, and the atlantoaxial joint may be destroyed by inflammatory pannus. Normal flexion movements of the head then result in subluxation due to separation between the anterior arch of the atlas and the odontoid peg of the axis vertebra. The odontoid peg may cause backward pressure on the cervical cord. In more advanced cases, there may be upward subluxation of the odontoid peg into the foramen magnum as the head settles down on the neck. Subluxation at subaxial levels is also important, and because there is relatively less room for the cervical cord in the midcervical region, even minor degrees may cause neurological lesions. Any patient with rheumatoid arthritis who develops cervical spine symptoms should be carefully assessed for cervical subluxation.

1. Epidemiology and Natural History of Rheumatoid Cervical Subluxation

Cervical subluxation in rheumatoid arthritis (RA) is associated with a more destructive disease and tends to be cumulative with time. Between 30% and 40% of patients with established RA have cervical spine involvement radiologically, and 5% of these have neurological lesions. Long-term studies of the natural history have shown that in many of these patients the lesion progresses only slowly, if at all. However, in a significant proportion, the lesion is progressive and may result in life-threatening neurological complications.

2. Clinical Presentation and Diagnosis

Patients with significant neck symptoms should undergo careful neurological assessment. The pain may be felt in the back of the neck and often radiates to the occiput. Alternatively, it may radiate into the upper limbs. Sensory disturbances such as parasthesiae and feelings of running water in arms are not uncommon. The patient and examiner may notice marked weakness of the upper limbs. A common presentation is for the patient to "go off their legs." This is usually due to proprioceptive sensory loss consequent to posterior column involvement. Sometimes patients may feel overtly dizzy or ataxic. The clinical assessment should include a search for disturbances of cranial nerve function (usually a late development and associated with vertical subluxation of the odontoid causing pressure on the medulla oblongata). In the upper limbs, there may be marked weakness, and the changes of a lower motorneurone lesion or an upper motorneurone lesion may be observed. In the lower limbs the common findings are spasticity with hyperreflexia and upgoing plantar responses, as well as loss of posterior column sensation, including joint position sense and vibration sense. The patient may be ataxic if observed attempting to walk. Sphincter disturbance and incontinence of micturition is a late and serious finding. The mandatory early investigation of patients with involvement of the cervical spine is lateral radiography of the neck in extension and flexion, which shows the unstable subluxation on the flexion radiograph.

3. Management of Rheumatoid Cervical Subluxation

In the absence of neurological symptoms and signs, the patient should be warned about sudden trauma to the neck, especially in motor vehicles. A soft collar can be provided for comfort and partial immobilization (and to remind medical attendants that there is a potential problem!). If there are clinically significant symptoms or signs, the patient should be referred for MRI of the cervical spine and given a firm collar to prevent more than minimal flexion of the head. These are more comfortable if molded to fit the individual patient, and various suitable plastic materials, such as plaster zote, are available. The further management of patients with significant cervical myelopathy will depend on an expert neurosurgical assessment. A number of surgical procedures to relieve pressure on the cervical cord and stabilize the neck are now used; the technical details are beyond the scope of this chapter.

4. Other Connective Tissue Diseases

Although back pain may occur in other connective tissue diseases, especially inflammatory systemic lupus erythematosus, this is rarely of major clinical significance and can be treated by simple symptomatic measures. It should be noted that vertebral osteoporosis is more common in all the inflammatory rheumatic disorders and may be a secondary cause of back pain.

IV. NONINFLAMMATORY SKELETAL DISEASES OF THE SPINE

A. Spondylosis

This is the most common disorder of the spine; it affects the majority of the population who are middle aged and older. Spondylosis is essentially a radiological diagnosis and comprises, to a variable degree, narrowing of the intravertebral discs, reactive osteophytosis at the vertebral margins, and osteoarthritis of the posterior facet joints. Both noninflammatory low back pain and radiological spondylosis are very common in the population but the correlation between them is poorly defined and their interrelationship is not clear. However, factors that appear to predispose to both low back pain and radiological spondylosis include genetic and developmental influences and occupational issues, including previous injury. Some minor vertebral anomalies may occur in families. Individuals who do heavy manual labor develop the features of spondylosis more than those in sedentary occupations; these changes are more common in men than women. The condition known as juvenile osteochondrosis or Scheuermann's disease appears to predispose to spondylosis in later life and is often associated with an increased thoracic kyphosis and with thoracolumbar back pain in younger people. In this condition, there appears to be a developmental abnormality of the intervertebral discs and vertebral endplates which results in premature disc narrowing and kyphosis in the thoracic spine and Schmorl's nodes and premature disc degeneration in the lumbar spine. Schmorl's nodes are vertical disc herniations through the adjacent vertebral plate.

The treatment of spondylosis is essentially symptomatic. The wide variety of orthodox and heterodox health practitioners who treat low back pain is evidence for the lack of clear understanding about the underlying pathology, but many patients have radiological spondylosis as well as a history of episodes of back strain. Among the more rational approaches to the treatment are regular exercise programs that maintain spinal posture and muscle strength, attention to appropriate posture and mobility at work, and avoidance of inappropriate lifting and other strains. Local treatment such as steroid and anesthetic injections to facet joints can be given when these are identified as a source of pain, and epidural injections when there is significant referred pain to a lower limb. In addition, various manipulative techniques have been shown to relieve episodes of acute back pain that often occur in patients with spondylosis.

B. Intervertebral Disc Lesions

Acute and chronic lesions of intervertebral discs are very common, especially in the lumbar spine. The typical clinical features of an acute lumbar disc protrusion are well known and described elsewhere in this book. Chronic intervertebral disc lesions are features of spondylosis and spinal stenosis and are referred to in sections of this chapter dealing with these conditions.

C. Spondylolysis and Spondylolisthesis

Spondylolysis is a condition in which there is a defect in the pars intra-articularis of the neural arch of the vertebra. When this is present, it is usually in the lumbar lower vertebrae. It is sometimes found in young adults and may come to attention when back pain develops, for example in an athlete. It is more common in older people in association with spondylosis and spondylolisthesis. It is a matter of controversy whether the lesion in young people is primarily congenital, or secondary to trauma in the form of a stress fracture. Whatever the cause, it predisposes to severe attacks of back pain and also to spondylolisthesis. In severe cases, it may be treated surgically.

Spondylolisthesis is a condition in which there is anteroposterior malalignment of one vertebra on an adjacent vertebra. Usually the upper vertebra slips forward from the lower, but occasionally the slip is reversed (known as a retrolisthesis). Spondylolisthesis is most commonly found in one of the lower lumbar segments in older people and is associated with severe changes of spondylosis. It may also occur in young people in association with spondylolysis. In severe cases, spinal stenosis may occur secondary to the malalignment and the proliferative bony changes of the associated spondylosis. Spondylolisthesis usually presents with low back pain and on examination, this pain may be exacerbated by extension. There may be tenderness locally at the affected segment. It is one of the few situations in which a spinal corset may be valuable to help control the instability, and a variety of other symptomatic conservative and rehabilitative treatment is used. In severe cases, consideration can be given to spinal fusion at the affected level.

D. Spinal Stenosis

Spinal stenosis is most common in the lumbar spine. It is a condition in which the spinal canal is either locally or diffusely sufficiently narrow to cause pressure on the cauda equina. It is either constitutional due to a congenitally narrow spinal canal or more commonly, secondary to proliferative bone changes associated with spondylosis and previous disc degeneration or to spondylolisthesis. The clinical picture is characteristic in that the patient complains of back and leg pain specifically provoked by physical activity. Unlike the pain felt in the lower leg of vascular claudication due to atherosclerosis in the lower limb arteries, the leg pain associated with lumbar stenosis is felt in the buttocks and thighs. It is relieved by rest. In addition, the patient will often adopt a flexed posture to diminish pain by maximizing the space in the spinal canal. The main differential diagnosis of the pain provoked by walking is vascular claudication due to ischemia of the cauda equina. It is usually necessary to undertake imaging by computed tomography (CT) or MRI to distinguish between these two conditions, but the cauda equina vascular claudication is often associated with widespread atherosclerosis elsewhere. Occasionally, surgical treatment may be offered to patients with lumbar stenosis, especially if it involves a localized area. There are reports that epidural injections may relieve the symptoms, at least temporarily. The treatment of vascular cauda equina claudication is generally disappointing.

E. Diffuse Idiopathic Skeletal Hyperostosis

Diffuse idiopathic skeletal hyperostosis (DISH) was originally described in the spine by Forrestier and is sometimes still known as Forrestier's disease. It is in fact a diffuse condition that also affects other parts of the skeleton. As far as the spine is concerned, the condition is characterized by pain and stiffness in the back that may be progressive and poorly responsive to treatment. All movements are very limited and the radiological features are characteristic. They comprise florid paravertebral ossification of characteristic pattern that is usually most prominent on the right side of the lower thoracic spine and thought to be inhibited on the left side by the presence of the aorta. Changes are also prominent in the lumbar region where they are more likely to be bilateral. The characteristic appearances are best seen on anteroposterior plain radiographs. The condition appears to be constitutional and no specific cause has been found. It is apparently noninflammatory in origin and no specific genetic marker has been identified. The process cannot be reversed and treatment is symptomatic.

F. Nonspecific Low Back Pain and Musculoligamental Lesions

This term is used to describe the common situation in which a patient complains of low back pain, but often no specific clinical or radiological signs are found. The complex interrelationship of psychic and somatic factors in such patients must be taken into consideration in the differential diagnosis of spinal symptoms, but a lengthy dissertation on the management of cases when specific causative pathology cannot be identified is beyond the scope of this chapter. On the other hand, many individuals experience acute self-limited episodes of spinal pain with local pain and tenderness, the precise pathology of which is unknown but which resolve spontaneously or with various conservative therapeutic approaches.

G. Spinal Dysraphism and Other Congenital Abnormalities

Spina bifida and other abnormalities of embryological development may give rise to skeletal symptoms as well as neurological lesions. They are dealt with in other chapters in this book.

V. INTRINSIC BONE DISEASE OF THE SPINE

A. Osteoporosis

The spine is one of the sites of predilection of this increasingly recognized and common condition. It is particularly common in postmenopausal women in whom it is associated with declining estrogen levels after menopause. Bone mass diminishes by about 1% per annum after achieving its peak at the age of approximately 30 years and this loss may accelerate up to 5% in some individuals in the period immediately after menopause. For epidemiological purposes, osteoporosis has been defined by the World Health Organization as a condition in which bone mineral density is 2.5 standard deviations (SD) or more below the young adult mean. Lesser degrees of bone loss, 1–2.5 SD below the mean, are defined as osteopenia. In patients who undergo an early menopause for whatever reason, estrogen levels decline at an earlier age and these individuals are more likely to develop osteoporosis. Other contributory factors include a family genetic background contributing to low peak bone mass, lifelong low levels of physical activity, poor nutrition, smoking, and the nulliparous state. A comprehensive discussion of the epidemiology, pathology, and treatment of this condition exceeds the scope of this book.

Insofar as the spine is affected, the condition may be asymptomatic but the common modes of clinical presentation include: (1) progressive loss of height and increasing thoracic kyphosis and (2) the acute vertebral crush syndrome. The first presentation may be insidious, noticed only when the patient is made aware of a change in height or posture by relatives or friends. The acute presentation characteristically involves the sudden onset of severe spinal pain after a trivial injury, or even spontaneously. The lower thoracic vertebrae are most often affected, followed by the upper lumbar vertebrae. The pain is characteristically fairly localized and referred anteriorally in a girdle distribution and will be exacerbated by standing, bending, or coughing. The pain may be excruciating in the acute phases and all voluntary movement impossible. Examination may show local tenderness over the affected vertebrae, as well as the change in posture and loss of movement in the spine. The diagnosis depends on the clinical signs and characteristic radiological changes, including anterior wedge or codfish-shaped vertebral compression fractures. The finding of reduced bone density in the lumbar spine by absorption photometry can confirm the diagnosis of osteoporosis. However, in a patient presenting with an acute vertebral crush fracture, especially older patients, other causes must be excluded and it is appropriate to check the full blood count, ESR, and serum chemistry, including alkaline phosphatase. If a metastasis is suspected, then an isotope scintiscan should be done after a clinical check for primary lesions. If the ESR is elevated, the immunoglobulin profile and urine Bence Jones protein should be measured for possible myeloma.

Effective long-term pharmacological treatment is now available for osteoporosis, especially bisphosphonates, and to a lesser extent, vitamin D analogs and calcitonin. Hormone replacement therapy is protective against osteoporosis in postmenopausal women. The intense pain of the acute vertebral crush syndrome may need, in addition to analgesics, a course of calcitonin injections or intravenous infusions of a bisphosphonate.

B. Paget's Disease

Osteoitis deformans, also known as Paget's disease, is an intrinsic disorder of bone metabolism that presents in older age groups and has an irregular geographic distribution. The cause is unknown. This disease usually presents in a long limb bone or the pelvis but the spine is also commonly involved. It is an infrequent cause of back pain and the diagnosis is usually made on the radiological appearances. The vertebral bodies expand when affected by Paget's osteitis and very rarely, this may encroach on the spinal canal to cause myelopathy or cauda equina lesions. Paget's disease cannot be reversed but the progression of the disease can be halted or slowed by bisphosphonate treatment. This treatment also improves the bone pain of Paget's disease, which may occur at rest and disturb sleep. Paget's disease weakens the bone and increases susceptibility to pathological fractures, but these rarely affect the spine.

C. Osteomalacia

Osteomalacia is now uncommon in the western world and when it does occur, is often associated with disorders in which malabsorption is present. Osteomalacia can also occur after the use of certain anticonvulsant drugs in epilepsy, the best known being phenytoin. Osteomalacia results in diminished bone mineral density and can therefore result in loss of vertebral height and crush fractures, as in osteoporosis. The diagnosis depends on the appropriate biochemical changes including hypocalcemia, raised alkaline phosphatase, and often low vitamin D levels but a bone biopsy may be needed to establish the diagnosis. The treatment depends on appropriate replacement therapy.

D. Metastatic Bone Disease of the Spine

Although primary malignant neoplasms are rare in the skeleton, including the spine, secondary malignancy is common in the vertebrae and should always be suspected where there is an inappropriate localized vertebral lesion, especially a pathological fracture. Such lesions may be painful, with or without fracture, and a high index of suspicion for primary neoplasms that metastasize to the spine should be kept in mind. Primary tumors that metastasize to bone include breast, prostate, thyroid, kidney, and lung, but almost any primary tumor can do so. Hematological malignancy, especially myeloma, commonly affects the vertebral bodies, as well as other parts of the skeleton, and may present with diminished bone density and vertebral crush fractures. Detailed diagnosis and management of such lesions are outside the scope of this chapter.

VI. SUMMARY

The spine is commonly involved in a wide variety of rheumatological disorders, and the spinal cord may be involved secondarily. These disorders range from primary inflammatory diseases, especially AS and related conditions, to the very widespread and common noninflammatory structural disorders of the spine, as well as intrinsic bone disease. The practitioner dealing with spinal cord lesions must be aware of the various ways in which the vertebral column can be involved in disease and the potential secondary effects of such lesions on the spinal cord.

19

Spinal Vascular Disease

W. Louis Merton

St. Mary's Hospital and Portsmouth Hospitals NHS Trust, Portsmouth, England

Vascular compromise of the spinal cord and roots is, in the vast majority of cases, due to degenerative or traumatic change in the supporting structures that make up the vertebral column. The presentation, neurological sequelae, and management of these are covered in other chapters.

Cord ischemia or infarction due to intraluminal vascular occlusion within the spinal column is uncommon, the usual explanation being anterior spinal artery syndrome. Similarly it is a rare presenting feature of thoracic or abdominal pathologies that interfere with the arterial supply, or even less commonly, with venous drainage of the cord. Aortic surgery to correct some of these gives rise to cord infarction surprisingly rarely, especially when one considers the porridge-like consistency of atheroma associated with aneurysms and the relatively small caliber of vessels feeding the cord.

I. ANATOMY

The arterial supply of the spinal cord is composed of two longitudinal systems. The anterior spinal artery arises from the fusion of ventral radicular branch arteries and runs along the ventral surface of the cord overlaying the central sulcus. There are two posterior spinal arteries that lie over the dorsal surface, arising from the dorsal radicular branch arteries and at times, these form a plexus small vessels. There are also circumflex vessels that connect the two systems.

The anterior spinal artery is formed rostrally from branches of both vertebral arteries. In the cervical region, there is a rich supply of branches from the
costocervical, thyrocervical, and extracranial vertebral arteries, as well as from
the occipital branch of the external carotid artery. Below this level, the radicular
branches of segmental arteries gain access to the spinal column running along-
side the anterior nerve roots via the intervertebral foramina. There are more
radicular branches feeding the cervical and lumbar enlargements. The thoracic
cord is supplied by few radicular arteries, presumably reflecting the reduced
metabolic requirements as there is less gray matter. The anterior spinal artery
may be discontinuous in these regions. Another important factor is the switch
from the subclavian artery feeding the radicular arteries to direct aortic supply
in the upper thoracic region. This tenuous arterial supply to upper and midthoracic levels represents a watershed area vulnerable to systemic hypotension or
occlusion of a single vessel. From lower thoracic to upper lumbar regions, the
much larger radicular artery of Adamkiewicz supplies the anterior spinal artery.
It accompanies the left T10 anterior root in 30% of patients and in the remainder, any root from T9 to L1 (3). At the level of the conus, there is an anasto-
motic ring comprising segmental branches of lumbar and iliolumbar arteries
joining the anterior and posterior arterial systems.

The posterior spinal arteries, which are affected much less often than the
anterior system, also arise from the vertebral arteries rostrally, with further contributions from the dorsal radicular branches at each level.

The anterior spinal arteries supply most of the spinal gray matter via sulcal
central arteries that pass posteriorly through the anterior median sulcus before
deviating laterally to supply one-half of the cord at each level. The posterior
spinal artery supplies approximately one-third of the cord, and in particular the
posterior columns, via the pial arterial plexus penetrating from the surface of
the cord. The peripheral white matter in the anterior spinal artery territory is
similarly supplied.

The venous drainage of the ventral cord tends to accompany the anterior
spinal artery. Posteriorly, the more prominent veins run separately to the spinal
arteries, draining into posterior radicular veins with every second or third root.
The venus plexus is particularly prominent at the lumbar enlargement.

II. ISCHEMIC MYELOPATHY

The clinical presentation of spinal ischemia ranges from the abrupt onset of
what is essentially a spinal stroke with features of a transverse myelopathy, to
involvement of a more restricted vascular territory, e.g., anterior spinal artery,
to the more ingravescent myelopathy that can be associated with a dural arteriovenous fistula.

The isolated "neurological" presentation of paraparesis or tetraparesis, sometimes with a brief radicular pain at onset, coming on in minutes or hours and associated with loss of sphincter control and spinothalamic sensation, but with preserved dorsal column function, can be easily categorized as an anterior spinal artery event. Spinal shock usually predominates, in which initial limb areflexia gives way to later pyramidal signs. Myelography and magnetic resonance imaging (MRI) show an expanded cord in the acute phase, whereas later MRI studies may show a more discrete area of abnormal signal in the cord compatible with infarction. As a general rule, anterior spinal artery syndrome is a clinical diagnosis and is managed conservatively, but if the report of Baba et al. (2), which details perfusion of the radicular artery of Adamkiewicz with dexamethasone and urokinase in three patients resulting in neurological improvement, is replicated, then more active management may have to be considered.

Posterior spinal artery occlusion is much rarer and presents with anesthesia below the affected cord level if the dorsal horn involvement predominates, or paraesthesiae if it is the posterior columns. In the acute phase, pyramidal signs and even spinothalamic involvement may develop, possibly reflecting cord edema rather than more extensive vascular occlusion, as these features can recover completely.

III. MANAGEMENT AND OUTCOME

Treatment is essentially supportive, with initial high-quality nursing care giving way to the multidisciplinary involvement of physiotherapists, occupational therapists, and social workers. Investigation of the presenting syndrome and the search for associated conditions that may be treatable are based on a careful history, clinical examination, and a range of clinical investigations, in particular imaging.

There are few follow-up studies of patients after spinal infarction. In a study from the Netherlands, 10 patients were reviewed (5). All of the eight survivors had some residual leg weakness, with seven living at home with no professional help. Seven suffered continuous disabling pain unrelated to the degree of weakness.

IV. SYMPTOMATIC SPINAL ISCHEMIA

The cause of cord ischemia can be divided into four main groups. In what I term "neurological myelopathy," there may be no certain etiology for what is essentially an isolated neurological syndrome. This group has already been covered by the syndromes relating to spinal vascular territory. The other two major groups are those in which ischemia is a resultant or concomitant feature of extraspinal disease, e.g., aortic dissection, or in which it is a complication of treatment, e.g., cross-clamping the aorta above the renal arteries. Finally with greater radiological and surgical skills, therapeutic ischemia should be considered in relation to arteriovenous malformations.

The range of extraspinal diseases that cause spinal ischemia is extensive. Atherosclerotic change in the aorta is by far the most common, manifesting as either a dissecting or a nondissecting aneurysm. In the acute phase, systemic hypotension is usually an important factor over and above occlusion of segmental arteries by thrombus, atheroma, or the dissecting aortic wall. Elective repair of an abdominal aortic aneurysm where cross-clamping is possible below the renal arteries is associated with the lowest risk of cord ischaemia (down to 0.25%), whereas with incipient rupture or dissection of thoracic or thoracoabdominal aorta, the risk rises to more than 10% in survivors. The presence of neurological dysfunction at presentation in one series (4) was associated with a mortality rate of 54%.

Adult-type co-arctation of the aorta can present as a progressive upper thoracic myelopathy, with neurogenic intermittent claudication being one manifestation. Usually the aberrant circulation is via the enlarged vertebral, thyrocervical, and costocervical arteries to the anterior spinal arteries, with retrograde flow through radicular and then intercostal vessels to the aorta below the coarct. The dilatation and increased tortuosity of the anterior spinal artery may exert a direct pressure on the cord, or ischemia may be due to a "steal phenomenon." Other aortic diseases in the form of distal occlusion or aortitis (Takayasu's or giant cell arteritis) can result in myelopathy. In the preantibiotic era, syphilitic aortitis was an important possibility. Cord ischemia/infarction due to single-vessel involvement may be seen after local trauma such as a stab wound affecting the radicular artery of Adamkiewicz, dissection of a vertebral artery, or thoracic wall surgery in which a critical radicular artery is tied off. Atheromatous emboli are rare and, even when present at postmortem, may not have been clinically significant.

Various interventions are rarely associated with spinal ischemia. Angiography (aortic or bronchial) is now less likely to cause cord damage, because contrast agents have been modified over the years and more selective studies are performed. Bronchial tree embolization is also a potential hazard. The use of a balloon pump in cardiac surgery has been implicated, but the need for its use in the first place indicates that the patient has systemic hypotension that may be implicated as well. The greater the degree of instrumentation in scoliosis surgery, the greater the intraoperative risk of myelopathy; in particular, the tightening of laminar wires is the period of greatest risk when monitoring cord function. Complications are also more likely when there is greater initial neurological involvement, i.e., severe learning disabilities with limited or no ability to walk.

Radiation induced myelopathy is now very rare. There were more problems in treating patients with teratomas prior to the introduction of chemotherapy, as quite high-dose para-aortic fields were used. In some patients with Hodgkin's disease a transient myelitis, usually manifesting with sensory symptoms, may be seen about 8 weeks after ceasing treatment. As a general rule, the reduced total radiation dose and increased fractionation avoid damage to the neuraxis in survivors.

Disease of the vertebral column can present in unusual ways. Myelopathy due to a steal syndrome is a rare feature of Paget's disease of bone affecting the spinal column, with reports that treating the bone disease reverses the neurology (7). Nucleus pulposus embolism, usually affecting the cervical cord, is often only recognized at postmortem.

Small-vessel disease is most likely to be due to immune-mediated vasculitis, with rare reports of polyartertis nodosa, rheumatoid arthritis, and Sjögren's syndrome causing myelopathy.

The pathology of the myelopathy associated with systemic lupus erythematosus (SLE) is surprising. Provenzale and Bouldin (6) argue that there are three different pathological presentations. A transverse myelitis with infarction/ischemia limited to one level of the cord is associated with a vasculitis. In patients whose myelopathy is due to a large subdural hematoma, there is no associated inflammatory change in small vessels. It is speculated that there may be some other form of localized small-vessel disease or that there is a coagulopathy, i.e., lupus anticoagulant. Thirdly, there is the group in which patchy vacuolar change is seen in the peripheral white matter at multiple levels of the cord in the absence of vasculitis. Not surprisingly, the symptoms and signs in these cases are quite varied with some showing no obvious sensory deficit and a varied array of brisk, reduced or absent reflexes at different cord levels.

Granulomatous angiitis usually manifests as cerebral disease, but when presenting with spinal involvement, fatal cerebral involvement will follow (if steroids and cytotoxic therapy are not initiated).

As recreational diving increases in popularity, decompression sickness, often manifesting with cord symptoms or signs, is not uncommon. Rapid transfer to a center with a decompression chamber, with a full clinical assessment prior to treatment, is the ideal management (see Chapter 20).

V. ARTERIOVENOUS MALFORMATIONS

The presentation of angiomata relates to their position and the type of manifesting complication. Thoracolumbar angiomata are much more common, show a significant predominance in males, usually lie posteriorly, and are less likely to have a significant intramedullary component. Whereas the posterior spinal arteries may be involved, the feeder vessels often do not arise from vessels normally supplying the cord. In the cervical region, intramedullary involvement is much more common, presentation is earlier, and the sex ratio 1:1.

Hemorrhage is the most common acute presentation and can be indistinguishable from subarachnoid hemorrhage arising from cerebral vessels. It has been shown that hemorrhage can arise from an associated aneurysm rather than the angioma itself. In the 1% of patients presenting with subarachnoid hemorrhage in which four-vessel cerebral angiography shows no apparent abnormality, a spinal angioma should be considered. A bruit over the spinal column, although rare, is highly suggestive. Local meningism can be prominent, and in one case I have seen, marked retrocollis was evident with little or no cerebral involvement. The differential diagnosis of spinal hemorrhage, with or without bleeding into the CSF, is limited. Other forms of hamartoma or tumor in the absence of trauma are possible, whereas coagulopathy or vasculitis needs to be considered.

Infarction may explain stepwise deteriorations, but pathological specimens often show no evidence of infarction. The more ingravescent presentation may be the result of cord compression due to a mass effect, or ischemia. The latter may be related to exercise, i.e., cord or cauda equina claudication or posture. Traditionally, a vascular steal syndrome has been postulated to explain cord ischemia but Aminoff (1) questions this explanation. As already indicated, thoracolumbar arteriovenous malformations (AVMs) may not share any circulation with the cord. Secondly, Aminoff offers a compelling explanation in the form of reduced intramedullary perfusion pressure due to a reduced arteriovenous pressure difference caused by relatively high local venous pressure. This would explain why ligating an arteriovenous fistula reverses local ischemia.

Magnetic resonance imaging and selective angiographic studies are the mainstays of diagnosis and evaluation of angiomata. Depending on position and type, surgery or embolization may be considered. In the more recently recognized dural arteriovenous fistulas, in which there is little in the way of additional abnormal vessels, reports of successful surgical ligation with marked improvement in neurology are increasingly reported. It is felt that this remediable condition is underdiagnosed in the elderly.

REFERENCES

1. Aminoff MJ. Spinal vascular disease. In: Disease of Spinal Cord. Critchley E, Elsen A, eds. Springer, 1992.

2. Baba H, Tomita K, Kawagishi T, Imura S. Anterior spinal artery syndrome. International Orthopedics 1993; 17(6):353–356.
3. Hughes JT. Vascular diseases of the spinal cord. In: Handbook of Clinical Neurology. Vol. 55. Vascular diseases, part III. Vinken PJ, Bruyn GW, Klawans HL, eds. Elsevier, 1989.
4. Lynch DR, Dawson TM, Raps EC, Galetta SL. Risk factors for the neurologic complications associated with aortic aneurysms. Arch Neurol 1992; 49(3):284–288.
5. Pelser H, Van Gijn J. Spinal infarction: A follow-up study. Stroke 1993; 24(6):896–898.
6. Provenzale J, Bouldin TW. Lupus-related myelopathy: Report of three cases and review of the literature. J Neurol Neurosurg Psychiatry 1992; 55(9):747–862.
7. Yost JH, Spencer-Green G, Krant JD. Vascular steal mimicking compression myelopathy in Paget's disease of bone: Rapid reversal with calcitonin and systemic steroids. J Rheumatol 1993; 20(6):1064–1065.

20

Decompression Illness

A. W. Murrison
Institute of Naval Medicine, Alverstoke, Hants, England

T. James R. Francis
Naval Submarine Medical Research Laboratory, Groton, Connecticut

E. M. Sedgwick
University of Southampton, Southampton, Hampshire, England

I. INTRODUCTION

When decompression illness (DCI) affects the nervous system, the spinal cord is involved in more than 75% of cases. When correct diving procedures are strictly applied, DCI is largely preventable. The Norwegian experience has been a reduction of DCI incidents among professional divers operating in the North Sea from 54 per annum in 1978 to 0 in 1992 when 2850 dives were logged. In the United Kingdom, there were 1386 registered professional divers in 1992 but probably 50,000 recreational divers undertaking 1–2 million dives per year. Sykes (1989) estimated that there were about 200 instances of DCI per annum in the UK of which 5–10% were fatal.

The symptoms of DCI are protean, but a history of diving during the previous 24 hours should alert the physician to the possible diagnosis. The initial symptoms of DCI may seem trivial, such as tingling and a little numbness. Such symptoms may quickly develop into severe neurological deficits. Divers also commonly experience hypothermia and dehydration, to which one may be tempted to attribute minor symptoms. No time can be allowed for any diagnostic confirmatory tests, nor should one be tempted to "wait and see" in case the symptoms abate. No harm can result from instituting recompression therapy, but paraplegia may be the result of delaying it. The onset of symptoms is usually within 1 hour of surfacing from a dive; the onset is delayed longer than

1 hour in only 15% of cases. Treatment by recompression must commence as soon as possible. The longer the delay before recompression, the less likely is a successful outcome. It has been estimated that 90% of patients obtain relief if recompression begins within half an hour of surfacing, whereas only 50% are relieved if the delay is 6 hours. After 12 hours, the results of recompression are poor.

The diving community is alert to the risks, but delays in diagnosis commonly occur when a diver moves away from his "buddy" into a nondiving environment, e.g., a hotel or airport. The symptoms may be brought on, or made worse, by flying. Passenger aircraft cabins are pressurized to 5–8,000 feet which adds to the divers decompression. It is recommended that diving activity ceases 24 hours before flying, but enthusiastic scuba divers have been known to overlook this.

The wise physician will not disregard a likely diagnosis of DCI on learning that the dive has been properly conducted with appropriate decompression stops during ascent. Even short and shallow dives can produce bubbles in the bloodstream, and ascent schedules have evolved on the low probability rather than the impossibility of developing DCI. There is also the human fallibility with respect to the truth that should be taken into account.

II. TERMINOLOGY

Traditionally, the decompression disorders have been classified, as shown in Table 1 (Elliott and Moon, 1993). The subclassification of decompression sickness was based upon the observations of Golding et al. (1960). However, it has

Table 1 Traditional Classification of the Decompression Disorders

Decompression Sickness	
Type I	Type II
Musculoskeletal	Neurological
Skin	Cardiorespiratory ("chokes")
Lymphatic	Vestibular/auditory
Fatigue	Shock
	Arterial Gas Embolism
	Barotrauma

Source: Elliott and Moon, 1993.

recently become recognized that such an approach may be misleading because, in practice, it may be very difficult to classify cases correctly. This is particularly the case in distinguishing between arterial gas embolism and neurological decompression sickness, where the former diagnosis is presumptive in the absence of evidence of pulmonary barotrauma (Harker et al., 1993), except in exceptional circumstances of very short or shallow dives (Benton et al., 1994). Furthermore, the mechanisms underlying decompression sickness and arterial gas embolism may occur within the same patient (Neuman and Bove, 1990) and the pathology of the two conditions is reported to be similar (Bridgwater et al., 1991). Distinguishing between inner ear barotrauma and vestibular decompression sickness is also notoriously difficult (Talmi et al., 1991). A further difficulty is that, as yet, there is no definitive diagnostic test for decompression sickness. It is perhaps not surprising, therefore, that studies have shown a poor concordance between experienced physicians making these diagnoses (Smith et al., 1992; Kempner et al., 1992; Kumar et al., 1994). For these reasons, a descriptive approach to classifying a unified condition of decompression illness has been proposed (Table 2), which is becoming widely accepted (Bennett and Elliott, 1993; Murrison and Francis, 1991).

Table 2 Descriptive Terminology for Decompression Illness

Evolution	Manifestations
Progressive	Pain
Static	Limb pain
Spontaneously improving	Girdle pain
Relapsing	Cutaneous
	Neurological
	Audiovestibular
	Pulmonary
	Lymphatic
	Constitutional
	Hypotensive

Source: Francis and Smith (1991).

The general form of the terminology is: Acute [*evolution term*], [*manifestation term(s)*].

In decompression illness, additional information that should be recorded is the time of onset; inert gas burden (depth-time profile), and evidence of barotrauma (Francis and Smith, 1991).

III. MECHANISMS OF NEUROLOGICAL DECOMPRESSION ILLNESS

Decompression illness is a condition which has long been thought to be initiated by the presence of gas bubbles within tissues (Bert, 1878). The dysfunction that results from the presence of these bubbles may be as a result of both their physical presence within the tissue and the highly complex inflammatory responses they are capable of initiating.

A. Origins of Bubbles

There are two principal mechanisms by which bubbles may be released into tissues as a result of decompression. The most frequent mechanism is thought to be as a result of inert gas (normally nitrogen) dissolved in tissues becoming sufficiently supersaturated during decompression that bubbles begin to form. This may occur in a wide variety of tissues, particularly in those with a high affinity for nitrogen (which generally have a high lipid content (Weathersby and Homer, 1980) and a relatively low perfusion, which limits the rate at which the dissolved gas can be removed in solution by the cardiopulmonary system. The solubility of nitrogen is five times greater in fat than in water. Once these bubbles are formed, they may induce tissue dysfunction at their site of formation—so called autochthonous bubbles or, after their redistribution as emboli via the circulation, cause dysfunction in other tissues. Factors associated with the generation of DCI include: the dive or decompression profile (Weathersby, et al., 1986) and, in aviators, whether the prebreathing of oxygen has been employed (Waligora, et al., 1987); previous dive profiles [there is good evidence that divers and compressed-air workers who are "worked up" experience a lower frequency of DCI than those who are not (Walder, 1968; Thalmann, 1986; Lam and Yau, 1988)]; and exercise taken while under pressure (Van Der Aue, et al., 1951) or after decompression (Van Der Aue et al., 1949; Cook, 1951). Additional factors have also been implicated, but their effect is either relatively small or questionable. These include age (Bradley, 1987; Lam and Yau, 1989), body fat content (Lam and Yau, 1989, Curley et al., 1989), and the effects of immersion in water and cold (Weathersby et al., 1990; Thalmann, 1985; Mekjavic and Kakitsuba, 1989). The complex interactions of numerous potential predisposing factors have made their identification and quantification difficult. It is not, therefore, surprising that cases of DCI commonly occur unexpectedly.

It is recognized that the human can tolerate a certain burden of venous gas emboli. Doppler studies have shown that they may arise from apparently innocuous dives in asymptomatic divers (Pilmanis, 1976; Eckenhoff et al., 1990). It is apparent that this is possible because the lungs are highly efficient filters of gas emboli (Butler and Hills, 1979). However, if this filter is overwhelmed by extensive bubbling (Butler and Hills, 1985; Vik et al., 1990) or if there is a right to left shunt, then bubbles may enter the arterial circulation and provoke symptoms. There is evidence from cross-sectional studies in man that a higher proportion of divers who have suffered DCI have an intracardiac shunt than divers who have not or the general adult population (Moon and Camporesi, 1989; Wilmshurst et al., 1989). However, the significance of this finding has yet to be fully evaluated. There are anecdotal reports of experienced divers who have never suffered DCI, yet have apparently substantial intracardiac shunts (Cross et al., 1992). To date, no longitudinal study exists to assess whether divers with a patent foramen ovale (PFO) succumb to DCI with a greater frequency than divers who have no such shunt. However, the evidence in pigs indicates that the presence of a PFO is associated with the right-to-left shunting of bubbles (Vik et al., 1993).

Less commonly, bubbles are driven into the bloodstream as a result of pulmonary barotrauma, a condition in which gas escapes from the pulmonary air spaces and enters the pulmonary venous circulation. This condition is only recognized with any frequency in divers, being very rare in aviators or compressed-air workers. Pulmonary barotrauma is frequently associated with rapid decompression, such as occurs in a diver who surfaces rapidly in an emergency, and with breath-holding on ascent. In such circumstances, the expanding gas in the pulmonary air spaces achieves an overpressure that is sufficient to cause the lung to rupture (Malhotra and Wright, 1961). However, it has also been described in cases of pre-existing pulmonary disease (Jenkins et al., 1993) and may occur for no apparent reason (Gorman, 1984). Although the precise mechanisms involved in lung rupture have yet to be elucidated in cases where there was no apparent breath-holding, traditional concepts of subclinical airway obstruction are being questioned, and evidence for the role of small lungs and altered compliance is accumulating (Brooks et al., 1988; Colebatch and Ng, 1991; Benton et al., 1994).

B. Consequences of Bubbles

1. Autochthonous Bubbles

The discovery of autochthonous bubbles in spinal cord white matter was first made in an experimental study early this century (Boycott et al., 1908). However, the authors were of the opinion that the principle mechanism of bubble-induced spinal cord injury in DCI was embolic. Although occasional reports of autochthonous bubble injury to the spinal cord in both animal studies and man were made subsequently (Clay, 1963; Kitano et al., 1977), it was not until the late 1980s that this was studied systematically. In order for bubbles to form and grow in the spinal cord, there must be a sufficient inert gas tension (Francis et al., 1990a). This is only likely to occur after relatively deep dives with a short decompression time, and the onset of symptoms is likely to be rapid, because the washout of gas from the cord will progress quickly once the decompression is completed (Francis, 1990).

It is pertinent that, in both animals and man, neurological DCI tends to occur after short, deep dives (Lehner and Lanphier, 1989; Aharon-Peretz et al., 1993) and tends to have a short latency (Francis et al., 1988a; Francis et al., 1988b). However, it is clear that cases of neurological DCI occur with a longer latency than can be readily explained by autochthonous bubbles. Hence, more than one mechanism is likely to be involved (Francis et al., 1988a). Once formed, autochthonous bubbles are thought to provoke tissue dysfunction in a number of ways. Most obvious is the disruption of tissue architecture, both as a result of the disintegration of axons at the site of bubble formation and the distortion of those displaced by bubble growth. There is also evidence that the architecture of myelin may also be disrupted (Sykes and Yaffe, 1985). However, these effects are likely to account for only a small proportion of the observed loss of function (Francis et al., 1990b).

Other mechanisms that may be involved are ischemia, caused by the disruption of the local microcirculation, and biochemical tissue-bubble interactions akin to those described between bubbles and blood (Hallenbeck and Andersen, 1982). It is unlikely in most circumstances that the extent of bubbles formation is sufficient to provoke a global spinal cord ischemia, as postulated by Hills and James (1982). After a brief period of growth, these bubbles begin to shrink, as the gas they contain diffuses down a pressure gradient to be cleared by the circulation. As local tissue pressure is relieved, blood flow is restored to the disrupted microcirculation and petechial hemorrhages are found at the sites of bubble formation. It has recently been shown that the extent of the hemorrhage correlates inversely with recovery from DCI (Broome et al., 1994).

2. Embolic Bubbles

Although autochthonous bubbles are likely to play an important role in the onset of DCI affecting the spinal cord, particularly where the onset is rapid, there is almost certainly a role for intravascular bubbles. One possible mechanism is for venous gas emboli to accumulate in the epidural vertebral venous plexus. It has been argued that the slow-moving blood flow in these vascular channels provides an environment conducive to the blood-bubble interactions mentioned above (which include the activation of Hageman factor), thus promoting coagulation and infarction of the spinal cord as a result of obstruction of the venous outflow (Hallenbeck et al., 1975). However, the histology of venous infarction of the spinal cord—predominantly central, hemorrhagic infarction—differs substantially from the punctate, white matter hemorrhage generally seen in DCI (Hughes, 1971; Palmer, 1986). Furthermore, venous infarction is a very rare condition of the spinal cord. Thus arterial emboli are now considered to be more likely to initiate spinal cord DCI, particularly when the onset is delayed. In the brain, however, it is almost universally accepted that arterial gas emboli are the mediators of DCI. The mechanisms involved in arterial gas embolism of the spinal cord are likely to be very similar to those in the brain, which have been the subject of recent study.

It is used to be considered that arterial bubble emboli inflicted an obstructive ischemic injury on the brain in a similar manner to solid emboli. However, it would now appear that this is not the case. During their passage along cerebral arterioles, spherical bubbles elongate to become cylindrical. They only arrest in the circulation if the resistance between them and the vessel wall exceeds the perfusion pressure. Commonly, cerebral arterial gas embolism is associated with an increased systemic blood pressure, which is probably of brainstem origin (Evans et al., 1981). Furthermore, the response of cerebral arteries to embolism is a maximal vasodilatation that may also be a result of brainstem reflexes, although it is now thought to be a local endothelial response (Helps et al., 1990a,b). As a result of these reflexes, most bubbles pass through the cerebral circulation either immediately or after only a short delay (Gorman and Browning, 1986; Gorman et al., 1987). During their passage through the cerebral circulation, bubbles inflict endothelial injury by stripping endothelial cells away from their basement membrane (Haller et al., 1987; Drewry, 1992). It has also been reported that they remove surfactant layers from endothelial cells, rendering them increasingly permeable to proteins (Hills and James, 1991). As a consequence, there is a loss of integrity of the blood-brain barrier and a loss of vascular autoregulation (Persson et al., 1978; Nishimoto et al., 1978; Fritz and Hossman, 1979). The subsequent accumulation of leucocytes at the sites of embolic injury is associated with a loss of both cerebral blood flow and function (Hallenbeck et al., 1986; Dutka et al., 1989; Helps and Gorman, 1991).

IV. MANAGEMENT OF NEUROLOGICAL DECOMPRESSION ILLNESS

Management of DCI starts with a correct dive plan that allows enough time and air for the specified decompression stops during ascent. The development of time-depth recorders worn by divers should help to determine how closely the diver is able to adhere to his plan.

A recommended and widely used recompression schedule is Table RN62 shown in Figure 1. Note that the duration of therapy is 4.5 hours, during which the patient is relatively isolated from conventional medical intensive care. Most

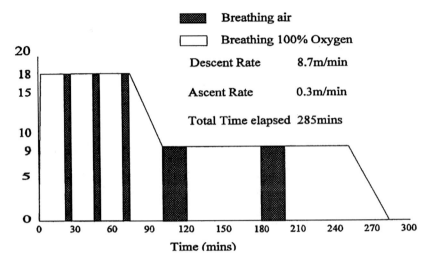

Figure 1 A diagram of the recompression schedule of Table RN62. The ordinate is pressure measured in meters of sea water: 9 meters of sea water = 1 atmosphere pressure. Pressure in the chamber is 2 atmospheres above normal or 3 atmospheres absolute (ATA). The air-breathing intervals prevent any toxic effects of pure oxygen.

recompression chambers are large enough to accommodate a support technician who may enter or leave by an airlock. Necessary drugs, intravenous fluids, etc., have to be passed in through an airlock. No electrical equipment is permitted because of the fire risk in an environment with a raised pressure of oxygen.

The management of DCI is based on the clinical observation that symptoms are ameliorated by the recompression of victims and subsequent slow decompression. The duration of treatments and the therapeutic gases used together with pressures applied and adjunctive therapies have been refined through clinical experience and on the basis of results from animal modeling of the disease.

A. Therapeutic Recompression

Empiricism in the management of DCI was reduced by the development of a dog model of DCI affecting the spinal cord (Leitch and Hallenbeck, 1984a, 1984b) and of cerebral arterial gas embolism (CAGE) (Leitch et al., 1984a, 1984b). These relied upon the juxtaposition of percutaneous needles against spinal cord and brain respectively to record somato-sensory evoked potentials (SEPs) after the stimulation of peripheral nerves.

Summed peak-to-peak SEP amplitudes were used to monitor the course of DCI affecting the spinal cord, and it was found that their reduction correlated with a reduction in spinal cord blood flow (Leitch and Hallenbeck 1984a). Subsequently, the model's neurophysiological response to a range of treatment profiles was recorded. It was shown that the delay between disease onset and the start of recompression was a crucial determinant of neurophysiological recovery (Leitch and Hallenbeck 1985a), a finding that concurred with clinical experience (Rivera 1964). In the model, the maximum effect of treatment was seen 25 minutes after the onset of recompression (Sykes et al., 1986).

Although it followed from Boyle's Law that, in the treatment of DCI as much pressure as possible should be applied, a therapeutic advantage was not discerned on exceeding ambient pressures of 3.0ATA (Leitch and Hallenbeck 1985a). This was also the experience in the CAGE model (Leitch et al., 1984a, 1984b; Dutka et al. 1987).

If DCI fails to improve after conventional short, oxygen-based protocols, it is usual to consider the prescription of deep or prolonged recompressions. Also, algorithms in which inert gases other than nitrogen are used may be tried. The efficacy of these remains largely anecdotal. The therapeutic use of an inert gas (usually helium) other than the one breathed prior to the onset of DCI (usually the nitrogen in air) has theoretical advantages and is considered if treatment is envisaged at pressures that exceed the safe limits for the use of 100% oxygen. The argument for this approach is that, if the rate of transport of inert gas from offending bubbles exceeds the rate at which the therapeutic inert gas replaces it, then accelerated bubble shrinkage may be achieved. In animal studies, helium-oxygen mixtures have resulted in faster bubble shrinkage in adipose tissue, spinal cord white matter, and tendon than that observed when air or 100% oxygen is breathed. However, the clinical advantage of recompression with a helium-oxygen gas mixture instead of pure oxygen, which was claimed by James (1981) and by Douglas and Robinson (1988) was not supported experimentally using the Leitch dog model of DCI (Pearson et al., 1991).

B. Adjuvants to Recompression Therapy

The Leitch dog model of CAGE was used to revoke the standard practice of placing victims in the head-down position in the hope that bubbles would shift caudally by virtue of their buoyancy. Dutka et al. (1990) demonstrated impaired recovery in terms of SEP amplitude as a result of placing dogs with CAGE in the head-down position and, in the same model, Polychronidis, et al., (1990) found that the head-down position compromised the blood-brain barrier and elevated intracranial pressure. Consequently, it was recommended that patients with CAGE should be transported in the horizontal or even sitting position (Dutka, 1990), a conclusion that has met with general acceptance.

Dutka (1990) reported that fluid replacement in the Leitch dog model of CAGE led to an improved neurophysiological outcome. This concurs with the improved survival noted among hamsters with DCI when treated with parenteral normal saline (Lynch et al., 1989). Clinically, fluid administration is likely to be especially important because of the diuresis and decrease in blood volume caused by immersion (Deuster et al., 1989) and consequent rise in hematocrit with resulting reduction in cerebral blood flow (Thomas et al., 1977).

The administration of lidocaine has been shown to be advantageous in terms of SEP recovery in a cat model of CAGE (McDermott et al., 1990) and in a dog model of the disease (Evans et al., 1984). However, Gelb et al. (1987) reported that, although SEPs recovered acutely to a greater degree if lidocaine was administered to cats that had been subjected to focal cerebral ischemia, the advantage was no longer evident after 30 minutes and was not apparent histopathologically. The only clinical report of the use of membrane stabilizers in the treatment of DCI is that of Drewry and Gorman (1992) who described a case that appeared to respond to lidocaine after a suboptimal response to recompression.

The Leitch animal model has been used to determine that conventional doses of corticosteroids are unlikely to be beneficial in the management of acute DCI (Francis et al., 1987). Furthermore, Francis and Dutka (1989) demonstrated that SEP amplitude recovery could not be expected in DCI affecting the canine spinal cord from treatment with a single "mega-dose" of methylprednisolone (20 mg/kg). Failure to achieve therapeutic benefit from glucocorticoids in this model was consistent with the lack of support available for steroid treatment in non–diving-related spinal cord injury in humans (Bracken et al., 1984, 1985, 1990). However, the regimen used by Francis and Dutka (1989) fell short of the 30 mg/kg dose of methylprednisolone at which the drug's anti-inflammatory action is joined by the neuroprotective effects provided by oxygen-free radical scavenging and maximal inhibition of lipid peroxidation (Hall and Braughler, 1982; 1986). This might explain Young's (1992) finding that treatment with very high doses of methylprednisolone (15–30 mg/kg) resulted in improved white matter blood flow and SEPs in severely contused cat spinal cords. Furthermore, it has been increasingly recognized that the classic view of neurological DCI as a spinal condition is untenable and that the brain is often involved. The improved cerebral blood flow from the administration of high-dose steroid soon after the induction of experimental occlusive stroke suggests that some central benefit may be obtained from steroid usage in acute DCI (de Courten-Myers et al., 1994). The promising use of gangliosides in the acute phase of spinal cord injury (Young, 1992) and their less impressive impact in stroke (Argentino et al., 1989; Braune, 1991; Hernandez et al., 1994) have yet to be assessed in neurological DCI.

V. LONG-TERM NEUROLOGICAL CONSEQUENCES OF DIVING

For some years now, concern has been expressed that there may be long-term neurological consequences of deep diving and a recent conference examined the evidence and concluded as follows:

> There is evidence that changes in bone, the central nervous system, and the lung can be demonstrated in some divers who have not experienced a diving accident, or other established environmental hazard. The changes are, in most cases, minor and do not influence a diver's quality of life. However, the changes are of a nature that may influence the diver's future health. The scientific evidence is limited and future research is required to obtain adequate answers to the questions of long-term health effects of diving (Hope et al., 1994).

Historically, divers have been low status, poorly paid manual workers enjoying little statutory employment health protection. Decompression illness was regarded as an unavoidable occupational hazard and the failure of intellectual capacity in divers of longstanding ("divers' dementia") became part of diving folklore. However, improved diving practices, supported by health and safety legislation, have promoted the physical health of divers and reduced the likelihood that diving might cause a "punch drunk" syndrome of the sort reported in boxers (Corsellis, 1989). Nonetheless, concern remains in the diving community over the possibility of insidious, diving-related damage to nervous tissue. This fear has been heightened by reports of brain involvement in what was previously understood to be largely a condition of the spinal cord.

The ultrasonographic demonstration of bubbles in the bloodstream after apparently innocuous dive profiles (Spencer et al., 1969) and the association between DCI and the interatrial shunts that are present in a quarter of the population (Wilmshurst et al., 1989; Moon et al., 1991) may be associated with cerebral insults, since bubbles have been shown to compromise the blood-brain barrier in animals (Hallenbeck and Andersen, 1982; Hills and James, 1991).

Reports of long-term nervous system damage in hyperbaric workers resulted from the uncontrolled studies of Rozsahegyi (1959) and Rozsahegyi and Roth (1966). Of particular importance was their identification of a widespread, insidious, cognitive impairment in workers who had suffered from decompression illness while engaged in the construction of the Budapest metro under what would today be regarded as poor working conditions. On following up patients for 2–5 years, a mixture of physical and mental improvements and deteriorations was found, although it seems likely that it was, at least in part, the result of subsequent hyperbaric exposure with or without further DCI.

Psychological and neurological difficulties after DCI have been reported by Kelly and Peters (1975), Levin (1975), Peters et al. (1977), and Vaernes and Eidsvik (1982). These accounts, which appear to be based on the same small population of divers, also reported a correlation between the possession of neurological features and psychological deficits. Patients were characterized as having both neurological and psychological findings that suggested multifocal disease. The divers used were mostly plaintiffs awaiting litigation and this might have influenced their symptomatology, their performance on psychological testing, and the detection of "soft" neurological signs. It has been pointed out by Edmonds (1994) that, as subjects were assigned to the control group if they were found to have normal psychometric results, the difference between controls and divers was unremarkable. Vaernes and Eidsvik (1982) reported psychological deficits, mainly problems with memory, in nine divers who had experienced "near miss" diving accidents, compared with 15 incident-free divers and an age-matched nondiver control group. The nature of the incidents supposed to have caused the deficits is not clear; reference is made to carbon dioxide poisoning, hypoxia, "bends," and emboli.

Hoiberg and Blood (1985) reported that divers with histories of DCI were more likely to be hospitalized and to suffer from vascular diseases and headaches. A large number of United States Navy diving officers without histories of DCI were also studied, and it was found that they had significantly higher hospitalization rates than controls for diseases of the joints and nervous system (Hoiberg, 1986). The validity of Hoiberg's findings was challenged by Dembert (1987) on the grounds of inadequately matched controls. Similarly, Edmonds and Boughton's report (1985) of psychometric impairment in abalone divers, who accepted DCI as an occupational hazard, was questioned by subsequent work (Edmonds and Hayward, 1987; Williamson and Clarke, 1986; Andrews et al., 1986). Williamson et al. (1987) found that abalone divers scored better on some aspects of behavioral tests and worse on others compared with nondivers. This was compatible, predictably, with "risk-taking" personalities.

Various neurological phenomena are peculiar to hyperbaric exposure, but they are generally held to be physiological and entirely reversible. In particular, the incapacitating effects of inert gas narcosis effectively sets the maximum depth for air diving. High pressure neurological (nervous) syndrome (HPNS) is seen at great depth while breathing man-made gas mixtures. Its manifestations include tremor, dizziness, nausea and vomiting, sleep pattern changes, poor performance on psychometric testing, and reduced alpha and increased theta electroencephalographical activity. Todnem et al. (1989) examined participants before and after a deep saturation dive and found, as already described (Aarli et al., 1985; Vaernes et al., 1987; Stoudemire et al., 1984), a miscellany of minor neurological and neurophysiological abnormalities immediately after the dive. These generally resolved but in some cases, they took several months to do so. Those with a past history of diving or non–diving-related central nervous system injury appeared to be more likely to have abnormalities after the dive. Vaenes et al. (1989) claimed, on the basis of neuropsychological testing before and after deep saturation diving, that repeated deep diving may lead to certain long-term neuropsychological abnormalities of a type that implicated phylogenetically older structures in the brain. Divers who underwent shallower saturation exposure were also found to be at risk but needed to dive over a protracted period of time to suffer the same ill effects. The nonblind study of Todnem et al. (1990) found that the prevalence of neurological and psychological symptoms and signs in commercial divers was significantly greater than that found in nondiver controls. Further, abnormalities in general were independently positively correlated with dive exposure, prevalence of decompression illness, and age.

Several neuroimaging techniques have been used to investigate the possibility of diving-related cerebral changes. Adkisson et al. (1989), using ^{99}TC[1] labeled hexamethylpropyleneamine oxime (HMPAO) to perform single photon emission tomography (SPET), studied cerebral perfusion in cases of neurological DCI and, on the basis of the distribution of the perfusion deficits revealed, suggested that the condition was a manifestation of a more diffuse, multifocal insult than had previously been recognized. This was later questioned by Hodgson et al.'s (1991) study using HMPAO-SPET in cases of neurological DCI, which differed from Adkisson et al.'s (1989) in having more satisfactory control data. Hodgson, et al. (1988) found that there was no correlation between computed tomographic (CT) abnormalities and clinical status in an uncontrolled sample of 47 divers. Cerebral abnormalities on magnetic resonance imaging (MRI) were found to be more plentiful in nondiver controls than in professional divers, and their prevalence correlated inversely with length of diving experience. There was no correlation with history of DCI (Todnem et al., 1991; Rinck et al., 1991). Abnormalities consisted of unidentified bright objects (UBOs), which were felt to be mainly a manifestation of degenerated myelin and axons together with areas of gliosis in relation to damaged blood vessels. These could be the result of vascular insufficiency over a protracted period (Kirkpatrick and Hayman, 1987). However, the MRI studies performed on divers are open to criticism on the grounds of the confounding factors operating in controls. Indeed, when the same divers were compared with a group of office workers, it emerged that diving was positively related to the presence of UBOs (Brubakk, 1994). The absence of a consistent relationship between the prevalence of MRI changes and DCI is unremarkable if, as seems likely, the diagnosis was assigned on the basis of vague autonomic symptoms. Brubakk (1994) suggested that the inverse relationship between diving experience and the prevalence of MRI changes might be explained by divers with changes leaving the occupation early. Positron-emission tomography (PET), a high resolution functional cerebral imaging modality, failed to support the hypothesis that regional brain abnormalities may occur in the absence of neurological signs in DCI (Moon et al., 1991).

Pathological studies in man are rare, but Palmer et al. (1987) found significant degenerative change in the spinal white matter of 8 of 11 divers who had never suffered episodes of DCI and who had died suddenly. All the divers were within 38 weeks of an annual medical examination as required by U.K. law and had been passed as fit. Spinal cords were examined by the Marchi stain, which is not normally used by neuropathologists but it, and its derivatives, are used in neuroanatomy. Osmium in the Marchi stain becomes attached to globules of degenerating myelin of axons undergoing Wallerian degeneration. The reaction begins some 7–10 days after the damage has occurred, and the osmium is seen intracellularly in macrophages at 10 weeks and remains for an indeterminate but long (possibly years) time afterward. Degeneration was present in the posterior funiculi and, to a lesser extent, in the anterior and lateral funiculi. This study has been criticized, as the delay between death and fixation of the tissue was not recorded and long delays are thought likely to lead to artifacts (Mork et al., 1994). Mork's own examination of 20 spinal cords from amateur, professional, and saturation divers failed to demonstrate histopathological or immunocytochemical evidence of damage.

Palmer et al. (1992) reported cerebral vasculopathy with perivascular lacunae, hyalinization of vessel walls, perivascular white matter vacuolation, and necrotic foci in the gray matter at postmortem in divers without documented histories of neurological DCI. The suggestion was made that these changes were consistent with intravascular gas bubble formation. This was compatible with Palmer et al.'s earlier description of spinal cord lesions in divers without histories of decompression illness (1987).

Palmer's (1992) description of cerebral vasculopathy may concur with the demonstration of retinal pigment and microvascular defects seen in divers on retinal angiography by Polkinghorne et al. (1988). It was observed that these changes, which correlated with exposure to diving and to histories of DCI, were compatible with vascular obstruction such as might be produced by gas bubble occlusion. However, in a similar study, Murrison (1994) failed to identify differences on retinal flourescein angiography between professional divers and nondiver controls and found no relationship between the prevalence of changes and dive exposure or history of diving-related illness.

In a clinical setting, somato-sensory evoked potentials are a very sensitive method for detecting myelopathy, even subclinical lesions as occur in multiple sclerosis. The early changes of DCI involve splitting of the myelin laminae on the cord, so the use of evoked potentials to detect and monitor DCI has a sound experimental basis (Sykes and Yaffe, 1985). Changes in SEPs are known to occur in spinal cord DCI and have even been monitored during recompression

(Murrison et al., 1993; Moon et al., 1987). Recompression itself does not alter normal SEPs.

Somato-sensory evoked potentials from the tibial nerve of a group of 71 divers who had suffered DCI 1 month to 4 years previously showed no abnormality in 38 who had made a complete recovery and who were clinically normal. There was a clear difference between divers recovered from DCI and those with definite residual neurological abnormalities, and even divers left with only subjective residuals such as sensory changes and complaints of weakness undetectable on clinical examination showed a difference from the recovered divers. No abnormalities were detected in the SEPs from the median nerve of any group. Although not definitive, this suggests that the lesions may be multifocal in the cord and that the longer the path traversed in the neuroaxis, the more likely it is that abnormality will be detected (Murrison et al., 1994).

A further study of spinal cord function as assessed by clinical neurological examination and by SEP evoked by stimulating the posterior tibial nerve was done in 32 very experienced professional divers who had never had DCI, were medically fit to dive, and confirmed as neurologically normal. All had done at least 50 dives to 30 m or deeper, or 50 days of saturation diving. Twelve of 32 had an SEP P40 latency longer than two standard deviations of normal. (Statistically one might expect one or two subjects to fall beyond 2 standard deviations).

This study and Palmer's postmortem studies on fit, healthy divers suggest that some subclinical deterioration occurs in the spinal cord. It clearly has no effect on the subject's lifestyle, at least up to the point of retirement (usually 45–50 years of age) from diving, when annual medicals cease. Follow-up studies will be necessary to determine whether divers are more prone to spinal problems later in life.

In the field of long-term health effects, an important dichotomy in scientific approach becomes apparent. Psychology has become adept at searching for behavioral changes, while medical science is developing sophisticated imaging techniques to examine brain function. Philosophically most scientists now accept what Francis Crick called "The Astonishing Hypothesis,"—that every conscious, mental, or behavioral event is the result of activity in the nervous system that obeys physicochemical laws (Crick, 1994). Imperfections in psychological and medical methodologies do not at present allow for interchangeability of findings. Nevertheless, because the physical brain is responsible for our "being," it is our responsibility to protect it from damage.

VI. SUMMARY

Prevention of spinal cord damage due to DCI depends on divers themselves and on strict application of regulations and recommendations. Accidents in European waters are now largely confined to leisure divers who are less regulated. There are areas in the world where unprofessional practices obtain and it is frequently from here that access to recompression treatment may be most difficult. The principal treatment is still the application of gas laws, which demand recompression. The method has been refined empirically, but promptness is the most important single factor for a good prognosis. General medical support must be applied as needed. The use of adjuvants remains experimental.

In the long term, there are some lingering doubts about the cumulative damage to the central nervous system but to date, no adverse effects on the quality of life have been demonstrated.

REFERENCES

Aarli JA, Vaernes R, Brubakk AO, Nyland H, Skeidsvoli H, Tonjum S. Central nervous dysfunction associated with deep sea diving. Acta Neurol Scand 1994; 71:2–10.

Adkisson GH, Hodgson M, Smith F, Torok Z, MacLeod MA, Sykes JJW, Strack C, Pearson RR. Cerebral perfusion deficits in dysbaric illness. Lancet 1989; ii:119–121.

Aharon-Peretz J, Adir Y, Gordon CR, Kol S, Gal N, Melamed Y. Spinal cord decompression sickness in sport diving. Arch Neurol 1993; 50:753–756.

Andrews G, Holt P, Edmonds C, Lowry C, Cistulli P, McKay B, Misra S, Sutton G. Does non-clinical decompression stress lead to brain damage in abalone divers? Med J Aust 1986; 144:399–401.

Argentino C, Sacchetti ML, Toni D, Savoini G, D'Arcangelo E, Erminio F, Federico F, Milone FF, Gallai V, Gambi D, et al. GM1 ganglioside therapy in acute ischemic stroke. Stroke 1989; 20(9):1143–1149.

Bennett PB, and Elliott DH. In: The physiology and medicine of diving. 4th ed. Bennett PB, Elliott DH, eds. London: Saunders, 1993; ix–x.

Benton PB, Woodfine JD, Francis TJR. A review of spirometry and UK submarine escape training tank incidents (1954–1993) using objective diagnostic criteria. Undersea and Hyperbaric Medicine 1994, 21(suppl):70.

Bert P. La pression barometrique: Recherches de physiologie experimentale. Paris: G Masson 1878. Translated by Hitchcock MA and Hitchcock FA. Columbus College Book Co., 1943. Republished by the Undersea Medical Society, Bethesda, MD, 1978.

Boycott AE, Damant GCC, Haldane JS. Prevention of compressed air illness. J Hyg (Camb), 1908; 8:342–443.

Bracken MB, Collins WF, Freeman DF, Efficacy of methylprednisolone in acute spinal cord injury. JAMA 1984; 251:45–52.

Bracken MB, Shepherd MJ, Collins WF,. A randomised controlled trial of methylprednisolone or naloxone in the treatment of acute spinal-cord injury: Results of the second national acute spinal cord injury study. N Engl J Med 1990; 322:1405–1411.

Bracken MB, Shepherd MJ, Hellenbrand KG, Methylprednisolone and neurological function 1 year after spinal cord injury. Results of the national acute spinal cord injury study. J Neurosurg 1985; 63:704–713.

Bradley ME. Metabolic considerations. In: Fitness to Dive. Linaweaver PG, Vorosmarti J, eds. Bethesda, MD: Undersea and Hyperbaric Medical Society, 1987; 98–103.

Braune S. Is ganglioside GMI effective in the treatment of stroke? Drugs-Aging 1991; 1(1):57–66.

Bridgwater BJM, Pezeshkpour GH, Pearson RR, Dutka AJ. The cerebral histopathology of acute experimental decompression illness. Undersea Biomed Res 1991; 18(suppl):25–26.

Brooks GJ, Pethybridge RJ, Pearson RR. Lung function reference values for FEV_1, FEV_1/FVC ratio and FEF_{75-85} derived from the results of screening 3788 Royal Navy submariners and submarine candidates by spirometry. Aberdeen: EUBS meeting, 1988.

Broome JR. Multifocal CNS haemorrhage as a cause of recompression treatment failure in a pig model of neurological decompression illness (DCI). Undersea and Hyperbaric Medicine 1994; 21(suppl):69–70.

Brubakk AO. Silent vascular gas bubbles—fact or fiction? In: Hope A, Lund T, Elliott DH, Halsey MJ, Wiig H, eds. Long Term Health Effects of Diving. University of Bergen, Bergen, Norway, 1994; 140–141.

Butler BD, Hills BA. The lung as a filter for microbubbles. J Appl Physiol 1979; 47:537–543.

Butler BD, Hills BA. Transpulmonary passage of venous air emboli. J Appl Physiol 1985; 59:543–547.

Clay JR. Histopathology of experimental decompression sickness. Aerospace Med 1963; 34:1107–1110.

Colebatch HJ, Ng CK. Decreased pulmonary distensibility and pulmonary barotrauma in divers. Respir Physiol 1991; 86:293–303.

Cook SF. Environmental factors affecting decompression sickness. Part II. Role of exercise, temperature, drugs and water balance in decompression sickness. In: Fulton JF, ed. Decompression Sickness. Philadelphia: WB Saunders, 1951; 223–241.

Corsellis JAN. Boxing and the brain. BMJ 1989; 298:105–109.

Crick F. The Astonishing Hypothesis. London: Simon & Schuster, 1994.

Cross SJ, Evans SA, Thomson LF, Lee HS, Jennings KP, Shields TG. Safety of subaqua diving with a patent foramen ovale. BMJ 1992; 304:481–482.

Curley MD, Robin GJ, Thalmamm ED. Percent body fat and human decompression sickness. Undersea Biomed Res 1989; 16(suppl):29.

de Courten-Myers GM, Kleinholz M, Wagner KR, Xi G, Myers RE. Efficacious experimental stroke treatment with high-dose methylprednisolone. Stroke 1994; 25(2):487–492.

Dembert ML. Long term health consequences of diving accidents. Undersea Biomed Res 1987; 14:372–373.

Deuster PA, Smith DJ, Smoak BL, Montgomery LC, Singh A, Doubt TJ. Prolonged whole-body cold water immersion: Fluid and ion shifts. J Appl Physiol 1989; 66:34–41.

Douglas JDM, Robinson C. Heliox treatment for spinal decompression sickness following air dives. Undersea Biomed Res 1988; 15:315–319.

Drewry A, Gorman DF. Lidocaine as an adjunct to hyperbaric therapy in decompression illness: A case report. Undersea Biomed Res 1992; 19:187–190.

Dutka AJ. Therapy for dysbaric central nervous system ischaemia: Adjuncts to recompression. In: Bennett PB, Moon RE, eds. Diving Accident Management, Bethesda, MD: Undersea and Hyperbaric Medical Society, 1990; 222–234.

Dutka AJ, Hallenbeck JM, Kockanek P. A brief episode of severe hypertension induces delayed deterioration of brain function and worsens blood flow after transient multifocal cerebral ischaemia. Stroke 1987; 18:386–395.

Dutka AJ, Kochanek PM, Hallenbeck JM. Influence of granulocytopaenia on canine cerebral ischaemia induced by air embolism. Stroke 1989; 20:390–395.

Dutka AJ, Polychronidis J, Mink RB, Hallenbeck JM. Head-down position after air embolism impairs recovery of brain function as measured by the somatosensory evoked response in canines. Undersea Biomed Res 1990; 17(suppl):64–65.

Eckenhoff RG, Olstad CS, Carrod G. Human dose-response relationship for decompression and endogenous bubble formation. J Appl Physiol 1990; 69:914–918.

Edmonds C. The mythology of diver's dementia. In: Hope A, Lund T, Elliott DH, Halsey MJ, Wiig H, eds. Long Term Health Effects of Diving. University of Bergen, Bergen, Norway, 1994; 140–141.

Edmonds C, Boughton J. Intellectual deterioration with excessive diving (punch drunk divers). Undersea Biomed Res 1985; 12:321–326.

Edmonds C, Hayward L. Intellectual impairment with diving: A review. In: Bove AA, Bachrach AJ, Greenbaum LJ, eds. Proceedings of the ninth Symposium on Underwater and Hyperbaric Physiology. Bethesda MD: Undersea and Hyperbaric Medical Society, 1987; 877–886.

Elliott DH, Moon RE. Manifestations of the decompression disorders. In: Bennett PB, Elliott DH, eds. The Physiology and Medicine of Diving. 4th ed. London: Saunders, 1993; 481–505.

Evans DE, Catron PW, McDermott JJ, Thomas LB, Kobrine Al, Flynn ET. Effect of lidocaine after experimental cerebral ischaemia induced by air embolism. J Neurosurg 1989; 70:97–102.

Evans DE, Kobrine Al, LeGrys DC, Bradley ME. Protective effect of lidocaine in acute cerebral ischaemia induced by air embolism. J Neurosurg 1984; 60:257–263.

Evans DE, Kobrine AI, Weathersby PK, Bradley ME. Cardiovascular effects of cerebral air embolism. Stroke 1981; 12:338–344.

Francis TJR. The Role of Autochthonous Bubbles in Acute Spinal Cord Decompression Sickness. Ph.D. thesis, University of London, 1990.

Francis TJR, Dutka AJ. Methylprednisolone in the treatment of acute spinal cord decompression sickness. Undersea Biomed Res 1989; 16(2):165–174.

Francis TJR, Dutka AJ, Clark JB. An evaluation of dexamethosone in the treatment of acute experimental spinal decompression sickness. Proceedings of the Ninth International Symposium on Underwater and Hyperbaric Physiology. Bethesda MD: Undersea and Hyperbaric Medical Society, 1987; 999–1013.

Francis TJR, Dutka AJ, Flynn ET. Experimental determination of latency, severity and outcome in CNS decompression sickness. Undersea Biomed Res 1988b, 15:419–427.

Francis TJR, Griffin JL, Homer LD, Pezeshkpour GH, Dutka AJ, Flynn ET. Bubble-induced dysfunction in acute spinal cord decompression sickness. J Appl Physiol 1990b; 68:1368–1375.

Francis TJR, Hardman JM, Beckman EL. A pressure threshold for in-situ bubble formation in the canine spinal cord. Undersea Biomed Res 1990a; 17(suppl):69.

Francis TJR, Pearson RR, Robertson AG, Hodgson M, Dutka AJ, Flynn ET. Central nervous system decompression sickness: Latency of 1070 human cases. Undersea Biomed Res 1988a; 15:403–417.

Francis TJR, Smith DJ, eds. Describing decompression illness. Bethesda, MD: Undersea and Hyperbaric Medical Society, 1991.

Fritz H, Hossman KA. Arterial air embolism in the cat brain. Stroke 1979; 10:581–589.

Gelb AW, Steinberg GK, Lam AM, Manniken PH, Peerless SJ, Neto AR. Lidocaine transiently protects in focal cerebral ischaemia. Stroke 1987; 18:278.

Golding F, Griffiths P, Hempleman HV, Paton WDM, Walder DN. Decompression sickness during construction of the Dartford Tunnel. Br J Indust Med 1960; 17:167–180.

Gorman DF, Arterial gas embolism as a consequence of pulmonary barotrauma. In: Desola J, ed. Diving and Hyperbaric Medicine. Barcelona: EUBS, 1984; 348–368.

Gorman DF, Browning DM, Parsons DW, Traugott FM. Distribution of arterial gas emboli in the pial circulation. SPUMS J 1987; 17:101–115.

Gorman DF, Browning DM. Cerebral vasoreactivity and arterial gas embolism. Undersea Biomed Res 1986; 13:317–335.

Hall ED, Braughler JM. Glucocorticoid mechanisms in acute spinal cord injury: A review and therapeutic rationale. Surg Neurol 1982; 18:320–327.

Hall ED, Braughler JM. Role of lipid peroxidation in post traumatic spinal cord degeneration: A review. Cent Nerv Syst Trauma 1986; 3:281–294.

Hallenbeck JM, Andersen JC. Pathogenesis of the decompression disorders. In: Bennett PB, Elliott DH, eds. The Physiology and Medicine of Diving. London: Balliere Tindall, 1982; 435–460.

Hallenbeck JM, Bove AA, Elliott DH. Mechanisms underlying spinal cord damage in decompression sickness. Neurology 1975; 25:308–316.

Hallenbeck JM, Andersen JC, eds. Pathogenesis of the decompression disorders. In: The Physiology and Medicine of Diving. 3rd ed. Bennett PB, Elliott DH, eds. San Pedro, CA: Best, 1982; 425–460.

Hallenbeck JM, Dutka AJ, Tanashima T, Kochanek PM, Kumaroo KK, Thompson CB, Obrenovitch TP, Contreras TJ. Polymorphonuclear leucocyte accumulation in brain regions with low blood flow during the early postischemic period. Stroke 1986; 17:246–253.

Haller C, Sercombe R, Verrechia C, Fritsch H, Seylaz J, Kuschinsky W. Effect of the muscarinic agonist carbachol on pial arteries in vivo after endothelial damage by air embolism. J Cereb Blood Flow Metab 1987; 7:605–611.

Harker CP, Neuman TS, Olson LK, Jacoby I, Santos A. The roentgenographic findings associated with air embolism in sport scuba divers. J Emerg Med 1993; 11:443–449.

Helps SC, Parsons DW, Reilly PL, Gorman DF. The effect of gas emboli on rabbit cerebral blood flow. Stroke 1990a; 21:94–99.

Helps SC, Meyer-Witting M, Reilly PL, Gorman DF. Increasing doses of intracarotid air and cerebral blood flow in rabbits. Stroke 1990b; 21:1340–1345.

Helps SC & Gorman DF. Air embolism of the brain in rabbits pretreated with mechlorethamine. Stroke 1991; 22:351–354.

Hernandez NE, MacDonall JS, Stier CT Jr, Belmonte A, Fernandez R, Karpiak SE. GM1 ganglioside treatment of spontaneously hypertensive stroke prone rats. Exp Neurol 1994; 126(1):95–100.

Hills BA, James PB. Spinal decompression sickness. Mechanical studies and a model. Undersea Biomed Res 1982; 9:185–201.

Hills BA, James PB. Microbubble damage to the bloodbrain barrier: Relevance to decompression sickness. Undersea Biomed Res 1991; 18:111–116.

Hodgson M, Smith DJ, MacLeod MA, Houston AS, Francis TJR. Case control study of decompression illness using 99Tcm-HMPAO SPECT. Undersea Biomed Res 1991; 18(suppl):17.

Hodgson M, Beran RG, Shirtley G. The role of computerised tomography in the assessment of neurological sequelae of decompression sickness. Arch Neurol 1988; 45:1033–1035.

Hoiberg A. Consequences of US Navy diving mishaps: Decompression sickness. Undersea Biomed Res 1986; 13:383–394.

Hoiberg A, Blood C. Age-specific morbidity and mortality rates among US Navy enlisted divers and controls. Undersea Biomed Res 1985; 12:191–203.

Hope A, Lund T, Elliott DH, Halsey MJ, Wiig H, eds. Long term health effects of diving. University of Bergen, Bergen, Norway, 1994, 140–141.

Hughes JT. Venous infarction of the spinal cord. Neurology 1971; 21:794–800.

James PB. A review of neurological decompression illness. In: James PB, McCallum RI, Rawlins JSP, eds. Report of Proceedings of a Symposium on Decompression Sickness. Cambridge, England: European Undersea Biomedical Society, 1981;9–15.

Jenkins C, Anderson SD, Wong R, Veale A. Compressed air diving and respiratory disease. A discussion document of the Thoracic Society of Australia and New Zealand. Med J Aust 1993; 158:275–279.

Kelly PJ, Peters BH. The neurological manifestations of decompression accidents. In: Hong SK, ed. Man and the Sea. Bethesda MD: Undersea Medical Society, 1975; 227–232.

Kempner GB, Stegmann BJ, Pilmanis AA. Inconsistent classification and treatment of type I and type II decompression sickness. Aviat Space Environ Med 1992; 63:410.

Kirkpatrick JB, Hayman LA. White matter lesions in MR imaging of clinically healthy brains of elderly subjects: Possible pathological basis. Radiology 1987; 162:509–511.

Kitano M, Hayashi K, Kawashima M. Three autopsy cases of acute decompression sickness: Consideration of pathogenesis about spinal cord damage in decompression sickness. J West Jpn Orthop Traumatol 1977; 26:110–116.

Kumar KV, Billica RD, Powell R, Waligora JM. Symptom—based classification of decompression sickness—preliminary evaluation of a new system (LIP scheme). Undersea and Hyperbaric Medicine 1994; 21(suppl):64.

Lam TH, Yau KP. Analysis of some individual risk factors for decompression sickness in Hong Kong. Undersea Biomed Res 1989; 16:283–292.

Lam TH, Yau KP. Manifestations and treatment of 793 cases of decompression sickness in a compressed-air tunnelling project in Hong Kong. Undersea Biomed Res 1988; 15:377–388.

Lehner CE, Lanphier EH. Influence of pressure profile on DCS symptoms. In: Vann RD, ed. Bethesda, MD: Undersea and Hyperbaric Medical Society, 1989; 299–326.

Leitch DR, Greenbaum LR Jr, Hallenbeck JM. Cerebral arterial air embolism. II. Effect of pressure and time on cortical evoked potential recovery. Undersea Biomed Res 1984a; 11:237–248.

Leitch DR, Greenbaum LT Jr, Hallenbeck JM. Cerebral arterial air embolism. III. Cerebral blood flow after decompression from various pressure treatments. Undersea Biomed Res 1984b; 11:249–263.

Leitch DR, Hallenbeck JM. Somotosensory evoked potentials and neuraxial blood flow in central nervous system decompression sickness. Brain Res 1984a; 311:307–315.

Leitch DR, Hallenbeck JM. Remote monitoring of neuraxial function in anaesthetized dogs in compression chambers. Electroenceph Clin Neurophysiol 1984b; 57:548–560.

Leitch DR, Hallenbeck JM. Pressure in the treatment of spinal cord decompression sickness. Undersea Biomed Res 1985a; 12:291–305.

Leitch DR, Hallenbeck JM. A model of spinal cord dysbarism to study delayed treatment: II. Effects of treatment. Aviat Space Environ Med 1985b; 55:679–684.

Levin HW. Neuropsychological sequelae of diving accidents. In: Hong SK, ed. Man and the Sea. Bethesda MD: Undersea Medical Society, 1975; 232–241.

Lynch PR, Krasner LJ, Vinciquerra T, Shaffer TH. Effects of intravenous perfluorocarbon and oxygen breathing on acute decompression sickness in the hamster. Undersea Biomed Res 1989; 16:275–281.

Malhotra MC, Wright HC. The effects of raised intrapulmonary pressure on the lungs of fresh unchilled cadavers. J Pathol Bacteriol 1961; 82:198–202.

McDermott JJ, Dutka AJ, Evans DE, Flynn ET. Effects of treatment with lidocaine and hyperbaric oxygen in experimental cerebral ischemia induced by air embolism. Undersea Biomed Res 1990; 17(suppl):35–36.

Mekjavik IB, Kakitsuba N. Effect of peripheral temperature on the formation of venous gas bubbles. Undersea Biomed Res 1989; 16:391–401.

Moon RE, Campresi EM, Massey EW, Erwin CW, Djang WG. Functional imaging of the central nervous system (CT, MRI, xeon blood-flow) and use of evoked potentials during therapy of decompression sickness and arterial gas embolism. Proceedings of the ninth International Symposium on Underwater and Hyperbaric Physiology. Bethesda MD: Undersea and Hyperbaric Medical Society, 1987; 1015–1024.

Moon RE, Camporesi EM. Patent foramen ovale and decompression sickness in divers. Lancet 1989; 1:513–514.

Moon RE, Hoffman JM, Hanson MW, Reiman RE, Coleman RE, Theil DR, Fawsett TR, Francis JJ, Gorback MS, Massey EW. 18F-deoxyglucose positron emission tomography (PET) in the evaluation of neurological decompression illness. Undersea Biomed Res 1991; 18(suppl):18.

Mork SJ, Moorild I, Brubakk AO, Eidsvik S, Nyland H. A histopathologic and immuno-cytochemical study of the spinal cord in amateur and profession divers. Undersea and Hyperbaric Medicine 1994; 21:391–402.

Murrison AW. Ophthalmic defects in divers. In: Hope A, Lund T, Elliott DH, Halsey MJ, Wiig H, eds. Long Term Health Effects of Diving. University of Bergen, Bergen, Norway, 1994; 140–141.

Murrison AW, Francis TJR. An introduction to decompression illness. BJHM 1991; 46: 107–110.

Murrison AW, Glasspool E, Pethybridge RJ, Francis TJR, Sedgwick EM. Neurophysiological assessment of divers with medical histories of neurological decompression illness. Occup Environ Med 1994; 51:730–734.

Murrison AW, Glasspool E, Segwick EM. Neurophysiological monitoring of acute neurological decompression illness. Journal of the Royal Naval Medical Service 1993; 79:139–144.

Neuman TS, Bove AA. Combined arterial gas embolism and decompression sickness following no-stop dives. Undersea Biomed Res 1990; 17:429–436.

Nishimoto K, Wolman M, Spatz M, Klatzo I. Pathophysiologic correlations in the blood-brain barrier damage due to air embolism. Adv Neurol 1978; 20:237–244.

Palmer AC, Calder IM, Hughes JT. Spinal cord degeneration in divers. Lancet 1987; ii:1365–1366.

Palmer AC. The neuropathology of decompression sickness. In: Cavanagh JD, ed. Recent Advances in Neuropathology. Vol. 3. Edinburgh: Churchill Livingstone, 1986; 141–162.

Palmer AC, Calder JM, Yates PO. Cerebral vasculopathy in divers. Neuropathol Appl Neurobiol 1992; 18:113–124.

Pearson RR, Bridgewater BJM, Dutka AJ. Comparison of treatment of compressed air-induced decompression sickness by recompression to 6ATA breathing air and heliox. Undersea Biomed Res 1991; 18(suppl):25.

Persson LI, Johanasson BB, Hansson HA. Ultrastructural studies on blood-brain barrier dysfunction after cerebral air embolism in the rat. Acta Neuropathol (Berl) 1978; 44:53–56.

Peters BH, Levin HS, Kelly PJ. Neurologic and psychologic manifestations of decompression illness in divers. Neurology 1977; 27:125–127.

Pilmanis AA. Intravenous gas embolism in man after compressed air open water diving. Technical Report No. N00014-67-0269-0026. Washington DC: US Office of Naval Research, 1976.

Polkinghorne PJ, Cross MR, Sehmi K, Minassian D, Bird AC. Ocular fundus lesions in divers. Lancet 1988; ii:1381–1383.

Polychronidis JE, Dutka AJ, Mink RB, Hallenbeck JM. Head down position after cerebral air embolism: Effects of intracranial pressure, pressure volume index and blood-brain barrier. Undersea Biomed Res 1990; 17(suppl):99–100.

Rinck PA, Svihus R, de Francisco P. MR imaging of the central nervous system in diving. Journal of Magnetic Resonance Imaging 1991; 1:293–299.

Rivera JC. Decompression sickness among divers: An analysis of 935 cases. Mil Med 1964;129:314–334.

Rozsahegyi I. Late consequences of neurological forms of decompression sickness. Br J Indust Med 1959; 16:311–317.

Rozsahegyi I, Roth B. Participation of the central nervous system in decompression. Ind Med Surg 1966 ;35:101–110.

Smith DJ, Francis TJR, Pethybridge RJ, Wright JM, Sykes JJW. Concordance: A problem with the current classification of diving disorders. Undersea Biomed Res 1992; 19(suppl):40.

Spencer MP, Campbell SD, Sealey JL, Henry FC, Lindbuergh J. Experiments on decompression bubbles in circulation using ultrasonic and electromagnetic flowmeters. J Occup Med 1969; 11:238–244.

Stoudemire A, Miller J, Schmitt F. Development of an organic affective syndrome during a hyperbaric diving experiment. Am Psychiatry 1984; 80:333–340.

Sykes JJW, Yaffe LJ. Light and electron microscope alterations in spinal cord myelin sheaths after decompression sickness. Undersea Biomed Res 1985; 12:251–258.

Talmi YP, Finkelstein Y, Zohar Y. Decompression sickness induced hearing loss. A review. Scand Audiol 1991; 20:25–28.

Thalmann ED. Air-N_2O_2 decompression computer algorithm development. NEDU Report 8–85. Panama City, FL: US Navy Experimental Diving Unit, 1985.

Thalmann ED. Development of a decompression algorithm for constant 0.7 ATA oxygen partial pressure helium diving. NEDU Report 1–86. Panama City, FL: US Navy Experimental Diving Unit, 1986.

Thomas DJ, Marshall J, Ross Russell R, Wetherley-Mein G, DuBoulay GH, Pearson TC, Symon L, Zilkha E. Effects of haematocrit on cerebral blood flow in man. Lancet 1977; 2:941–943.

Todnem K, Nyland H, Dick APK, Lind O, Svihus R, Molvaer OL, Aarli JA. Immediate neurological effects of diving to a depth of 360 metres. Acta Neurol Scand 1989; 80:333–340.

Todnem K, Nyland H, Kambestad BK, Aarli JA. Influence of occupational diving upon the nervous system. Br J Ind Med 1990; 47:708–714.

Todnem K, Skeidsvoll H, Svihus R, Rinck P, Riise T, Kambestad BK, Aarli JA. Electroencephalography, evoked potentials and MRI brain scans in saturation divers: An experimental study. Electroencephalog Clin Neurophysiol 1991; 79:322–329.

Vaernes RJ, Eidsvik S. Central nervous system dysfunction after near-miss diving accidents. Aviat Space Environ Med 1982; 53:803–807.

Vaernes RJ, Kolve H, Ellertsen B. Neuropsychological effects of saturation diving. Undersea Biomed Res 1989; 16:233–251.

Vaernes RJ, Kolve H, Ursin H. Neuropsychological and neurophysiologic reactions during a heliox dive to 450msw. Ninth International Symposium on Underwater and Hyperbaric Medicine. Bethesda, MD: Undersea and Hyperbaric Medical Society, 1987; 565–572.

Van Der Aue OE, Keller RJ, and Brinton ES. The effect of exercise during decompression from increased barometric pressure on the incidence of decompression sickness in man. NEDU Report 8–49. Panama City, FL: US Navy Experimental Diving Unit, 1949.

Van Der Aue OE, Keller RJ, Brinton ES, Barron G, Gillam HD, Jones RJ. Calculation and testing of decompression tables for air dives employing the procedure of surface decompression and the use of oxygen. NEDU Report 13–15. Panama City, FL: US Navy Experimental Diving Unit, 1951.

Vik A, Brubakk AO, Hennessy TR, Jenssen BM, Ekker M, Slordahl SA. Venous air embolism in swine: Transport of gas bubbles through the pulmonary circulation. J Appl Physiol 1990; 69:237–244.

Vik A, Jenssen BM, Brubakk AO. Arterial gas bubbles after decompression in pigs with patent foramen ovale. Undersea and Hyperbaric Medine 1993; 20:121–131.

Walder DN. Adaptation to decompression sickness in caisson work. Biometerology 1968; 11:350–359.

Waligora JM, Horrigan DJ, Conkin J. The effect of extended O_2 pre-breathing on altitude decompression sickness and venous gas bubbles. Aviat Space Environ Med 1987; 58:A110–A112.

Weathersby PK, Homer LD. Solubility of inert gases in biological fluids and tissues. Undersea Biomed Res 1980; 7:277–296.

Weathersby PK, Survanshi SS, Hays JR, McCallum ME. Statistically based decompression tables III: Comparative risk using US navy, British and Canadian standard air schedules. NMRI Report 86–50 Bethseda, MD: Naval Medical Research Institute, 1986.

Weathersby PK, Survanshi SS, Nishi RY. Relative decompression risk of dry and wet chamber air dives. Undersea Biomed Res 1990; 17:333–352.

Williamson A, Clark B. The neuropbehavioural effects of professional abalone diving. In: Edmonds C, Ed. The Abalone Diver. National Safety Council of Australia, 1986.

Williamson A, Edmonds C, Clarke B. The neurobehavioral effects of professional abalone diving. Br J Indust Med 1987; 44:459–466.

Wilmshurst PT, Byrne JC, Webb-Pepploe MM. Relation between interatrial shunts and decompression sickness in divers. Lancet 1989; 2:1302–1306.

Young W. Medical treatments of acute spinal cord injury. J Neurol Neurosurg Psychiatry 1992; 55:635–639.

21

Cervical Spondylosis and Myelopathy

Jonathan Duffill and Fausto Iannotti

*University Clinical Neurological Sciences, Southampton General Hospital,
Southampton, England*

Cervical spondylosis is a degenerative condition affecting the discs, bones, and joints of the cervical spine. Fifty percent of the population have signs of spondylosis on plain radiographs by the fifth decade. The incidence increases to 97% of men and 93% of women by the seventh decade. In the majority of cases, these changes remain asymptomatic, but in a minority, involvement of the cervical spinal cord and/or nerve roots may cause neurological complications.

Brain, Northfield, and Wilkinson first recognized that myelopathy could be caused by degenerative cervical spondylosis rather than "chondromas" as previously thought (1). Since the recognition that compression due to spondylosis could cause myelopathy, surgery has been widely advocated as an effective treatment. A variety of operative procedures, using either anterior or posterior approaches and with or without fusion or instrumentation, have been developed to relieve cord compression. This chapter focuses on the pathology, diagnosis, natural history, and management of cervical spondylotic myelopathy.

I. ANATOMY

The cervical spinal is the most mobile segment of the spinal column. The discs, which account for 22% of the height of the spinal column, allow an increased range of movement between vertebrae. They also spread loading forces and provide a shock absorbing function for axial loading. Particular anatomical features of the discs and vertebrae allow for these functions but also help to explain the pathological changes that occur in spondylosis.

The annulus fibrosus, consisting of fibrocartilage arranged in a concentric lamellar fashion with each layer in a differing direction, is attached to the anterior and posterior longitudinal ligaments (2,3). The attachment to the posterior longitudinal ligament, however, becomes less secure with age. This, coupled with the predominantly vertical arrangement of annular fibers posteriorly may, in part, explain the predominance of posterior disc protrusions.

The nucleus pulposus is clearly distinct from the annulus at birth and accounts for 40% of the total disc cross-sectional area although only 15% by volume. The maximum diameter of a completely extruded nucleus has been calculated at 0.7 cm. The nucleus has a semigelatinous appearance and consists of collagen fibers and mucopolysaccharide ground substance. Several age-related changes occur within the disc. The number of cells decreases with aging and they become concentrated beneath the endplates. The nucleus also contains more fibrocartilaginous material and less mucopolysaccharide ground substance, and the water content falls from 88% to 70%. The water content of the annulus also falls.

The cartilage endplates are situated between the nucleus and the trabecular bone of the vertebral bodies and are 1 mm thick. Fibers pass from the endplates and into the nucleus, anchoring it between the middle third and posterior third of the disc. Small blood vessels also pass into the disc via the endplate, but these begin to close by 8 months of age and are closed completely by the age of 30. Small pores in the endplate allow nutrition of the disc by diffusion of water and metabolites; thus calcification of the endplate may interfere with disc nutrition.

II. PATHOPHYSIOLOGY

Cervical spondylosis is a degenerative condition accompanying aging and exacerbated by repetitive use. The changes begin in the disc with a reduction in the water content of the nucleus. It is thought that this decreased hydration leads to an inability of the disc to generate high intradiscal pressures and thus distribute normal loads. Annular fibrillation and weakness then predispose to nuclear herniation and/or annular protrusion, the former being more common in younger patients and after trauma. These changes are uncommon at the C2-3 level but are frequent below this and most often affect the C5-6 and C6-7 discs. A reduction of disc height follows and leads to loss of the normal cervical lordosis, with compensatory hyperextension at other levels. Reactive processes are then responsible for the development of a decrease in the size of the spinal canal. A reactive hyperostosis causes a spondylotic bar to develop posteriorly as the bodies come closer together. The abnormal approximation of the vertebral bodies also leads to destruction of the uncovertebral joints, reactive hypertrophy resulting in osteophytes causing dorsolateral compression within the vertebral canal and compromise of the intervertebral foramen (4). Further reduction in mobility may result in degeneration and hypertrophy of the facet joints and ligamentum flavum causing posterior compression of the cord.

Experimentally, it has been demonstrated that these changes can be produced in the rabbit by repetitive flexion/extension of the cervical spine. The early onset of cervical spondylosis in some patients such as those with athetoid cerebral palsy may thus be an overuse phenomenon. Repetitive overuse may contribute to the early onset or progression of cervical spondylotic myelopathy (CSM) in some patients.

Although the changes of spondylosis cause a reduction, particularly in the anterior-posterior (A-P) diameter of the spinal canal, in the majority of cases neurological complications do not develop, so additional factors must therefore contribute to the onset of myelopathy. The initial constitutional diameter of the spinal canal is thought to be a significant factor. The normal canal diameter between C3 and C7 is 17–18 mm. If the acquired A-P diameter falls below a critical size of 11–13 mm then myelopathy is more likely to develop (5). Patients with a constitutionally narrow canal are thus more at risk of developing myelopathy with spondylotic reduction in the spinal canal diameter. There is, however, considerable overlap in the constitutional canal diameter between symptomatic and asymptomatic groups.

Normal and abnormal spinal movement also plays a role in the pathogenesis and progression of CSM. The center of rotation of the cervical spine is anterior to the vertebral bodies, so the length of the spinal cord increases in flexion and decreases in extension. It is proposed that stretching of the cord in flexion and movement against anterior spondylotic bars result in repeated cord trauma. The increase in cord cross-sectional area on extension, together with the concomitant reduction in canal cross-sectional area also causes intermittent pinching of the cord between anterior spondylotic bars and disc material and the posterior ligamentum flavum.

There is considerable debate as to whether myelopathy is the result of direct compression of neural tissue or a secondary effect caused by impairment of the vascular supply of the cord. The vascular theory was first proposed by Brain, and supported by Allen, who had noted blanching of the cord on flexion during surgery. The vascular supply of the anterior two-thirds of the spinal cord is from the anterior spinal artery via the central sulcal artery. The posterior horn and posterior columns are supplied by small dorsolateral arteries and from the pial plexus. Capillary anastomoses do connect the two systems, but a watershed zone is therefore present within the cord. The anterior spinal artery, a branch of the vertebral artery, is reinforced by variable cervical medullary arteries that enter the spinal canal via the intervertebral foramen. These vessels are most common at C6, followed by C3, C4, and C5. The number of vessels and the side from which they enter is highly variable. It has been suggested that myelopathy could result from compression of the anterior spinal artery or a cervical medullary vessel in the intervertebral foramen. Nurick, however, failed to demonstrate an association between generalised vascular disease and CSM (7). The syndrome of anterior spinal artery thrombosis, although reported in association with CSM, is rare. If compression of the medullary artery by narrowing or fibrosis in the intervertebral foramen is the cause of CSM, then the frequent lack of radicular symptoms in patients with CSM and the failure of patients with radiculopathy to go on to develop CSM is not adequately explained. It appears unlikely that major arterial compression plays a role in the majority of patients with CSM. It is more likely, however, that distortion and compression of the transverse intramedullary arteries after changes in cord length and area, as described above, result in ischemic damage to the cord (8).

The gross pathological changes in the cord are most marked at areas of maximal compression opposite spondylotic bars at the level of the intervertebral disc. The gray matter may show neuronal loss and ischemia, progressing to necrosis and cavitation. The white matter often shows minimal change but may show evidence of demyelination and necrosis.

Cervical spondylotic myelopathy is therefore due to multiple factors, including degenerative changes beginning in the disc leading to encroachment and narrowing superimposed on a narrow cervical canal. This may be exacerbated by movement of the cervical spine and cord. These changes result in cord and/or root dysfunction as a direct result of compression and indirectly occurring after ischemia caused by distortion of small intramedullary vessels.

III. SYMPTOMATOLOGY

The symptoms and signs of cervical spondylotic myelopathy involve both motor and sensory impairment, with variable, often mixed patterns of upper and lower motor neurone-type signs, spinothalamic and/or posterior column sensory loss, and cervical or upper limb pain. Sphincter disturbance may also be a feature. Gradual onset of spastic paraparesis with increased tone in the legs, clonus, and flexor spasms is a typical presentation. The symptoms are usually bilateral but may be asymmetrical. Weakness may not be marked but, if present, is usually most evident in hip flexion, knee flexion, and ankle dorsiflexion. The reflexes are brisk and the plantar responses extensor. The features in the upper limbs are often mixed with radicular symptoms at the level of the lesion and myelopathic symptoms below. For example there may be weakness with wasting and hyporeflexia in the C5 distribution but spasticity and increased reflexes in C7-T1 innervated muscles. Radiculopathy is present in 40–80% of patients with myelopathic signs in the legs. The pattern of sensory loss is also variable and depends on the site of compression, which may be the spinothalamic tract, the posterior columns, or the dorsal nerve root. Therefore, pain and temperature sensation may be lost, joint position sense and vibration may be affected leading to gait ataxia, or all sensory modalities may be impaired in the upper limb in a radicular distribution (9). The varied symptoms and signs in CSM can be categorized into five groups (10,11):

1. The transverse myelopathy syndrome, where corticospinal tracts and posterior columns or spinothalamic tracts are involved.
2. A group with principally motor symptoms of corticospinal tract damage with or without anterior horn cell involvement but in which sensory deficits are minimal.
3. A partial Brown-Séquard syndrome may be caused in CSM with ipsilateral motor loss and contralateral impairment of pain and temperature.
4. Symptoms of upper limb sensory loss and weakness with sparing of the legs due to a central cord syndrome.
5. Radiculopathy with variable myelopathic symptoms not classified above.

Cervical spine or radicular pain is not a prominent feature of CSM. In a number of series, it was present in only 10–19% (12). A typical feature of CSM is the "numb clumsy hand" in which the muscles are wasted and sensation is impaired. Other authors have described the amyotrophic hand in CSM, where there is no sensory impairment or increased tone; rather wasting and weakness are present.

Bladder disturbance in CSM commonly presents with irritative bladder symptoms, frequency, urgency and urge incontinence, with difficulty in voiding being less frequent. Tammela et al. found such symptoms of irritative bladder in 61% of patients with CSM and 46% had detrusor instability on urodynamic studies. This symptom is due to compression of the inhibitory pathways of the reticulospinal tract that pass superficially in the lateral columns (13).

Cervical spondylotic myelopathy may be difficult to distinguish from other neurological conditions and although improvements in imaging techniques and neurophysiology have improved the accurate diagnosis of this condition, it can still be difficult to confirm the diagnosis. The principal differential diagnoses that are often considered include other mass lesions causing cord compression such as extrinsic or intrinsic tumors and acute and chronic infection. These may be more easily excluded now using magnetic resonance (MR) scanning, but intrinsic cord tumurs may still prove a difficult diagnostic problem. Diagnostic problems may also occur in multiple sclerosis and motor neurone disease, which may both produce similar symptoms and signs to some cases of CSM. The emphasis must be on taking a meticulous history and examination together with MR imaging and, if doubt exists, examination of the cerebrospinal fluid (CSF) and where appropriate, neurophysiological tests of the sensory and motor pathways.

IV. NATURAL HISTORY

In making a decision whether conservative or surgical treatment is necessary, one needs to understand the natural history of a condition, then to establish that the results of treatment will lead to improvement. Unfortunately the natural history of CSM is poorly described. It had been generally accepted, since the original descriptions, that surgery was the treatment of choice, and long-term studies of the natural history in untreated cases were not performed. However, a few authors have attempted to look at this subject.

Lees and Aldren-Turner followed up 44 patients with CSM for between 1 and 32 years (14). Twenty-six patients were followed up for at least 5 years. The pattern of progression of the condition was an initial development of symptoms, precipitated by trauma in a small group, followed by long periods of static symptomatology or improvement. Further short exacerbations occurred at variable intervals over subsequent years, but were followed by further periods of stability or improvement. Very few patients had a progressive gradual deterioration. With respect to treatment, 28 patients were given a collar and of these, 17 improved, 7 remained unchanged, and 4 deteriorated. Eight patients had surgery, two improved, three remained unchanged, and one was made worse. In the 11 remaining cases, no treatment was given or the prescribed collar was not worn. These patients had a period of stable symptoms for between 2 and 30 years, and only 1 patient had a severe disability at the end of the follow-up period. Lees and Aldren-Turner concluded that CSM was a relatively benign condition in which progressive deterioration was rare and long periods of stable symptomatology occurred interspersed with short bouts of deterioration. They also noted that in a second group of 51 patients presenting with radiculopathy, only, there was no progression to myelopathy.

Nurick studied 91 patients and agreed that CSM was a generally benign and nonprogressive condition (15). He also reviewed the results of laminectomy for CSM published up to 1969 and found that they were not significantly different from the natural history of the condition. However, in his series patients treated by laminectomy did better than those treated conservatively although this did not reach statistical significance, and in the most severely affected patients the results were poor. In a small group of patients treated by Smith-

Robinson type anterior interbody fusion, the results of surgery were excellent in six of seven cases. Nurick found that age at presentation was a significant prognostic factor for subsequent deterioration, a factor not identified by Lees and Turner.

Symon and Lavender studied 48 cases of CSM treated surgically and compared them to Lees and Turner's patients. They found that 29 of 41 (70%) patients improved after cervical laminectomy. Although agreeing that those with mild disability remained unchanged and were not helped by surgery, they argued that with moderate or severe disability, significant improvement occurred as a result of surgery (16).

Phillips found 73% of cases had a sustained improvement after surgery (Cloward's procedure—see later) and results were best in those with less than 1 year's history of symptoms. He argued that Lees and Turner's series had a bias toward mild symptomatology and agreed that these cases were adequately treated with conservative measures. However, Phillips concluded that surgery should be performed before severe disability occurred or when moderate disability had been present for only a short time (17).

Clarke and Robinson found that although there were intermittent episodes of worsening in 75% of cases, there was a gradual progression of symptoms and signs between these episodes in two-thirds of patients. In only one-third was the condition stable between acute episodes. They also found that spontaneous improvement was rare (18). This view of a steady deterioration after presentation, with little spontaneous improvement is the typical experience of the majority of recent authors.

A number of authors have reviewed the issue recently (12,19–21) and concluded that there is a need to compare the various surgical procedures performed for CSM and the natural history of the condition. It would seem that, although desirable, this sort of study is unlikely to occur. The overwhelming surgical view is that surgery is beneficial and it would be ethically difficult to randomize a patient with severe disability or progressive deterioration into a study with a conservative or no treatment arm.

V. INVESTIGATION

The radiological investigation in suspected cases of CSM should include plain radiographs of the neck in flexion and the extension and an MR scan including T1- and T2-weighted images. In selected cases, computed tomography (CT) and/or myelography still have a role, particularly in the demonstration of calcification in soft tissues or bone abnormalities (22,23).

On plain radiography, the common features are loss of disc space height and osteophytes. Loss of the normal cervical lordosis may also be demonstrated and measurement of the A-P diameter of the canal is also useful. To avoid magnification errors it can be useful to express this as the ratio of the A-P diameter of the vertebral body compared to the canal at the same level (the Pavlov ratio). This ratio is approximately 1 in the normal population, and values less than 0.8 indicate a narrowed spinal canal. Dynamic studies in flexion and extension will demonstrate abnormal movement, which may influence the decision to operate and the type of procedure to be performed.

Magnetic resonance imaging is a safe noninvasive investigation that has the advantage of allowing visualization of the cord as well as the bones, discs, and ligaments. Images can be obtained in three planes and the whole length of the spinal canal and the brain can easily be imaged if necessary. Magnetic resonance imaging accurately identifies the level of maximal compression in CSM and whether this is anterior or posterior. Some osteophytes may not be adequately shown on MR but will be seen on plain radiography. In difficult cases where further information about bone or calcified soft tissues is required, fine-cut axial CT scans remain useful. Myelography with postmyelography CT, the previous mainstay of investigation, may still be used in a minority of cases when MR is contraindicated or degraded by artifact.

The ability of MR to image the spinal cord has allowed the demonstration of signal changes within the substance of the cord (Fig. 1). This was first reported, in association with compression in CSM by Takahashi, et al. in 1987 (24). In 128 patients with compressive lesions of the cervical cord, high signal on T2 images was seen in 18.8%. In those with herniated discs, this rose to 32.4%. Spinal cord constriction or narrowing was the most important associated finding. It was suggested that the signal change represented myelomalacia or cord gliosis secondary to compression (24,25). Experimentally it has been shown in animals that cord edema is seen as high signal on T2 images. Haupts and Haan favored a shear/stress hypothesis as a cause of the signal change (26). In a study of 29 patients with CSM treated by anterior spinal fusion, there was abnormal signal on T2 in 12 patients. The preoperative and postoperative disability of this group was greater than it was in the 17 with no cord signal change.

After surgery postoperative recovery was better in the five patients in whom the signal intensity decreased on postoperative MR. The possible prognostic significance of signal change has been confirmed in other series. Mehalic et al. found that the intensity of the signal change may also be significant (27). Patients with an intense but focal signal change did better than those with mild signal change who also tended to show cord atrophy. The suggestion was that intense signal change represents a reversible pathological process such as inflammation or edema, whereas mild signal change and atrophy represent irreversible gliosis. Yone et al. failed to find any relationship between signal change, disability, or postoperative outcome in patients with CSM even in those

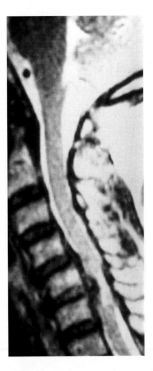

Figure 1 Sagittal T2-weighted MR scan demonstrating a large disc prolapse at C5-6 with significant cord compression and high signal within the spinal cord.

where the signal change resolved after surgery (28). The occurrence of signal change that is not congruent with areas of compression or is unduly extensive should raise the possibility of other pathologies, including spinal cord tumor and demyelination (Fig. 2).

It is also important to remember that changes attributable to CSM are found in a significant number of asymptomatic patients. Pallis, et al. found signs of cord or root compression in 50% of a group of patients with asymptomatic canal narrowing on x-ray and in 75% of those older than age 65 (29). Teresi, et al. looked at the cervical spine in 100 patients who had an MR for laryngeal disease. Disc protrusion was seen in 57% of patients older than 64 years of age and 20% of those aged 45–54 years. Cord compression was present in 7 of the 100 patients, although the reduction of cord area averaged 7% and did not exceed 16% (30).

Magnetic resonance imaging also has a useful role in the postoperative assessment of patients with CSM and this aspect is discussed later.

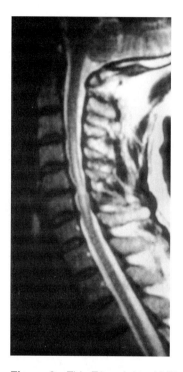

Figure 2 This T2-weighted MR scan shows extensive signal change within the spinal cord extending from C3-4 to C6-7. There is a disc protusion at C5-6. The extent of signal change raised the possibility of an alternative diagnosis including demyelination. Investigations were negative and the patient was treated by anterior cervical discectomy.

VI. NEUROPHYSIOLOGY

Neurophysiological assessment in CSM can be used as an aid in the diagnostic process or for intraoperative monitoring. In electrical diagnosis of radiculopathy and myelopathy, nerve conduction studies electromyograms (EMG) and evoked potential studies may be used. The former two techniques aid differentiation between peripheral nerve entrapment and neuropathy (a not uncommon source of confusion), radiculopathy (with lower motor neuron findings on EMG), and myelopathy. Somato-sensory evoked potentials (SEP) can also be useful. Median and ulnar SEP theoretically allow discrimination between plexopathy, radiculopathy, and myelopathy, although practically, the utility of such techniques can be disappointing. This can occasionally be due to coexistent pathologies. Yu and Jones found median nerve abnormalities in only in 5 of 21 cases of CSM and ulnar nerve abnormalities in 10 (31). Similarly, de Noordhoot et al.

found median nerve abnormalities in 25% of cases, and magnetic stimulation proved a more sensitive investigation of their patients with CSM (32).

Measurement of motor pathways is now also possible. Percutaneous magnetic stimulation, developed by Barker, et al., is a painless, safe technique that stimulates the motor cortex or nerve root at the intervertebral exit foramen and allows investigation of the motor evoked potential (MEP) and measurement of the motor conduction time of the corticospinal tract (33). The technique was first used in multiple sclerosis and motor neuron disease (MND) and has increasingly been reported in CSM (32,34–37).

The procedure initially involved assessment of the MEP to upper limb muscles. Subtraction of the conduction time during stimulation over the neck from conduction time during cortical stimulation gives the motor conduction time (MCT). This is the conduction time from the cortex to the anterior horn cell plus a short length of the motor root from the anterior horn cell to the intervertebral foramen. The true central motor conduction time (CMCT) can be calculated using the cortical motor latency and the F and M response obtained by electrical stimulation using the formula:

$$CMCT = \text{cortical latency} - (F + M - 1)/2$$

Measurements are usually made in the abductor pollicis brevis (APB) or abductor digiti minimi (ADM) but any upper limb muscle can be used. Brunholz and Claus also studied magnetic stimulation to the leg area and found that the CMCT to the tibialis anterior (TA) was a more sensitive indicator of extramedullary cervical cord compression (35). The CMCT to the TA was abnormal in 70% of cases but only 51% when measured to ADM. Subclinical lesions were also detected in 41% of patients who had prolonged CMCT with radiological evidence of cord compression but who had not yet developed clinical signs.

A study of clinical findings, SEP and magnetic stimulation found that the MEP was a sensitive indicator of spinal cord dysfunction (34). Magnetic stimulation detected abnormalities in 84% of patients with radiological evidence of cord compression, whereas SEP demonstrated abnormalities in only 25%. It was also found that a number of patients had subclinical abnormalities on magnetic stimulation before clinical disabilities developed. However postoperative improvement in clinical signs was not matched by normalization of the CMCT. Jaskolski, et al. did not detect subclinical lesions but did find that a postoperative clinical improvement was matched by an improvement in the motor conduction time (34). Abnormalities of the MEP are found in approximately 50% of patients with CSM. The role of magnetic stimulation in CSM is not yet established and the relationship between MR appearances, particularly cord signal change and delayed CMCT, is yet to be established. The significance of subclinical abnormalities and whether these should influence the decision to operate also remain open.

VII.   TREATMENT

The nonsurgical treatment of CSM may involve either simple observation and monitoring of the patient or treatment with a soft or hard collar. Although the use of a collar is widespread, the type of collar used and length of time it is worn vary. The collar should be fitted to hold the neck in the neutral or slightly flexed position. It should be remembered that patient compliance with an uncomfortable and restrictive treatment is often poor. Medical treatment of CSM may also include analgesia with nonsteroidal anti-inflammatory drugs; antispasmodic drugs are used in some cases.

In patients with moderate to severe neurological deficits and/or progressive disease, surgical intervention is common. The aim of surgical intervention for CSM is to relieve the narrowing of the cervical canal and to stabilize the vertebral column where abnormal mobility is present. Before surgery is contemplated, an unequivocal diagnosis of CSM must be made on the basis of a careful clinical history, examination, and imaging. The surgical procedures can be performed via a posterior or anterior approach.

The earliest procedure performed for CSM was cervical laminectomy. This operation remains appropriate in those with extensive multiple-level narrowing of the cervical canal and particularly when significant posterior compression is present due to hypertrophy or buckling of the ligamentum flavum. It is essential that the normal cervical lordosis is present, and cervical laminectomy is contraindicated in those with a kyphotic deformity. The presence of cervical instability is a second contraindication to surgery although in a small group, laminectomy after anterior cervical fusion may be appropriate. A laminectomy is performed at the affected level and at the levels above and below. In many cases, a C3 to C7 laminectomy is performed and this may be supplemented by foramenotomies at selected levels if radicular symptoms are also a feature.

The procedure is performed under general anesthesia and it is essential to take great care during induction and intubation to avoid forcible hyperextension of the neck and the risk of neurological injury. Awake, endoscopic intubation is often appropriate. The patient is positioned either prone or sitting. The sitting position, although popular with some surgeons because it allows a dry field, carries the risk of air embolism. Other surgeons find it uncomfortable. The patient should be positioned with the neck in neutral to avoid excessive stretching of the cord over any anteriorly placed discs or osteophytes. The skin and paraspinal muscles are infiltrated with lignocaine and adrenaline to provide postoperative analgesia and reduce blood loss. A laminectomy is then performed at the appropriate levels, taking care not to further compress the dural sac. Hypertrophied ligamentum flavum is also removed. In patients with a normal cervical lordosis once an adequate decompression has been performed, the dural sac bulges posteriorly. In cases with radiculopathy, a partial medial facet-ectomy and foraminal decompression can be performed to relieve nerve root compression (38). Previously additional maneuvers, including opening of the dura, dura grafting, sectioning of the dentate ligaments, and removal of anteriorly placed disc or osteophyte were performed. These procedures carry increased risks of cord injury and have not been shown to improve outcome. It has since been demonstrated that the dentate ligament does not hold the cord against any anterior compressive factors but transmits cephalocaudal stresses between cord and dura. After cervical laminectomy, early mobilization is encouraged, and a soft collar may be worn for comfort but is not essential. The typical hospital stay is 5 to 7 days.

The anterior approach for decompression and fusion of the cervical spine in CSM was developed simultaneously by a number of authors in the late 1950s (39–41). The rationale behind the approach was to provide a simple technique allowing access to and removal of anteriorly placed prolapsed disc and osteophyte with simultaneous fusion of the vertebral bodies. Since the initial introduction of this approach, it has steadily gained in popularity and various modifications have been introduced. A wide variety of procedures are now performed although the superiority of one technique over another has not been proven. An anterior cervical approach is most suited to cases in which compression is limited to one or two levels, although surgery can be performed at three or, very rarely, four levels. Instability, if present, can be dealt with by a simultaneous fusion procedure.

The operation is performed with the patient supine under general anesthesia with the same care taken at induction as mentioned above for cervical laminectomy. A skin crease incision is made extending from the midline to the anterior border of the sternomastoid muscle on one side (usually the right). A plane can then be established with the sternomastoid muscle and carotid sheath laterally and the larynx and pharynx medially leading to the vertebral column. Confirmation that the appropriate level has been identified is obtained by intraoperative x-ray screening of a spinal needle inserted into the disc space. This approach can provide access to up to three adjacent intervertebral discs between C3-4 and C7-T1. With minor modifications C2-3 and T1-T2 may be reached. Although the approach to the vertebral column is relatively standard with only minor differences between surgeons, the treatment of the disc, osteophytes, and the attitude to fusion varies considerably.

In the original description by Smith and Robinson, the disc and endplates were removed with no attempt to decompress the cord by removal of osteophytes (40). A wedge-shaped bone graft was tailored to fit the interspace to produce fusion. Cloward developed a technique that improved access by drilling out a cylindrical hole centerd on the disc. Prolapsed disc and osteophytes are removed and the cord decompressed. A dowel of bone is then cut to insert into the interspace to promote fusion, although other shapes of graft are also used (39). The aim of fusion in this procedure is to abolish abnormal movement and so reduce pain. Repeated spinal cord injury due to excessive movement is also prevented. Loss of disc space height, which may cause narrowing of the nerve root exit canals, is also avoided by immediate fusion. In addition fusion may promote resorption of osteophytes and for this reason some surgeons do not routinely excise osteophytes at the time of surgery (42). However, resorption may take several years and the majority of surgeons, having gained access to the disc space, proceed to remove significant posterior or posterolateral osteophytes using curettes, micropunches, or high speed drills. It is undoubtedly safer to perform such surgery under microscopic control. The use of the operative microscope with its good light source, appreciation of depth, and magnification allows adequate decompression of the cord and roots via the disc space without undue risk of injury. This technical advance means the bone exposure performed in a Cloward or Smith-Robinson procedure is not always required.

Further divergence of opinion is evident with regard to the posterior longitudinal ligament (PLL). Whereas some surgeons always leave this structure intact, others believe it should be opened and excised to expose the dura. Opening the PLL allows prolapsed disc that has protruded through an opening to be identified and removed, a finding in 5–35% of cases. This procedure also prevents buckling or nipping of the PLL, a possible cause of postoperative pain. If the PLL is opened, particular care must be taken not to injure the dural sac.

Whereas earlier operations always involved fusion, there has been a more recent move to anterior spinal decompression without fusion. Fusion using autologous bone usually means taking an iliac graft. This produces a 20% incidence of complications, commonly pain, which makes it unpopular with patients. Other graft sites previously used include tibia and the fibula for strut grafts in trench procedures (see below). Bone may also be used from bone banks, and xenografts with calf bone are also available. Nonbiological graft materials include methylmethacrylate, hydroxyapatite, and biopolymer. These materials do not produce superior results to bone but do avoid the possibility of donor site complications. Insertion of a graft provides stability and promotes fusion. However the results of surgery have not been shown to be influenced by the fusion rate. Using iliac bone fusion occurs in 70–100% of cases. Even in series when no graft has been inserted, the fusion rate is 74–100%.

The successful use of anterior cervical decompression without fusion was first reported in 1960. This procedure was initially used for acute soft disc protrusions causing radiculopathy or myelopathy when the osteophytic changes of established spondylosis are minimal. The disc is incised and removed, thus decompressing the cord or root, and the space left empty. This procedure produces excellent results in acute soft disc prolapse (43). When used in myelopathy due to CSM, osteophytes are also excised and the posterior border of the adjacent vertebrae may be removed to provide a more extensive decompression. The lateral extent of decompression is limited by the vertebral arteries. Some authors have found this procedure to be inferior to decompression and fusion. Yamamoto noted initial improvement in all patients but this was maintained in only 47% (44). Patients developed recurrent symptoms, new symptoms due to adjacent spur formation, or severe interscapular or cervical pain. An interbody fusion was added as a second procedure in four cases. More recently, Maurice-Williams and Dorward reported on 291 operations for CSM treated by single-level anterior cervical decompression without fusion in 92% of cases (45). In 21% of those cases, osteophytes alone caused the compression whereas in 79%, soft disc prolapse was significant. At early follow-up, only 4% were unchanged or worse and improvement in neurological symptoms was found in 94%. Neck pain was a postoperative problem in only 1%. Lesonin, et al. also found discectomy without fusion to be advantageous and preferred it to the Cloward procedure (46). Patients had less complications, a shorter postoperative stay, and were able to return to work earlier.

The complications of cervical surgery include the general complications of any operation such as chest infection or atelectasis, cardiac disorders, deep vein thrombosis, and pulmonary embolism. The mortality rate for anterior surgery is 0.3–1.5%. The soft tissue complications of anterior surgery include injury to the esophagus or trachea, pneumothorax, and thoracic duct injury. Vessels at risk are the carotid and vertebral arteries and the jugular vein. Hematoma may occur superficially in the neck, and extradural hematomas have been reported. Infection may be superficial and a minor problem but discitis can cause severe, prolonged pain. Neural structures that may be injured, other than the cord and roots, include the superior and recurrent laryngeal nerves and the sympathetic chain. Dural injury may result in a CSF fistula or meningitis.

The incidence of neurological deficit due to cord or root injury was 1.04% over a 5-year period covering 5,356 procedures of which 64% were anterior (47). Neurological complications were more common in posterior procedures compared to anterior, and the cord was more at risk during a posterior procedure. Others quote the rate of neurological complications at 2–8% for cervical laminectomy. Root symptoms after laminectomy may be due to traction secondary to dorsal displacement of the dural sac and cord after decompression. Complications due to anterior bone grafts include displacement and nonunion. At the donor site, infection, hematoma, and pain may ensue. The lateral cutaneous nerve of the thigh may be injured while taking iliac grafts.

Further surgical development has led to the operation of vertebrectomy with strut grafting. In this procedure a central gutter or trench is drilled out of the affected vertebral bodies extending across the disc spaces. After decompression the vertebral column is reconstructed with a long iliac, rib, or fibula graft. This operation is used for patients with severe multilevel disease (Fig. 3). Some

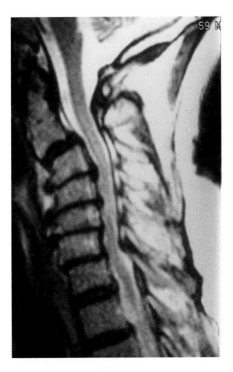

Figure 3 A T2-weighted MR showing multiple degenerative discs, loss of the normal cervical lordosis, and cord compression from C3-4 to C6-7.

authors have compared laminectomy, anterior decompression, and fusion and vertebrectomy with strut graft and found the latter procedure to produce superior results. Improvement in 70–80% of cases has been reported.

Instrumentation to provide more immediate stability is also used in some cases. Use of the Caspar system and anterior titanium plating has produced good results. The Caspar system requires bilaminar screw insertion and therefore carries a risk of cord or root injury, although this is not high in expert hands. The titanium anterior locking plate with cancellous screws avoids this risk and does not require intraoperative screening. Titanium also has the advantage of MR compatibility, allowing good-quality postoperative imaging if required.

VIII. RESULTS

The results of surgery for CSM are difficult to assess and compare for a number of reasons. Many of the studies are retrospective and include a wide range of cases from single-level acute soft disc prolapse in younger patients to elderly disabled patients with extensive multilevel spondylotic changes. The assessment of improvement is also variable. Three main scales are used (Odum, Nurick, and Japanese Orthopaedic Association [JOA]). The scale proposed by the JOA is increasingly used and benefits from assessing upper and lower limb function as well as bladder symptoms (48). The Nurick scale is an assessment of walking and is easy to apply (15). The outcome as assessed by Odum, et al. is graded from excellent to poor (49).

The published results of surgery vary widely for both posterior and anterior procedures. In the 45 cases first reported by Brain, et al., 21 had a posterior decompression (1). Improvement was noted in 16 cases although this was of moderate or marked degree in only 8. In 5 patients there was no change. Patients did better if they were younger than age 50 or had symptoms of less than 2 years' duration. Clarke and Robinson reported surgical results in 32 patients. Seventeen patients improved or stabilized but immediate deterioration occurred in five and a further six experienced longer-term deterioration. Although patients younger than 50 years tended to do better, this was not significant and the duration of symptoms was not found to be a factor. Nurick reviewed 474 cases reported to 1969 and found 56% improved, 25% remained unchanged, and 19% were worse. These results failed to suggest a significant benefit from posterior decompression when compared to conservative treatment. In 45 patients treated by laminectomy in his series, Nurick found 14 were improved, 21 were unchanged, and 10 were worse. In the conservatively treated group, 8 of 37 patients improved, 16 were unchanged, and 13 were worse. Other reports give better results from posterior surgery. Epstein found improvement in 80–85% of cases. In Hakuda's series of the patients treated by laminectomy or laminoplasty, symptoms recurred in only 10.5% (50). Symon and Lavender reported 60 cases of whom 48 improved, 10 remained unchanged, and only 2 were worse as a result of surgery (16). In a review of 1,000 cases by Lesonin, only 10 % had a deterioration during a 20-year follow-up period (46). Some of the earlier poor results may have been due to attempts to remove anterior osteophytes via a laminectomy or opening of the dura and section of the dentate ligaments, procedures that carry a higher risk of neurological injury. In a recent report of 100 cases of CSM treated between 1978 and 1988, 51 cases had a laminectomy. Although early (1 month) results were good with 66.6% improving, 21.6% unchanged, and 9.8% worse, late deterioration occurred and at last follow-up 37.3% had improved, 25.5% were unchanged, and 37.2% were worse. The only factor associated with a worse outcome was the preoperative duration of symptoms.

The published outcomes for anterior surgery in CSM have a similar wide range of results. Nurick reported that 55% of patients improved after anterior cervical decompression and fusion, 41% were unchanged, and 4% were worse.

A number of authors have found improvement in 70–94% of cases. Less favorable results have also been reported, where improvement occurs in only 50% of cases. A variety of surgical procedures were used in these series without influencing the outcome. A number of authors have found that early improvement may be lost and results at long-term follow-up are often worse. Various factors that have been found to influence outcome in some series include age, duration of symptoms, severity of symptoms, the involvement of the legs, and presence of bladder symptoms. The duration of symptoms before surgery is the most consistently significant factor.

The increased use of noninvasive imaging in CSM using MR has lead to the investigation of the causes of failure to improve after surgery. Clifton examined 56 patients with cervical spondylosis who had a poor result after surgery (51). Thirty-seven had myelopathy and nineteen a pure radiculopathy. Magnetic resonance imaging and computed myelography were used to assess the adequacy of surgery. In eight cases, an alternative diagnosis was reached. Only 12 of 56 cases had an adequate decompression at the correct level. Inadequate surgery was found in 32 cases due to residual compression at the operated level or failure to operate at other significantly compressed levels. Batzdorf and Flannigan evaluated 22 patients, of whom 12 were assessed as having had an adequate decompression (52). In the remaining 10 cases, cord compression persisted Harada reported better results in 51 patients with myelopathy due to spondylosis or calcification of the posterior longitudinal ligament (53). In only three was the degree of cord compression, unchanged although it had only partially resolved in 23. The degree of neurological recovery was worse in the three patients in whom a significant decompression was not achieved. These reports reinforce the need for accurate diagnosis and an adequate decompression performed at the correct level via the appropriate approach.

IX. CONCLUSION

Cervical spondylosis is a common degenerative condition that produces neurological complications of radiculopathy or myelopathy. These complications occur due to compression of the nerve roots or spinal cord in those with a narrowed spinal canal and are exacerbated by normal and abnormal movements. Secondary ischemia in the watershed zone due to narrowing of intramedullary vessels probably plays a role in the pathogenesis of myelopathy.

Patients present with varied symptoms and signs, and the degree of disability and the pattern of disease progression is variable. Investigation with plain radiographs and MR is appropriate, with CT in a minority. Treatment is conservative in those with minimal symptoms and stable disease. Surgery is indicated in those with more severe disability and when the condition is deteriorating. An anterior approach with or without grafting and fusion is appropriate for anteriorly placed lesions at one to three levels. More extensive disease and severe canal stenosis are amenable to posterior decompression by laminectomy. The results of surgery are variable and in some series do not differ greatly from the natural progression of the disease. Prognostic factors have yet to be identified, although increasing age of the patient and length of history are commonly associated with poor outcome. The significance of cord signal change on MRI and the role of magnetic stimulation and somato-sensory evoked potentials is not established. In view of the increasing age of the population, this condition is going to become more prevalent. Additional research needs to be directed to better patient selection for surgery and tailoring of treatment to the patient. Thus research should attempt to identify prognostic factors; also better outcome measures are needed if we are to improve the results of surgical intervention in this condition.

REFERENCES

1. Brain WR, Northfield D, Wilkinson M. The neurological manifestations of cervical spondylosis. Brain 1952; 75:187–225.
2. Lestini WF, Wicsel SW. The pathogenesis of cervical spondylosis. Clin Orthop 1980; 239:69–93.
3. Coventry MB. Anatomy of the intervertebral disk. Clin Orthop 1969;67:9–15.
4. Al-Mefty O, Harkey HL, Marawi I. Experimental chronic compressive myelopathy. J Neurosurg 1993; 79:550–561.
5. Bohlman HH, Emery SE. The pathophysiology of cervical spondylosis and myelopathy. Spine 1988; 13:843–846.
6. Barnes MP, Saunders M. The effect of cervical mobility on the natural history of cervical spondylotic myelopathy. J Neurol Neurosurg Psychiatry 1984; 47:17–20.
7. Nurick S. The pathogenesis of the spinal cord disorder associated with cervical spondylosis. Brain 1972; 92:87–100.
8. Brieg A, Turnbull I, Hassler O. Effects of mechanical stress on the spinal cord in cervical spondylosis. A study on fresh cadaver material. J Neurosurg 1966; 25:45–56.
9. Clark CR. Cervical spondylotic myelopathy: History and physical findings. Spine 1988; 13:847–849.
10. Crandall PH, Batzdorf U. Cervical spondylotic myelopathy. J Neurosurg 1966; 25:57–66.
11. Gregorius KF, Estrin T, Crandall PH. Cervical spondylotic radiculopathy and myelopathy. Arch Neurol 1976; 33:618–625.
12. Rowland PL. Surgical treatment of cervical spondylotic myelopathy: Time for a controlled trial. Neurology 1992; 42:5–13.
13. Tammela TLJ, Heiskari MJ, Lukkarinen OA. Voiding dysfunction and urodynamic

findings in patients with cervical spondylotic spinal stenosis compared with severity of the disease. Br J Urol 1992; 70:144–148.

14. Lees F, Aldren-Turner JW. Natural history and prognosis of cervical spondylosis. BMJ 1963; 92:1607–1610.

15. Nurick S. The natural history and the results of surgical treatment of the spinal cord disorder associated with cervical spondylosis. Brain 1972; 95:101–108.

16. Symon L, Lavender P. The surgical treatment of cervical spondylotic myelopathy. Neurology 1967; 17:117–121.

17. Phillips DG. Surgical treatment of myelopathy with cervical spondylosis. J Neurol Neurosurg Psychiatry 1973; 36:879–884.

18. Clarke E, Robinson PK. Cervical myelopathy. A complication of cervical spondylosis. Brain 1956; 79:483.

19. Uttley D, Monro P. Neurosurgery for cervical spondylosis. Br J Hosp Med 1989; 42:62–70.

20. LaRocca H. Cervical spondylotic myelopathy: Natural history. Spine 1988; 13:854–855.

21. Editorial. Management of cervical spondylotic myelopathy and radiculopathy. J Neurol Neurosurg Psychiatry 1994; 57:257–263.

22. Statham PF, Hadley DM, Macpherson P. MRI in the management of suspected cervical spondylotic myelopathy. J Neurol Neurosurg Psychiatry 1991; 54:484–489.

23. Alker G. Neuroradiology of cervical spondylotic myelopathy. Spine 1988; 13:850–853.

24. Takahashi M, Sakamoto Y, Miyawaki M, Bussaka H. Increased signal intensity secondary to chronic cervical cord compression. Neuroradiology 1987; 29:550–556.

25. Matsuda Y, Miyazaki K, Tada K, Yasuda A, Nakayama T, Murakami H, Matsuo M. Increased MR signal intensity due to cervical myelopathy. J Neurosurg 1991; 74:887–892.

26. Haupts M, Haan J. Further aspects of MR-signal enhancements in stenosis of the cervical spine. Neuroradiology 1988; 30:545–546.

27. Mehalie TF, Pezzuti RT, Applebaum BI. Magnetic resonance imaging and cervical spondylotic myelopathy. Neurosurgery 1990; 26:

28. Yone K, Sakou T, Yanase M, Yanase M, Ijiri K. Preoperative and postoperative magnetic resonance image evaluations of the spinal cord in cervical myelopathy. Spine 1992; 17:S387–S392.

29. Pallis C, Jones AM, Spillane JD. Cervical spondylosis. Incidence and complications. Brain 1954; 77:274–289.

30. Teresi LM, Kulkin RB, Reicher MA, Moffit BJ, Vinuela FU, Wilson GM, Bentson JR, Hanafee WN. Asymptomatic degenerative disc disease and spondylosis of the cervical spine: MR imaging. Radiology 1987; 164:83–88.

31. Yu YL, Jones SJ. Somatosensory evoked potentials in cervical spondylosis. Brain 1985; 108:273–300.

32. deNoordhoot M, Remacle JM, Pepin JL. Magnetic stimulation of the motor cortex in cervical spondylosis. Neurology 1991; 41:75–80.

33. Barker AT, Freeston IL, Jalinous R, Jarret JA. Clinical evaluation of conduction

time measurements in central motor pathways using magnetic stimulation of human brain. Lancet 1986; 1:1325–1326.
34. Dvorak J, Herdmann J, Janssen, Theiler R, Grob D. Motor-evoked potentials in patients with cervical spine disorders. Spine 1990; 15:1013–1016.
35. Brunholzl C, Claus D. Central motor conduction time to upper and lower limbs in cervical cord lesions. Arch Neurol 1994; 51:245–249.
36. Jaskolski DJ, Laing RJ, Jarratt JA, Jakubowski J. Pre- and postoperative motor conduction times, measured using magnetic stimulation, in patients with cervical spondylosis. Br J Neurosurg 1990; 4:187–192.
37. Herdmann J, Dvorak J, Vohanka S. Neurophysiological evaluation of disorders and procedures affecting the spinal cord and the cauda equina. Curr Opin Neurol Neurosurg 1992; 5:544–548.
38. Epstein JA. The surgical management of cervical spinal stenosis, spondylosis and myeloradiculopathy by means of the posterior approach. Spine 1988; 13:864–869.
39. Cloward R. The anterior approach for the removal of ruptured cervical discs. J Neurosurg 1958; 15:602–617.
40. Smith GW, Robinson RA. The treatment of certain spine disorders by anterior removal of the intervertebral disc and interbody fusion. J Bone Joint Surg (Am) 1958; 40:607–624.
41. Whitecloud TS III. Anterior surgery for cervical spondylotic myelopathy. Smith-Robinson, Cloward and vertebrectomy. Spine 1988; 13:861–863.
42. Gore DR, Sopie SB. Anterior cervical fusion for degenerated or protruded discs. Spine 1984; 9:667–671.
43. Bollati A, Galli G, Gandolfini M, Marini G, Gatta G. Microsurgical anterior cervical disc removal without interbody fusion. Surg Neurol 1983; 19:329–333.
44. Yammamoto I, Ikeda A, Shibuya N, Tsugane R, Sato O. Clinical long-term results of anterior discectomy without interbody fusion for cervical disease. Spine 1991; 16:272–279.
45. Maurice-Williams, Dorward N. Extended anterior cervical discectomy without fusion: A simple and sufficient operation for most cases of cervical degenerative disease. J Neurol Neurosurg Psychiatry 1995; 59:212.
46. Lesonin P, Bouasako N, Clarisse J, Rousseaux M, Tomin M. Results of surgical treatment of myeloradiculopathy caused by cervical arthrosis based on 1000 operations. Surg Neurol 1985; 23:350–355.
47. Graham JJ. Complications of cervical spine surgery. Spine 1989; 14:1046–1050.
48. Hirabayashi K, Miyakawa J, Stamoki K, Maruyama T, Wakano K. Operative results and post-operative progression of ossification among patients with ossification of the posterior longitudinal ligament. Spine 1981; 6:354–364.
49. Odum GL, Finney W, Woodall B. Cervical disk lesions. JAMA 1958; 166:23–28.
50. Hukuda S, Mochizuki T, Ogata M, Shichikawa K, Shimomura Y. Operations for cervical spondylotic myelopathy. A comparison of the results of anterior and posterior procedures. J Bone Joint Surg [Br] 1985; 67:609–615.
51. Clifton AG, Stevens JM, Whitear P, Kendall BE. Identifiable causes for poor outcome in surgery for cervical spondylosis. Neuroradiology 1990; 32:450–455.
52. Batzdorf U, Flannigan B. Surgical decompressive procedures for cervical spondy-

lotic myelopathy. A study using magnetic resonance imaging. Spine 1991; 16:123–127.

53. Harada A, Mimatsu K. Postoperative changes in the spinal cord in cervical myelopathy demonstrated by magnetic resonance imaging. Spine 1992; 17:1275–1280.

22

Ossification of the Posterior Longitudinal Ligament

Robert Jeffrey Martin

Harbin Clinic, Rome, Georgia

Christopher S. Kent

Navy Regional Medical Center, San Diego, California

I. INTRODUCTION

Ossification of the posterior longitudinal ligament (OPLL) is a progressive, degenerative disease of the spine, distinct from spondylosis, that is becoming more widely recognized as a cause of cervical myelopathy. Originally described in two patients by Key in 1838 in England, it wasn't until 1960 that an autopsy description made by Tsukimoto sparked interest in OPLL as a cause of cervical myelopathy (16). After some initial reports in the literature from Japan (28,38,42), OPLL was thought to be a rare cause of myelopathy restricted to persons of Mongolian Asian descent. However, with increased awareness this "Japanese disease" has become frequently recognized in non-Japanese patients (8,17). Because the management of OPLL may vary from that of degenerative spondylosis, the recognition of OPLL is important.

II. ANATOMY AND BIOMECHANICS

The PLL is formed from the mesodermally derived mesenchymal sclerotomes between the sixth and ninth week (2,18). The PLL extends on the dorsal surface of the vertebral body from the axis, where it is contiguous with the tectorial membrane, to the sacrum. It is wider cranially, tapers caudally, and is thickest in the thoracic region (30). The PLL is wider over the intervertebral disc and the contiguous margin of the vertebral bodies. It is narrow and more loosely adherent over the center of the vertebral bodies, from which it is separated by the basivertebral veins (6). It is formed from two layers; the superficial layer forms a strap that spans several vertebral bodies, whereas the deeper layer spans only two vertebral bodies and constitutes the lateral expansion at each intervertebral disc. As opposed to the anterior longitudinal ligament (ALL), the PLL is smaller in cross-sectional area but the fibers of the PLL are more compact (45).

The PLL has similar material properties to the ALL but as it is smaller in cross-sectional area, the average tensile load-to-failure of the PLL in the lower cervical spine is 74.5 Newtons (N), whereas that of the ALL is 111.5 N. The difference is even greater in the thoracic spine with the load-to-failure being 106 N for the PLL and 295.5 N for the ALL (45).

Similar to ligaments elsewhere in the body, the PLL is a uniaxial structure that functions to resist tensile loads. Ligaments are best able to resist loads applied in a direction parallel to their fibers and offer no resistance to compression. The PLL, because of its anatomical orientation, is best able to bear loads in flexion and shares in the resistance-to-flexion moments with the other posterior ligaments, such as the interspinous, supraspinous, and ligamentum flavum.

The loads to which the PLL is subjected in vivo is a complicated function of the orientation of its fibers and the movement of the vertebra. The load to which it is subjected in flexion will vary depending on the amount of movement and the distance from the instantaneous axis of rotation (IAR) in the sagittal plane of the vertebra that is being stabilized. A longer lever arm will give the ligament a mechanical advantage, and the physiological loads are less likely to exceed the biomechanical limits of the ligament. The greatest range of movement in the lower cervical spine occurs at C5 (45) and although the exact IAR of the cervical vertebra in flexion is unclear, it is thought to lie in the posterior inferior border of the subjacent vertebra for C2 and progressively move superior and anteriorly as one descends to the lower cervical spine (45). Thus, the PLL would be better able to resist flexion in the lower cervical spine than the upper cervical spine, and similarly, flexion is more likely to exceed load capabilities of the PLL in the upper cervical spine than the lower cervical spine. It is interesting to note that OPLL is frequently most severe at the C4 and C5 (15,27) level and commonly progresses in a cephalad direction (10). In addition, after laminectomy, which removes the other flexion load-bearing ligaments, the progression of OPLL increases (9). In laminoplasty, the rate of progression is reported to be less than it is after laminectomy (9) but there is a decrease in the range of movement, which would result in less stress on the PLL.

III. PATHOLOGY

The pathophysiological development of OPLL is similar to that seen in ectopic bone formation elsewhere in the body. Initially, the ossification presents as a proliferation of cartilaginous tissue where the PLL has fibrous connections with adjacent periosteal tissue (15,31). The cartilaginous tissue then begins to calcify by the process of endochondral ossification. This process then extends through the PLL and may involve, and erode through, the dura mater. As these foci of ossification become continuous, mature lamellar bone is formed, complete with haversian canals and marrow formation.

Although OPLL can occur at any point along the spine, from 70–95% of cases are found in the cervical spine (4,26,27). The rest are found in the upper T-spine and the upper L-spine. Cervical OPLL originates at higher levels than most other degenerative spine diseases, usually at C5, but frequently extends in the cephalad direction. This cephalad-caudad progression occurs at an average rate of 4 mm/year, whereas the ossification increases in the anteroposterior (AP) direction at 0.67 mm/year on average (4,11). OPLL also involves several vertebral levels, spanning 2.7–4.0 levels in various series (11,46). Most series report a male predominance; however Epstein and Kojima did not find a significant male preponderance (4,15). The incidence increases with age, peaking in the sixth decade, similar to spondylosis (4,51).

Genetic factors in the development OPLL have long been hypothesized, given the relatively high incidence in the Japanese and the increased incidence of OPLL within patients' families. Taketomi et al. (39) have reported OPLL in a set of monozygotic twins. Tanikawa et al. (40) and Terayama (41) both proposed a possible autosomal dominant mode of inheritance. Terayama studied the cervical x-rays of 1,030 relatives of 347 OPLL patients. He found that 28.89% of siblings and 26.15% of parents also had OPLL. He found no statistical sex difference.

As reported by Terayama (41), studies have investigated patients with OPLL to assess the correlation with human leukocyte antigens (HLA). These studies indicate that the inheritance pattern is complex, and they were unable to identify a single specific locus of HLA that was characteristic of OPLL. However, Sakou, et al. (33), in a family pedigree study, examined HLA haplotypes in 112 relatives of 33 patients with OPLL. They found that certain HLA antigens formed clusters, and when both sets of haplotypes were inherited, there was a 56% incidence of OPLL. When only one or no haplotype cluster was inherited, OPLL was not found. Their impression, and others (31), is that OPLL has a genetic predisposition, but that it is manifested in the presence of several other factors, such as aging, environmental factors, and vertebral instability.

Immunohistochemical studies of the PLL in cases of OPLL have shown bone morphogenetic protein-2 (BMP-2) and transforming growth factor-beta in the regions of calcification but not in the uninvolved areas (14). These growth factors can induce ectopic ossification that can progress to de novo bone formation in several in vivo models. It is still unclear what initiates the biosynthesis of these growth factors or even if they play a causal role in the pathophysiology of OPLL.

Recently, serum growth hormone binding protein (GHBP), which is believed to be a circulating fraction of the growth hormone membrane receptor, has been shown to be increased in OPLL (12). This may lead to a heightened osteoblastic response to normal circulating growth hormone levels. The search for a link with OPLL and growth hormone was prompted by the association of an increased incidence of OPLL in acromegalics. There are several other conditions associated with an increased incidence of OPLL but the pathophysiologic basis remains unclear (43).

Using cultured cells, Ishida attempted to identify differences between the ligamentous tissue in OPLL and normal PLL (13). He found that the ossification group consisted primarily of osteogenic primitive mesenchymal cells, whereas the normal group contained primarily fibroblast-like cells. The conclusion was that the PLL in the ossification group had a highly osteogenic potential and that this was a major factor in the development of OPLL.

Patients with OPLL are frequently asymptomatic. However with progressive compression of the spinal cord, symptoms develop because of vascular compromise. There seems to be a critical amount of canal compression before this occurs. In Harsh's series (8), the critical canal diameter was 9–10 mm. Abe used a stenosis ratio (A-P diameter of ossification/A-P diameter of canal $\times$ 100) to assess the critical amount of stenosis (1). Although a larger stenosis index is more likely to be associated with symptomatology, the absolute residual canal diameter is the more important number. Canals that have already been compromised by congenital stenosis or spondylosis are more likely to become symptomatic with concomitant OPLL than a canal with a normal diameter.

The histological damage is seen primarily in the gray matter (19,23). As the cord becomes compressed by the ossified ligament, the anterior horn appears flattened and there is a progressive loss of neurons, particularly in the middle of the central gray to the ventral aspect of the posterior columns. This area is a watershed region between the central artery, which comes from the anterior spinal artery, and the posterior spinal arterial system. That makes this area extremely susceptible to ischemic events. Mizuno, et al. (19) have proposed a staging system for spinal cord damage secondary to OPLL (Table 1).

Neuronal loss in the anterior horn occurs in stage 2–3; at this point, the damage done to the cord is irreversible. It is therefore important to recognize

Table 1 Pathological Stages from Compression by OPLL

Stage	
0	Normal or mild compression of the anterior horn without neuronal loss
1	Mild compression of the anterior horn with partial neuronal loss
2	Marked deformity of the anterior horn with severe neuronal loss
3	Severe spinal cord damage with cystic cavitation

Source: Ref. 19.

the disease as early as possible. The white matter is also involved as there may be myelin loss with destruction of axons that eventually leads to cavitation (22).

In addition to the myelopathy, patients may have radicular signs secondary to nerve root atrophy and axonal loss where the nerve roots are stretched over the ossified mass. The damage is most evident where the roots exit the cord and pierce the dura (4).

IV. RADIOLOGY

Radiographic diagnosis of OPLL is an integral part of the therapy, as it helps to show the degree of cord damage, the extent of the ossified mass, and helps in planning the surgical intervention. Based on the radiographic findings, OPLL is commonly divided into four subtypes according to Hirabayashi: segmental (39%), which is limited by the vertebral bodies; continuous (27%), which crosses multiple levels and disc spaces; mixed (29%), which has features of both segmental and continuous; and other (or localized) (7.5%), where the ossification is found over the disc spaces (9) (Fig. 1). In addition, Epstein has proposed a separate category called OPLL in evolution (OEV), consisting of varied early changes of calcification and hypertrophy of the PLL at the disc spaces and disc margins (4). Ossification of the posterior longitudinal ligament can further be classified based on axial images such as square, mushroom, or hill-type (10) (Fig. 2).

Lateral cervical x-ray may be useful in diagnosing OPLL by showing a bony density posterior to the vertebral bodies (Fig. 3). In a study by Ohtsuka (27), cervical OPLL was found in 3.2% of asymptomatic Japanese more than 50 years old, whereas Hirabayashi (10) reported a 1.7% incidence on cervical x-rays in outpatients. In the presence of myelopathy, recent estimates of the prevalence of OPLL on plain radiographs have been as high as 27% in Japan and 23% in the United States (4,17). However, plain x-ray can often miss mild

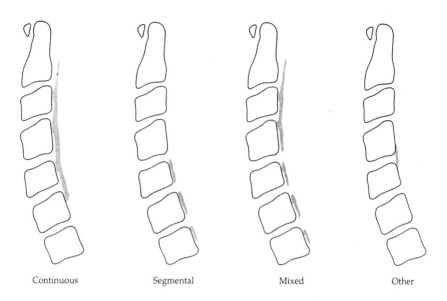

Figure 1 The classification of OPLL into four subtypes as described by Hira-bayashi. (From Ref. 9.)

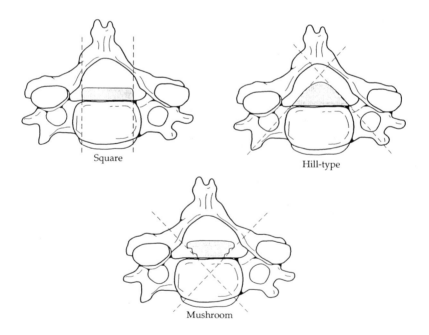

Figure 2 The classification of OPLL into three subtypes based on axial images. (From Ref. 9.)

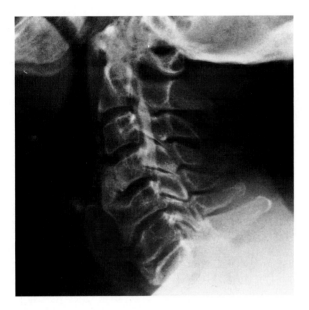

Figure 3 Plain film, with OPLL in the upper cervical spine clearly visible.

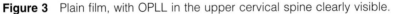

OPLL and small osteophytes and may fail to show the extension to the calcification behind the vertebral bodies that is diagnostic for OPLL. This would lead to the misdiagnosis of spondylosis.

Computed tomography (CT); myelo-CT, and polytomography can best fully define the extent of the ossified mass in OPLL. Computed tomography is able to detect OPLL when it is not visible on plain x-ray. Myelo-CT can also add to the information by delineating the amount of canal narrowing and cord compression. The ossification typically appears as an ovoid or oblong midline mass on axial images and may be separated from the vertebral body on some images, usually in the area removed from the disc space. This may represent the deep layer of the PLL that has not yet ossified (20,21). Hyperextension of the neck during CT-myelography should be avoided as it can exacerbate symptoms by further narrowing the canal and increasing the compression of the spinal cord.

Magnetic resonance imaging (MRI) has been shown to have increasing importance in the diagnosis of OPLL. On all spin echo (SE) images, OPLL appears as a low signal because of the lack of mobile protons in the cortical bone (Fig. 4). This can make visualization of OPLL on these types of images difficult (20). Although the average thickness of the ossified ligament is 6 mm in the continuous type and 3 mm in the segmental type, MRI is able to detect most cervical ossifications greater than 3.2 mm. With the development of fatty marrow in the ossification, one may see increased signal on T1 images making the diagnosis more apparent (32). This finding has been reported in 56% of the continuous type of OPLL[29] and in 11% of the segmental type (47). Signal changes within the spinal cord itself in areas of chronic compression on T2 or proton density images may be seen. This may represent either edema, demyelination, gliosis, or necrosis and correlates with the degree of clinical myelopathy as well as being a poor prognostic indicator. An increased T2 signal in the cord has been reported in 34% of patients with continuous OPLL and in 16% of those with the segmental type (47). This finding correlated to the thickness of the ossified ligament and the degree of spinal cord compression (29).

As MRI technology improves, more authors contend that MRI is an indispensable tool for diagnosis. McAfee, in a study of 106 cervical MRIs, concluded that MRI is advantageous over CT for several reasons, including noninvasiveness, no radiation exposure, ease of obtaining multiple images in various planes, ease of dynamic (flexion/extension) cord imaging, and better view of the cervicothoracic junction (17). Axial images are needed in cases of thinly ossified OPLL, as they can be easily missed on sagittal section.

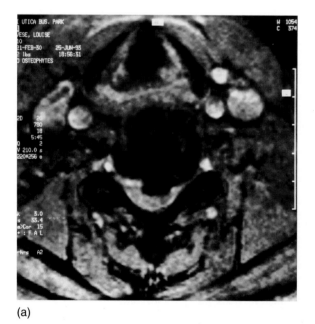

(a)

Figure 4   (a,b) Axial and (c) sagittal MRI images demonstrating the T2 low-signal intensity from OPLL.

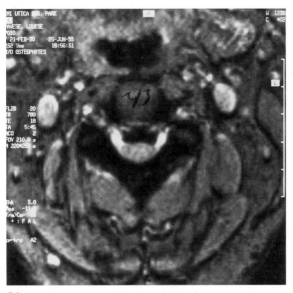

(b)

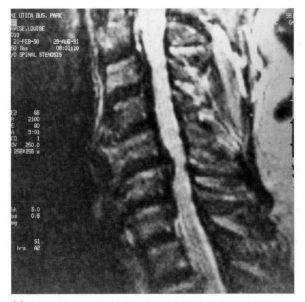

(c)

V. PRESENTATION AND THERAPY

Although most cases of OPLL remain asymptomatic, the onset of symptoms in those patients that do become symptomatic is usually gradual (24). In 80% there is no precipitating factor. Trauma leads to symptoms referable to OPLL in only 20% of patients (43,44). In Hirabayashi's accumulated cases of 2,162 patients, 47.7% presented with pain or dysesthesias of the upper limb, 41.9% had neck pain, 19% had pain in the lower limbs, 15.4% had motor disturbances of the lower limbs, 10.4% had motor disability in the upper limb, and only 1.0% presented with bladder dysfunction (Table 2) (10). In Harsh's series of 20 patients, the most common presentation was spastic quadraparesis, and the interval between initial symptoms and diagnosis was 7.5 months (8).

There are two approaches to the treatment of patients with OPLL, either conservative or surgical. A course of conservative management consisting of immobilization and bed rest, except in patients with a rapidly evolving myelopathy, is indicated. Those patients who are asymptomatic or present with only minimal deficits do well with conservative care (43). In a 5-year follow-up study of patients with only mild neurological deficits treated conservatively, 26.7% improved, 54.8% were unchanged, and only 18.5% deteriorated (10). However, OPLL is a slowly progressive disease and these patients need to be monitored closely to detect the onset of a rapid deterioration. Patients in whom surgical therapy is being considered may also benefit from a course of conservative management to reduce cord edema preoperatively.

Patients who present with severe myelopathy or who show deterioration of their neurological function require surgical decompression. We routinely give perioperative steroids, as these patients frequently have marked spinal cord compromise. Once the decision to operate has been arrived at, the choice of approach, either anterior, posterior, or both must be made. In the past, posterior approaches were preferred as OPLL frequently involves multiple levels, which increases the complexity of anterior operations. However the results from lami-

Table 2 Symptoms at Presentation of 2,162 Patients in Hirabayashi's Series

Pain/dysesthesias in upper extremities	47.7%
Neck pain	41.9%
Pain/dysesthesia in lower extremities	19.0%
Weakness—upper extremities	10.4%
Weakness—lower extremities	15.4%
Bladder dysfunction	1.0%

Source: Ref. 10.

nectomy are mixed, with reports of increased neurological deficits, such as nerve root palsies (3,49). These are thought to be secondary to traction on the roots with posterior migration of the cord. Also, the rate of progression of OPLL has been reported to increase after posterior decompressive procedures (9), possibly due to increased cervical mobility and increased biomechanical stress on the PLL. The increased rate of progression may be less with laminoplasty; however the open-door laminoplasty as described by Hirabayashi, et al. may reduce the cervical range of motion to one-half of the preoperative state (11). Numerous techniques of laminoplasty have now been described in the literature. Enlargement of the canal in the A-P diameter by 4–5 mm appears to be adequate for neurological improvement in most cases (11). There have been cases of the lamina collapsing and restenosing the canal, and careful attention to technique is required to prevent this (11,35). In addition, Nakano, et al. compared open-door laminoplasty to laminectomy and found no difference in clinical results (25).

The posterior approaches, however, do not directly address the anterior compressive bony mass on the spinal cord. As more experience with anterior multilevel corpectomies has been acquired, this now seems to be the preferred approach in terms of improvement of the neurological deficits and the prevention of further progression of the OPLL (1,15,48). However, anterior discectomies in the segmental type of OPLL may accelerate the ossification of the remaining PLL (9). The reports of serious complications with multilevel anterior corpectomies are low, but it is a technically demanding operation. One must be certain to perform a wide decompression to completely remove the ossified ligament. The lateral epidural veins are frequently a good landmark of the nerve roots emerging from the dural tube and bleeding from them is easily controlled with thrombin-soaked gelfoam. It is important though to work from the center laterally, especially in cases of thick or pedunculated OPLL so that the ossified ligament is not separated from the bony attachments to the vertebra and "floats" free. Drilling the ligament without causing further compression of the cord is then almost impossible, and peeling it up if it is still quite thick is difficult as it may torque into the cord causing further compression. Although leaving the ossified ligament and immobilizing the neck with a strut graft has been described with clinical improvement, in only 50% of cases did the ligament "float" away from the cord to achieve decompression (7). In certain instances, though, this may be preferable than continuing the attempt at a radical resection.

In 1/3 of the cases of OPLL, the dura is involved so that removal of the ossified ligament results in a dural defect (1). This may be repaired with an autogenous muscle or fascial graft along with postoperative lumbar cerebrospinal fluid (CSF) drainage, limitation of positive mechanical ventilation, and antiemetic medications (37).

Once the decompression is complete, the spine needs to be stabilized. Vascularized fibula grafts in the cervical spine that incorporate quickly have been described (5) but present obvious technical challenges, and their use in OPLL in most cases is unnecessary. Autogenous grafts fuse faster than allografts but, at least in single-level fusions, the clinical results are equivalent (50,52). If autogenous bone is selected, the iliac crest is simple to harvest and is practical for one-level to two-level corpectomies. If a longer strut graft is required, then the natural curve of the iliac crest may make this bone impractical. In that situation, the fibula may be used. An important consideration in the use of autogenous bone is the complications from the donor graft site. These include infection, hematoma, and persistent donor graft site pain. The use of allograft can avoid these potential problems (36). At our institution, allograft fibula has been used for several years with excellent clinical results.

With longer strut grafts, internal fixation is useful to prevent graft dislodgment and may avoid an external halo orthosis. The use of instrumentation is especially advisable when a posterior decompressive procedure has or will be performed. There is now a long experience with anterior cervical plates and, with adequate attention to detail, the complication rate is minimal.

Satomi and Hirabayashi have recommended both posterior and anterior procedures in cases of mixed-type OPLL that have a localized prominent ossification. The posterior decompression is done first to provide room for the cord, followed by the anterior decompression. The authors suggest waiting 3–6 weeks between operations (34).

VI. PROGNOSIS

The prognosis in OPLL is dependent on many factors. The most important is the neurological condition of the patient when the diagnosis is first made. Patients with neck pain, hand numbness, and/or urinary disturbances have reportedly fared best, whereas patients older than age 60, with myelopathy present for more than 2 years, or with more than 60% canal stenosis did not improve (9). Those patients with intrinsic spinal cord signal changes on MRI and presumably stage 2 or stage 3 injuries of the cord may not benefit from decompression other than possibly to avoid further deterioration (19).

So that although the natural history of OPLL is relatively benign, profound neurological deficits can and do occur. To prevent these deficits, more aggressive treatment directed at decompressing and stabilizing the spine is frequently indicated.

REFERENCES

1. Abe H, Tsuru M, Ito T, Iwaski Y, Koiwa M. Anterior decompression for ossification of the posterior longitudinal ligament of the cervical spine. Neurosurgery 1981; 55:108–116.
2. Bardeen CR, et al. In: *Manual of Human Embryology.* Vol. 1. Edit Keibel and Mall, eds. Philadelphia: J. B. Lippincott, 1910.
3. Correa A, Beasley B. Ossification of the posterior longitudinal ligament. NY State J Med 1980; 80:1972–4.
4. Epstein NE. Ossification of the posterior longitudinal ligament: Diagnosis and surgical management. Neurosurg Quarterly 1992; 2(3):223–241.
5. Friedberg S, Gumley G, Pfeifer B, Hybels R. Vascularized fibular graft to replace resected cervical vertebral bodies. Neurosurg 1989; 71:283–286.
6. Gray H. *Anatomy of the Human Body.* In: Goss CM, ed. 29th American ed. Lea and Febiger, 1973.
7. Hanai K, Inouye Y, Kawai K. Anterior decompression for myelopathy resulting from ossification of the posterior longitudinal ligament. J Bone Joint Surg 1982; 64 B:561–564.
8. Harsh GR, Sypert GW, Weinstein PR, Ross DA, Wilson CB. Cervical spine stenosis secondary to ossification of the posterior longitudinal ligament. J Neurosurg 1987; 67:349–357.
9. Hirabayashi K, Miyakawa J, Satomi K. Operative results and postoperative progression of ossification among the patients with ossification of cervical posterior longitudinal ligament. Spine 1981; 6:354–363.
10. Hirabayashi K, Satomi K, Sasaki T. Ossification of the posterior longitudinal ligament in the cervical spine. In: *The Cervical Spine.* 2nd ed. Philadelphia: J. B. Lippincott, 1989.
11. Hirabayashi K, Watanabe K, Suzuki N, Satomi K, Ishii Y. Expansive open door laminoplasty for cervical spinal stenotic myelopathy. Spine 1983; 8(7):693–699.
12. Ikegawa S, Kurokawa T, Hizuka N, Hoshino Y, Ohnishi I, Shizume K. Increase of serum growth hormone-binding protein in the patients with the ossification of the posterior longitudinal ligament of the spine. Spine 1993; 18(13):1757–1760.
13. Ishida Y. Studies on induction mechanism of ossification of the posterior longitudinal ligament of the spine, especially on the cultured cells from the human spinal ligament. J Jpn Orthop Assoc 1988; 62(11):1019–1027.
14. Kawaguchi H, Kurokawa T, Hoshino Y, Kawahara H, Oqata E, Matsumoto T. Immunohistochemical demonstration of bone morphogenetic protein-2 and transforming growth factor-B in the ossification of the posterior longitudinal ligament of the cervical spine. Spine 1992; 17(3S):S33–S35.
15. Kojima T, Wada S, Kubo Y, Kanamaru K, Shimosaka S, Shimizeu T. Anterior cervical vertebrectomy and interbody fusion for multi-level spondylosis and ossification of the posterior longitudinal ligament. Neurosurgery 1989; 24:864–872.
16. Lee T, Chacha PB, Khoo J. Ossification of posterior longitudinal ligament of the cervical spine in non-Japanese asians. Surg Neurol 1991; 35:40–44.

17. McAfee PC, Regan JJ, Bohlman HH. Cervical cord compression from ossification of the posterior longitudinal ligament in non-Orientals. J Bone Joint Surg 1987; 69B(4):569–575.

18. McLone DG. Development of the spine and spinal cord. In: *Neurosurgery. The Scientific Basis of Clinical Practice.* 2nd ed. Crockard A, Hayward R, Hoff JT, eds. 1992; 84–95. Blackwell Scientific Publication Boston:

19. Mizuno J, Nakagawa H, Iwata K, Hashizume Y. Pathology of spinal cord lesion caused by ossification of the posterior longitudinal ligament, with special reference to reversibility of the spinal cord. Neurol Res 1992; 14:312–314.

20. *MRI and CT of the Spine:* Case Study Approach. Kricun R, Kricun M, eds. New York: Raven Press, 1994.

21. Murakami J, Russell WJ, Hayabuchi N, Kimura S. Computed tomography of posterior longitudinal ligament ossification: Its appearance and diagnostic value with special reference to thoracic lesions J Comp Assist Tomogr 1982; 6(1):41–50.

22. Murakami N, Muroga T, Sobue I. Cervical myelopathy due to OPLL: A clinical pathology study. Arch Neurol 1978; 35:33.

23. Nakagawa H, Mizuno J. The pathophysiology and management of ossification of the posterior longitudinal ligament. Perspectives in Neurological Surgery 1992; 2(3):38–48.

24. Nakanishi T, Mannen T, Tokoyura Y. Asymptomatic ossification of the posterior longitudinal ligament of the cervical spine. Neurol Sci 1973; 19:375–381.

25. Nakano N, Nakano T, Nakano K. Comparison of the results of laminectomy and open-door laminoplasty for cervical spondylotic myeloradiculopathy and ossification of the posterior longitudinal ligament. Spine 1988; 13(7):792–794.

26. Nose T, Egashira T, Enomoto T, Maki Y. Ossification of the posterior longitudinal ligament: A clinico-radiological study of 74 cases. J Neurol Neurosurg Psychiatry 1987; 50:321–326.

27. Ohtsuka K, Terayama K, Yanagihava M, Wada K, Kasuga K, Machida T, Matsushima S. A radiological population study on the ossification of the posterior longitudinal ligament in the spine. Arch Orthop Trauma Surg 1987; 106:89–93.

28. Onji Y, Akiyama H, Shimomura Y, Ono K, Hukuda S, Mizuno S. Posterior paravertebral ossification causing cervical myelopathy: A report of eighteen cases. J Bone Joint Surg (AM) 1967; 49:1314–28.

29. Otake S, Matsuo M, Nishizawa S, Sano A, Kuroda Y. Ossification of the posterior longitudinal ligament: MR evaluation. AJNR 1992; 13:1059–1070.

30. Parke WW. Development of the spine. In: Rothman R, Simeone F, eds. *The Spine* 3rd ed. Philadelphia: W.B. Saunders Co., 1992.

31. Saika M. A morphological study on the etiology and growth of ossification of the posterior longitudinal ligament of the spine. J Jpn Orthop Assoc 1987; 61:1059–1072.

32. Sakamoto R, Ikata T, Murase M, Hasegawa T, Fukushima T, Hizawa K. Comparative study between magnetic resonance imaging and histopathologic finding in ossification or calcification of ligaments. Spine 1991; 16(11):1253–1261.

33. Sakou T, Taketomi E, Matsunaga S, Yamaquchi M, Sonoda S, Yashiki S. Genetic study of the ossification of the posterior longitudinal ligament in the cervical spine with human leukocyte antigen haplotype. Spine 1991; 16(11):1249–1252.

34. Satomi K, Hirabashi K. Ossification of the posterior longitudinal ligament. In: Rothman R, Simeone F eds *The Spine*. 3rd ed. Philadelphia: W.B. Saunders Co., 1992.

35. Satomi K, Nishu Y, Kohno T, Hiabayashi K. Long Term followup of the studies of the open door expansive laminoplasty for cervical stenotic myelopathy. Spine 1994; 19(5):507–510.

36. Segal HD, Harway RA. Orthop Rev 1992; 21:367–369.

37. Smith M, Bolesta MJ, Leventhal M, Bohlman HH. Postoperative cerebrospinal-fluid fistula associated with erosion of the dura. J Bone Joint Surg 1992; 74-A(2):270–277.

38. Suzak K, Udagawa E, Nagano M, Takada S. Ectopic calcification in the cervical epidural space and its clinical significance. J Jpn Orthop Assoc 1962; 36:256–261.

39. Taketomi E, Sakou T, Matsunaga S, Yamaguchi M. Family study of a twin with ossification of the posterior longitudinal in the cervical spine. Spine 1992; 17(3S):S55–S56.

40. Tanikawa E. Genetic study of OPLL. Bull Tokyo Med Dent Univ 1986; 33:117–128.

41. Terayama K, Furuya K, Nakajima H. Genetic studies on ossification of the posterior longitudinal ligament of the spine. Spine 1981; 14(11):1184–1191.

42. Terayama K, Maruyama S, Miyashita R, Mina K, Kinoshita M, Shimizu Y, Machizuki I. On the ossification of the ligament longitudinal posterior in the cervical spine. Orthop Surg Tokyo 1964; 15:1083–1095.

43. Trojan D, Pouchot J, Pokrupa R, Ford RM, Adamsbaum C, Hill RO, Esdaile JM. Diagnosis and treatment of ossification of the posterior longitudinal ligament of the spine. Amer J Med 1992; 92:269–306.

44. Tsuyama N, Terayama K, Ohtanik. The ossification of the posterior longitudinal ligament in the cervical spine (OPLL). J Jpn Ortho Assoc 1989; 55:425–440.

45. White AA, Panjabi MM. *Clinical Biomechanics of the Spine*. 2nd ed. Philadelphia: J.B. Lippincott Co., 1990.

46. Yamamoto I, Kageyama N, Nakamura K, Takahashi T. Computed tomography in ossification of the posterior longitudinal ligoma in the cervical spine. Surg Neurol 1979; 12:414–418.

47. Yamashita Y, Takahashi M, Matsuno Y, Sakamoto Y, Yoshizumi K, Oguni T, Kojima R. Spinal cord compression due to ossification of ligaments: MR imaging. Radiology 1990; 175(3):843–848.

48. Yang DY, Yang YC, Lee CS, Chou DY. Ossification of the posterior cervical longitudinal ligament. Acta Neuochir 1992; 115:15–19.

49. Yonenobu K, Hosono N, Iwasaki M, Asano M, Ono K. Neurologic complications of surgery for cervical compression myelopathy. Spine 1991; 16(11):1277–1282.

50. Young WF, Rosenwasser RH. An early comparative analysis of the use of fibular allograft versus autologous iliac crest graft for interbody fusion after anterior cervical discectomy. Spine 1993; 18(9):1123–1124.

51. Yu YL, Leong JC, Fang D, Woo E, Huang CY, Lau HK. Cervical myelopathy due to ossification of the posterior longitudinal ligament. Brain 1988; 111:769–783.

52. Zdeblick TA, Ducker TB. The use of freeze dried allograft bone for anterior cervical fusions. Spine 1991; 16:726–729.

23

Imaging of Spinal Disease

Simon Barker

Southampton General Hospital, Southampton, Hampshire, England

I. INTRODUCTION

The imaging of patients with spinal pathology was dominated by the use of plain radiographs and myelography in most neurological centers in the United Kingdom until the early 1990s. All of those centers now have access to magnetic resonance scanners and there has been a rapid and dramatic change in the method of examination of the majority of such patients. Additionally there have been changes in both the expectations of patients and in the threshold at which physicians will ask for radiological examination now that a noninvasive method of visualizing the spinal cord is available.

II. METHODS AVAILABLE FOR EXAMINATION

The methods available for examination of the spine are summarized in Table 1. Noninvasive techniques should be used initially to secure a diagnosis.

A. Plain Radiographs

Plain radiography remains the most common radiographic examination of the spine. The spine may be considered as six radiographic regions: atlanto-occipi-

Table 1 Main Techniques Used for
Diagnostic Imaging of the Spine

Plain radiography
Isotope bone scans
Myelography
Computed tomography
Magnetic resonance imaging
Spinal angiography
Discography and facet joint arthrography

---

tal, cervical, cervicothoracic, thoracic, lumbar, lumbosacral. The standard radiographic projections of each of these regions are anteroposterior (A–P) and lateral. In the cervical and lumbar regions, oblique projections allow visualization of the neural foramina and pars interarticulares. Lateral radiographs of the cervical and lumbar spine in flexion and extension after careful study of radiographs in standard projections may yield information about instability of the spine or the degree of movement possible.

Plain radiographs visualize the bones of the spine. They may provide limited information about large soft tissue masses arising inside the spinal canal or from the vertebral column. The normal intervertebral discs and contents of the spinal canal are not visualized.

B. Myelography

This involves the injection of contrast medium into the subarachnoid space and subsequent manipulation of the patient into a series of positions to obtain the optimum radiographic views of the spinal cord and/or nerve roots. Gas and oil contrast media have been superseded by water-soluble contrast media. Oil contrast media may produce a chronic inflammatory reaction in the leptomeninges (arachnoiditis), which is made worse by the presence of subarachnoid blood. The use of oil contrast media had been largely discontinued in the United Kingdom by the late 1970s; however, the side effects of their use continue to be of concern and importance in neurological practice. Of the water-soluble contrast media available, iopamidol and iohexol are the most widely used in the United Kingdom. They are both so called "nonionic" compounds and are relatively free from side effects.

Lumbar puncture is the usual site for the introduction of contrast medium. If this is carried out at L2-3 or L3-4, it avoids the normal spinal cord, which usually terminates at or above L1, and the most common sites of lumbar disc protrusions. The lumbar puncture may be carried out with the patient prone and a pillow under the abdomen to flex the lumbar spine, in the lateral decubitus position, or with the patient sitting with the back flexed. Lateral cervical puncture at the C1-2 level was introduced to overcome some of the initial difficulties experienced in obtaining good myelographic images of the cervical region with water-soluble contrast media. However there are potential hazards with this technique, particularly in patients with suspected lesions at or just below the foramen magnum or an expanded cervical cord (Fig. 1), and I always carry out myelography via lumbar puncture initially.

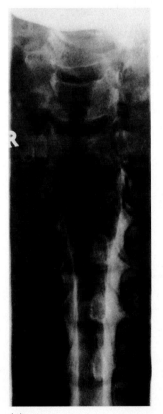

(a)

Figure 1 Spinal hemangioblastoma. (a) Myelography demonstrates expansion of the cervical cord seen as a filling defect in the contrast medium-filled subarachnoid space. (b) CT after myelography at the level of C1. An exophytic nodule (white arrow) protrudes posterolaterally on the right from the expanded cord. A thin rim of contrast medium is seen (black arrows). (c) Sagittal T1-weighted postgadolinium MRI. The enhancing nodule of the hemangioblastoma is seen at C1 (black arrowhead) and the associated syrinx (black arrow) extends down to the upper border of T1. The danger of a lateral cervical puncture for myelography in such a patient is obvious.

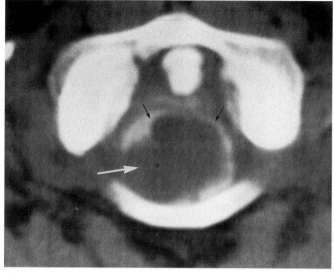

(b)

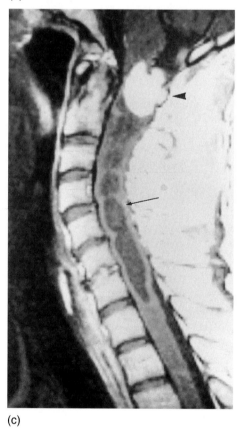

(c)

Figure 1 Continued

1. Complications of Myelography

Headache after lumbar puncture is common and its incidence and severity are reduced if a 22-gauge rather than a 20-gauge needle is used. Meningitis is very rare. Cervical puncture may damage the posterior inferior cerebellar artery, but this is very rare. Focal or generalized seizures may occur and are exacerbated by use of an excessive dose of contrast medium and uncontrolled flooding of it into the intracranial subarachnoid space. When there is partial or complete obstruction due to a compressive lesion in the spine, the removal of spinal fluid may worsen the patient's clinical condition.

C. Computed Tomography

Computed tomography (CT) uses a rotating x-ray tube together with a rotating or fixed set of detectors to obtain an image of a thin section of tissue. Multiple slices of tissue are scanned sequentially during a single study. The patient is usually supine in the scanner, as this is more comfortable than the prone position. The direct images of the spine are axial sections but coronal, sagittal, or oblique reformations are possible. There is inevitably some loss of contrast and spacial resolution when reformatted images are made.

Plain CT is good for visualizing the vertebral column (Fig. 2). The contents

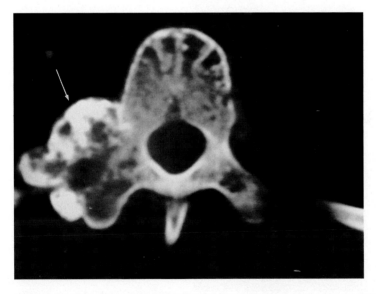

Figure 2 Osteochondroma. Axial CT scan through thoracic vertebra demonstrates exostosis arising from right transverse process (white arrow). The cortex of the exostosis and its medullary cavity are contiguous with that of the underlying bone.

of the spinal canal are relatively poorly seen, although epidural fat does help to outline the thecal sac. The spinal cord can be seen in the upper cervical region. Lumbosacral nerve roots are visualized, surrounded by epidural fat, in the intervertebral foramina. The addition of intrathecal contrast medium allows the whole of the spinal cord to be seen on CT. The cord has an elliptical shape in the cervical region and lies centrally in the canal. In the thoracic region, the cord has a more rounded appearance and lies anteriorly in the canal. Intrathecal nerve roots are also visible with intrathecal contrast, although demonstration of them in the cervical and thoracic region is variable. The nerve root sheaths fill with contrast in the lumbosacral region, and this can easily be seen on CT.

If CT is to be carried out after myelography, the patient is usually transferred to the scanner within 60 minutes of the initial procedure so that contrast medium has not dispersed. However there are some indications for delayed

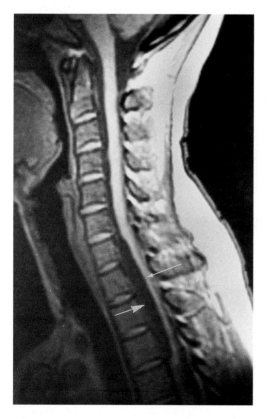

Figure 3 Arachnoid cyst. Sagittal T1-weighted MRI scan shows the cord (small white arrow) displaced posteriorly and compressed by an anterior intradural mass that is isointense to cerebrospinal fluid (large white arrow).

scanning. When a syrinx is suspected, scanning delayed for up to 36 hours may demonstrate contrast medium centrally within the cord. Spinal arachnoid cysts (Fig. 3) may be difficult to diagnose on myelography: the slower clearance of contrast medium from them than from the subarachnoid space may allow confirmation of this diagnosis by delayed scanning.

D. Magnetic Resonance Imaging

Magnetic resonance imaging (MRI) relies on the presence of MR-active nuclei in tissues, which align their rotational axis parallel or antiparallel to an external magnetic field. If an appropriate radiofrequency pulse is applied to these nuclei, they are displaced from their alignment and attain higher energy level. Once the radiofrequency pulse has stopped, the nuclei return to their original axis and in so doing, emit energy as a radiofrequency signal that can be detected. To be an MR-active nucleus, it is necessary to have an odd number of protons in the nucleus. Hydrogen is used for clinical MRI because of its abundance in the human body and large magnetic moment. Three parameters determine the images produced: proton density, T1 recovery and T2 decay of the tissue under scrutiny. The latter two are time constants. It is possible to obtain images *weighted* to each of these parameters and thus obtain three different types of image. This contrasts with CT, in which the image produced depends only on the electron density of the tissue examined, and so only a single type of image is available. It is possible to produce an image in any plane with the patient lying supine in the MR scanner. The sagittal plane is of obvious use in the spine. The high contrast resolution obtained in MRI allows direct visualization of the cord and cervical and lumbosacral nerve roots.

Contrast media may be used in MRI of the spine. They have in common the element gadolinium and are bound to one of a number of chelates to form a relatively safe water-soluble compound. These gadolinium chelates are paramagnetic substances that have a positive effect on magnetic susceptibility. At standard concentrations, they cause shortening of T1 and thereby increase, or brighten, the signal on T1-weighted images. The use of contrast medium in MR of the spine includes the improved detection of postsurgical epidural fibrosis, epidural abscess, and intramedullary and extramedullary tumor.

Not all patients are able to undergo MR scanning. Contraindications include intracranial aneurysm clips, cardiac pacemakers, cochlear implants, and neurostimulators. The safety of MRI for the fetus has not been established and so pregnancy, particularly the first trimester, is a relative contraindication.

E. Spinal Angiography

This is the study of the arterial supply of the vertebral column, meninges, and spinal cord. The indications include suspected spinal vascular malformations and demonstration of the angioarchitecture of vascular tumors of the cord, meninges, or vertebrae. If a vascular malformation is to be excluded, it is necessary to study all the vessels that may supply the spine. These include the vertebral, deep cervical, ascending cervical, intercostal, lumbar, and lateral and median sacral arteries. This can be technically demanding and is time consuming. We usually perform this examination under general anesthetic, which allows suspended ventilation during angiographic runs, essential for optimal image quality.

Given that there is a small but definite risk of paraplegia associated with this procedure, it should only be undertaken if the result will have a definite influence on the management of the patient. In the past, an abnormal myelogram was deemed necessary before proceeding to spinal angiography. Magnetic resonance imaging has taken over the role of myelography for spinal cord or vertebral column tumors but not completely for spinal vascular malformations, for which a myelogram may still be requested if there is an appropriate clinical history but negative MR scan.

F. Nuclear Medicine

Bone scintigraphy is usually carried out using a 99m technetium labeled phosphate complex. It has a half-life of 6.6 hours and allows high quality images of the skeleton to be obtained with relatively low radiation exposure. The phosphate complex leads to biodistribution in the skeleton. Scintigraphic lesions may be due to photon excess ("hot" spots) or photon deficiency ("cold" spots), the latter reflecting the inability of the tracer to reach the site of the lesion. Although useful in the detection of spinal metastases and osteomyelitis, the lack of anatomical detail and relatively low specificity limits the use of the bone scintigraphy in neurological units.

G. Discography

Water soluble contrast medium injected into the nucleus pulposus of cervical or lumbar discs may show abnormal morphology in a diseased disc and provoke the patient's symptoms. Much of the structural information can now be obtained by MRI. This technique is little used by neuroradiologists but is still employed in orthopaedic practice.

III. SPINAL PATHOLOGY

A. Trauma

Plain radiographs remain the initial investigation for patients with a history of trauma. Lateral and A–P radiographs can be obtained with the patient supine, they will show dislocation or fracture in approximately 90% of adults with major neurological deficits. Injuries of the spinal column predominate in the lower cervical region (30% of total) and the thoracolumbar (30% of total) region, with a smaller peak at the atlantoaxial level. In our unit, patients with major trauma to the head have an initial assessment of the cervical spine, where there may be associated injuries, by a single lateral radiograph. It is important, given the predominance of lower cervical injuries, to ensure that all seven cervical vertebrae and the first thoracic vertebra are included on this radiograph.

After plain radiography, CT may be indicated at those levels where significant bony or ligamentous injury has been shown. Computed tomography can be readily and swiftly performed in the supine position, even in patients with major trauma, to produce direct axial and reconstructed sagittal and coronal images. It provides additional information about bony alignment and fractures, in particular the presence of fractures of the posterior elements and encroachment on the canal or neural foramina by bone fragments. Such information allows decisions to be made on whether fracture reduction should be undertaken and whether it should be open or closed.

Current concepts of spinal instability are based on a three-column structure. The anterior column comprises the anterior longitudinal ligament, the anterior half of the vertebral body, and intervertebral disc; the middle column is made up of the posterior half of the vertebral body and intervertebral disc and the posterior longitudinal ligament; the posterior column is composed of the ligamentous complex and bony arch (including pedicles). Involvement of more than one column makes a spinal injury unstable. There are four common mechanisms of spinal injury: flexion, extension, vertical loading (compression), and rotation. Vertical distraction injuries are less common. More than one mechanism is often present in the injury of a particular patient. Flexion injuries are common in the cervical and thoracic spine and at the thoracolumbar junction (Fig. 4). If of moderate severity, they cause anterior vertebral body wedging and vertebral body fractures. More severe injuries disrupt the posterior annulus, posterior longitudinal ligament, and the posterior ligamentous complex. The addition of rotational forces may cause fractures of the neural arch and distraction or dislocation of the facet joints. Extension injuries are common in the cervical spine and cause fractures of the posterior bony elements. More severe injury disrupts the anterior longitudinal ligament and the intervertebral disc.

Compression injuries usually occur in the cervical spine and at the thoracolumbar junction. The former typically occur in diving injuries and the latter in jumping injuries. These usually result in burst fractures of the vertebral body that may be associated with retropulsion of bony fragments and/or disc into the spinal canal. Computed tomography has shown additional fractures of the posterior elements, particularly the articular pillars, not shown by plain radiographs.

Rotation injuries rarely occur alone but are usually in combination with flexion or extension. Fractures of the articular pillar and facet subluxation may follow rotation injury and in the cervical spine, uncovertebral fracture dislocation may occur.

Fractures occurring in the horizontal plane, such as a displaced horizontal fracture of the odontoid peg, will be difficult to demonstrate on axial CT and may, mistakenly, be thought due to patient movement and misregistration artefact. However these fractures should be readily visible on plain radiographs and CT sagittal reconstructions.

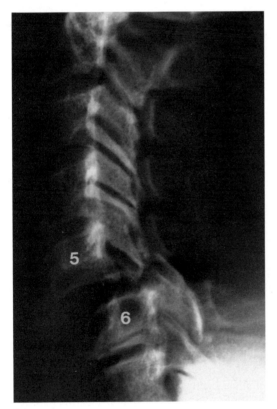

(a)

Figure 4 Hyperflexion injury resulting in bilateral facet dislocation at C5-6. (a) Lateral plain radiograph shows the C5 vertebra displaced anteriorly at least the distance of the A-P diameter of the articular pillar. (b) Sagittal T2-weighted MRI shows complete disruption of the intervertebral disc, the anterior and posterior longitudinal ligaments, and the posterior ligamentous complex. There is a faint high signal within the compressed cord consistent with contusion.

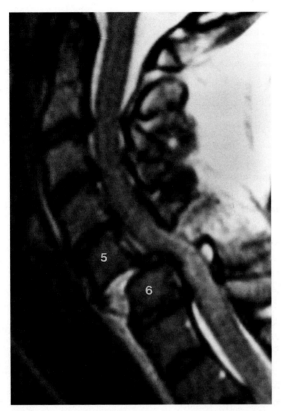

(b)

Significant spinal cord injury may sometimes occur without obvious fracture or dislocation, and this is more frequent in children than adults. Magnetic
resonance scanning is indicated when no injury has been demonstrated in a
patient with neurological deficit; when the demonstrable injury is at a level
inappropriate to the neurological deficit; or when an incomplete neurological
deficit is progressing. Unfortunately not all MR scanning facilities are set up to
provide a service for patients requiring ventilatory and other life support, although this should be a major priority in the planning of facilities expected to
serve patients with severe trauma.

Magnetic resonance scanning may show cord contusion (Fig. 4) and
edema, extradural hematoma, and traumatic disc prolapse. The ability to distinguish between intramedullary hemorrhage and edema in the cord is of prognostic value, but not of immediate management value. The late sequelae of trauma
to the spine, including cord transection, traumatic syrinx, myelomalacia, cord

tethering, meningocele, and accelerated spondylosis are all excellently demonstrated by MRI.

B. Degenerative Disease

Back pain is common, if not universal, in the adult population and fewer than 10% of patients complaining of back pain will have symptoms or signs of a nerve root lesion. As this symptom is so common, there are large numbers of requests for imaging of the spine. Plain radiographs are unfortunately of little positive benefit in management. Degenerative disease is so commonly seen on radiographs in patients older than age 50 that it may be regarded as normal; an acute lumbar disc protrusion often produces no significant plain radiographic abnormality.

Radiological investigation should be restricted to those whose back and leg pain does not respond to conservative measures or in whom there is abnormal neurology. In a small proportion of patients, plain radiographs will show unexpected pathology such as metastases, hemangioma, osteoid osteoma, Paget's disease, or infection. Computed tomography has been, and continues to be, used as the main method of investigation for lumbar disc disease or spinal stenosis in some centers. This has particularly found favor with orthopedic surgeons but less so with neurosurgeons. A prolapsed central or centrolateral lumbar disc typically appears as a convex soft tissue mass that effaces the epidural fat and displaces the thecal sac. Sometimes such disc material is calcified. It should be appreciated that the normal shape of the nonprolapsed L5-S1 disc is slightly convex.

A number of problems exist with the use of CT scanning in the lumbar spine:

1. Approximately 90–95% of lumbar disc prolapses occur at L4-5 and L5-S1. A high proportion of the remainder occur at L3-4. As a result, the usual practice is to scan at the lowest three mobile disc spaces. After such a protocol, no information is obtained about possible disc or stenotic disease at higher disc levels, and no information is obtained about the conus medullaris and proximal cauda equina, lesions of which may mimic low lumbar disc protrusions.
2. The relatively poor soft tissue contrast resolution within the spinal canal means that intrathecal pathology, e.g., a lumbar ependymoma, may be completely missed.
3. A very large disc prolapse, virtually obliterating the thecal sac may be missed for the same reason as in (2). A clue to this diagnosis is the absence of epidural fat.

Stenosis of the lumbar canal may be congenital or acquired. In congenital stenosis, the pedicles are short and bulky and the facet joints are closer to each other than normal. These two factors diminish the A–P and transverse dimensions of the spinal canal. Acquired stenosis is due to hypertrophic degenerative change at the facet joints, thickening of the ligamentum flavum, and diffuse disc bulge. Computed tomography is excellent for the demonstration of canal stenosis.

Myelography has been largely superseded in the United Kingdom and United States for the demonstration of lumbar disc disease. The myelographic appearance will depend on the size and position of the disc. Central disc prolapse produces an anterior extradural deformity of the contrast medium at the level of the disc space. A very large disc may completely block the passage of contrast medium. Centrolateral disc prolapse (Fig. 5) may cause a double contour on the lateral projection, with a lateral extradural deformity on the A–P projection and underfilling, displacement, or distortion of nerve root sheaths.

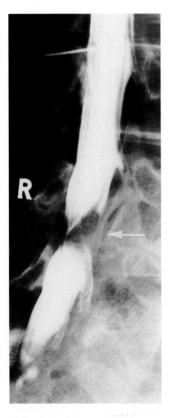

Figure 5 Disc protrusion on myelography. An oblique projection shows a left centrolateral disc prolapse at L4-5 seen as a lateral filling defect (white arrow). The left L5 nerve root is compressed.

Nerve roots may be swollen. Lateral disc prolapse may only affect a nerve root sheath with impaired filling, amputation, or displacement of it. Extraforaminal disc protrusion, which accounts for up to 4% of disc protrusions, usually produces no myelographic abnormality. Myelography may be technically difficult in the patient with lumbar stenosis and if disease is severe, there may be complete block to the flow of contrast, thereby preventing a full examination. Magnetic resonance imaging is now the prime method of radiological investigation of lumbar disc and stenotic disease. Magnetic resonance imaging allows direct visualization of the disc (Fig. 6) and its relationship to adjacent soft tissues. It provides morphological information about the disc and excellent delineation of disc prolapse because of the good soft tissue contrast resolution. Virtually all prolapsed discs show evidence of degeneration seen as decreased signal inten-

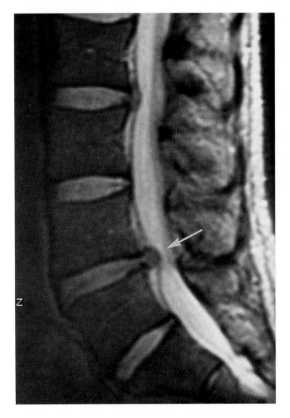

Figure 6   Sagittal T2-weighted MRI scan showing a central L4-5 disc protrusion (white arrow). There is some loss of disc height but no evidence of disc dehydration.

sity on T2-weighted images. There may be accompanying, and variable, signal change in the adjacent endplates and subchondral bone. Thecal sac narrowing in spinal stenosis is well seen in the sagittal and axial planes on MRI. Obliteration of epidural fat is best seen on T1-weighted images, but bone detail is probably best seen on T2-weighted gradient echo sequences.

The postoperative lumbar spine is a common clinical problem. Some epidural fibrosis occurs in most postoperative spines and can be seen on both CT and MRI. The thecal sac tends to be retracted toward the fibrotic tissue, which enhances immediately and uniformly after contrast administration. The degree of enhancement will depend on the interval since surgery.

Recurrent disc material (Fig. 7) exhibits mass effect displacing and compressing the thecal sac. It is often contiguous with the disc space and demonstrates peripheral enhancement, which may be delayed in its appearance after injection of the contrast medium. Recurrent disc and epidural fibrosis can be distinguished in 80% of patients on contrast enhanced CT and 90–95% on precontrast and postcontrast MR scans.

Many of the comments applied to plain radiography of the lumbar spine are also applicable to the cervical spine. There is often no clear correlation between radiographic appearance and symptoms or signs. Elderly patients with

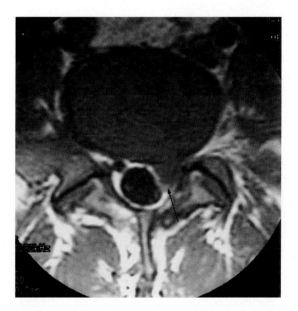

Figure 7 Recurrent disc herniation. Axial T1-weighted MRI scan postgadolinium at level of the disc space. Left recurrent disc herniation compresses the thecal sac and demonstrates peripheral enhancement (black arrow).

marked degenerative changes may be completely asymptomatic. Magnetic resonance imaging has become the screening method for imaging the cervical spine (Fig. 8). Cervical cord compression due to disc or osteophyte is excellently visualized. However there remain questions about the ability to evaluate radiculopathy and foraminal stenosis. Computed tomography has been regarded as the primary method for diagnosing foraminal stenosis because bone detail is so well delineated. Newer MRI techniques, including volume 3D gradient echo imaging, allow thin slice evaluation of the foramina and are probably as accurate as high-resolution CT with intrathecal contrast. Mild nerve root sheath defects on myelography may not produce a corresponding abnormality on MRI. However, this should be seen in the clinical context: asymptomatic or clinically irrelevant nerve root sheath defects are commonly present on myelography.

Notwithstanding the above comments, plain lateral radiographs in flexion and extension are an essential adjunct to MRI in those patients with significant cervical disease prior to surgery to assess for instability.

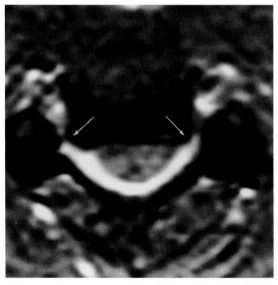

(a)

Figure 8 Cervical osteophytes. (a) Axial T2-weighted MRI scan shows posterolateral osteophytes narrowing the neural foramina (white arrows). (b) Sagittal T2-weighted MRI scan confirms that the cord is not compressed by these osteophytes (small white arrow). There is loss of height and dehydration of the disc (white arrowheads).

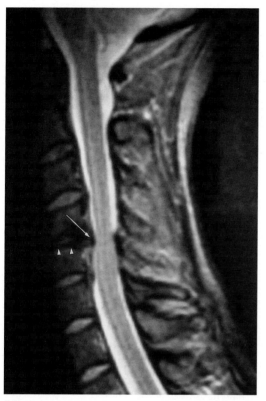

(b)

C. Spinal Cord Compression

The causes of spinal cord compression have traditionally been divided into extradural and intradural extramedullary on the basis of their myelographic appearance as a starting point toward the diagnosis. This classification has ignored the considerably less common subdural masses that are very similar in myelographic appearance to the extradural lesions. Figure 9 illustrates the myelographic appearance of extradural, intradural extramedullary, and intramedullary pathology. Extradural masses displace the contrast medium-filled subarachnoid space away from the bony margins of the spinal canal. Intradural extramedullary lesions displace the spinal cord, enlarging the ipsilateral subarachnoid space and forming a sharp crescentic interface between the contrast column and upper and lower surfaces of the mass. Intramedullary masses typically produce

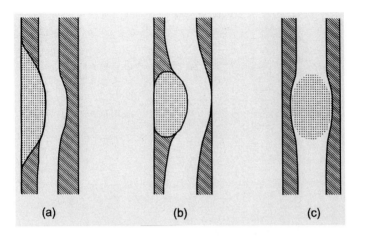

Figure 9 Diagrammatic representation of the myelographic appearance of (a) extradural, (b) intradural extramedullary, and (c) intramedullary pathology. The hatched areas represent the subarachnoid space filled with contrast medium. The dotted areas represent the pathological lesion. See text for further explanation.

fusiform expansion of the cord within the subarachnoid space in both A–P and lateral projections. It is important not to confuse an intramedullary lesion with an extradural lesion, which flattens the cord and so produces apparent expansion of the cord in one plane but flattening of it in the other.

Prior to MRI the investigation of a patient presenting with acute compression of the spinal cord was plain radiography of the chest and spine and then myelography. The majority of such patients have either metastatic or infective disease of the spinal column, hence the usefulness of the plain radiography.

Computed tomography may be useful after myelography as the small amounts of contrast medium flowing beyond a myelographic 'block' may not be seen on plain radiographs but are nearly always seen on CT, and so the upper extent of the pathology can be visualised. It also provides more accurate information about paraspinal soft tissue masses and involvement of the bony posterior elements by tumour.

All of the information required by a surgeon is excellently demonstrated by MRI. A longitudinal series of oil capsules taped to the patient's back can be used to locate the appropriate site for a skin marker at the pathological level prior to surgery. Table 2 lists the anatomical location of some common spinal lesions. By far the most common malignant neoplasm is metastasis. Bone scintigraphy is very sensitive in the detection of metastases but lacks specificity. Magnetic resonance imaging has now shown itself to be more sensitive than

Table 2 Anatomical Location of Some Common
Spinal Lesions

Extradural	Intradural/Extramedullary
Benign	Neurofibroma
Disc prolapse	Meningioma
Abscess	Dermoid/epidermoid
Neurofibroma	Lipoma
Hematoma	Metastases in CSF
Hemangioma	Intramedullary
Malignant	Tumors
Metastasis	Ependymoma
Lymphoma	Astrocytoma
Myeloma	Hemangioblastoma
	Syringomyelia
	Myelitis

scintigraphy. Metastases (Fig. 10) and lymphoma may be indistinguishable on MRI although the latter tends to produce less bone destruction. The majority of metastases are lytic and are low-signal intensity on T1 and high-signal intensity on T2 images. Spinal cord compression by benign tumors of the vertebral column, for example aneurysmal bone cyst, is uncommon.

Pyogenic infection of the extradural components of the spine most often starts in the vertebral body in adults, commencing in the subchondral portion and spreading to the disc space and further along the vertebral body. As the infection progresses, there may be paraspinal and epidural extension. In children, the richly vascularized intervertebral disc may be the primary site of infection. Tuberculous spondylitis may spare the intervertebral disc space and is frequently associated with large paraspinal masses that are out of proportion to the amount of bone destruction. The posterior bony elements are commonly involved. Nerve sheath tumors and meningiomas account for more than 90% of all intradural extramedullary neoplasms. Both categories may have combined intradural and extradural components ("dumbbell tumor"), but this is more usually a feature of nerve sheath tumors. Meningiomas (Fig. 11) are isointense to the spinal cord on both T1 and T2 images, whereas nerve sheath tumor tend to be isointense on T1 and hyperintense on T2 images. They all enhance. Classically, spinal meningiomas occur in the thoracic spine in middle-aged women. Of the intramedullary mass lesions that are tumors, 95% are gliomas, the majority being ependymomas or low-grade astrocytomas. Ependymomas occur most often in the conus medullaris and filum terminale and then in the cervical cord. Astrocytomas are most common in the cervical and then thoracic cord. Distinction between the two tumors may not be possible on MRI, although ependymomas often hemorrhage. Tumor cysts or an associated syrinx may be seen. Virtually all spinal cord tumors enhance on MRI, in contradistinction to intracranial primary intra-axial tumors (Fig. 1). This is important when considering the etiology of a syrinx: if there is no enhancement, then it is not due to tumor. Plaques of demyelination are another cause of focal expansion of the cord. Early MRI scanners did not easily detect these, but current scanners do. Spinal cord plaques may be seen in the absence of demonstrable brain lesions. They appear as elongated, poorly defined hyperintense areas on T2 with mass effect in the acute phase. Intramedullary metastases and intramedullary abscesses were considered rare prior to MRI but are now increasingly recognized.

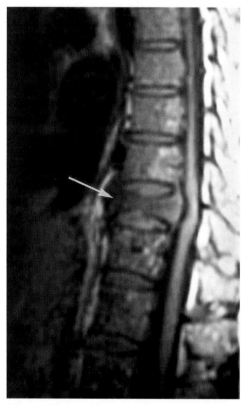

(a)

Figure 10 Metastasis from carcinoma of bronchus. (a) Sagittal T1 MRI scan shows pathological compression fracture of vertebral body (white arrow) and cord compression. (b) Axial T1 MRI scan demonstrates the extent of intraspinal soft tissue (small white arrows) and the compressed cord (black arrowhead).

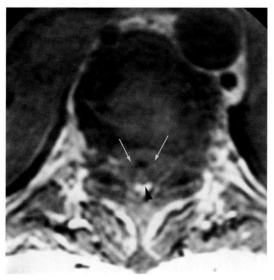

(b)

Figure 10 Continued

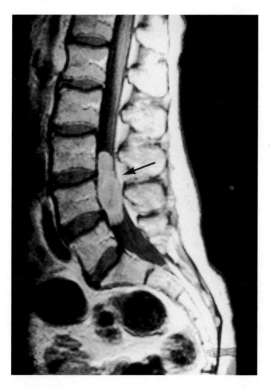

Figure 11 Lumbar meningioma. Sagittal T1-weighted MRI scan postgadolinium demonstrates an enhancing intradural mass (black arrow).

D. Vascular Malformations

These comprise arteriovenous malformations (AVM), arteriovenous fistulae, cavernous angiomas (Fig. 12) and capillary telangiectasias. Spinal arteriovenous malformations are intramedullary AVMs with a localized nidus supplied by multiple feeders from the anterior or posterior spinal arteries. They drain into tortuous dilated veins surrounding the spinal cord. Intramedullary AVMs usually present with acute neurological deficit due to hemorrhage, occur in children and young adults, and are often situated in the cervical or upper thoracic region. Both the multiple arterial feeders and the dilated veins are responsible for ser-

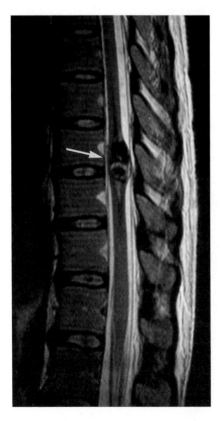

Figure 12 Sagittal T2-weighted MRI scan of intramedullary cavernous angioma (white arrow). There is focal expansion of the cord with mixed hypointense and hyperintense signal due to a mixture of blood breakdown products. Edema (hyperintense signal) is seen extending longitudinally within the cord above and below the lesion.

piginous filling defects visible on myelography and signal voids on MRI (Fig. 13). Spinal dural arteriovenous fistulae usually consist of a single transdural arterial feeder, the fistula located in the dural sleeve, and draining into perimedullary veins. In these patients, the dilated veins are visible on myelography. On MRI, in addition to venous signal voids anterior and posterior to the cord, high signal may be seen within the cord on T2 images: this is due to edema secondary to venous hypertension. These patients tend to be middle-aged and elderly men and they present with progressive neurological deterioration. The fistulae are usually in the lower thoracic region. Whereas negative full-length

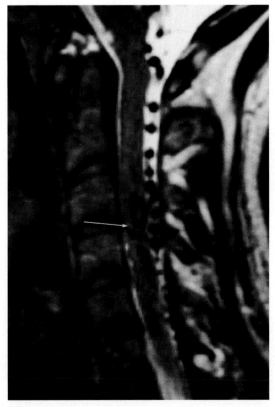

(a)

Figure 13 Intramedullary arteriovenous malformation. (a) Sagittal T2-weighted MRI shows signal void due to dilated arteries and veins in the subarachnoid space and within the cord (white arrow) due to the nidus. (b) Vertebral angiogram showing nidus (white arrow).

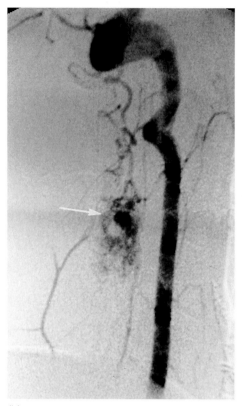

(b)

Figure 13 Continued

myelogram excludes a spinal AVM or AV fistula, a negative MRI does not do
so.

IV. CONCLUSION

Spinal imaging has become more sensitive, more specific, and less invasive
with the introduction of MRI. Exciting work is now being done on cerebrospinal fluid flow patterns detectable by MRI, which may increase our understanding of conditions such as syringomyelia. Our ability to detect flow within the
spinal arteries and veins by MRI needs to be improved before we can assign
spinal angiography to a purely therapeutic rather than diagnostic role.

FURTHER READING

1. Atlas SW, ed. Magnetic Resonance Imaging of the Brain and Spine. Raven Press, 1991.
2. Berenstein A, Lasjaunias P. Surgical Neuroangiography, Vol. 3, Functional vascular anatomy of the brain, spinal cord, and spine. Springer Verlag, 1990.
3. Berenstein A, Lasjaunias P. Surgical Neuroangiography. Vol. 5. Endovascular treatment of spine and spinal cord lesions. Springer Verlag, 1992.
4. Osborn, AG. Diagnostic Neuroradiology. Mosby, 1994.

24

Clinical Neurophysiology of Spinal Cord Disorders

W. Louis Merton
St. Mary's Hospital and Portsmouth Hospitals NHS Trust, Portsmouth, England

Jonathan Cole
Southampton General Hospital, Southampton, Hampshire, and Poole Hospital, Poole, Dorset, England

I. INTRODUCTION

The present chapter gives a resume of the techniques routinely available in clinical neurophysiology laboratories and discusses those spinal cord conditions in which such techniques are most useful. Clinical neurophysiology techniques may be viewed as having two aims: the assessment of function in the peripheral and central nervous system, and the localization and quantification of any abnormality found. Neurophysiological investigations are useful in spinal disease both in excluding peripheral nerve problems and in localizing physiologically— and occasionally anatomically—the source and type of lesion.

There are, however, several limitations to the stimulation parameters used. Peripheral nerves are conventionally divided into sensory and motor fibers, and in terms of axonal size, into large and small myelinated fibers and unmyelinated fibers. These different populations convey impulses concerned with touch, movement and position sense, temperature sensation, and pain respectively. Electrical stimulation of peripheral nerves or of skin itself activates only the largest of the large myelinated fibers, perhaps 2–4% of a peripheral nerve's sensory fibers. Although much useful information can be gained from study of these cell populations, we should be aware of the smallness of sample they represent. Smaller peripheral nerves could be activated by electrical stimulation, but this would be too painful for patients. Other more recent techniques do assess small fiber functions, e.g., laser evoked potentials and thermal psycho-physics (see below), but these are not in general use.

We also use tests with little direct knowledge of the percentage of abnor-mal fibers needed before physiological tests are definitely abnormal. In spinal cord monitoring in the UK, conventional wisdom is that if the evoked potential falls below 50% during a scoliosis operation, then the patient's likelihood of having a subsequent motor weakness rises, and the surgeon will take appro-priate action. Leaving aside the matter that the evoked potential is measuring a dorsal column sensory function and not a lateral column motor one, (which is the critical clinical function), it is not known how many of the large sensory fibers have to be affected before the evoked potential falls by this amount.

Despite these limitations clinical neurophysiology does produce objective data on the functioning of the spinal cord, and so is useful in the diagnosis of many clinical syndromes. Evoked potentials may also, for instance, be of im-portance in cases of hysterical or "functional" disorders in which the preserva-tion of sensory evoked potentials can have important implications.

II. TECHNIQUES

A. Peripheral Studies

1. Nerve Conduction Studies

In this technique, peripheral nerves are stimulated with surface electrodes rest-ing on the skin over a nerve. Sensory responses may be recorded from the surface overlying a nerve at a distance from the stimulation site, either ortho-dromically or antidromically, by averaging techniques (Fig. 1). The two mea-sures most useful are the amplitude of either the purely sensory nerve action potential (SNAP), or the compound action potential (CAP) from antidromic stimulation of a mixed nerve, and the conduction velocity determined by the latency of onset of an averaged response from a nerve after stimulation, with the distance between stimulation and recording sites being measured over the surface of the limb. (For fuller accounts, see Brown and Bolton, 1993; Kimura, 1993; and Binnie, et al., 1995).

An important aspect of sensory nerve conduction studies (NCS) reflects functional anatomy. The SNAP depends on the integrity of the sensory axon, whose cell body lies in the dorsal root ganglion. This is located between the spinal cord and the lateral spinous process at the level of the exit foramen. Classically in root pathology, the SNAPs are preserved, whereas motor conduc-tion and/or EMG shows evidence of dysfunction, although matters are fre-quently more complicated, especially in lumbosacral radiculopathy.

Motor responses are recorded from electrodes over the relevant muscle. The latency from stimulation to the onset of these motor action potentials

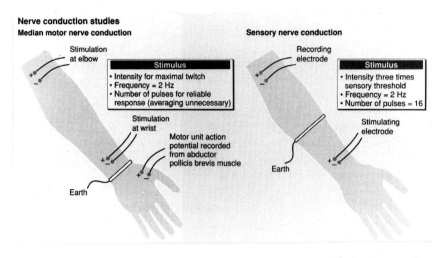

Figure 1 Technique of motor and sensory nerve conduction for the median nerve in the forearm. (Reproduced with permission from Cole J. Clinical neurophysiological testing. Surgery 1993; 11: 563–566.)

(MAPs) and the conduction velocity along a nerve from stimulation at two sites at varying distances from the peripheral muscle can be determined. This allows the determination of whether there is a peripheral entrapment neuropathy or a generalized neuropathy. This forms an important part of the differential diagnosis in radiculopathies, which can be mimicked by distal problems, e.g., carpal tunnel syndrome or a peroneal nerve lesion.

Further information about the degree of axonal loss can be estimated from amplitude measurements, whereas evidence of focal demyelination may be estimated by slowing and/or conduction block, which may be estimated from the area under the curve of a MAP.

There are reasonably well-established normative values for motor and sensory nerve conduction velocities and amplitudes, allowing the diagnosis of motor and sensory neuropathies. This, in turn, allows the exclusion of these diagnoses when spinal cord disease or radiculopathy is considered, although a limitation in studying elderly patients is that the loss of SNAPs from the feet is not necessarily pathological.

2. Segmental Reflexes

Late responses can be recorded from surface electromyograms (EMG) after peripheral activation. These are due to antidromic volleys passing along a mixed nerve to and from the cord. The F response is considered to arise from a small number of motor neurons in the motor neuron pool being close to firing threshold. The antidromic volley in motor nerves then causes these neurons to fire a second time, resulting in a small MAP recorded peripherally with a latency equal to the conduction time to and from the cord via the ventral root. The H response is considered to be a monosynaptic reflex, the afferent arc of which is via the sensory dorsal root and which is likely to activate fibers from muscle spindles. By computation of slowing in these two reflex responses, relative to any peripheral nerve slowing, information about delays due to dorsal and ventral root pathology is available. A limitation is that these reflexes can only be elicited by stimulation of a limited number of peripheral nerves.

More complex measurements of F wave temporal dispersion have been measured, and it has been suggested that they may allow more accurate information about both peripheral and radicular pathology (Panayiotopoulos, 1979). More complex measures of segmental reflexes have been investigated (see Burke, et al., 1992), although such tests are not used routinely in clinical medicine and are outside the scope of the present chapter.

3. Electromyography

Electromyography (EMG) is the recording of electrical activity in a muscle using a needle inserted into that muscle. The EMG is both viewed on a screen and heard on a loudspeaker. At rest, a muscle is silent except in the region of the neuromuscular junction. When a muscle is activated by the patient, the EMG recording becomes flooded by the discharge of motor units, usually with a peak-to-peak amplitude of 2–5 mV. In denervated muscles, spontaneous activity is recorded as individual muscle fibers fire (fibrillations and positive sharp waves), or as motor units fire (fasciculation). In situations where there has been reinnervation (sometimes called chronic partial denervation), spontaneous activity is no longer seen; however, those remaining motor units under voluntary control are larger than normal and may be more complex (polyphasic) and longer in duration, reflecting the takeover of muscle fibers by sprouting from a reduced number of motor axons (Fig. 2). A further characteristic is the increased variability in timing between different components that make up the more complex waveform (instability).

This technique can therefore determine the extent and severity of a lower motor neuron lesion, although it cannot strictly determine its site. It may occasionally be difficult to distinguish a motor neuropathy from a radiculopathy, or even from anterior horn cell disease from EMG alone. In such circumstances, EMG must be considered with other investigations. EMG can also give some evidence of an upper motor neuron lesion; in this circumstance, voluntary activity may be reduced, reflecting weakness, but the motor units recorded on EMG are normal, since there has been no lower motor neuron reorganization.

EMG activity

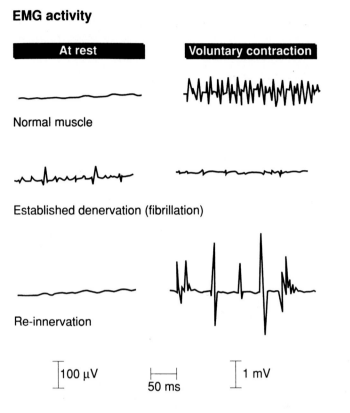

Figure 2 Diagram of concentric needle EMG, with the changes seen after denervation and reinnervation change. (From Cole, 1993.)

4. Tests of Small Fiber Function

There are no simple ways to record from small fibers. There are, however, tests that give information about function in this group of fibers. Cutaneous temperature perception may be assessed with surface pads that heat and cool the skin in a very accurate and reproducible manner, either determining the onset of the perception of a change in sensation or the method of limits, or asking for forced choice responses to small preset alterations in stimulus temperature, the method of levels, (for a fuller discussion see Binnie et al., 1995, pp 253–269). This psychophysical technique has been used thus far mainly in patients with small fiber peripheral neuropathies, (Fowler et al., 1987; Jamal et al., 1987), although it provides useful results in subjects with spinal pathology like syringomelia too.

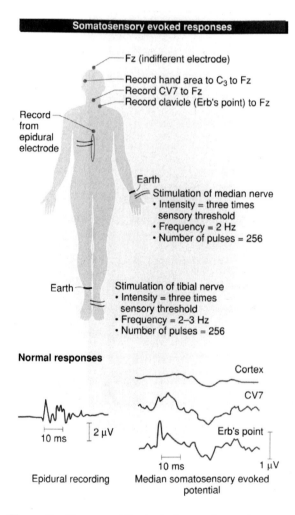

Figure 3 Diagram of the techniques of somatosensory evoked potentials, stimulating the median and tibial peripheral nerve and recording from the contralateral cortex and from the spinal cord. (From Cole, 1993.)

A clinically useful and more physiological test that has been available for many years is the histamine flare test of Lewis. This measures the integrity of the postdorsal root sympathetic system and is therefore important when sensory nerve action potentials are absent or not accessible on tests of nerve conduction (due to the age of the patient or the site of interest). It is not, however, used widely in clinical practice because of problems in execution, interpretation, and utility.

Microneurography has allowed the direct recording from a very limited number of small fibers, concerned both with afferent conduction of pain and autonomic function. In this painstaking but not painful technique, microelectrodes are inserted through the skin into peripheral nerves, and single and groups of axons recorded directly in conscious and cooperative subjects. It has provided evidence of independent control of muscle and skin vasoconstriction and so shifted thinking toward sympathetic function being different in those two organs (Vallbo et al., 1979). The technique is not easily applied to clinical practice, although it has provided a fascinating wealth of results on the pathophysiology of many diseases including those of the spinal cord (Wallin and Fagius, 1988).

B. Studies of Central Pathway Function

For the most part these techniques, which assess conduction in large fibers in the ascending and descending pathways of the cord, require activation of peripheral nerve fibers, so it is not always possible to determine central function in the presence of a significant peripheral abnormality.

1. Somatosensory Evoked Potentials

A peripheral nerve is stimulated in a similar way as for NCS, while averaged responses are recorded from a number of sites both peripherally and centrally. For instance in cervical somatosensory evoked potentials (SEPs), a peripheral nerve is stimulated, e.g., the median nerve at the wrist, and the traveling volley is recorded from overlying the middle third of the clavicle (Erb's potential), the seventh cervical vertebrae, the second cervical vertebra, and the contralateral scalp overlying the contralateral sensorimotor cortex. This allows measurement of peripheral nerve conduction, conduction to the root entry zone of the dorsal spinal cord, from dorsal root entry zone to the upper cervical cord, and from there to the primary receiving area of the sensory cortex. Any delay or deficit in amplitude may be localized as well as quantified (Fig. 3).

For SEPs from the legs, usually recorded after stimulation of the tibial nerve at the ankle, there is no easily recorded potential available until the cortical volley. This means that it can be difficult to localize a deficit along the pathway, although in practice other clinical and neurophysiological clues allow one to deduce the likely level of the lesion(s). For a fuller discussion, see Jones 1993a, b and Dimitrijevic and Halter, 1995.

Sensory evoked potentials have another increasingly important role, for they can be recorded from the cord itself as well as from the scalp if one uses an electrode close to the source of the traveling wave. In operations on the

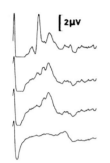

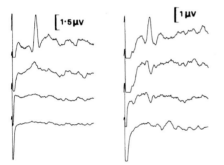

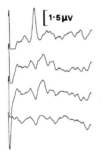

Figure 4 Median nerve somatosensory evoked potential (time base 50 ms). Top, Normal subject with recordings from Erb's point, CV7, CV2 and from over the contralateral sensorimotor cortex. Middle, Patient with multiple sclerois manifest as unsteadiness of gait and sensory disturbance in the hands (right more than left). Note the virtual absence of the cervical responses on both sides and the absent cortical response to right median nerve stimulation. Bottom, Patient with a possible local recurrence of spinal tumor near the foramen magnum. He presented with a gradual loss of sensation in the hands for 2 years, with normal peripheral nerve conduction. The top trace shows a normal Erb's potential. Subsequent traces were recorded over CV7, CV5, and CV2, and show marked attenuation of the traveling wave at this level.

vertebral column, mainly to correct scoliosis, an electrode may be placed by the surgeon above the level of the operative site and the SEP recorded to follow stimulation of a peripheral nerve. During these operations the cord is under threat of ischemia and other damage from distraction and tightening of the fixation by wire. Monitoring of spinal cord potentials continuously during the operation allows instantaneous, constantly upgraded information about the state of conduction in the dorsal column system, which has been found to correlate well with pyramidal tract function and hence with movement (see below).

2. Motor Evoked Potentials

More recently assessment of conduction along central motor pathways has been possible by transcutaneous electrical and magnetic stimulation (Merton et al., 1982; Rossini and Marsden, 1988). Short, high-intensity magnetic or electrical fields are passed via a surface coil through the skull to excite nervous tissue below. Electrical stimulation is uncomfortable and so little used in conscious subjects. Being painless, magnetic stimulation is used far more, although electrical stimulation has some advantages during surgery in activation of the cortex and subcortical neurons (Burke et al., 1993). Both of these techniques activate corticospinal tract neurons directly or indirectly, and so lead to twitch movements in the musculature of the limbs. Magnetic stimulation may be used at a cord and peripheral nerve level, although because its site of activation is not always known precisely, it is less useful in the latter.

With this technique it has been possible to measure the conduction velocity in the pyramidal pathways and spinal roots in a number of conditions, such as cervical spondylosis, multiple sclerosis, spinal injury, motor radiculopathy and neuropathy, including pudendal problems leading to neurogenic impotence and incontinence (Murray, 1990; Snooks et al., 1984; Swash, 1985; and for reviews see Rossini and Marsden, 1988, and Halliday, 1993). In some of these conditions central motor conduction time has been shown to be delayed as might have been expected when other techniques were also abnormal, e.g., in multiple sclerosis. In some cases of multiple sclerosis, clinically "silent" lesions have been detected in motor pathways but at a smaller frequency than silent abnormalities in sensory pathways determined by the use of SEPs.

It has proved possible, however, to detect those rare patients in whom there is chronic demyelinating peripheral neuropathy associated with multifocal central nervous system demyelination (Mills and Murray, 1986). Magnetic stimulation has also proved useful in the detection of delays associated with cervical spondylosis (Thompson et al., 1987) and in prolapsed disc disease (Ludolph et al., 1988).

3. Laser Evoked Potentials

Large myelinated nerve fibers can be activated by electrical stimulation, which is slightly uncomfortable at times, but tolerable. Stimulation of smaller fibers, particularly the A-delta class is not possible by this means; it is too painful because of the high currents required. However one would expect that these fibers could be activated in man by rapid heat stimuli if a fast and transient enough stimulus were available.

This has proved to be the case by using a CO_2 laser. Reliable cortical waves have been shown after cutaneous laser pulses applied to the skin. It is thought that the wave represents a primary incoming volley in A-delta fiber pathways (Bromm and Treede, 1991). It has shown a dissociation of laser and somatosensory EPs in syringomyelia and may become more useful in the assessment of lesions associated with hyperalgesia and hypoalgesia. As yet the technique has only been used to pick up cortical EPs, but efforts are underway to assess the effectiveness of dorsal root entry zone lesions in peripheral pain, and so to record A–delta-dependent responses in the dorsal horn itself.

C. Uses of Clinical Neurophysiology in Spinal Disorders

This volume contains an overview of conditions of the spinal cord, in most of which neurophysiological abnormalities may be found. It is not suggested, however, that in all such cases these techniques should be used. In complete spinal cord injury, for instance, it would seem inappropriate to perform SEP or motor EP in the absence of sensation or movement. This section will instead consider those situations in which the authors have found neurophysiological information most useful to the clinician.

1. Differential Diagnosis of Peripheral, Radicular, and Spinal Disease

Although one would imagine that there was little difficulty in distinguishing between a neuropathy, a radiculopathy, and a cord problem clinically, in practice there can be confusion, particularly in the elderly population. In our practice, it is not uncommon to be asked if the subject has a neuropathy or a radiculopathy in the legs, and in such cases peripheral nerve conduction may allow this distinction to be made. If the sensory responses are present, this allows the exclusion of a mixed neuropathy, although if they are absent this is of little discriminative value, as they can be absent in those who are asymptomatic. In these cases it is often useful to investigate sensory nerves in the arms. Motor conduction and EMG often show some change in the elderly and so do not allow differentiation between a motor neuropathy and a radiculopathy very easily. Sensory evoked potentials and F waves can be useful, however, in showing delays that are larger than one would expect from the motor nerve conduction velocities.

Surgeons who act on anatomical problems prefer a magnetic resonance image (MRI) or computed tomographic (CT) image of a root problem to a neurophysiological report. Not infrequently, however, MRI may show a mild disc protrusion or root encroachment, which the surgeons may be unsure is sufficient to explain the patient's symptoms. In this situation it can be reassuring to know physiologically that there is a dysfunction in a root, to say which root is most affected, and on occasions, to quantify the severity of the abnormality. The demonstration by EMG of unexpected denervation in a given myotome may add some urgency to proceedings, whereas less acute neuropathic change may offer further neurophysiological support for a motor radiculopathy. If widespread it may be the first indicator of anterior horn cell disease.

It is, however, to SEPs that neurophysiologists have turned to try to assess individual root function more selectively. In lumbosacral root lesions, the utility of SEPs has remained controversial. Katifi and Sedgwick (1986, 1987) suggested that SEPs were selective and specific for root lesions, if dermatomal cutaneous stimulation was used and various careful conditions and criteria for abnormality were met. In contrast, Aminoff, et al. (1985 a,b) were less enthusiastic about the findings of their study. The present authors' experience has been that following Katifi and Sedgwick's protocol can produce useful information about root lesions although our surgical colleagues still prefer, and require, to see nerve root compression before they believe it.

Cervical radiculopathies are a more difficult area for clinical neurophysiology. There is so much overlap between peripheral nerves, plexus, and roots that F waves and SEPs are frequently of little value. Careful EMG examination can show those roots that are most affected, but this often mirrors clinical weakness and so is only extending that examination. In cases of cervical radiculomyelopathy, posterior tibial SEPs can be as useful as median and ulnar ones. For by showing delayed and/or small/absent responses from the legs, one can say that there is a significant myelopathy (for discussion see Halliday, 1993).

Although rare, cervical myelopathies above the level of the cervical outflow can be diagnosed with the help of neurophysiology. The median SEP is recorded from a peripheral site, Erb's point, as well as from overlying the root entry zone, the scalp and from the high cervical region. Disappearance of potentials after Cv7 gives evidence of the high lesion (Fig. 4).

Neurophysiology can also be useful in cervical problems where the diagnosis may be a root avulsion or a plexopathy. By a combination of nerve conduction and SEP techniques, it can be shown whether the lesion is predorsal or postdorsal root ganglion. In some cervical spinal cord injuries too there can be doubt as to whether a problem is due to a peripheral ulnar nerve lesion, a plexus problem, or a cord problem. By a combination of techniques, neurophysiology can reveal the site or sites of pathology. In this situation a neurophysiologist may be able to give an opinion based in part on the clinical examination and in part on the results of several tests and relative weights given to them.

Sensory EPs can also be useful, showing that a presumed hysterical sensory loss does have an organic basis. Normal SEPs in the face of a clear loss of sensation in the affected part are some evidence against organic pathology too.

2. Anterior Horn Cell Disease

In the United Kingdom, it is likely that most, if not all, cases of motor neuron disease (MND), synonymous with amyotrophic lateral sclerosis (ALS) and progressive muscular atrophy (PMA), will be seen by a clinical neurophysiologist. The examination seeks to exclude a sensory neuropathy, show preserved or slightly abnormal motor conduction (due to large fiber dropout), and to show degeneration and partial reinnervation of the lower motor neuron. This may be expressed as either fibrillation or fasciculation. These findings are not specific for MND and can be seen in multifocal motor neuropathy (MMN) with conduction block, and in some cases of radiculopathy. Careful analysis of motor conduction in several nerves at several points helps the exclusion or confirmation of MMN (Binnie et al., 1995; Van den Bergh et al., 1989).

The combination of lower motor neuron abnormalities with hyperreflexia allows more certainty in the diagnosis of MND, though even that does not completely exclude MMN. Occasionally sensory nerve amplitudes can be slightly reduced. This should not be used to exclude the diagnosis in the presence of the other more definite findings.

Whereas MND is a disease that can affect both the upper and lower motor neurons, poliomyelitis affects the lower motor neuron alone. We have no experience of acute polio; however we do see patients with increasing weakness many years later. An EMG in postpolio syndrome (PPS) usually shows evidence of chronic denervation and reinnervation change with very large motor units, representing extensive reinnervation, together with fasciculation, positive sharp waves and fibrillation, supposedly representing decompensation of the remaining motor neurons. However, similar findings have been found in patients who have had polio but do not have the progressive weakness characterising PPS (Ravits et al., 1990), so one must be cautious in making a diagnosis of PPS on the basis of EMG alone, as one is with the diagnosis of other diseases. In our experience these findings occur in more muscles than the subject claims were affected by the original attack of polio, and one is frequently surprised by the mismatch between the level of functioning patients enjoy and their marked neuropathic EMG findings.

3. Acute Inflammatory Demyelinating Polyneuropathies

Electromyograms and nerve conduction have an important role in both the diagnosis of and the estimation of prognosis in this range of conditions that include combinations of demyelinating and axonal damage, of which the most frequently seen is Guillain-Barré syndrome.

The hallmarks of this condition include evidence of peripheral demyelination with block in conduction. Electromyogram may show either denervation or absence of fibrillation without any ability to contract the muscle voluntarily and with preservation of muscle bulk, which probably represents proximal block. Sensory conduction is usually far less affected in the early stage than is motor conduction, and indeed a syndrome in which sensory nerves are affected more than motor nerves may make one doubt the diagnosis of GBS. Two weeks after the onset of florid symptoms in GBS, however, it is likely that sensory nerve conduction will be abolished or severely depressed.

The temptation in GBS is to perform EMG as soon as the diagnosis is suspected. However, as in other conditions, the changes in nerve conduction and in EMG may take several days to become apparent, so it is usually better to wait 5–7 days before investigating, just as, after complete nerve transection, changes reflecting denervation take several days to be seen in a peripheral muscle.

There is often pressure to confirm the diagnosis early, before plasmapheresis or immunoglobulin treatment is started. In those cases neurophysiology may show subtle changes that may offer some support for the diagnosis. This can be confirmed at a later date. There are several useful tricks: if the sensory conduction in the arms is more affected than in the legs, a reversal of the normal aging affect, then this is in favor of the diagnosis. It is often necessary to measure conduction in several nerves, for the disease presents in a patchy manner.

At a suitable time (2–3 weeks after disease onset), EMG showing marked axonal damage carries a more serious prognosis than one showing proximal block. Sequential studies may suggest worsening of the neurophysiology when the patient is improving, reflecting this delay of several days between neurophysiological and clinical findings.

The almost routine use of immunoglobulin therapy has modified the usual progression of neurophysiological changes seen in acute and chronic inflammatory demyelinating neuropathies. In particular, there is evidence of reversal of peripheral conduction block at the most peripheral sites at rates faster than can be explained by reinnervation.

4. Syrinx

When the presenting clinical picture is typical of a syrinx with dissociated sensory loss, then neurophysiology has little part to play. Rarely, however, cases present without obvious sensory symptoms, with progressive weakness mimicking a radicular syndrome. In these patients who are often young or middle aged, the syrinx may have been present for many years. Neurophysiology may take place before MRI, simply because the diagnosis is not suspected, and the neurophysiologist, in showing a more widespread neuropathic pattern than expected, may be in a position to suggest that the problem is not confined to a single root.

5. Multiple Sclerosis

In cases in which the only clinical manifestation of multiple sclerosis is spinal, in showing multiple delays in visual and brainstem auditory evoked potentials, neurophysiological tests can point toward multiple pathology, which nowadays would be investigated in greater detail with MR scanning (Ormerod et al., 1987). A danger that should never be forgotten is that pathology may coexist: the presence of delayed visual EPs does not mean that the spinal lesion has to be demyelination, and occasional compressive lesions are missed for this reason.

In rare cases in which pain is a major feature of the presentation in multiple sclerosis, there may be pathology in the dorsal root ganglion and commensurate reduction in sensory nerve conduction.

6. Hereditary Motor Neuropathy or Spinal Muscular Atrophy

Although characteristic EMG features are described in hereditary motor neuropathy with very large voluntarily activated motor units, this pattern is by no means typical. The EMG may show a gradation from a neuropathic pattern, through a nonspecific mixture of large, normal, and small units to a more uniform myopathic pattern with small units seen often with marked polyphasia and with a reduced interference pattern. Thus neurophysiology can show a lower motor neuron problem in such cases, which can be of importance, but is not often diagnostic.

7. Spinal Cord Monitoring

It is beyond the scope of this chapter to go into the details of spinal monitoring. Some of the general aspects will, however, be considered. Unlike in most uses of neurophysiology—diagnosis of pathology—the aim in monitoring is to predict when damage may be occurring to allow the surgeon or anesthetist a chance to reverse it.

The techniques used thus far in spinal monitoring have been varied. Somato-sensory EPs have been used in three main ways. Peripheral nerve stimulation and recording of the resultant wave from the cerebral cortex or the cord rostral to the site of operation was the earliest technique used (Engler et al.,

1978, and Jones et al., 1982, respectively). Spinal cord evoked potentials (SCEPs) are recorded by placing an electrode close to the cord, e.g., in the epidural space and stimulating the sensory pathway beyond the operative site. They may be recorded proximal to the operative site after stimulation of a peripheral nerve, e.g., the tibial nerve in thoracic operations, or by stimulating the cord with a second epidural electrode. Alternatively antidromic sensory potentials may be recorded below the operative site from stimulation of the cord above it (Tamaki, 1989; and chapters in Dimitrijevic and Halter, 1995). Motor tracts above the operative site may be stimulated either by magnetic or electrical pulses and recordings taken from either muscles below the level at risk or, if paralyzing agents are used, by recording directly from the cord below the site (Boyd et al., 1986; Levy et al., 1987; Shields et al., 1990).

In the United Kingdom at present, SEPs are probably the most widely used. Decreases of 50% or more in the spinal EP are considered significant and sufficient for the surgeon to relax the distraction. This simple technique has reduced the need for a wake-up test and has become almost mandatory for medicolegal purposes (Forbes et al., 1991, Ashkenaze et al., 1993; Jones, 1993c). In a large series of 754 patients, 14 developed postoperative complications and in all of these, their SEPs had fallen by 50% at some stage during the operation and could not be restored quickly. In common with others' experience, the time during operation that this drop occurred most was during insertion or tightening of sublaminar wires (Waller et al., 1991).

Cortical recordings suffer from the disadvantage that potentials are depressed by anesthesia, especially the volatile halogenated agents, and by hypotension (Taylor et al., 1994). They are, however, less invasive than the other two methods. Spinal cord EPs are more resistant to the type of anesthetic used and because the cord pathway between stimulus and recording sites is short and the spinal cord fibers are able to follow higher stimulation frequencies than cortical potentials, averages may be built up very quickly (for more details, see Dimitrijevic and Halter, 1995).

Motor evoked potentials (MEPs) have been used in a variety of spinal operations and with a number of techniques, including electrical and magnetic stimulation of the cortex and spinal cord above the operative site/lesion and recording from spinal cord, peripheral nerve, and muscle (Boyd et al., 1986; Levy et al., 1987; Shields et al., 1990, together with articles in Jones, et al., 1994; and Dimitrijevic and Halter, 1995).

At present, different groups of researchers are exploring the use of SEPs, SCEPs and MEPs, stimulating and recording from various sites and sometimes using combinations of these techniques. Although different laboratories have different preferences, it is abundantly clear that neurophysiological monitoring during spinal surgery has significant advantages. Allowing the surgeon security that he has not caused damage to the long tracts of the spinal cord and circumventing wake-up test monitoring paves the way for more radical surgery. In the near future these techniques will be more refined and more widely available.

III. CONCLUSIONS

Clinical neurophysiologists should give a report that combines a consideration of the electrical findings along with the clinical history and examination. Cardinal error is to suggest a finding that is clinically unlikely, although findings may not infrequently be unsuspected, e.g., a carpal tunnel syndrome previously not detected. The report should seek to interpret the findings in light of the history and to answer the question posed by the referring doctor according to the level of neurological understanding of that doctor.

Clinical neurophysiologists may be used as auxiliary neurologists by their nonneurological colleagues. Thus they may pick up a case of MND referred as a dropped foot or a radiculopathy, or a cervical root syndrome may turn out to be a brachial neuritis. Rarely, more important and unsuspected pathologies may be found. Thus one of the authors was referred a case of a cervical fracture with weakness in the arms and legs. Neurophysiology showed a mild lower motor neuron problem in both limbs that was considered insufficient to explain the clinical weakness. There was also hyperreflexia, and MRI showed a previously unsuspected C1 instability that had been present for some years and which required fixation. Neurophysiologists are used to give their clinical opinion as well as to give interpretations of specialized tests.

It is also important for negative findings to be interpreted accurately. Normal findings in a case of pain due to a cervical injury do not exclude a significant root or cord syndrome and are a great frustration in whiplash injuries. Normal findings do, however, make a diagnosis of a neuropathy very difficult to sustain and, by exclusion, might suggest a diagnosis of a radiculopathy.

In the course of an EMG and NCS, the doctor may be with the patient for 45 minutes or more, longer than most other doctors ever spend with them. This allows the neurophysiologist time to elicit a feeling for the case. They can then give the patient a summary of the findings, dependent on the patient's perceived expectations and the diagnosis. Although no neurophysiologist would tell a patient that he or she had a terminal illness after a single visit, nor wish to explain prognosis and other details that the referring clinician would be expected to discuss, it would seem reasonable to give patients knowledge of a neuropathy or radiculopathy, as well as some idea of the next step in investigation and treatment.

Lastly neurophysiologists are becoming required not simply to perform diagnostic tests but to monitor during surgical procedures. Evoked potentials, which a few years ago were used in support of diagnoses like demyelination, have found another wide area of usefulness in an acute surgical rather than a medical setting, and this use is likely to increase in the years to come.

REFERENCES

Aminoff MJ, Godin DS, Barbaro NM, Weinstein PR, Rosenblum ML. 1985a Dermatomal somatosensory evoked potentials in unilateral radiculopathy. Ann Neurology 1985a; 17:171–176.

Aminoff MJ, Godin DS, Parry GJ, Barbaro NM, Weinstein PR, Rosenblum ML. Electrophysiologic evaluation of lumbosacral radiculopathies: electromyography, late responses and somatosensory evoked potentials. Neurology 1985b; 35:1514–1518.

Ashkenaze D, Mudiyam R, Boachie-Adjei O, Gilbert C. Efficacy of spinal cord monitoring in neuromuscular scoliosis. Spine 1993; 18(12):1627–1633. 15.

Binnie CB, Cooper R, Fowler CJ, Mauguiere F, Prior PF, Osselton JW. Clinical Neurophysiology: EMG, Nerve Conduction and Evoked Potentials. London: Butterworth Heinemann, 1995.

Boyd SG, Rothwell JC, Cowan JMA, Webb PJ, Morley TP, Asselman P, Marsden CD. A method of monitoring function in corticospinal pathways during scoliosis surgery with a note on motor conduction velocities. J Neurol Neurosurg Psychiatry 1986; 49:251–257.

Bromm B, Treede R-D. Laser-evoked cerebral potentials in the assessment of cutaneous pain sensitivity in normal subjects and patients. Rev Neurol 1991; 147(10):625–643.

Brown WF, Bolton CE. Clinical Electromyography. 2nd ed. Stoneham, MA: Butterworth-Heinemann, 1993.

Burke D, Gracies JM, Mazevet D, Meunier S, Pierrot-Deseilligny E. Convergence of descending and various peripheral inputs onto common propriospinal-like neurons in man. J Physiol 1992; 449:655–671.

Burke D, Hicks R, Gandevia SC, Stephen J, Woodforth I, Crawford M, Gandevia SC, Stephen J, Woodforth I, Crawford M. Direct comparison of corticospinal volleys in human subjects to transcranial magnetic and electrical stimulation. J Physiol (London) 1993; 470:383–393.

Cole JD. Clinical neurophysiological testing. Surgery 1993; 11:563–566.

Dimitrijevic MR, Halter JA. Atlas of Human Spinal Cord Evoked Potentials, Boston: Butterworth-Heinemann, 1995.

Engler GL, Spielholtz NI, Bernhard WN, Danziger F, Merkin H, Wolf T. Somatosensory evoked potentials during Harrington instrumentation for scoliosis. J Bone Joint Surg 1978; 60A:528–532.

Forbes HJ, Allen PW, Waller CS, Jones SJ, Edgar MA, Webb PJ, Ransford AO. Spinal cord monitoring in scoliosis surgery. Experience with 1168 cases. J Bone Joint Surg (British Volume) 1991; 73(3):487–91.

Fowler CJ, Carroll MB, Burns D, Howe N, Robinson K. A portable system for measuring cutaneous thresholds for warming and cooling. J Neurol Neurosurg Psychiatry 1987; 50:1211–1215.

Halliday AM. Transcutaneous stimulation and the measurement of central conduction time. In: Halliday AM, ed. Evoked Potentials in Clinical Testing. London: Churchill Livingstone, 1993; 359–564.

Jamal GA, Hansen S, Weir AI, Ballantyne JP. The neurophysiological investigation of small fiber neuropathies. Muscle Nerve 1987; 10:537–454.

Jones SJ. Clinical applications of short-latency somatosensory evoked potentials. Ann NY Acad Sci 1982; 338:517–530.

Jones SJ. Somatosensory evoked potentials I: Methodology, generators and special techniques. In: Halliday AM, ed. Evoked Potentials in Clinical Testing. London: Churchill Livingstone, 1993a; 383–420.

Jones SJ. Somatosensory evoked potentials I: Clinical observations and applications. In: Halliday AM, ed. Evoked Potentials in Clinical Testing. London: Churchill Livingstone, 1993b; 421–466.

Jones SJ. Evoked potentials in intraoperative monitoring. In: Halliday AM, ed. Evoked Potentials in Clinical Testing. London: Churchill Livingstone, 1993c; 421–466.

Jones SJ, Boyd S, Hetreed M, Smith NJ. Handbook of Spinal Cord Monitoring. Proceedings of the Fifth International Symposium, London, 1992. London: Kluwer Academic, 1994.

Katifi HA, Sedgwick EM. Somatosensory evoked potentials from posterior tibial nerve and lumbosacral dermatomes. Electroencephalogr Clin Neurophysiol 1986; 65:249–259.

Katifi HA, Sedgwick EM. Evaluation of the dermatomal somatosensory evoked potential in the diagnosis of lumbo-sacral root compression. J Neurol Neurosurg Psychiatry 1987; 50:1204–1210.

Kimura J. Electrodiagnosis in Diseases of Nerve and Muscle, Philadelphia: FA Davis, 1993.

Levy WJ, McCaffrey M, Hagichi S. Motor evoked potential as a predictor of recovery in chronic spinal cord injury. Neurosurgery 1987; 20:138–142.

Ludolph AC, Spille M, Masur H, Elger CE. Befunde im periphermotorichen System nach Stimulation der motorischen Wurzein: Polyradikulitis, amyotrophe Lateralsklerose und Polyneuropathie. Zeitschrift fur EEG EMG 1988; 19:255–259.

Merton PA, Hill DK, Morton HB, Marsden CD. Scope of a technique for electrical stimulation of human brain, spinal cord and muscle, Lancet 1982; 2:597–600.

Mills KR, Murray NMF. Neurophysiological evaluation of associated demyelinating peripheral neuropathy and multiple sclerosis: A case report. J Neurol Neurosurg Psychiatry 1985; 49:320–323.

Murray NMF. Magnetic stimulation of the brain: Clinical applications. In: Magnetic Stimulation in Clinical Practice, ed. Chokroverty S. London: Butterworths, 1990; 205–231.

Ormerod IEC, Miller DH, McDonald WI, du Boulay EPG, Rudge P, Kendall BE, Moseley IF, Johnson G, Tofts PS, Halliday AM, Bronstein AM, Scaravilli F, Harding AE, Barnes D, Zilka K.J. The role of NMR imaging in the assessment of multiple sclerosis and isolated neurological lesions: A quantitative study. Brain 1987; 110:1579–1616.

Panayiotopoulos CP. F-chronodispersion: A new electrophysiologic method. Muscle Nerve 1979; 2:68–72.

Ravits J, Hallett M, Baker N, Nilsson J, Dalakas M. Clinical and electromyographic studies of postpoliomyelitis muscular atrophy. Muscle Nerve 1990; 13:667–674.

Rossini PM, Marsden CD, eds. Non-invasive Stimulation of Brain and Spinal Cord. Neurology and Neurobiology. Vol 41. New York: Alan Liss, 1988.

Shields CB, Palmeimo MPJ, Backman MH, Edmonds HL Jr, Johnson JR. Intraoperative use of transcranial magnetic motor evoked potentials. In: Magnetic Stimulation in Clinical Neurophysiology, Chokroverty S., ed. London: Butterworths, 1990; 173–184.

Snooks SJ, Barnes PRH, Swash M. Damage to the innervation of the voluntary anal and periurethral striated sphincter musculature in incontinence: An electrophysiological study. J Neurol Neurosurg Psychiatry 1984; 47:1269–1273.

Swash M. New concepts in incontinence. BMJ 1985; 290:4–5.

Tamaki T. Spinal cord monitoring with spinal potentials evoked by direct stimulation of the spinal cord. In: Desmedt JE, ed. Neuromonitoring in Surgery. Clinical Neurophysiology Updates 1. Amsterdam: Elsevier, 1989; 139–150.

Taylor BA, Webb PJ, Hetreed M, Mulukutla RD, Farrell J. Delayed postoperative paraplegia with hypotension in adult revision scoliosis surgery. Spine 1994; 19(4):470–474.

Thompson PD, Dick JPR, Asselman P, Griffin GB, Day BL, Rothwell JC, Sheehy MP, Marsden CD. Examination of motor function in lesions of the spinal cord by stimulation of the motor cortex. Ann Neurol 1987; 21:389–396.

Vallbo AB, Hagbarth KE, Torebjork HE, Wallin BG. Somatosensory, proprioceptive, and sympathetic activity in human peripheral nerves. Physiological Reviews 1979; 59:919–957.

Van Den Burgh P, Logigian EL, Kelly JJ. Motor neuropathy with multifocal conduction blocks. Muscle Nerve 1989; 12:26–31.

Waller CS, Paterson JMH, Edgar MA, Jones SJ. Incidence of spinal cord impairment related to extent of SEP decline and recovery, aetiology and instrumentation in operations for scoliosis. In: Shimoji K, Kurokawa T, Tamaki T, Willis WD Jr, eds. Spinal cord monitoring and electrodiagnosis. Berlin: Springer-Verlag, 1991; 353–359.

Wallin BG, Fagius J. Peripheral sympathetic neural activity in conscious humans. Annual Review of Physiology 1988; 50:567–576.

25

Urological Aspects of Spinal Cord Disease

Vijay Chandiramani
University Hospital of South Manchester, Manchester, England

David Thomas
Lodge Moor Hospital, Sheffield, England

Clare J. Fowler
Institute of Neurology, London, England

I. INTRODUCTION

Normal bladder control is a severe test of the integrity of the spinal cord. In humans and in many other mammals, the decision when to empty the bladder is under voluntary control: to exercise this control requires intact neural connections between the medial aspects of the frontal lobes and the most caudal part of the spinal cord. Any disruption of these pathways inevitably impairs the two functions of the bladder—storage and emptying.

II. NEUROLOGICAL CONTROL OF THE BLADDER IN SPINAL HEALTH

In health, the bladder acts as a reservoir to store the urine continually excreted by the kidneys. The bladder exists in its storage mode for approximately 99% of the time and then, at a convenient moment, through a series of coordinated activities, contracts to produce complete elimination of its contents. de Groat has argued that because the two activities, storage and voiding, are mutually exclusive, the pontine micturition center can be considered to act as a switch, switching neural pathways between the two conditions (1). Higher centers determine which condition the bladder should be in, but it is pathways that descend from the pontine micturition center in the dorsal tegmentum of the pons to the sacral spinal cord that affect the bladder's activity.

A. Storage

Figure 1 shows the state of the bladder and outlet mechanism and its innervation, during storage. Parasympathetic activity, which innervates the detrusor muscle, is inhibited by descending inhibitory pathways from the pontine micturition center (2). The bladder neck outlet mechanism and the striated muscle of the urethral sphincter and pelvic floor are held in a state of contraction, the former probably through tonic sympathetic activity originating from the thoracolumbo sympathetic outflow (T12–L2), the latter from tonic activity from the anterior horn cells in Onuf's nucleus (S2–S4), which innervates the striated muscle of the sphincter. Continence is achieved by maintaining a higher pressure in the urethra than in the bladder.

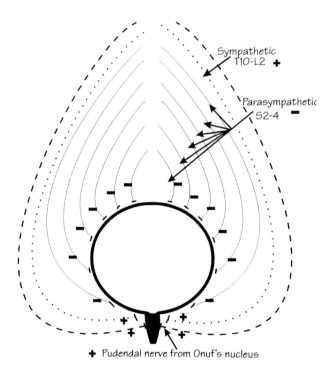

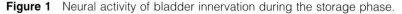

Figure 1 Neural activity of bladder innervation during the storage phase.

The intravesical pressure should not rise more than 10 cm of water during filling despite an increase in volume from 0 to between 450–550 ml. This is achieved not only by inhibition of the parasympathetic activity but also by an active process of relaxation of the detrusor muscle, which produces the phenomenon of "bladder compliance." The neural pathways that determine these various coordinated activities descend from the pontine micturition center through spinal pathways.

B. Emptying

The physiological trigger for bladder emptying is a sense of fullness. The afferent fibers that mediate this sensation are, at least in the cat and probably also in humans, A-delta myelinated fibers. These afferent fibers pass from the lower urinary tract to the spinal cord through nerves conveying all three types of afferent fibers, i.e., parasympathetic, sympathetic, and somatic. There is probably some synaptic connection between afferent and efferent fibers at a sacral spinal level but in health, this is of relatively minor significance compared to the major routing of the afferent traffic to the pontine micturition center and to "consciousness."

When bladder fullness is sensed, a continent individual makes the necessary social arrangements to void. When preparations are complete, higher centers are thought to "switch" the neural mechanisms in the pontine micturition center from the storage to the emptying program.

The first recordable event of voiding is electrical silence and relaxation of the usually tonically firing striated muscle of the urethral sphincter and pelvic floor (3). This means that voiding is achieved by an active process of relaxation, a rather unusual neurological event. The detrusor contraction follows some seconds later (Fig. 2). The spinal pathways by which these events are achieved are uncertain, but intact connections between the sacral spinal cord and pontine micturition center are critical for their coordinated activity.

III. CHANGES IN BLADDER BEHAVIOR AFTER A SPINAL CORD LESION

It is clear from the foregoing description that the controlling influence of the pontine micturition center is of paramount importance for physiological bladder control. Spinal cord disease interrupts both the afferent ascending pathways to this center, as well as the descending efferent pathways. Both physiological actions of the bladder are impaired, with the result that it neither stores nor eliminates effectively.

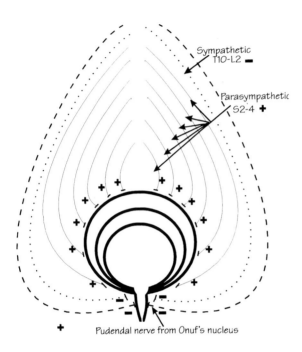

Figure 2   Neural activity of bladder innervation during the voiding phase.

A.   Failure of Storage

Failure of storage results in incontinence. The various mechanisms that operate (as shown in Figure 1) to achieve storage fail, mainly through lack of inhibition of detrusor activity. The detrusor muscle becomes overactive so that the bladder develops spontaneous contractions over which the patient has no control.

Figure 3a shows the normal routing of afferent activity from the bladder in the intact spinal cord, and Figure 3b shows the changes that occur after interruption of the afferent pathways between the sacral spinal cord and the pontine micturition center. The major change that has been demonstrated in experimental animals is the emergence of a new afferent reflex arc (4). In spinal health the afferent fibers are unmyelinated A-delta fibers but after disconnection from the pons, unmyelinated C-fibers emerge as the predominant afferents from the lower urinary tract. These are thought to be present in spinally intact animals, but their emergence as the controlling afferents after spinal cord disease is thought to be an example of a neural plasticity. Immediately after spinal cord injury the bladder is inactive and this condition may persist anywhere from 6 weeks to several months. Toward the end of that period, the bladder usually

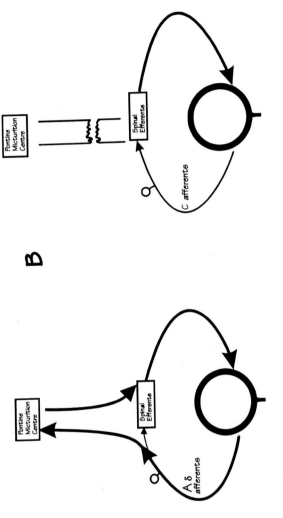

Figure 3 Changes in bladder afferents after a spinal cord lesion. (A) A = δ fibers are the predominant afferents from the lower urinary tract under normal conditions. (B) After interruption of spinobulbospinal pathways, unmyelinated C fibers emerge as the predominant afferents.

develops volume-determined reflex contractions, and it may well be that these are due to the establishment of the emerging reflex.

Extensive animal experiments have shown that the C-fibers that subserve volume-determined bladder voids are sensitive to capsaicin (5). This means they may be stimulated by the initial irritant effect of applied capsaicin but are also sensitive to its selective neurotoxic effects. The success of treating some patients with partial spinal cord lesions and troublesome detrusor hyperreflexia with intravesical capsaicin suggests that the emergent C-fiber reflex is important in humans also (6).

B. Failure of Emptying

The physiological coordination of the outlet mechanism, i.e., bladder neck and striated urethral sphincter, together with the detrusor muscle, is lost after disconnection from the pons. The normally coordinated activity is replaced by a disordered action known as "detrusor sphincter dyssynergia"—when the detrusor muscle develops a volume determined contraction, the sphincter contracts simultaneously (7). This may lead to abnormally high pressures in the bladder and incomplete bladder emptying. The patient is aware of difficulty with micturition and an interrupted stream. The tendency for incomplete bladder emptying is probably further exacerbated by the lack of normal parasympathetic drive from the descending bulbospinal pathways that, under physiological circumstances, maintain the detrusor contraction throughout voiding.

IV. CLINICAL CONSEQUENCES OF SPINAL CORD DISEASE FOR BLADDER BEHAVIOR

Patients with partial progressive spinal cord disease usually report bladder symptoms together with a deterioration of lower limb function. This is to be expected, because any lesion above the level of the lumbar cord affecting the innervation of the legs is likely to disrupt the connections between the pons and the sacral spinal cord.

Most commonly patients with spinal pathology causing a disturbance of bladder control complain of urgency. From the preceding paragraphs it will be apparent that this is due to the development of detrusor hyperreflexia, consequent to the neurological changes illustrated in Figure 3b.

Detrusor hyperreflexia can be readily demonstrated by urodynamic studies, and Figure 4 shows a typical trace. On filling to volumes well under the normal capacity of 400 ml, the bladder develops spontaneous rises in pressure that the patient is unable to suppress. These may occur at very low volumes, under 100 ml, and whether they produce incontinence depends somewhat on the extent of

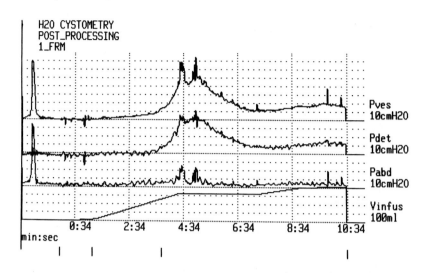

Figure 4 Cystometric tracing showing detrusor hyperreflexia.

the pressure rise. The patient reports a feeling of urinary urgency and imminent micturition just as the detrusor pressure begins to rise.

Frequency often accompanies the complaint of urgency, due to the hyper-reflexic nature of the detrusor and the reduced capacity of the bladder. However, frequency is not inevitably associated with urgency and in many ways, unpredictable urgency causing urge incontinence can be just as disruptive to normal life as a combination of urinary frequency and urgency.

A. Voiding Disorders and Incomplete Emptying

Patients with spinal cord disease complain most of incontinence and it may only be on direct questioning that they admit to disorders of voiding. However, incomplete voiding can seriously exacerbate the difficulties of bladder storage and should not be overlooked. With a relatively minor spinal cord lesion, the patient may complain of difficulty initiating micturition and an interrupted stream.

The extent to which patients are aware that their bladder is emptying incompletely is very variable. Not infrequently, a patient who has a postmicturition residual volume of between 100 and 200 ml may be surprised by the discovery because he or she feels the bladder is not full. Others however may deduce the existence of a significant postmicturition residual volume from the fact that they can pass urine, albeit with difficulty, and then return to the toilet

5 minutes later and pass the same amount again. In a study of a series of patients with multiple sclerosis and spinal cord disease, we discovered that those patients who thought they might not be emptying their bladder were usually correct, whereas half those who thought they were emptying their bladder to completion were incorrect (8). This has important consequences for management.

Patients with complete or near-complete spinal cord lesions are unable to initiate any sort of voluntary micturition. Voiding occurs either when the bladder reaches a particular volume, or if the patient discovers some maneuvre that triggers reflex bladder emptying.

B. Autonomic Dysreflexia

An uncommon but life-threatening disorder, autonomic dysreflexia, may occur after spinal cord trauma to levels above T6. This is an exaggerated sympathetic response to stimuli below the level of the lesion, particularly from sensory input through the sacral cord segment. The most powerful stimulation comes from the bladder and urethra, producing a sudden rise of blood pressure with a severe headache and sweating in the normally innervated segments of the head and neck. Removal of the stimulating cause (e.g., full bladder) will lead to a quick resolution of the symptoms but if left unrelieved, the huge rise of blood pressure may lead to cerebrovascular complications and death. Local anesthetic spinal blockade will prevent autonomic symptoms arising during surgical manipulation of the bladder and urethra.

V. SPINAL CAUSES OF BLADDER DISORDERS

Table 1 lists various causes of spinal cord disease, most of which have been described in detail in other parts of this book.

In general, in all these conditions the extent of bladder dysfunction mirrors the severity of paraparesis or paraplegia evident in the lower limbs. This can be clearly seen in patients with multiple sclerosis who initially may have only mild spinal cord disease that is evident while walking distances or at speed. These patients usually have mild urgency and frequency without incontinence. As their lower limb disability progresses, they become dependent on an aid for walking and may develop worsening urgency and urge incontinence. By the time walking has become difficult, a failure of emptying is a prominent part of their bladder dysfunction; when they become chair-bound, medical management of their bladder may be difficult. Once unable to stand unaided or transfer, an indwelling catheter is likely to be necessary.

Figure 5 shows the correlation between deteriorating mobility as estimated by the Kurtzke expanded disability status score (EDSS) and bladder dysfunc-

Table 1 Spinal Cord Disease
Causing Bladder Dysfunction

Traumatic spinal cord injury
Multiple sclerosis
Neoplasms—metastatic, primary
Tropical spastic paraparesis
Arteriovenous malformations
Cervical myelopathy
Tethered cord
Spina bifida

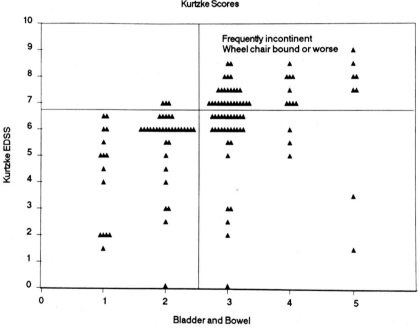

Figure 5 Kurtzke EDSS in 135 patients with multiple sclerosis showing a correlation between deteriorating lower limb function and bladder control. The graph is based on data described in a paper by Betts et al. (1992). Patients with higher Kurtzke scores, especially those who are wheelchair-bound, often have troublesome frequency, urgency, and incontinence.

tion in a series of patients with multiple sclerosis. It is evident from this that by the time a patient is wheelchair-bound, i.e., EDSS higher than 6.5, they are likely to be frequently incontinent.

An important but as yet unexplained phenomenon is that, whereas after spinal cord injury, upper urinary tract disease is a real and serious possible complication, the same does not seem to occur in nontraumatic spinal cord disease despite what may be a similar level of spasticity affecting the lower limbs. Upper urinary tract disease developing due to a combination of high bladder pressure during detrusor contractions or poor compliance, together with incomplete emptying and recurrent urinary tract infections, can "blow up" the ureters, leading to hydronephrosis and renal failure. This can occur insidiously in patients who have suffered a traumatic paraplegia at a time when they seem otherwise well. It is for this reason that such patients must remain under close urological supervision throughout their lives. By contrast renal failure in patients with nontraumatic spinal cord disease is exceedingly rare. Although there have been reports of patients with multiple sclerosis and spinal cord disease developing urological complications (9), renal failure is rarely listed among causes of death in patients with multiple sclerosis (10). In our own experience of many hundreds of patients with multiple sclerosis and bladder dysfunction, very few have been observed to have developed significant renal impairment (8). If this does occur, it seems to be in elderly men who had indwelling catheters for some years and been subject to recurrent urinary tract infections. Much the same seems to pertain to other "medical" causes of spinal cord disease.

One consequence of this fortunate but unexplained phenomenon ought to be that neurologists should interest themselves in their patients' incontinence. There is undoubtedly a tendency among nonurologists to consider that all bladder symptoms are outside their province. This is partly due to the fact that many physicians are haunted by the specter of upper tract damage in patients with traumatic spinal cord disease, as well as the fact that formerly, urodynamic studies were emphasized as being essential for management of neurogenic bladder disorders and that the facility for these investigations usually exist only within the urology department. A further contributing factor regrettably, has been a lack of concern by the medical profession for what they may hitherto have referred to as "nursing problems."

There is undoubtedly a great deal that nonurologists can do to improve the management of patients with bladder disorders due to spinal cord disease, based on some very simple principles.

VI. MANAGEMENT OF BLADDER DYSFUNCTION DUE TO SPINAL CORD DISEASE

The two disorders of bladder function, i.e., disordered storage and emptying that result from spinal cord disease, must be dealt with separately. The primary aims of management of a patient with a neurogenic bladder disorder is to achieve urinary continence and preserve renal function.

A. Investigations

The extent of incomplete emptying is unpredictable, both from the history and clinical estimate of severity of neurological deficit, and may play an important part in contributing to disorders of storage. In all patients who give a history suggesting a disorder of voiding, a measurement should be made of the post-micturition residual volume. This can either be done with ultrasound or by performing a catheterization after the patient has tried to void. In health, the postmicturition residual volume is negligible, and it is generally agreed that a volume of more than 100 ml is likely to contribute to bladder dysfunction. In those patients known to be at risk of developing upper tract disease, i.e., those with spinal cord injury or spina bifida, an assessment of the upper tracts with an intravenous urogram and follow-up isotope renograms is essential.

Urodynamics are useful in demonstrating abnormal detrusor behavior. The terminology used to describe the procedures and the measurements have been recommended by the Standardization Committee of the International Conti-nence Society (11). The tests range from simple frequency/volume voiding charts that record the fluid intake and volume voided per 24-hour period, to measurements of the pressure volume relationships during bladder filling and micturition, as documented by the filling cystometrogram and the voiding study. A complete cystometrogram is important in patients with spinal cord injury and myelodysplasia but may not always be necessary in patients with progressive neurological disease.

B. Therapy

Several factors must be considered when recommending a plan of bladder man-agement to a patient. Decisions may be influenced by medical criteria, i.e., prevention of deterioration in upper tract function, inadequate storage or empty-ing, poor sphincter control, recurrent urinary tract infections, as well as the patient's mental state and attitude, manual dexterity, motivation, and desire to remain free of an incontinence appliance.

1. Intermittent Catheterization

There is currently no effective oral medication for improving bladder emptying, and some physical means of achieving complete elimination is necessary. This can either be done by a permanent indwelling catheter or by teaching the patient to perform intermittent self-catheterization. The latter, if possible, is preferable for both bladder health and the patient's self-esteem.

Sterile, nontouch intermittent catheterization as a reliable and low-risk alternative to an indwelling catheter was introduced by Sir Ludwig Guttmann (12) after an 11-year study on the early management of voiding dysfunction in patients with spinal cord injury. He recommended an aseptic technique performed by medical staff. Subsequently, Lapides, et al. (13) popularized the idea of *clean* rather than sterile intermittent self-catheterization based on the theory that local host resistance (i.e., maintainence of a good blood supply to the bladder by avoiding overdistension) was a more important factor in preventing urinary tract infection than the risk of introducing bacteria at the time of catheterization. The technique of clean, intermittent self-catheterization has since transformed the management of neuropathic bladder dysfunction and is the treatment of choice in most patients who are unable to empty their bladder.

Intermittent catheterization is highly beneficial in controlling or alleviating urinary incontinence and is suitable for patients who have a significant residual due to impaired voiding. The incidence of recurrent urinary tract infections associated with incomplete bladder emptying is markedly reduced (14). Those with poor bladder compliance and detrusor hyperreflexia compromising the storage function of the bladder require additional treatment, usually anticholinergic drugs rather than surgery, along with intermittent catheterization.

At the first consultation, the reasons for introducing self-catheterization must be clearly explained. The logic of intermittent catheterization is not always obvious to a patient unaware of their incomplete emptying. Although many patients react with distaste to the idea of self-catheterization, most of them are pleasantly surprised at the ease with which they get accustomed to the technique and the overall benefits it achieves. It is best if a specialist urological nurse or continence advisor instructs the patient on the technique and provides continued support to deal with the queries that may arise.

A small-size (10–14) PVC catheter, Nelaton or Scott type, is usually used. Patients are advised to pass urine, then wash their hands with soap, rinse, and dry them prior to handling the catheter. Lubricating jelly is used on the tip of the catheter to aid insertion. It is generally recommended that intermittent catheterization be carried out between three to five times over a 24-hour period, although the frequency is best determined by the fluid intake and the volume of residual urine drained (15). Patients should keep a record of the residual urine drained from time to time. The incidence of bacteriuria rises if the catheterized volume is greater than 400 ml and hence, the frequency must be adjusted accordingly (16).

Maynard and Diokno (17) reported that although chronic bacteriuria is frequently found in urine from patients on intermittent catheterization, it does not cause any serious consequence in the urinary tract, provided there is no vesicoureteral reflux. Asymptomatic bacteriuria alone is not an indication for antibiotic treatment (18). Fortunately, symptomatic urinary tract infection is not common and when it does occur, usually responds to a short course of an antibiotic (19). The prevalence of urinary tract infection is increased if the catheterization is performed by a caregiver rather than the patient and if an external appliance, e.g., condom drainage, is used between catheterizations. Bladder calculus, prostatitis, and improper catheterization technique lead to persistent chronic infection and must be dealt with appropriately. The incidence of urethral complications, i.e., urethritis, stricture, and false passage, although low, seems to rise in patients using intermittent catheterization for more than 5 years. In a retrospective study of long-term, clean intermittent catheterization in 75 patients for a mean duration of 7 years (maximum 12 years), Wyndaele and Maes (20) noted that upper tract dilatation had improved in the majority of cases. Their recommendation of close surveillance in patients using intermittent catheterization to detect changes in neuropathic bladder dysfunction, in particular reduced bladder compliance leading to hydronephrosis, was subsequently confirmed by Perkash and Giroux (21). This is perhaps more relevant to patients with spinal cord injury and myelodysplasia than multiple sclerosis, in as much as in the former group, continence does not necessarily imply that storage and voiding are occurring in a urodynamically safe environment.

C. Detrusor Hyperreflexia

The mainstay of treatment of hyperreflexia is drugs. Normal bladder contraction is mediated by the release of acetylcholine at postganglionic parasympathetic receptor sites. Logical pharmacotherapeutic approaches therefore include blocking the stimulus for contraction or interfering with the ability of the detrusor to respond to such a stimulus. The drugs used can be classified as anticholinergics, such as atropine and propantheline; musculotropics such as oxybutynin, dicyclomine, flavoxate; and tricyclic antidepressants, such as imipramine. The two main objectives achieved by pharmacological manipulation are improvement in the symptom complex associated with detrusor hyperreflexia and lowering of the intravesical pressure.

Anticholinergic agents act by competitive inhibition of acetylcholine at the muscarinic receptor sites. Propantheline was the most commonly used drug to reduce detrusor hyperreflexia, and Blaivas, et al. (22) documented its therapeutic effect in reducing involuntary detrusor contractions in patients with multiple sclerosis. The side effects, which are due to its antimuscarinic action and common to most anticholinergics in varying proportions, include dry mouth, blurred vision for near objects, tachycardia, constipation, and drowsiness and it is contraindicated in narrow-angle glaucoma.

Musculotropic drugs possess direct smooth muscle relaxant properties and therefore act on sites distal to the cholinergic receptor mechanism. Oxybutynin hydrochloride is a musculotropic but has additional antimuscaranic and local anesthetic properties. Several studies have shown its effectiveness in controlling detrusor hyperreflexia (23–25). The starting dose is 2.5 or 3 mg b.d. and any increase in dosage must be gradual. It is commonly said that if the side effect of a dry mouth is not experienced by the patient, then the drug level is not within the therapeutic range. Tricyclic antidepressants decrease smooth muscle contractility and increase bladder outlet resistance. Imipramine is occasionally used in the management of detrusor hyperreflexia. Calcium influx is important in the excitation-contraction coupling of the smooth muscle of the detrusor (26). Theoretically, a combination of anticholinergic and calcium antagonistic actions would not only be more effective in combating detrusor hyperreflexia but also decrease the side effects occurring with therapeutic doses of anticholinergics and calcium antigonists (27). Terodiline was an agent in this class, but it was withdrawn due to cardiac side effects. A suitable alternative is awaited.

Before beginning anticholinergic therapy, a measurement should be made of the patient's postvoid residual urine volume. If a significant residue is present, then the patient must be taught clean intermittent self-catheterization, inasmuch as in addition to reducing hyperreflexia, anticholinergics have the effect of lessening the efficiency of bladder emptying. For the same reason, deterioration in the initial beneficial effect of anticholinergics suggests incomplete bladder emptying, and hence follow-up of such patients should include an ultrasound scan for postmicturition residual.

Intravesical instillation of oxybutynin is a safe and effective alternative for patients who cannot tolerate oral oxybutynin. The patient must be performing intermittent self-catheterization and the best results are obtained in those who have retained some bladder sensation and have good sphincter control. Intravesical oxybutynin has been shown to increase bladder capacity and volume when the first hyperreflexic contraction appeared while decreasing the magnitude of the filling pressures (28). Earlier reports (29) indicated that the use of intravesical oxybutynin was without systemic anticholinergic side effects, except in patients who had undergone some form of augmentation cystoplasty procedure previously (30). However it is absorbed into the systemic circulation in significant amounts and a recent study (31) has shown that some patients may have anticholinergic side effects, mainly dry mouth.

D. Desmopressin

In spinal cord disease, nocturia and ennuresis are a consequence of reduced bladder capacity and an overactive detrusor. Desmopressin (DDAVP), an analogue of the natural pituitary hormone vasopressin, has an antidiuretic effect, increasing reabsorption of water by the kidney and temporarily decreasing urine production. Desmopressin, thus transiently circumvents the problem of volume-determined detrusor hyperreflexic. It has a more pronounced antidiuretic effect and a longer duration of action than vasopressin; unlike vasopressin it has no vasoconstrictor action. Although hyponatremia and water intoxication causing confusion, headaches, and a general malaise are reported side effects, they are not common. Desmopressin spray given intranasally in a dose of 20 μg has been found to be very beneficial in decreasing nocturnal polyuria in patients suffering from multiple sclerosis (32). Patients are advised to use it only once in a 24-hour period. If the patient does not report any lessening of voiding frequency after treatment with DDAVP, the postmicturition residual should be measured.

E. Capsaicin

Most of the patients with urinary incontinence can be managed with a combination of anticholinergic medication and intermittent self-catheterization, but a proportion are so severely hyperreflexia that their incontinence is intractable and they can only be offered either long-term catheterization, a urosheath (in men), or major reconstructive or diversion surgery. All these treatments have potential major short-term and long-term side effects.

After a spinal cord lesion interrupts the spinobulbar pathways, a new sacral reflex emerges (Fig. 3), the afferent neurons of which are unmyelinated C fibers (4). This C-fiber mediated sacral reflex replaces the normal A-delta afferent supraspinal reflex pathway and is the afferent system for volume-determined detrusor contractions.

Capsaicin is the pungent ingredient of red peppers and is used extensively in neuroscience research because of its selective section on small unmyelinated sensory neurones (C fibers). Animal experiments have shown that the immediate effect of capsaicin is stimulatory, with transmission of sensory impulses sensed as painful irritation and a release from the peripheral nerve terminals of neuropeptides including substance P and CGRP. This is followed by a long-lasting impairment of certain sensory functions, mediated by bladder afferents (mainly unmyelinated C fibers) leading to an increased bladder capacity (33).

Based on this theory, an intravesical instillation of 100 ml of 1 or 2 mmol capsaicin has been used in a small number of patients to lessen detrusor hyperreflexia and improve incontinence (34). Subjective improvement noted as decreased number of incontinence episodes, freedom from use of incontinence appliances, and decreased frequency/urgency of micturition has been seen. The best responses have been in patients with some residual neurological function in their lower limbs, rather than those totally bed-bound. Urodynamic studies in these patients corroborate the symptomatic improvement, and an increase in bladder volume at first detrusor hyperreflexia and decreased magnitude of these contractions can be demonstrated. The duration of benefit is variable but improvement, if it occurs, usually lasts for several months. The instillation then needs to be repeated (35).

F. Surgical Management

Applying the functional classification of voiding dysfunction (36), operative treatment can be based on whether bladder abnormality is due to failure to store or failure to empty, either because of the bladder or the outlet (Table 2). Deteriorating renal function and persistent urinary incontinence in a patient with otherwise good prognosis are the most appropriate indications for operative intervention.

External sphincterotomy gives the best results in a male patient with a suprasacral cord lesion causing incomplete emptying of the bladder and involuntary detrusor contractions, who is prepared to use a continous external collecting device. A clam enterocystoplasty converts a high-pressure urinary bladder into a low-pressure urinary reservoir using bowel. To perform this oper-

Table 2 Operative Treatment

Failure to empty
  Because of the bladder
    Brindley anterior sacral root stimulator
    Suprapubic catheterization
  Because of the outlet
    External sphincterotomy
Failure to store
  Because of the bladder
    Augmentation ("clam") cystoplasty
    Bladder transection
    Posterior root section
  Because of the outlet
    Artificial urinary sphincter
Other procedures
  Urinary diversion
  Chronic indwelling catheter

ation, the bladder is opened in the sagittal or coronal plane (hence, "clam") so that the detrusor is no longer able to generate a contraction, and small bowel that has been opened on its antimesenteric border is sutured to fill the defect and increase the bladder capacity.

VII. CONCLUSION

Spinal cord disease commonly has a profound effect on bladder function. Two disorders are likely to result: detrusor hyperreflexia and incomplete emptying. The extent to which these two disorders exist is variable but as a general rule, each becomes worse with deteriorating spinal function. The two types of dysfunction must be managed separately; the first line therapy for detrusor hyperreflexia is anticholinergic medication, and incomplete emptying must be managed by some physical means of improving drainage, preferably intermittent catheterization. In patients with partial spinal cord lesions, successful bladder management restoring continence can usually be achieved by simple medical measures and physicians should be aware of the available options.

REFERENCES

1. de Groat WC. Central neural control of the lower urinary tract. In: Bock G, Whelan J, eds. Neurobiology of Incontinence. Chichester: John Wiley & Sons, 1990; 27–56.
2. Blaivas JG. The neurophysiology of micturition: A clinical study of 550 patients. J Urol 1982; 127:958–963.
3. Tanagho EA, Miller ER. Initiation of voiding. Br J Urol 1970; 42:175–183.
4. de Groat WC, Kawatani T, Hisamitsu T, et al. Mechanisms underlying the recovery of urinary bladder function following spinal cord injury. J Auton Nerv Sys 1990; 30:S71–S78.
5. Maggi CA, Santicioli P, Borsini F, Giuliani S, Meli A. The role of the capsaicin-sensitive innervation of the rat urinary bladder in the activation of micturition reflex. Naunyn-Schmiedeberg's Arch Pharmacol 1986; 322:276–283.
6. Fowler C, Jewkes D, McDonald W, Lynn B, deGroat W. Intravesical capsaicin for neurogenic bladder dysfunction (letter). Lancet 1992; 339:1239.
7. Blaivas JG, Sinha HP, Zayed AAH, Labib LB. Detrusor-external sphincter dyssynergia. J Urol 1981; 125:542–544.
8. Betts CD, D'Mellow MT, Fowler CJ. Urinary symptoms and the neurological features of bladder dysfunction in multiple sclerosis. J Neurol Neurosurg Psychiatry 1993; 56:245–250.
9. Samellas W, Rubin B. Management of upper tract complications in multiple sclerosis by means of urinary diversion to an ileal conduit. J Urol 1965; 93:548–552.

10. Phadke JG. Survival pattern and cause of death in patients with multiple sclerosis: Results from an epidemiological survey in north east Scotland. J Neurol Neurosurg Psychiatry 1987; 50:523–531.

11. Abrams P, Blaivas JG, Stanton SL, Andersen JT. The standardization of terminology of lower urinary tract function. Scand J Urol Nephrol 1988; suppl 114:5–19.

12. Guttman L, Frankel H. The value of intermittent catheterisation in the early management of traumatic paraplegia and tetraplegia. Paraplegia 1966; 4:63–84.

13. Lapides J, Diokno AC, Silber SJ, Lowe BS. Clean, intermittent self-catheterization in the treatment of urinary tract disease. J Urol 1972; 107:458–461.

14. Lapides J, Diokno AC, Gould FR, Lowe BS. Further observations on self-catheterization. J Urol 1976; 116:169–171.

15. Anderson RU. Prophylaxis of bacteriuria during intermittent catheterisation of the acute neurogenic bladder. J Urol 1980; 123:364–366.

16. Bakke A. Physical and psychological complications in patients treated with clean intermittent catheterization. Scand J Urol Nephrol 1993; suppl 150, 1–69.

17. Maynard FM, Diokono AC. Clean intermittent catheterization for spinal cord injury patients. J Urol 1982; 128:477–480.

18. Lewis RI, Carrion HM, Lockhart JL, Politano VA. Significance of asymptomatic bacteriuria in neurogenic bladder disease. Urology 1984; 23:343–347.

19. Mohler JL, Cowen DL, Flanigan RC. Suppression and treatment of urinary tract infection in patients with an intermittently catheterized neurogenic bladder. J Urol 1987; 138:336–340.

20. Wyndaele J, Maes D. Clean intermittent self-catheterization: A 12-year followup. J Urol 1990; 143:906–908.

21. Perkash I, Giroux J. Clean intermittent catheterization in spinal cord injury patients: A followup study. J Urol 1993; 149:1068–1071.

22. Blaivas JG. Management of bladder dysfunction in multiple sclerosis. Neurology 1980; 30(12):12–18.

23. Gajewski JB, Awad SA. Oxybutynin versus propantheline in patients with multiple sclerosis and detrusor hyperreflexia. J Urol 1986; 135:966–968.

24. Diokno AC, Lapides J. Oxybutynin: A new drug with analgesic and anticholinergic properties. J Urol 1972; 108:307–309.

25. Brooks ME, Braf ZF. Oxybutynin hydrochloride (ditropan)—Clinical uses and limitations. Paraplegia 1980; 18:64–68.

26. Forman A, Andersson KE, Henriksson L, Rud T, Ulmsten U. Effects of nifedipine on the smooth muscle of the human urinary tract in vitro and in vivo. Acta Pharmacologica et Toxicologica 1978; 43:111–118.

27. Andersson KE, Sjogren C. Aspects on the physiology and pharmacology of the bladder and urethra. Prog Neurobiol 1982; 19:71–89.

28. Brendler CB, Radebaugh LC, Mohler JL. Topical oxybutynin chloride for relaxation of dysfunctional bladders. J Urol 1989; 141:1350–1354.

29. Madersbacher H, Jilg G. Control of detrusor hyperreflexia by intravesical instillation of oxybutynin hydrochloride. Paraplegia 1991; 29:84–90.

30. Massad CA, Kogan BA, Trigo-Rocha FE. The pharmacokinetics of intravesical and oral oxybutynin chloride. J Urol 1992; 148:595–597.

31. Kasabian NG, Vlachiotis JD, Lais A, et al. The use of intravesical oxybutynin chloride in patients with detrusor hypertonicity and detrusor hyperreflexia. J Urol 1994; 151:944–945.
32. Hilton P, Hertogs K, Stanton SL. The use of desmopressin (DDAVP) for nocturia in women with multiple sclerosis. J Neurol Neurosurg Psychiatry 1983; 46:854–855.
33. Maggi CA. The role of neuropeptides in the regulation of the micturition reflex: An update. Gen Pharmacol 1991; 22(1):1–24.
34. Fowler CJ, Beck RO, Gerrard S, Betts CD, Fowler CG. Intravesical capsaicin for treatment of detrusor hyperreflexia. J Neurol Neurosurg Psychiatry 1994; 57:169–173.
35. Chandiramani VA, Peterson T, Beck RO, Fowler CJ. Lessons learnt from 44 intravesical instillations of capsaicin. Neurourol Urodyn 1994; 13(4):3–4.
36. Wein AJ. Classification of voiding dysfunction: A simple approach. In: Barrett DM, Wein AJ, eds. Controversies in Neuro-Urology. New York: Churchill Livingstone, 1984; 239–250.

26

Omental Transposition in Spinal Cord Injury

C. J. Gerber and Glenn Neil-Dwyer
Southampton General Hospital, Southampton, Hampshire, England

Dorothy A. Lang
Southampton University Hospitals Trust, Southampton, Hampshire, England

I. BACKGROUND

The unique properties of the omentum and its ability to produce neovascularization has been recognized for many years. In spinal cord injury, its use has attracted much attention in the medical literature and popular press with occasional reports of outstanding results after omental transposition.

In the United Kingdom, the incidence of spinal injury is approximately 15 per million population per year. The usual cause is indirect violence; road traffic accidents account for 55% of admissions to a spinal injury unit, whereas domestic, industrial, and sports injuries are responsible for most of the remainder (19). The majority of patients affected are young males. The prognosis for recovery depends on the amount of damage sustained by the cord at the time of injury; recent reports suggest an increased incidence of cervical spine injuries (19). Although with modern treatment the mortality is in the order of 10% (2), only 14% regain independence, with the degree of dependence depending on the level of the lesion. More than 40% will require rehousing and only a third of patients are capable of returning to their previous employment (19). In addition, the financial burden to society has been estimated to amount to approximately nearly £1 million in terms of lost earnings and lifetime medical support.

II. PATHOPHYSIOLOGY

Spinal cord injury and the resultant neurological deficit can be explained by a series of structural, vascular, physiological, and biochemical processes that are thought to be irreversible and influenced by the degree of injury (1,4–6,8,31–34). There are two principle mechanisms of injury: the primary mechanical injury and a secondary injury analogous to that which occurs after head injury (Table 1). Theoretically, these secondary phenomena are potentially preventable or reversible. After acute spinal cord injury, sequential histological changes are seen, including hemorrhage, edema, axonal and neuronal necrosis, demyelination with cyst formation, and infarction (1). These can be seen within 5 minutes of cord injury using electron microscopy (6).

Three clinical syndromes of cord injury are recognized. Concussion involves transient loss of cord function and although no structural cause has been identified, an increase in extracellular potassium may be responsible. Contusion of the spinal cord results in a sequential chain of events altering cord function, and transection results in immediate functional loss, both complete and permanent (8).

After experimental cord injury, spinal cord blood flow falls, resulting in progressive posttraumatic ischemia in the first few hours after the injury. These changes are thought to be due to a loss of local autoregulation, and secondary cord damage is exacerbated by the frequent accompanying hypotension (5,6,33–36). Interestingly, experimental hypertension after a cord injury does not return local spinal cord blood flow to normal and is not associated with improved outcome (20).

Spinal cord injury results in an increase in central reflex excitability and an alteration in sympathetic control of blood pressure and temperature regulation (36,39,40). Dopamine, noradrenaline, and serotonin levels have been shown to be decreased below the level of cord injury, whereas proximally concentrations appear to be increased (10,27). Naftchi in 1985 demonstrated a global decrease in activity of the hypothalamic pituitary adrenal axis in tetraplegic patients (26). Acute spinal cord injury results in an increase in plasma and cerebrospinal fluid concentrations of endorphins, possibly resulting in altered local spinal blood flow (9,10).

III. RECOVERY AFTER SPINAL CORD INJURY

Historically spinal cord injury has been recognized as a condition with a very high mortality. In World War I, approximately 90% of patients with a spinal cord injury died (19). However with modern management, the mortality is about 10% (2,3). Most patients (75–85%) have a complete neurological deficit

Table 1 Primary and Secondary Mechanisms of
Spinal Cord Injury

Primary Injury
  Acute compression
  Impact
  Missile
  Distraction
  Laceration
  Shear
Secondary Injury
  Vascular changes
    loss of autoregulation
    systemic hypotension (neurogenic shock)
    hemorrhage
    loss of microcirculation
    reduction in blood flow
    vasospasm
    thrombosis
  Electrolyte changes
    increased intracellular calcium
    increased extracellular potassium
    increased sodium permeability
  Biochemical changes
    neurotransmitter accumulation
      catecholamines
      excitotoxic amino acids
    arachidonic acid release
    free radical production
    eicosanoid production
      prostaglandins
    lipid peroxidation
    endogenous opioids
  Edema
  Loss of energy metabolism
    decreased adenosine triphosphate production

immediately after the injury. Fifteen percent of patients with a cervical spine injury that is initially complete will make some motor recovery and 3% become ambulatory at 1 year. The outcome with paraplegics is worse, with 5% of patients making some motor recovery or becoming ambulatory (7). Outcome is irrespective of operative or nonoperative treatment. Any patient who remains complete at 1 week essentially has no chance of walking independently. The picture with incomplete lesions is less clear and depends on the extent of the injury.

Until recently, little in the way of intervention was shown to improve functional outcome in patients with a spinal cord injury. However, the results of the NASCIS 2 study suggest that high-dose methylprednisolone given within 8 hours of spinal cord injury will lessen the resultant deficit (3). This study has been strongly criticized for its methodology and the way in which the results were interpreted, but the fact that some improvement occurred lends credence to the secondary injury hypothesis of spinal cord injury (42).

A. The Use of Omentum

The omentum majus consists of a fold of peritoneum, containing fat and the gastroepiploic vessels, arising from the greater curvature of the stomach. It is well known to have unique properties and its ability to produce vascular connections has been known for many years. In 1906, Morison considered the capacity of the omentum to form new vascular attachments of great surgical importance, and he coined the term "the abdominal policeman," because its properties helped to promote healing and prevent perforation of inflamed bowel (25).

O'Shaughnessy, in 1936, showed that the omentum could be used to provide collateral circulation to ischemic hearts in greyhounds. He was able to demonstrate new vascular connections with particles of ink appearing within the myocardium, the chambers of the heart, and in the aorta after the injection of India ink suspension into the omental graft artery (29). The next year he reported that omental transposition to the heart resulted in improvement of angina in three of six patients (30). This operation was popularized by Vineberg in the 1960s when it was combined with internal mammary implantation (37). It has since been superseded by the advent of coronary artery bypass grafting.

The omentum has been used clinically to improve lymphatic drainage of an area (i.e., in limbs with chronic lymphedema after surgery) after experimental work demonstrated new lymphatic channels developing between tissues of an extremity and a pedicled omental graft (12). It has been shown experimentally to be capable of cerebrospinal fluid absorption and was proposed as a possible treatment for hydrocephalus (21,41).

In 1973, vascular anastomoses were demonstrated between transposed omentum and the brain. These anastomoses have been shown to prevent the occurrence of experimentally induced infarction (13,14). The success of various experimental models led to omental transposition being used in a number of patients who had stable neurological deficits after a stroke with varying results.

Currently it is used in the treatment of moyamoya disease with encouraging results (24).

In 1975, Goldsmith reported revascularization of the spinal cord using intact omentum with maintenance of spinal cord blood flow and preservation of cord function with the immediate application of the omentum after acute spinal cord trauma in cats. In addition he showed that the omentum increased blood flow to the distal segment of the transected cord. The increased blood flow was dependent on the patency of the omental vessels (15,16). A lipid angiogenic factor isolated from omental tissue was felt to explain its facility to promote new vessels (17).

The omentum has been reported to contain dopamine, noradrenaline, adrenaline, choline acetyltransferase, gastric polypeptides and more recently, a neural growth factor (18). It is, however, unclear whether the omentum produces, concentrates, or simply serves as a conduit for these neurochemicals. Additionally the omentum has been shown to reduce scarring after spinal cord injury (16). Theoretically any of these factors could be beneficial to spinal injured patients.

B. Technique of Omental Transposition

The operation is performed concurrently by two teams of surgeons. The first step of the operation is to separate the omentum from the transverse colon. The omentum is then removed from the distal two-thirds of its attachment to the greater curvature of the stomach maintaining a vascularized pedicle based on the gastroepiploic vessels. At this stage, the omentum must be lengthened, usually by dividing the left gastroepiploic artery, which is smaller than the right, and then by dividing the arcades within the omentum while preserving the arterial supply primarily along the periphery of the omentum. The omentum can be lengthened to reach the brain in all patients and can extend as far as the hallux in some!

Once the omentum is lengthened sufficiently to be applied to the area of the damaged spinal cord without tension, it is passed subcutaneously to the region of the spinal injury, where the second team of surgeons have performed a laminectomy and exposed the damaged cord. The arachnoid is dissected off the cord, occasionally using the microscope. The omentum is then stitched to the underside of the dura so that it is closely applied to the spinal cord bridging the damaged segment. The wounds are then closed. The patients usually have a mild postoperative ileus that lasts 24–48 hours. Other potential complications of the surgery are a Cerebrospinal Fluid (CSF) leak that usually settles spontaneously, presumably because of the ability of the omentum to absorb CSF.

C. Preliminary Studies

1. The Brook Hospital Study

There are a few reports of patients' neurological states being improved by omental transposition. Unfortunately these cases are anecdotal and little attention was paid to conducting a detailed study until the Brook Hospital study (28). It was felt appropriate to follow the extensive experimental work carried out during a 25-year period with a careful study into the effects of omental transposition on patients with a chronic spinal injury. This study was performed nearly 10 years ago. The patients involved had sustained an isolated spinal cord injury. Patients had to show some initial recovery in function, implying that the cord was not transsected, but their neurological deficit had to be fixed for at least 1 year prior to surgery. Consent was obtained over a period of time from the patients and their relatives, who understood that the surgery was experimental, had no guarantee of success and carried a possible risk of deterioration after surgery. Prior to operation, all the patients had detailed clinical and functional assessments. In addition sensory evoked potentials were performed, each patient had a computed tomography (CT) scan or a magnetic resonance imaging (MRI) scan performed to localize accurately the damaged area and confirm continuity of the spinal cord.

2. Results

Ten patients were involved in this study. Six patients had sustained a cervical cord injury, and the remainder had injuries in the thoracolumbar region.

Three patients developed a CSF fluid leak from the laminectomy wound, but this stopped within days. Two patients developed chest infections that responded to physical and antibiotic therapy. Six patients developed urinary tract infections that responded to the appropriate antibiotic therapy.

No patient deteriorated after surgery.

Two of the six cervical patients had demonstrable improvement in function. Of the four patients with a thoracolumbar injury, one improved. The case histories of the patients who improved are briefly described.

Case 1

A 16-year-old boy sustained a fracture dislocation of D10-11 that required a fusion 3 years before omental transposition. He was wheelchair-bound but independent for all transfers. He used a standing frame but had poor three-point ambulation. He catheterized himself 5 hourly, had little rectal sensation, and was fecally incontinent. He had a sensory level at T10-11 with flaccid legs and grade 3 hip flexion. He underwent omental transposition from T9-L1.

One year after the operation he had increased movement around the hip and some movement at the knee. However, the major improvements were that some rectal sensation had returned so that he was no longer fecally incontinent. He was also able to perform four-point ambulation. These improvements led to the patient regarding himself as more socially acceptable and enabled him to return to school.

Case 2

A 37-year-old man sustained a fracture dislocation, resulting in quadriplegia, at C5-6. He had an anterior fusion at that level. He subsequently developed a posttraumatic syrinx that was initially treated by an anterior decompression, followed 2 years later by a myelotomy and cyst drainage. He continued to deteriorate slowly neurologically. When assessed for omental transposition 6 years after his injury, he was in a wheelchair and needed assistance for transfers. He triggered his bladder and bowels, and had poor temperature control, with severe spasms in his legs. He had a sensory level at C6, good shoulder power bilaterally with elbow flexion, but only a flicker of extension bilaterally. There was some movement of his thumb and index finger on the left, but none on the right.

He underwent omental transposition from C4-7. Two years postoperatively, he had improved function in both hands, being able to hold a tumbler with the right hand and feed himself. His leg spasms improved and he felt his temperature control to be better. There had been no alteration in spasticity or bladder and bowel function.

Case 3

This 18-year-old gymnast sustained a C4-5 fracture dislocation while performing a floor exercise. He was immediately tetraplegic. He had an anterior decompression and fusion performed at the time. Two years later, he presented for omental transposition. At that time, he was able to feed himself with assistance. He had to be strapped into his chair because of poor balance. His temperature control was grossly impaired. His bladder was automatic and he needed suppositories for his bowels. There was a sensory level at C4-5. He was able to shrug his left shoulder with grade 3 movement in the right, grade 4 flexion in the elbow bilaterally but no extension. He underwent omental transposition from C3-7.

After 2 years' follow-up, he had improved function in his right arm and hand. His writing, which had previously been indecipherable, became progressively more legible. He had some function in his left arm and shoulder and was thus able to balance himself in his wheelchair, which he was able to push with his right arm. There was improvement in his spasms and the patient said that he had good temperature control. There was no other discernible change, but the changes were such that he was able to return to work and teach gymnastics.

All three patients sustained low-velocity injuries. Although this study suggested that omental transposition may have a place in the treatment of patients with a chronic spinal injury, it failed to address many questions. How is improved neurological function achieved? Does the omentum increase spinal blood flow to the damaged area, and if so, is increased flow related to improved neurological function? Is ischemia or the concept of neuronal idling the essential pathology behind the demonstrable recovery? Is the improvement in temperature control described by patients with a cervical cord injury due to an improvement in autonomic function? Are some of these changes explicable by the delivery of neurotransmitters to the area of damaged cord by the omentum?

To attempt to answer some of these questions, a more detailed and exhaustive study was designed.

3. The Wessex Study

The same selection criteria in the Brook study were used for the selection of patients. To objectively test whether the omental transposition was the cause of improvement, the study was designed as a multiple baseline across-subjects study, with at least three preoperative assessments. The assessments used were very rigorous, the most important being the clinical and functional assessments. These consisted of grading the patient's motor and sensory deficits, as well as the application of well-established assessments of disability and handicap (Table 2). All patients underwent an MRI scan to show physical continuity of the cord, localize the area of damage, and exclude secondary features of cord injury such as a syrinx. Videourodynamics were performed to assess bladder function and the electrophysiological assessments included motor and somato-sensory evoked potentials (22,35). Dynamic thermography and Doppler skin blood flow measurements were performed to assess any changes in temperature regulation. The most important assessments were the clinical and functional assessments.

Eighteen patients have been enrolled into the study. Follow-up has not been completed at the time of writing and the full results will be published in approximately 1 year. However the preliminary results are encouraging. In two paraplegics, there has been some improvement in hip function and some return of sensation in the lower limbs. One patient with a high cervical cord injury

Table 2 Assessments of Disability and Handicap

Modified Ashworth scale for spasticity
Rivermead mobility index
Wheelchair mobility index
Barthel activities of daily living (ADL) index
Frenchay activities index
Nottingham extended ADL index

(C4-5) had some increased power in wrist extension. One patient deteriorated a few months after surgery, and this deterioration was mirrored by changes in thermoregulation. Her condition subsequently improved and 2 years after surgery, she has almost returned to her preoperative state. One patient died of recurrence of lymphoma 10 months after surgery.

IV. OMENTAL TRANSPOSITION—THE FUTURE?

These studies have demonstrated that, in patients with a fixed deficit, improvement is possible after omental transposition. What is uncertain is how this is achieved. It is attractive to postulate that the revascularization of a chronically ischemic cord may reactivate idling neurones. Another possibility is the delivery of neurotransmitters and neural growth factors to an area of injured cord produces a stimulatory effect. However, the detailed results of this study are necessary before any constructive arguments can be offered.

These preliminary results do open the debate on the question of early omental transposition in acute spinal cord injury. Experimentally, omental transposition will reduce the formation of scar tissue in an acutely damaged spinal cord and, as Marquis and Siek have shown, will promote and channel the growth of sprouting axons through the area of damaged cord (23). Whether this regrowth is sufficiently organized to restore function is not yet clear.

The omentum may have a unique role to play in the management of patients with a spinal injury. The ultimate aim of our investigations will be to minimize the acute effects of a spinal cord injury by the use of omental transposition, so that a significant and sustained improvement in function is achieved.

REFERENCES

1. Allen AR. Remarks on the histopathological changes in the spinal cord due to impact. An experimental study. Journal of Mental and Nervous Disorders 1914; 41:141–147.
2. Bracken MB, Freeman DH Jr, Hellenbrand K. Incidence of acute traumatic hospitalized spinal cord injury in the United States, 1970–1977. Am J Epidemiol 1981; 13:615–622.
3. Bracken MB, Shepherd MJ, Collins WF. A randomized controlled trial of methyl prednisolone or naloxone in the treatment of acute spinal-cord injury: Results of the second acute spinal cord injury study. New Engl J Med 1990; 322:1405–1411.
4. Collins WF. A review and update of experiment and clinical studies of spinal cord injury. Paraplegia 1983; 21:204–219.
5. Dohrmann GJ, Allen WE. Microcirculation of traumatized spinal cord. A correla-

tion of microangiography and blood flow patterns in transitory and permanent paraplegia. J Trauma 1975; 15:1003–1013.

6. Dohrmann GJ, Wagner FC Jr, Bucy PC. The microvasculature in transitory traumatic paraplegia. An electron microscopic study in the monkey. J Neurosurg 1971; 35:263–271.

7. Ducker TB, Lucas JT, Wallace CA. Recovery from spinal cord injury. Clin Neurosurg 1983; 30:495–513.

8. Eidelberg E. The pathophysiology of spinal cord injury. Radiol Clin N Amer 1987; 15:241–246.

9. Faden AI, Holaday JW. Endorphins in traumatic spinal cord injury. Pathophysiological studies and clinical implications. Mod Probl Pharmacopsychiatry 1981; 17:158–74.

10. Faden AI, Jacobs TP, Smith GP. Neuropeptides in spinal cord injury: Comparative experimental models. Peptides 1983; 4:631–634.

11. Foy PM, Findlay GFG. Spinal injury. In: Miller JD, ed. Northfield's Surgery of the Central Nervous System. London 1987; 871–893.

12. Goldsmith HS, De Los Santos R, Beattie EA Jr. Relief of chronic lymphedema by omental transposition. Ann Surgery 1967; 166:573–585.

13. Goldsmith HS, Chen WF, Duckett S: Brain vascularisation by intact omentum. Arch Surg 1973; 106:695–698.

14. Goldsmith HS, Duckett S, Chen WF. Prevention of cerebral infarction in the dog by intact omentum. Am J Surg 1975; 129:262–265.

15. Goldsmith HS, Duckett S, Chen WF. Spinal cord revascularisation by intact omentum. Am J Surg 1975; 129:262–265.

16. Goldsmith HS, Steward E, Chen WF, Duckett S: Application of intact omentum to the normal and traumatised spinal cord. Spinal Cord Reconstruction 1983; 43:235–243.

17. Goldsmith HS, Griffith AL, Kupferman A, Catsimpoolas N. Lipid angiogenic factor from omentum. JAMA 1984; 15:2034–2036.

18. Goldsmith HS, McIntosh T, Vezina RM, Colton T. Vasoactive neurochemicals identified in omentum: A preliminary report. Br J Neurosurg 1987; 1:359–364.

19. Grundy D, Russell J, Swain A. ABC of spinal cord injury. Br Med J 1986.

20. Guha A, Tator CH, Rochon J. Spinal cord blood flow and systemic blood pressure after experimental spinal cord injury in rats. Stroke 1989; 20:372–377.

21. Levander B, Zwetnau NN. Bulk flow of CSF through a lumbo-omental graft in the dog. Archives of Neurochirurgie 1975; 41:147–155.

22. Levy WJ, McCaffrey M, Hagichi S. Motor evoked potentials as a predictor of recovery in chronic spinal cord injury. Neurosurgery 1987; 20:138–142.

23. Marquis JK, Siek GL. Neurotrophic substances present in omental tissue. First International Congress on the Omentum, 1988.

24. Miyamoto S, Kikuchi H, Karasawa J, Nagata I, Ikara I, Yamagata S. Study of the posterior circulation in moyamoya disease. Part 2. Visual disturbance and surgical treatment. J Neurosurg 1986; 65:454–460.

25. Morison R. Remarks on some functions of the omentum. Br Med J 1906; 1:76–78.

26. Naftchi NE. Alterations of neuroendocrine functions in spinal cord injury. Peptides 1985; 6(1):85–94.

27. Naftchi NE, Wooten EW. The CNS and adrenal tyrosine hydroxylase activity and norepinephrine, serotonin, and histamine in the spinal cord after transection. Federal Proceedings 1972; 31:832.
28. Neil-Dwyer G. A pilot study of the effect of omental transposition on patients with a traumatic chronic spinal injury. J Neurol Neurosurg Psychiatry 1989; 2:924.
29. O'Shaughnessy L. An experimental method of providing a collateral circulation to the heart. Br J Surg 1936; 23:665–670.
30. O'Shaughnessy L. Surgical treatment of cardiac ischaemia. Lancet 1937; 1:185.
31. Osterholm JC. The pathophysiologic response to spinal cord injury: The current status of related research. J Neurosurg 1974; 40:5–33.
32. Sandler AN, Tator CH. Review of the effect of spinal cord trauma on the vessels and blood flow in the spinal cord. J Neurosurg 1976; 45:638–646.
33. Tator CH. Vascular effects and blood flow in acute spinal injuries. J Neurosurg Sci 1984; 28:115–119.
34. Tator CH, Fehlings MG. Review of the secondary injury theory of acute spinal cord trauma with emphasis on vascular mechanisms. J Neurosurg 1991; 75:15–26.
35. Taylor S, Ashby P, Verrier M. Neurophysiological changes following traumatic spinal lesions in man. J Neurol Neurosurg Psychiatry 1984; 47:1102–1108.
36. Tsai S, Shih C, Shyy T, Liu J. Recovery of vasomotor response in human spinal cord transection. J Neurosurg 1980; 52:808–811.
37. Vineberg AM. The bloodless greater omentum for myocardial revascularisation. Diseases of the Chest 1968; 54:315–322.
38. Wallace CM, Tator CH. Spinal blood flow measured with microspheres following spinal cord injury in the rat. Can J Neurol Sci 1986; 13:91–96.
39. Wallin BG, Stjernberg L. Sympathetic activity in man after spinal cord injury. Brain 1984; 107:183–198.
40. Wallin G. Abnormalities of sympathetic regulation after cervical cord lesions. Acta Neurochir 1986; 36(suppl):123–124.
41. Yonekawa Y. Experimental intracranial transplantation of the omentum majus in dogs: A tentative new treatment for hydrocephalus and cerebral ischaemia. Archives of Japanese Chirurgie 1977; 47:3–17.
42. Young W. Medical treatments of acute spinal cord injury. J Neurol Neurosurg Psychiatry 1977; 55:635–639.

27

Pain Associated with Disease of the Spinal Cord

Jonathan Cole

Southampton University Hospital, Southampton, Hampshire, and Poole Hospital, Poole, Dorset, England

I. INTRODUCTION

It may legitimately be asked why a chapter dedicated to pain alone should be included in this volume. Pain, after all, is only a symptom and a few books would have a chapter, say, on spasticity or hyperreflexia. It is, however, because pain is only a symptom, and has no signs, that it can frequently be overlooked or inadequately treated. The purely symptomatic nature of pain was emphasized by the I.A.S.B. committee for taxonomy that defined it as "An unpleasant sensory and emotional experience associated with actual or potential tissue damage, or described in terms of such damage."

They continued that, "Pain is always subjective. Each individual learns the application of the word through experiences related to injury in early life (36)."

Without wishing to enter into too great a definitional controversy, the above definition has relied on not only pain's perception and experience but also on a measure of communication of the unpleasantness. It should not be forgotten that in some cases, specifically children or those who are suffering from learning disabilities or senile dementias, this element of reportage is not always present (1). Having accepted that this description of pain is not always possible, there is now much information on those words used to describe the sensory quality of pain, together with its more emotional parts, and to describe the overall intensity of the total pain experience (31,32).

This questionnaire and others have been used quite extensively, although not always with uniform results. Melzack has suggested that the most severe pains, apart from labor pain, are causalgias. On a linear analog scale, causalgia might reach around 42 in pain after accidental amputation of a digit; just below that would be childbirth at 30–40, and then chronic back pain and phantom limb pain between 25 and 27. Arthritis would be rated as 19(34). In another study however, it was found, using the McGill questionnaire, the Sternbach Pain Index, and the Zung Pain and Distress Index, that pain associated with chronic spinal cord injury rated equal to or worse than pain from cancer, childbirth, or phantom limbs (13).

As many have suggested there are profound differences between the acute severe pain, which the normal population may experience, and chronic debilitating pain, which alters the quality of pain and has effects on the individual at many levels. This chapter will consider some of the syndromes associated with spinal cord disease that lead to pain, their incidence, their pathophysiology, and possible methods of treatment. It will focus on spinal cord injury because the chronic pain associated with this condition has been underestimated in the past. Also, this pain, in being resistant to most treatment, acts as a challenge at therapeutic and pathophysiological levels, and so is a model for spinal pain associated with other diseases.

II. THE RELATION OF PAIN TO SPINAL CORD DISEASE

Pain may be divided conveniently, although rather simplistically, into neuropathic pain and neurogenic pain. Injury or damage to peripheral tissues evokes activation of free nerve endings, which leads to the perception of neurogenic pain. Whether due to a cut, bruise, or fracture, this is the pain most of us experience at some time in our lives. In contrast, neuropathic pain is perceived due to abnormal functioning within nerve cells at some level of the neuraxis. Within neuropathic pain, differentiation may be made between that originating from peripheral abnormal function, e.g., neuralgia after peripheral nerve injury or postherpetic neuralgia, where abnormal firing may occur in dorsal root ganglion cells, and central neuropathic pain, where the pain generator is considered to be within the brain and spinal cord. As will be seen, these anatomical divisions merge in the pathophysiology of pain.

A. Neuropathic Pain

Some spinal cord pain syndromes are likely to include more than one of these mechanisms in their origin. In spinal cord injury, for instance, multiple origins for pain may be apparent. Acutely, there is usually damage to the bones, muscles, and ligaments surrounding the cord at the level of the injury. Pain also may be the result of associated nerve root pressure and be projected into the limbs, in a way similar to sciatica. Lastly, and often emerging far later, is "central" or dysesthetic pain, which is comparatively common in the chronically spinal cord-injured population.

The classification of pain associated with spinal cord injury has recently been reviewed by Siddall et al. (47). They suggested the following terms, based on the system involved: musculoskeletal, visceral, neuropathic, and other types. We are particularly concerned with the neuropathic pain. Siddall, et al. subdivided this in two ways: first by the site of the presumed origin of pain, neuropathic at the level of the injury and below the level, and second, in terms of likely causation, either radicular or central. Thus pain at the level of the injury arising from nerve root damage and with increased pain on movement would be "neuropathic at-level radicular pain." Pain felt bilaterally below the level and in an insentient part of the body would be "neuropathic below-level central pain."

Although some relatively early reports discussed the incidence of central pain associated with spinal cord injury (6,14,39), these findings did not perhaps receive sufficient notice, in Britain at least, probably because of the ineffectiveness of treatment and the legitimate desire to use distraction therapy. This is despite the fact that central pain after spinal cord injury was probably first described by Holmes in soldiers of the First World War (21). He described the pain as starting shortly after the injury and subsiding after about 1 month, although it is generally agreed that central pain can be much more longlasting than this.

However, more recently both within the United Kingdom and elsewhere, the prevalence and incidence of this sort of pain has become more apparent. A more recent review of the literature, for instance, suggested that of those with spinal cord injury, 34–94% experienced pain, of whom one-third considered it severe (5). Such wide variability suggests methodological and definitional differences. To try to obviate such objections, Rose et al. (41), in a postal survey, asked not about pain per se but about the effect that pain had on daily living activities. They found that in 98 out of 885 respondents with pain, it was their pain rather than immobility that stopped them from working. Of those in work, 83% said that pain interfered with their work; in 118 it stopped social activity.

Although spinal cord-injured patients comprise a large percentage of those living with chronic pain secondary to spinal cord disease, it is apparent that central pain may be a consequence of lesions at any level of the spinal cord (as well, of course as more centrally). Any cause of myelopathy can be associated with pain. Thus vascular lesions of the cord [infarction, hemorrhage, or arteriovenous malformation (AVN)], multiple sclerosis (MS), transverse myelitis, syringomyelia, and any vascular insult to the cord may have pain as a significant part of their clinical syndrome.

Pain in MS has also been neglected. However 29–58% of people with MS have pain; in 32%, pain was their worst symptom (48). In some cases painful stiffness associated with spasticity may be accompanied by back pain, probably due to local mechanical causes. Root pain, and in some cases more central dysesthetic pain, may also occur. Although syringomyelia is classically known to present with loss of pain sensation, diffuse central pain can be a sufficiently large part of the syndrome that the diagnosis is delayed. Such pain may be due to central cord disturbance secondary to the syrinx itself. Acute transverse myelopathy, in contrast, is often recognized as a spinal cord syndrome because of the development of paresthesia—reduction in sensation in an area projected below the level of spinal involvement—or by a most severe back or supposedly root pain, which is usually around the higher level of the cord affected.

Although the most common symptom in patients with tumors of the spinal cord is pain, the type, the site, and projection of that pain depend on the location of the tumor itself. Not surprisingly, root pain is associated most frequently with extradural tumor and often involves more than one root. In contrast, pain associated with very rare spinal meningiomas may be bilateral. Intraspinal tumor rarely produce root pain except in the lumbosacral segments (for obvious reasons). Intramedullary spinal cord tumors may be associated with less clearly localized pain that has a dull, aching, and unpleasant quality.

If spinal cord injury central pain is due to deafferentation, then it is not surprising that such pain can arise, unfortunately, after cordotomy. The pain may arise months after the surgery, however, which makes this procedure one of near-last resort except in those with terminal illness. Lastly, although uncommon, severe lightning pain in tabes dorsalis associated with syphilis is likely to be due to intrinsic spinal cord dysfunction.

B. Peripheral Neurogenic Pain

In addition to central pain syndromes associated with spinal cord disease, there are a number of conditions in which pain is associated with abnormalities at the roots or just beyond.

One of the most important medical, surgical, and social problems in the Western world is nerve root compression in the low back which produces pain localized to the low back and projected down into one of the legs. This topic is of course a huge one and beyond the scope of the present chapter. The importance of accurate diagnosis that distinguishes root compression due to a disc, a facet joint syndrome, or epidural fibrosis cannot be overestimated. In some cases, although not all, the type, characteristics, and location of the pain can be helpful in determining the diagnosis. Certainly, the location of the pain is a prognostic factor if surgery is to be considered. Pain felt diffusely in the back carries a worse prognosis for root decompression than more clearly lateralized and projected pain into a limb. The importance of selective operation in such patients is highlighted by the frequency of the so-called failed back syndrome in which subjects have persistent low back pain after a variety of surgical operations for a number of different pathologies (54).

If the exact site and type of pathology are frequently poorly understood in low back syndromes, the opposite is the case in two other severe pain syndromes associated with afferent radiculopathy or ganglionopathy. Whereas cervical root compression is associated with pain, paresthesia, and weakness similar to compression of lumbosacral roots, central pain is associated with traumatic avulsion of the cervical nerve roots. Wynn Parry (55) found that 98 out of 108 cases of brachial plexus avulsion suffered significant pain, whereas pain was less of a problem in 167 patients with a brachial plexus lesion distal to the dorsal root ganglion. The pain was very different than cervical disc protrusion. Although the pain was projected in a dermatomal distribution, it was described as being hot or burning. It would frequently be perceived constantly but with severe paroxysms. Despite the lesion being peripheral to the central nervous system, the pain has many characteristics of so-called central pain. There is also a not inconsiderable incidence of brachial plexus and root lesions associated with cervical spinal cord injury that is not always recognized.

Lastly, postherpetic neuralgia is usually expected to begin 3 months after the onset of acute shingles. The pain, often remarkably similar to some brachial avulsions, is described as being continuously burning or raw, with superimposed paroxysmal increases, and in a dermatomal distribution. In addition, whereas the scars of infection may be hypoesthetic, hyperesthesia and hyperpathia may also occur. Conventionally the site of abnormal neural discharge is considered to be the sensory nerve bodies of the dorsal root ganglion. It might therefore be considered an example of a peripheral neurogenic pain. However, such anatomical divisions, as suggested above, even in this condition, are oversimplified. Watson et al. (53) examined the spinal cord, dorsal root ganglion, dorsal root, and peripheral nerve from five patients, three with severe posthepatic neuralgia and two without pain.

Three cases had severe postherpetic neuralgia with constant pain with exacerbations, and two had no persistent pain. In both groups, there was marked loss of myelin and axons in the affected nerve or sensory root. However, only in those with chronic pain was dorsal horn atrophy and cell axon and myelin loss with fibrosis observed in the relevant sensory ganglion. It is likely therefore that a complex interaction between dorsal root ganglion, dorsal horn, and possibly central areas of the neuraxis was responsible for the chronic pain syndrome.

III. PATHOPHYSIOLOGY OF PAIN ASSOCIATED WITH THE SPINAL CORD

Understanding the pathophysiology of pain is not simply an intellectual exercise, for it allows the potential for physiological treatments. The failure to understand the complex nature of particularly chronic pain has, in the past, led to erroneous and often irreversible treatments, such as neurectomy and cordotomy.

A. Neurogenic Pain

In the classical physiological model, peripheral nociceptors associated with free nerve endings are activated by peripheral tissue damage and impulses are transmitted to the spinal cord through C-fiber and A-delta nerves. After synapsing in the dorsal horn (usually in the superficial laminae), impulses are transmitted rostrally through the contralateral spinothalamic tract to wide areas of the brainstem and brain. Even in comparatively simple, peripherally originating, nociception, however, simple stimulus response relationships do not hold. The phenomenon of hyperalgesia, in which the threshold for pain is lowered and pain increased for suprathreshold stimuli, occurs after most peripheral injury. This perceptual event is thought to be due to the peripheral nerve fibers having a decreased threshold for response, an increased response to suprathreshold stimulus, and in some cases spontaneous activity (27,29).

However, hyperalgesia is not solely due to peripheral sensitization. Secondary hyperalgesia also occurs in the area surrounding the original insult, and this has been shown to be due to a central effect in which increasingly secure synaptic links develop between those nociceptive pathways and pathways that previously may not have been involved in the perception of pain.

This secondary hyperalgesia leads to a small area around the tissue damage in which stroking can evoke a painful perception. This phenomenon, also known as allodynia, suggests synaptic contacts between low-threshold peripheral mechanic receptors, normally associated with touch perception, and nociceptive pathways. That such a mechanism does exist has received clinical evidence from Cole, et al. (9), who showed that spinal cord stimulation of dorsal column fibers centrally in the cord evoked severe pain in a subject with allodynia.

The arcane details of hyperalgesia are less important to the argument than the fact that even in comparatively simple peripherally originating pain, central synaptic plasticity may lead to altered input/output relations in the nociceptive pathway, probably at a dorsal horn level. Such reorganization has indeed been shown in an animal model by Asada et al. (3).

B. Neuropathic Pain

Several mechanisms have been suggested for the development of neuropathic pain, including "local irritation at the site of injury," activation of alternative pathways inside or outside the spinal cord, biochemical changes, abnormal firing and reorganization of deafferented neurons, and loss of descending inhibition (46).

It seems likely that a central phenomenon in this pain is ectopic and inappropriate generation of nociceptive input to the central pain perception mechanism, although the underlying pathophysiology remains unclear. Evidence comes from a number of sources. In central thalamic pain, damage to neurones may lead to ectopic discharge associated with pain. In some forms of central pain associated with spinal cord injury it is thought that a spontaneous discharge may arise at the level of the stump. The lack of exact localization of such pain arises because of the deafferentation that is involved in the origin of the pain, although neurons of the neural stump have been shown to be tonically discharging (28). In a patient with phantom foot pain, Nystrom and Hagbarth (37) recorded ongoing discharge in the peroneal nerve. Percussion of the stump neuroma led to pain and ongoing spike activity. Perhaps surprisingly though, peripheral local anesthetic blocked the neuroma but did not reduce the ongoing discharge, suggesting that in phantom limb pain, the ectopic discharges may be at the level of the dorsal root ganglion or even more central.

It will have become apparent that most neuropathic pains, either peripheral or central, are associated not only with ectopic discharge, but with a degree of deafferentation. The most obvious example is in spinal cord injury but a degree of deafferentation may also occur in a number of other central pains, including postherpetic neuralgia. The mechanisms of generation of such pain are likely to differ from those that are involved in peripherally originated hypersensitivity, inasmuch as the latter appears almost instantaneously whereas central deafferentation pain may take months to develop. Some form of slow plastic reorganization appears likely, something that will be considered in more detail later.

1. The Quality of Chronic Neuropathic Pain

Pain that is endured over time, often for years, comes to have a different quality than that which we may experience acutely. Because those with this chronic pain have an experience we have not shared, their descriptions strain at what can be expressed. Patients describe their pain as being continuous and as having little relation to any stimulation. It is poorly localized and often described in terms of cramping, aching, burning, or stabbing. Although continuous, it can be worse paroxysmally. Whereas the words used to explain chronic pain are familiar to us all, the quality of this pain is probably quite different than the pain we may have acutely (4). In spinal cord injury, or say brachial root avulsion, the pain is often projected to the deafferented part, making it homologous to phantom limb pain even though the limb remains.

IV. TREATMENT OF PAIN ASSOCIATED WITH SPINAL CORD DISEASE

A. Neuropathic Pain

1. Medical Treatments

For neurogenic pain associated with spinal cord disease, treatment depends on its cause. Radiculopathy, for instance, may respond to operative intervention. Although not especially effective, such patients also usually receive a variety of oral analgesics. Although not always simple to treat, such pains may in general be less resistant to treatment than the neuropathic pains that will be considered.

Despite increasing recognition of neuropathic pain resulting from spinal cord injury, there have been very few properly controlled trials of drug medications. For most patients, a slowly increasingly cascade of oral analgesics will have been tried with, on the whole, disappointing or mixed results. It is often difficult to distinguish between placebo effects and real ones, and of course individual pain syndromes and individual subjects' responsiveness to various drugs may differ too. A large scale postal survey found that of their sample of 885, 232 had taken drugs, including a few who had tried opiates but discontinued them as being ineffective (41). Only 162 took drugs regularly, mostly aspirin and paracetamol. This reflected not the trivial nature of their pain, but rather the ineffectiveness of analgesics in this condition. Interestingly 132 found that alcohol did alleviate their pain significantly, and more than one respondent had been concerned about the risks of addiction because of this. They found that many patients with spinal cord injury and central pain had tried opioids, but few continued. This has been considered evidence, erroneously in the author's opinion, that these subjects' pain is not severe. Trials of opioids in patients with central pain have provided evidence that such pains have a very low sensitivity to such drugs (2).

Antidepressant drugs, both the older adrenergic and newer selective serotonin reuptake inhibitors, have been used with some success in chronic, otherwise intractable, central pain, independent of any antidepressant effect. However, this trial was in central postoperative pain and such favorable results have not been evident in pain secondary to spinal cord injury. It is the impression that, to be effective, antidepressants must be given in fairly large doses and that the analgesic properties correlate with plasma concentrations of the drug (7).

Antiepileptic drugs are also widely used for central neurogenic pain, despite the absence of good double blind control trials. Carbamazepine, phenytoin, sodium valproate, and clonazepam are among those used. The rationale is that antiepileptic drugs suppress atopic discharge neurones in epilepsy and may therefore dampen pain arising from spontaneous ectopic discharges. However once again, double blind cross-over trials are few. In one recent study, sodium valproate was not found to be useful in relieving central pain in 20 people with spinal cord injury (16).

In view of the relative ineffectiveness of these drugs, combination therapy was suggested by Sandford, et al. (43) after their success in a single tetraplegic subject in whom carbamazepine and amitryptiline were ineffective singly, but did have a significant analgesic effect when taken together. It is a little depressing that such examples seem so few and far between, and are at the level of single case studies.

If the primary central generator of central pain is, say, at the stump of an injured spinal cord, the logical treatment might be to deliver local anesthetic to that area. Success in relieving spasticity with this technique has led us to use in pain. Siddall, et al. (45) showed a combination of clonidine and morphine to be effective when morphine alone was not useful in the treatment of neuropathic below-level spinal cord pain, in a single case study. Unfortunately intrathecal delivery of analgesics, although effective in some cases, has many complications and long-term side effects and is not in widespread use. Chronic intraspinal opioid and local anesthetic mixtures appear to be limited at the moment to use in those with terminal illness (26).

Despite all these therapeutic measures, it is the unfortunate experience of those with spinal cord injury chronic central pain that they find most analgesics are of little value. This may reveal something about the pathogenesis of chronic central pain, as will be considered later.

The classical liberal approach to any problem is to try to avoid the situation that brought about the deleterious event in the first place. This approach is also physiologically logical in pain. If complex and long-lasting hypersensitivity can result from the long-term effects of even a comparatively trivial peripheral nociceptive input, then the obvious solution is to reduce that input. Thus in 1988 Wall argued for preventing postoperative pain by local anesthesia to the spinal cord receiving nociceptive input from the operative site (52). Clinical trials of such an approach have been begun (30,50). Tverskoy et al. (50) found that postoperative pain after hernia repairs was significantly reduced in a group who had spinal anesthesia, or general plus local anesthesia, compared to those who had general anesthesia alone. Neural blockade at the time of surgery, when nociceptive impulses are presumed to enter the central nervous system, may reduce the significance of postoperative pain by suppressing the original stimulus for a more sustained hyperexcitability state.

It will be particularly interesting to see whether incidents of such catastrophic events as phantom limb pain can be reduced in those cases where limb amputation was performed under spinal as well as general anesthesia.

2. Neurostimulation Techniques

Where an obvious peripheral cause of pain is present then removal or reduction of the original stimulus will reduce the pain. What is intellectually simple may of course be technically very difficult. It is known, however, that in pain due to nerve root entrapment, decompression can lead to almost immediate resolution of the pain. The situation is far more complex in the chronic pain syndromes that we are, for the most part, concerned with.

In cases where no continuing tissue damage or entrapment is known to cause the pain, the therapeutic options alter. Some pains involving partial deafferentation may respond by altering the balance between nociceptive and low-threshold inputs. Such a theoretical justification underlies the introduction of transcutaneous electrical nerve stimulation (TENS). Some postherpetic neuralgia, causalgias, and radiculopathies respond in part to TENS. In general, chronic pain states are less easily treated with TENS, as one would have expected.

After the introduction of TENS, the next logical step was to stimulate low-threshold afferents directly in the spinal cord via dorsal column stimulation. The procedure is usually done as a trial at first, with a temporary percutaneous electrode placed under x-ray control in the epidural space above the dorsal columns. There is agreement among workers in the field that for pain relief to be successful and sustained, the area of stimulator sensation, or a warm paresthesia, has to cover the area of projected pain. If pain relief is reasonable for several days to weeks, the next stage is to implant the system below the surface of the skin with a radio receiver. The procedure has now been evaluated for more than 20 years. Although it may be fair to say that the initial enthusiasm has been tempered by long-term experience, it is a useful procedure in a number of conditions like incomplete plexus lesions, postamputation pain, and some peripheral nerve lesions. It has proved of particular value, surprisingly, in ischemic pain due to peripheral vascular disease.

It is not surprising that stimulation over the dorsal aspect of the cord has proved to be ineffective in complete transverse lesion of the spinal cord and deafferentation pain due to spinal root avulsion (10,15,25,40). In a recent trial, only 20% of subjects claimed a pain relief of 50% after 3 years (8,46). In these conditions stimulator sensation does not overlap the painful area, probably because of the pathophysiology of the pain. Deafferentation has abolished the dorsal column input from the painful area by definition, and the pain is likely to be rising from ectopic discharge, possibly in the deafferented dorsal column with rostral projection through spinothalamic tracts. Without primary or secondary dorsal column afferents to stimulate, there is no possibility of segmental interaction between dorsal column and spinothalamic systems.

This, incidentally, is the reverse of the situation in allodynia in which dorsal column stimulation may make the pain worse, showing that in allodynia, activation of afferents from low-threshold cutaneous receptors leads to pain due to altered central connections (9).

In one case of postamputation pain, spinal cord stimulation was successful for several years; then, despite recurrent attempts, stimulation no longer led to sensation in the phantom. It was concluded that this may have been due to transganglionic degeneration in the secondary dorsal column fibers secondary to long-term deafferentation (11,12).

Proximal brain stimulation for intractable pain has been tried to a number of areas, mainly in the thalamus. It is obviously a procedure that is greatly invasive and one of last resort. A detailed discussion of this is outside the scope of this volume.

3. Neurosurgical Procedures

If one views the nociceptor pathways as beginning in the periphery and ending somewhere in the brain, then it may seem logical, if ectopic discharges are occurring at one level peripherally, to cut that ectopic generator off from the more rostral structures in the hope of reducing the perception of pain.

As has been seen, however, even in the simplest peripheral pain syndromes, central effects also occur and the history of neurosurgical ablations has at best been mixed. Three main kinds of spinal cord surgical lesion have been tried in the treatment of central pain: anterolateral cordotomy to remove the crossed spinothalamic tract, dorsal root entry zone (DREZ) lesions to remove the dorsal horn and Lissauer tract, and cordotomy. All these procedures have some success in relieving pain, at around 50%, and may also relieve pain for weeks and months after the operation.

Dorsal root entry zone ablations have been found most effective in radicular pain. In one review, Sampson et al. (42) found that of 39 patients with pain associated with cauda equina and conus lesions, 54% were pain free with 20% requiring nonopioids afterward. The frequency of complications was 21%.

It should be understood that neurosurgical patient techniques are a method of last resort, and that most of these patients will have had chronic pain for some time so that the population in whom this approach is used are a very difficult group to treat. Many also have a limited life expectancy (because of cancer, etc.), so that a period of 3–6 months without pain may be eagerly accepted. Having said that, a cordomyelotomy, which is designed to preserve descending inhibitory tracts, has been found in 2 out of 3 patients to be at least very effective in relieving pain for more than 10 years (38).

V. CONCLUSIONS

Unfortunately, despite all the above methods of treatment, chronic pain associated with spinal cord injury remains, like most forms of chronic pain, most difficult to treat. One hopes that from this we can learn something of the pathophysiological nature of such pain, and so design logical treatments.

In most cases in which it is effective, both TENS and spinal cord stimulation appear to work by stimulation of large myelinated afferents that, it is known, can reduce the segmental and possibly the suprasegmental transmission of nociceptive information in a way similar to that described in Melzack and Wall's gate theory (35).

Although some patients have obtained good pain relief from partial deafferentation lesions with such stimulation techniques, on the whole experience suggests that there is a slow deterioration in the efficacy of such treatments. This in turn parallels the unfortunately common experience that once severe acute pain has become chronic, it then becomes extraordinarily difficult to relieve. It will be remembered, for instance, that lateral cordotomies for central spinal cord injury pain are effective for a few months but then gradually the pain returns.

Once established within the central nervous system, chronic pain may not behave in a simple manner. It is probably simplistic to think that central pain originates chronically from an ectopic generator, say in the base of the stump of the spinal cord, and that if that stump is removed the pain will be abolished. Rather, it appears that just as "simple" peripheral neurogenic pain produces central sensitization at a dorsal horn level, so chronic pain originating within that dorsal horn may produce prolonged and widespread changes within the brain itself, at thalamic and multiple cortical levels.

It was in part the disappointment of ablative procedures and the behavior of chronic pain that led Melzack to propose his neuromatrix model for central pain (33). In this he suggested that phantom limb phenomena and chronic pain may be represented in a widespread net of neurons extending throughout the brain. Thalamocortical and limbic loops may diverge to allow parallel processing of differing components of the neuromatrix and then converge to allow interaction between inputs and outputs. This, as stated, is a rather vague hypothesis, without more anatomical details. However with position emission tomography (PET) techniques, multiple areas involved in pain perception are being delineated (20). The therapeutic implications of such a model, in which widespread areas of the brain interact to produce chronic pain once pain is established, might at first sight be considered bleak. They do certainly suggest that attempts at the lower parts of the neuraxis to relieve pain by ablation are doomed to long-term failure, but this has proved clinically to be the case for some time. It is possible, however, if there are multiple areas for processing of nociceptive perceptions, that selective ablations of such areas might be effective in relief of pain (see below).

Legitimate and parallel questions are why nociceptive input should behave like this; why a short stimulus should lead to such longlasting plastic alterations in the central nervous system; and why in some cases, as in the case of spinal cord injury pain, these alterations become apparently permanent. (Rose, et al. (41) found no evidence that chronic pain after spinal cord injury lessened with time.) Whereas there is a good evolutionary reason for pain, to alert to damage and to protect during healing, there seems no use to chronic debilitating pain such as many have to live with. One could answer that any animal with damage severe enough that chronic pain resulted would have long been killed by predators. However such pain is reflecting a curious, even mysterious, aspect of the organization of the nociceptive/pain mechanism.

Another and possibly related question is why peripheral nerves require such a large percentage of small myelinated and unmyelinated fibers (about 80%) to input temperature, autonomic functions, muscle fatigue, and pain that is perceived usually very infrequently. An answer to this question may be related to the mechanisms of plastic and permanent change in central synaptic efficiency. Some time ago, Wall suggested that one function of such small fibers might be to set the boundaries of synaptic territories of the larger myelinated fiber inputs, which are under competition with each other for transmission of their inputs (18).

Evidence for this theory has recently come from experiments investigating the alteration in localization of cutaneous sensation after limb amputation (19,24). The authors found that reorganization of cutaneous inputs and perception after amputation correlated with the presence of phantom pain from that area, suggesting that this plasticity was related to nociceptor input. "The greater the cortical reorganisation after amputation the more likely painful stimuli will be mislocated into the phantom limb and the more likely patients will suffer phantom limb pain." (24)

Further evidence for the involvement of nociceptive input comes from work on individuals with chronic pain. Katz and Melzack (23) found evidence for the expansion of cortical receptive fields and for referred sensation in people with chronic pain without amputation.

As we have seen, once chronic pain is established, it is very difficult to remove and one is left with exploring strategies for living with it. How people actually do this has been studied by a number of workers (17,22,44). There is beginning to be a consensus that people have two broad coping strategies. Some people live with the expectation that they will receive help with the pain that has been imposed on them, whereas others believe that they can control their pain themselves. They avoid "catastrophizing" their pain and refuse to believe they are severely disabled by it. Not surprisingly, those who actively manage their pain do better than those who are more passive. It is likely that premorbid personality in part determines these responses. A realistic self-evaluation of pain and goals in life is also important. If no effective treatment is likely, then further work in this field is necessary to determine those factors that allow some people to cope better.

In the long term, however, one would like not to study how subjects cope with pain but to reduce or remove it. This still seems a long way off. It may be possible to develop selective drugs that are particularly effective in certain areas of the brain concerned with either the representation of nociceptor input or even with perception of pain itself. These areas are becoming delineated now using functional imaging techniques like PET (20). It is perhaps falsely optimistic though to expect selective "magic bullet" neurotransmitter inhibitors for such a system. Alternatively the realization that small areas of cortex are involved in pain perception may allow experiments with highly selective neurosurgical ablation based on coregistration of magnetic resonance imaging (MRI), functional MRI, and say, PET scanning. Certainly more selective thalamotomies for intractable tremor and dyskinesiae are showing encouraging results in Parkinson's as we learn more about the physiology and anatomy of that disease. The same may be the case with chronic pain, and past failures should not prevent trials in the future. Such small selective ablations were suggested by Melzack (33) and indeed some encouraging experimental evidence from animal experiments was cited (49,51).

Finally, as so often is the case prevention is better than cure and a realization of the mechanism, evolution, and incidence of chronic pain after deafferentation may lead to new therapeutic interventions. In low spinal cord injury for instance, which is initially painless, might the incidence of subsequent chronic dysesthetic pain be reduced by early use of intrathecal low-dose analgesia?

REFERENCES

1. Anand KJS, Craig KD. New perspectives on the definition of pain. Pain 1996; 67:3–6.
2. Arner S, Meyerson BA. Genuine resistance to opioids—Fact or Fiction? Pain 1991; 47:116–118.
3. Asada H, Yasum W, Yamaguchi Y. Properties of hyperactive cells in rat spinal cord after peripheral nerve section. Pain 1990; Suppl 5:S22.
4. Bennett JG. Neuropathic pain. In: Wall, PD, Melzack, R. Textbook of Pain. London and Edinburgh: Churchill Livingstone, 1994; 201–224.
5. Bonica JJ, Introduction: Semantic, Epidemiologic and Educational issues. In: Casey KL, Ed. Pain and Central Nervous System Disease: The Central Pain Syndromes. New York: Raven Press, 1991; 31–29.

6. Botterell EH, Callaghan JC, Soussi AT. Pain in paraplegia: Clinical management and surgical treatment. Proc Royal Soc Med 1953; 47:281–288.
7. Bovie J. Central pain. In: Wall BD, Melzack R. Textbook of Pain. London and Edinburgh: Churchill Livingstone, 1994; 871–902.
8. Cioni B, Meglio M, Pentamalli L, Visocchi M. Spinal cord stimulation in the treatment of paraplegic pain. Neurosurg 1995; 82:35–39.
9. Cole JD, Illis LS, Sedgwick EM. Pain produced by spinal cord stimulation in a patient with allodynia and pseudotabes. J Neurol Neurosurg Psychiatry 1987; 50:1083–1084.
10. Cole JD, Illis LS, Sedgwick EM. Intractable central pain in spinal cord injury is not relieved by spinal cord stimulation. Paraplegia 1991; 29:167–172.
11. Cole JD, Illis LS, Sedgwick EM. On the late failure of spinal cord stimulation for deafferentation pain. Restorative Neurology and Neuroscience 1992; 4:345–347.
12. Csillik B, Knyih-Csillik E. Transganglionic degeneration. In: Adelman G. Encyclopaedia of Neuroscience. Boston: Burkhauser, 1987; 306–307.
13. Davidoff G, Roth E, Guarraeini M, Sliusa J, Yarkony G. Function limiting dysethetic pain syndrome among traumatic spinal cord injury patients: A cross sectional study. Pain 1987; 29:39–48.
14. Davis L, Martin J. Studies upon spinal cord injuries. J Neurosurg 1947; 4:483–491.
15. Davis R, Lentini R. Transcutaneous nerve stimulation for treatment of patients with spinal cord injury. Surg Neurol 1975; 4:100–101.
16. Drewes AM, Andreasen A, Poulsen LH. Valproate for treatment of chronic central pain after spinal cord injury. Paraplegia 1994; 32:565–569.
17. Ecclestone C. The attentional control of pain: Methodological and theoretical concerns. Pain 1995; 63:3–10.
18. Edelman GM. Neural Darwinism. New York: Basic Books, 1988.
19. Elbert T, Flor H, Birbaumer N, Knecht S, Hampson S, Larbig W, et al. Extensive reorganisation of the somatosensory cortex in adult humans after nervous system injury. Neuroreport 1994; 5:2593–2597.
20. Hseih J-C, Belfrage M, Stone-Elander J, Hansson P, Ingvar M. Central representation of chronic ongoing neuropathic pain studied by positive emission tomography. Pain 1995; 64:303–314.
21. Holmes G. 1919, Pain of central origin. In: Osler W, ed. Contributions to Medical and Biological Research. New York: Paul B Hoeber, 1919; 235–246.
22. Jensen MP, Turner JA, Romano JM, Karoly P. Coping with chronic pain: A critical review of the literature. Pain 1991; 249–283.
23. Katz J, Melzack R. Referred sensations in chronic pain patients. Pain 1987; 28:51–59.
24. Knecht S, Henringen H, Elbert T, Flor H, Hohling C, Paner C, Taub E. Reorganisation and perceptual changes after amputation. Brain 1996; 119:1213–1219.
25. Krainick J-U, Thoten U. Spinal cord stimulation. In: Melzack R, Wall BD. Textbook of Pain. London and Edinburgh: Churchill Livingstone, 1994; 1219–1223.
26. Krames ES. The chronic intraspinal use of opioid and local anaesthetic in mixtures for the relief of intractable pain: When all else fails! Pain 1993; 55:1–4.
27. LaMotte RH, Shain CN, Simone DA, Tsaie F-P. Neurogenic hyperalgesia: Psychophysical studies of underlying mechanisms. J Neurophysiol 1991; 66:190–211.

28. Loeser JD, Ward AA, White LE. Chronic deafferentation of human spinal cord neurones. J Neurosurg 1968; 29:48–50.

29. Mayer RA, Campbell JN. Myelinated nociceptive afferents account for the hyperalgesia that follows a burn to the hand. Science 1981; 213:1527–1529.

30. McQuay HJ, Carroll D, Moore RA. Post-operative orthopaedic pain—the effect of opiate premedication and local anaesthetic blocks. Pain 1988; 33:291–295.

31. Melzack R. Pain Measurement and Assessment. New York: Raven Press, 1983.

32. Melzack R. The short form McGill Pain Questionnaire. Pain 1987; 30:191–197.

33. Melzack R. Phantom limbs and the concept of a neuromatrix. Trends in Neuroscience 1988; 13:88–92.

34. Melzack R, Katz J. Pain measurement in persons in pain. 3rd ed. In: Wall BD, Melzack R. Textbook of Pain. London and Edinburgh: Churchill Livingstone, 1994; 337–351.

35. Melzack R, Wall BD. Pain Mechanisms: A New Theory. Science 1965; 150:971–978.

36. Merskey H. The definition of pain. Eur J Psychiatry 1991; 6:153–159.

37. Nystrom B, Hagbarth KE. Microelectrode recordings from transected nerves in amputees with phantom limb pain. Neuroscience letters 1981; 27:211–216.

38. Pagni CA, Canavero S. Cordomyelotomy in the treatment of paraplegia pain—experience in two cases with long-term results. Acta Neurol Belg 1995; 95:33–36.

39. Pollock LJ, Brown M, Boshes B, Finkelman I, Chor H, Arief AJ, Finkle JR. Pain below the level of injury of the spinal cord. Arch Neurol Neurosurg Psychiatry 1951; 319–322.

40. Richardson RR, Meyer PR, Cerullo LJ. Neurostimulation in the modulation of intractable paraplegic and traumatic neuroma pains. Pain 1980; 8:75–84.

41. Rose M, Robinson J, Ells J, Cole JD. Pain following spinal cord injury: Results from a postal survey. Pain 1988; 34:101–102.

42. Sampson JH, Cashman RE, Nashold BS Jr, Friedman AH. Dorsal root entry zone lesions for intractable pain after trauma to the conus medullaris and cauda equina. J Neurosurg 1995; 82:28–34.

43. Sandford PR, Lindblom LB, Haddox J. Amitryptiline and carbamazepine in the treatment of dysethetic pain in spinal cord injury. Arch Phys Med Rehab 1992; 73:300–301.

44. Schmitz U, Saile H, Nilges P. Coping with chronic pain: Flexible goal adjustment as an interactive buffer against pain related distress. Pain 1996; 67:41–51.

45. Siddall PJ, Gray M, Rutlowski S, Cousins MJ. Intrathecal morphine and clonidine in the management of spinal cord injury pain: A case report. Paraplegia 194; 59:147–148.

46. Siddall PJ, Taylor DA, Cousins MJ. Pain associated with spinal cord injury. Curr Opin Neurol 1995; 8:447–450.

47. Siddall PJ, Taylor DA, Cousins MJ. Classification of pain following spinal cord injury. Spinal Cord 1997; 35:69–75.

48. Stenager E, Knudsen L, Jensen K. Acute and chronic pain syndromes in multiple sclerosis. Acta Neurol Scand 1991; 84:197–200.

49. Tasker RAR, Choiniere M, Libman SM, Melzack R. Analgesia produced by injection of lidocaine into the anterior cingulum bundle of the rat. Pain 1989; 31:237–248.

50. Tverskoy TM, Cozacovcahayche M, Bradley EL, Kissin I. Postoperative pain after inguinal herniorrhaphy with different types of anaesthesia. Anesth Analg 1990; 70:29–35.

51. Vaccarino AL, Melzack R. Analgesia produced by injection of lidocaine into the lateral hypothalamus. Pain 1989; 39:213–219.

52. Wall PD. The prevention of post-operative pain. Pain 1988; 33:289–290.

53. Watson CBN, Deck JH, Morshead C, Van der Koog D, Evans R. Post-herpetic neuralgia: Further post-mortem studies of cases with and without pain. Pain 1991; 44:105–117.

54. Wynn Parry CB. The failed back. In: Wall BD, Melzack R. Textbook of Pain. London and Edinburgh: Churchill Livingstone, 1994; 1075–1094.

55. Wynn Parry CB. Pain in avulsion lesions of the brachial plexus. Pain 1980; 9:41–53.

28

Sexual Problems Associated with Spinal Cord Disease

Anthony Matthew Tromans

Duke of Cornwall Spinal Treatment Centre, Salisbury District Hospital, Salisbury, Wiltshire, England

Jonathan Cole

Southampton University Hospital, Southampton, Hampshire, and Poole Hospital, Poole, Dorset, England

There are few, if any, problems in which bodily dysfunction and psychological effect are as intimately related as in disturbances of sexual function. When one adds the differences between male and female physiology and anatomy at one level and experience and perception at another, then the area becomes both daunting and fascinating. It is also an essentially personal area that is often approached, at least in the United Kingdom, diffidently and poorly. Although this chapter cannot claim to be comprehensive, it does point the way to a consideration that sexuality, however defined and however experienced, is as important a part of the lives of those with spinal injury as it is in others' lives.

Sexual dysfunction is a disturbance in any of the facets of sexual activity and may present in a patient with a disability in many ways, from the "low level"—altered function in the sex organs—to the "highest level"—where a person's confidence and very identity may be placed in jeopardy. The disabled group to be considered are those with spinal cord injuries (SCI), but the problems and solutions discussed may be relevant to other groups of disabled patients as well.

Many people find discussing sex, sexual activities, and the intimate details of a person's sex life difficult. This may be the case not only for patients but also for their professional caregivers. One of us, a doctor working in physical medicine, has had no formal training in sexual counseling. Any medical professional expertise lies principally in overcoming the mechanical problems of penile erectile and ejaculatory dysfunction; the wider problems of sexual dysfunction are only encountered when we are approached by a patient. Whether this is a personal failure, a failure of training, or inadequate resourcing to provide an appropriate counselor is open to debate. Our preferred approach has been to raise the topic of erections, fertility, and contraception when seeing patients in clinic, hoping to allow them to take the discussion further if they want.

Sexuality, however, is a complex topic, and despite knowing our patients well, we often do not progress beyond the medical problem of erection, fertility, or contraception. Perhaps it is because as their doctors, we tend to have known a person for several months from their initial injury, so that our relationship has become too close for such a topic to be discussed. Patients might find it easier to discuss such matters with a specialist nurse.

Spinal injuries are often divided into two groups: paraplegia (with a cord injury below the first thoracic vertebrae and therefore normal arm function); and tetraplegia (injury of the first thoracic vertebrae or above and therefore some loss of upper limb function). These are two very crude and diverse categories, inasmuch as independence of movement is related to many components including the total amount of body control, trunk stability (for ease of sitting), and the presence of spasticity, which may interfere with positioning of paralyzed limbs, produce troublesome involuntary movements, or occasionally aid transfer and some movement. Spinal injuries may also be incomplete, with preservation of sensation or voluntary movement below the level of the injury leading to enhanced function and independence, or complete. Factors other than sensation and movement may be relevant: for instance, chronic neurogenic pain (not uncommon after spinal cord injury) may be both a great emotional drain and reduce independence. Mobility and independence are important in that they allow and enable disabled individuals to take a lead and control the physical aspects of their relationships.

Although admittedly, this is a somewhat arbitrary method, we will now discuss problems with the sexual organs and with sexuality from the "lower level" upward. Men and women need to be considered separately because their problems are different, particularly at the lower level.

I. MALE SEX ORGAN FUNCTION

His physical problems concern penile sensation, erection, and ejaculation, with complex interactions between these three.

A. Sensation

Sensation from the glans is conveyed through the nerves to the sacral roots, then through the cord to the brain. It may be normal, altered, or absent after

SCI. Sensory problems cannot be influenced medically, unless there is penile hypersensitivity that interferes with function, a rare cause of male dyspareunia or unpleasant/painful sexual intercourse. The only solution is to anesthetize the penis by local nerve block—a last course of action that may be unacceptable to the patient.

Penile sensation may be separate from ejaculatory and orgasmic sensation. Some patients have the normal sensation of ejaculation whether antegrade (leading to the ejaculate being jettisoned from the penis) or retrograde (into the bladder). It is likely that any physical sensation of stimulation of the penis, ejaculation, or of indirect awareness of these will enhance the derived pleasure from intercourse. Sensation, however, may not be necessary for sexual pleasure and fulfillment. Many patients also experience indirect sensations from which they will derive pleasure. Although they may not feel penile sensation, its stimulation causes spasms or changes in blood pressure, flushing, and goose bumps (dysreflexic symptoms), which come to be interpreted, in the correct physical context, pleasurably. Others experience spasms or dysreflexic symptoms at the time of ejaculation that are also pleasurable.

The neurophysiology of the spinal cord is poorly understood and either as a result of incomplete transection of the cord with sparing of a sensory pathway in an apparently asentient person, or possibly because of a vagal mechanism, there may be direct physical pleasure in those with an apparently complete cord lesion (at least in women) (1). There is, of course, pleasure to be gained from engaging in a sexual relationship, something that will be considered in more detail later.

B. Erection

The neurological pathway enabling penile erection is parasympathetic and, like penile sensation, is through the sacral nerve roots (principally the second). The parasympathetic nervous system controls the penile blood flow and when stimulated, there is vasodilatation of the arterioles with increased blood flow inflating the corpora cavernosa. Their engorgement leads to penile enlargement and partial obstruction of venous return to achieve a full erection.

Erections may be reflex (by stimulating the penis directly), or psychogenic (due to thoughts of a sexual nature). In health, during sexual intercourse, the erection is maintained by both mechanisms, so that when one's thoughts stray to other matters, such as football, the erection is not lost. Some spinally injured patients will only experience psychogenic erections, and distraction due to pain or physical problems, such as moving back and forth, may result in the erection being lost.

In some patients, stimulation of the penis directly may cause an erection, for example, during manual handling during preparation for penetration, but this may then be lost as the vagina fails to maintain an adequate level of physical stimulation, a frustrating and dispiriting course of events. Alternatively, the duration of the erection may not be sufficient to complete intercourse, being adequate for penetration but becoming flaccid before fulfilment. The penile erection may be incomplete, so the glans penis does not engorge, although the shaft is turgid, or worse still, the shaft may remain pliable and so never achieve sufficient stiffness for penetration. Or there may be a complete absence of erectile function, made more frustrating during sexual activities, despite there being an ample erection in association with a full bladder (a reflex that may occur in non-spinally injured males and possibly accounting for early morning erection).

C. Erection Enhancement

Therapy to provide and maintain erection has four basic mechanisms.

1. Mechanically Assisted Engorgement and Its Maintenance

If the penis can be encouraged to fill with blood and the blood trapped, it should be possible to have penetrative intercourse. This may be helped by a tube that fits over the penis making an air tight seal at the pubis that can then be vacuumed. The penis fills with blood to occupy the vacuum expanding to fill the tube. A rubber ring placed over the end of the tube is slipped off to constrict the base of the penis, preventing the blood from escaping and maintaining the erection once the vacuum is released and the tube removed. (Such devices have been available in sex shops for many years to enhance penile size). Intercourse may then take place. Some people who can achieve an adequate erection but are unable to maintain it may just use constrictor bands around the base of the penis.

These systems are not infallible, and to achieve an air tight seal it is necessary to use a lubricant and possibly to shave the pubic hairs. The constrictor band may fail to maintain the erection or may be too tight, needing a lubricant to facilitate removal. It is also possible to damage the penis, especially if accidentally left in place.

For some couples, these devices are very successful, whereas others find they intrude into their intimacy. For some they can enhance foreplay and can be used as a sex toy. As in so many areas of rehabilitation medicine, the individual's preferences are of great importance.

2. Pharmacological Assistance

Vasoactive drugs (the nitrates) may cause penile engorgement and erection. If given systematically, however, they have unacceptable systemic side effects, such as hypotension and vasodilatory headaches that may interfere with the use of any erection achieved.

Drugs delivered directly into the penis by injection may avoid systemic side effects. The principal drugs used include papaverine, phentolamine, and alprostadil. Papaverine is an alpha-adrenergic antagonist that, if injected in doses of 20–120 mg, can give a useful erection. Phentolamine, another alpha-adrenergic antagonist, may be used in conjunction with papaverine injected into the penis. Neither papaverine or phentolamine are licensed for this usage in the United Kingdom and are often only available through a hospital pharmacy. Alprostadil is a synthetic prostaglandin that is commercially available (Upjohn Ltd.) as a kit and licensed for intracavernosal injection in erectile dysfunction.

Intracavernosal injections have potential side effects; the patient must also be taught under medical supervision. Injection into a vascular organ like the penis may result in a dramatic hematoma. There is also a risk of introducing infection and of causing penile fibrosis.

The most serious risk, however, is of priapism (prolonged erection), requiring the patient to seek medical help if present for more than 6 hours. Priapism may cause severe penile damage, the stagnant blood becoming hypoxic, with clotting leading to fibrosis and obliteration of the corpora. Its treatment includes aspiration of blood from the penis to allow the corpora to collapse through the administration of alpha-adrenergic stimulants such as aramine or adrenaline by injection into the penis. This needs to be undertaken carefully with monitoring to avoid local and systemic effects. Rectal diazepam may also be of some benefit.

Not all patients are prepared to use injections. It does reduce the spontaneity of intercourse and it is difficult to think of the syringe as a sex toy. The partner may also need to undertake the injection if the male has poor hand function. However for some couples the technique has proved useful. There are continuing developments pharmacologically, and it is likely that a safe oral medication to enhance erectile function will be soon available.

3. Mechanically Achieved and Maintained Erections

Penile implants, devices inserted at operation into the corpora cavernosae, can be used to provide an erect phallus. There are three basic types. With flexible semirigid rods, the erection is permanent, with the drawback that the penis is susceptible to trauma and the possibility of erosion and extrusion of the implants. Helical springs, which bend in one direction to become rigid and flaccid in the other are outside our experience. Hydrodynamic implants, in which the corpora are replaced with deflated tubes and a fluid-filled reservoir is placed intra-abdominally, have a pump in the scrotum that, when pressed, moves fluid from the reservoir into the implants and so erects the penis. Such devices are sophisticated, expensive, and prone to mechanical failure.

All penile implants need to be inserted at open operation, are susceptible to infection and mechanical failure, and their removal often results in fibrosis obliterating the corpora making further surgery difficult. This in turn prevents alternative means of achieving an erection.

4. Electrically Achieved Erections

The sacral anterior root stimulator—the Brindley Bladder Stimulator—electrically stimulates the motor branches of the sacral nerve roots to cause and maintain an erection. Because there is no preoperative test to demonstrate its ability to lead to an erection, it is never implanted solely to provide erections. Its main purpose is to treat urinary continence. Once bladder control is achieved the stimulation parameters for erection may be sought. Unfortunately the patient may sometimes experience disturbing rhythmical movements of the legs during usage as a result of skeletal muscle stimulation. An additional inconvenience is that the surface transmitter has to be held over the receiver for the duration of stimulation.

D. Preparing for Intercourse

Most spinally injured people do not have control over their bladder and rely on a drainage mechanism such as a urethral catheter or condom urinal. They may have to empty the bladder with a catheter to avoid embarrassing urinary incontinence. (Fecal incontinence is less of a problem in men.) Some authors describe the use of the urethral catheter as a penile splint, with it being pulled down the side of the penis and held in place by a condom. Most people, however, remove the catheter and use a towel to soak up any leakage.

The mechanics of intercourse depend not only on the disability but on the imagination. A double bed is easier both for undressing and for coping with spasm. Different positions will have to tried: the partner will generally have to be on top and may have had to assist with the mechanics of the erection and be prepared to stop at any time because of spasm or, more importantly, dysreflexia.

The higher the spinal lesion, the greater the likelihood of adequate and spontaneous erectile function and ejaculation. With intact local spinal reflexes at a sacral level, the tetraplegic often requires less assistance with sexual function than the paraplegic. Unfortunately the tetraplegic is also susceptible to autonomic dysreflexia. The lower thoracic paraplegic may have lost all spontaneous erectile potential due to damage to the lower motor neurons of the sacral nerve roots, although paradoxically, they may have intact ejaculatory function as this occurs at the tenth thoracic segment. Ejaculation will be psychogenic in origin as the sensory pathway is disrupted.

E. Ejaculation

There are no means of improving ejaculation for pleasure, and therefore the therapies are to assist with conception. Some patients will spontaneously, but unreliably, ejaculate during intercourse. Often the vagina does not provide an adequate physical stimulus and more vigorous means of stimulation are required. Manual stimulation may be sufficient but often mechanical stimulation with a vibrator is necessary. People who ejaculate reflexly often cannot ejaculate again for several days or up to 2 weeks. We know of no logical explanation for this.

Some of those spinally injured men who cannot reflexly ejaculate may benefit from electrical stimulation, either transrectally or by implantation of electrodes onto the hypogastric plexus. The sympathetic nerves involved in ejaculation leave the spinal cord at the tenth thoracic vertebrae and travel through the sympathetic chain to cross the pelvic brim in the hypogastric plexus, where they are accessible to the surgeon for the implantation of electrodes.

Transrectal stimulation relies on one of two modes with the first, Brindley, relying on the intact reflex and the other, Seager, directly stimulating the musculature of the seminal vesicles, leading to a more reliable but less powerful trickling emission.

The semen is caught in a receiver and if it is of good quality, simple intravaginal insemination may achieve pregnancy. The quality of the sperm may be altered and it may need preparation prior to being used for fertilization. The reasons for this are diverse: it is thought that there may be testicular damage due to alteration of temperature either because it is trapped between the legs in the seated position, or as a result of altered blood flow secondary to nerve damage. The presence of an indwelling catheter or recurrent urinary tract infections may cause occult damage to the mechanism of spermatogenesis. Lastly there may have been episodes of orchitis leading to frank testicular damage and atrophy.

With poor quality semen, or when sperm can only be obtained by testicular or epididymal aspiration, advanced assisted fertility techniques are required such as in vitro fertilization (IVF) or intracytoplasmic sperm injection (ICSI). Ejaculation may also be retrograde, necessitating retrieval of semen from the bladder and separation from urine with resuspension in a sperm culture media prior to fertilization. Microbiological examination of semen is essential as occult infection is not uncommon and its introduction into the uterus may have devastating consequences.

The counseling of the spinally injured patient is often managed by their spinal physician as few infertility centers in the United Kingdom can manage ejaculatory disorders. Often, little thought is given either to consequences of conception (the ability of the disabled parent to care for a child) or of the psychological consequences of failure to be of assistance. It is, fortunately, becoming increasingly common to work in conjunction with an infertility unit, and there is increasing access to other professional counselors.

II. FEMALE SEX ORGAN FUNCTION

The sensory problems and their solutions, if any, are essentially similar to those found in the male. The problem of reduced perineal sensation after SCI has been considered recently by Whipple and Komisaruk, who started from their anecdotal experience that women with clinically complete SCI have reported having orgasms (1).

They divided a group of women into those with complete injury below T10, and those with injury above T10, the level at which the hypogastric nerves are reported to enter the cord. They found that in both groups women reported orgasm and had the autonomic alterations associated with orgasm after vaginal or cervical stimulation. They concluded that either—as can never be excluded—the injuries were not complete, or these changes were central image induced, (Women do consider themselves more imaginative), or that there may be sensory afferents ascending via the vagus nerve, for which there is neuroanatomical evidence in the rat.

There are, however, obvious differences in the requirements for tumescence between male and female. Whereas sexual intercourse for the female relies less on neurological function for alteration in the genitalia, the older ideas that the female sexual organs are passive during foreplay and orgasm need to be revised (2). In those with spinal injury, labial engorgement and mucous lubrication may be absent and a water-soluble gel may be needed.

A urethral catheter may be taped to one side in the groin out of the way, or removed. More commonly in the female, an indwelling catheter is placed suprapubically to avoid the problems of urethral damage and so does not directly interfere with intercourse.

In the noncatheterized individual, it may be necessary to catheterize temporarily and intermittently to avoid urinary incontinence. The vagina and the rectum are in intimate contact, and vaginal stimulation may initiate reflex rectal activity and result in fecal incontinence. It may therefore be necessary to perform a bowel evacuation prior to intercourse.

As discussed above, the sensory disturbances are similar to those of the male, and direct and indirect pleasurable sensations may be experienced. The risks of autonomic dysreflexia and spasms are also similar to the male. Positions for intercourse may have to be planned to cope with joint contractures and care taken, especially when trying to overcome the problems of hip adduction.

Excessive force in a moment of passion may result in bony fracture especially in the presence of disuse osteoporosis.

A. Fertility

The fertility of the female is less disturbed than that of the male. It is not uncommon for there to be a period of posttraumatic amenorrhea that may last for up to a year, but once resolved there are very few other insults to fertility. Pelvic inflammatory disease is uncommon despite the problems of urinary tract infection and a reduced ability to maintain perineal hygiene easily.

B.   Pregnancy

Once a woman is pregnant, there are the problems of mobility and self care with increasing abdominal size. Getting behind a steering wheel and lifting the wheelchair in and out of the car may become impossible. Urinary management may also become more difficult with reduced bladder volumes and the problems of reaching around the "bump" to intermittently catheterize.

Urinary infections are more common in the general population during pregnancy. Those with a neurogenic bladder are more vulnerable and the upper urinary tracts need to be monitored closely with ultrasound scans.

The onset of labor may be missed due to lack of sensation either of uterine contractions or even of the breaking of the waters. Those with neurological lesions above the sixth thoracic vertebrae may experience autonomic dysreflexia that are best controlled by an epidural anesthetic. Those who were spinally injured before skeletal maturity may have a small pelvis and may need an elective cesarean section. Spinally injured patients may need to be admitted to the hospital during the latter stages of their pregnancy, either for close monitoring for the onset of labor or for elective therapeutic interventions such as induction of labor or a cesarean section. The problems of a disabled mother coping with a child are beyond the scope and the remit of this book. These problems should neither be dismissed nor considered insuperable.

C.   Contraception

The choice of contraceptive is that of the patient but in the spinally injured, there are some further problems. If we assume it is the female partner who takes the precautions, then the oral contraceptive's risk of thromboembolism may be increased in those who are recumbent for most of their lives. It must not be overlooked that concomitant medication such as antibiotics may reduce the efficacy of contraceptives. Intrauterine devices may increase the risk of pelvic inflammatory disease secondary to urinary sepsis and may lead to heavier periods. There are theoretical advantages in depot injections of progesterone because of both the contraceptive effect and less frequent menstruation.

III. CENTRAL COMPONENTS OF SEXUAL DESIRE AND PLEASURE

Sexual appetite or libido is difficult to assess and of course varies over time and circumstances. It may be expressed in the frequency of sexual thoughts, intercourse, or masturbation. There are little data on the alteration on libido in patients with SCI.

Whipple et al. (3) found, not surprisingly, that initially after injury there was a "shutting down" of sexuality, associated with a belief, for women at least, that sexual pleasure was no longer possible, followed by a conscious decision not to consider their sexual nature. Later, after the immediate postinjury period, there was a suggestion of reawakening of sexuality and feeling, then a sense of being robbed of it. Later still in the rehabilitation process, a phase of sexual rediscovery was seen to emerge when a newfound resourcefulness allowed expression of recovered libido.

Although their work referred to women, it is likely that a similar passage of emotion and of libidinous thoughts occurs in men. Most of those who have SCI are fit young men whose preinjury libidos must have been high. After a period spent focusing on their injury, it is not surprising that their sexual appetite returns. Where practical, one imagines that some people will engage in self stimulation. However for full enjoyment, another person must be involved. The rest of the chapter will consider aspects of this.

A. Sexuality After Spinal Cord Injury

The complexities of social relationships and the contribution by sexuality to one's self-esteem are far too involved a subject to be dealt with in a short chapter. A few observations may be made, together with some data on such matters as the marriage and divorce rates after SCI.

After the occurrence of any disability, contact with people may present various degrees of difficulty. It may be easier to meet family and friends than to go out and meet new people. Familiar friends soon take you for a person and reduce the stigma of the disability. Newly met people tend to see the problem first, before focusing more slowly on the person themselves. Often for those with spinal injury, the first contact with the opposite sex occurs on the wards. Staff on the spinal injuries unit, while talking to patients, will compliment them on their appearance, even flirt with them gently, boosting their egos and treating them as fellow human beings. Relationships develop as friends, as like siblings, paternalistically, or even sexually. (It is not too uncommon for a female member of the staff to enter into a serious relationship with or marry a male patient.) Such early postinjury relationships reinforce male patients' sexuality and allow them at least to perceive the potential for developing more serious relationships in the future.

However the female patient is not so easily reassured. Male members of staff are rare and most are medical. For many reasons, including fear of being accused of sexual impropriety, male staff are less likely to pay appropriate compliments, flirt with, or cuddle the female patient. Male staff may fail to provide sufficient sexual attraction for the female to find their compliments worthwhile. Lastly it may be less likely that a man will become sexually attracted to a woman with spinal injury than for a woman to do so to a man, reflecting the differences in those factors rated as attractive and desirable between the two sexes. For whatever reason, we have never witnessed a relationship develop between a male member of staff and a female patient.

After several months on a ward surrounded by family, friends, and medical staff, patients are then discharged to the outside world where they may have to meet completely new sets of people, some or most of whom have little experience of SCI. It becomes up to the injured person to put such people at their ease socially. At such meetings, it is unlikely that a sexual dimension will be at the forefront. At some time however patients will begin thinking in such terms.

In some cases sex takes place inside a stable relationship; at other times it is more casual. The type of relationship depends on the individual's needs, some wishing to have "one night stands" with intimate sexual contact, others seeking friendship but not necessarily on a lasting basis.

For someone with SCI, there are obvious limitations to their ability to attract partners for these sorts of temporary relationships. It does occur however. One man stated that he had "pulled" more women since being in a chair than before his accident. Whether this is as a result of him trying to prove himself, pity on the part of his female contacts, or their ignorance, i.e., feeling sexually safe with a disabled person, is not known. This may be part of the patient's normal sexual maturation.

To make contact with others, a person needs to be mobile and independent. Mobility needs to be beyond the home so that aspects such as transport and access to public buildings are relevant. Independence is important, because the establishment of intimacy in the presence of a third party is not easy. Perhaps this is why it is not uncommon for a relationship to develop with a caregiver, as frequent encounters and privacy readily occur. These problems of reduced mobility and independence have often brought groups of disabled people together so that it is understandable that relationships develop. The spinally injured population is small, however, there being six to nine hundred new injuries a year in the United Kingdom spread over a wide range of ages and geographical areas. In addition only a small number of women are injured. These factors may account for it being relatively uncommon for relationships to develop between two members of a specific disabled population. It is also becoming more common to integrate disabled people into the community during their rehabilitation and rely less on communal housing, sheltered workshops, and day centers, which may reduce or remove one from social contact.

There are as many differing relationships and expectations from relationships as there are individuals. Such matters are of course very difficult to quantify. There are more solid data from marriage and divorce rates following SCI.

B.   Marriage and Divorce After SCI

Spinal cord injury has many ramifications—on employment and housing as well as on relationships. Although concerned with the latter in the present discussion and its dependence on sexuality, however loosely defined, we are not unaware that marriage depends on factors other than sexual or asexual relationships. With that proviso, it is illuminating to look at marriage and divorce rates associated with SCI and at the effect SCI has on partnerships.

As Dijkers et al. (4) point out, deductions in this field can be difficult to make. Spinal cord injury will place a strain on a marriage, but there will be other stressful factors that, are not exclusively related to SCI, including loss of job, loss of ability to housekeep and help with children, and reduced mobility throwing people together. Other variables like age (younger people tend to divorce more), must also be removed from the equations.

When such variables are considered, then studies thus far have been conflicting, some suggesting as increased divorce rate after SCI but others disagreeing.

There are more reliable data on the rate of marriages after SCI. In the first 3 years after SCI, it appears that marriage rates are lower than in a control population. Also the rate of marriage during that 3-year period declined, suggesting that marriages planned before the SCI still took place but few new ones occurred. Five years after injury, 88.5% of those single at the time of injury were still single compared with 65.4% of an age-matched control population. Of those married at the time of injury, 81.2% were still married 5 years later, compared with 88.7% of a control population. Of the postinjury marriages, 21.7% ended in divorce compared with 15.0% among a control population in 5 years. Other studies have suggested that marriages taking place after one partner has SCI fare better than those in which the marriage occurred preinjury. In one, the partner had accepted the injured spouse freely at the time of marriage and did not have the injury imposed on them. Those who marry after injury also appear more motivated and better adjusted psychologically.

Thus in each of these cohorts, there is a slight excess of failure of relationship, but, more optimistically, this excess is comparatively small given the large additional pressures those with SCI and their loved ones learn to live with. Figures have only been compiled for 5 years injury. Several observers suggest that it takes 7 years or more to learn to live with SCI, so that the figures for a longer period may be even more similar to controls.

C. Intimacy, Sexual Gratification, and Sense of Self

In the first part of this chapter we discussed sexual function in purely physiological terms. In reality of course, many levels of intimacy and subtlety enter into a relationship as personal as the sexual one.

Independence is not only a physical obstruction; it also provides a psychological barrier. This is so not only for the disabled person but also for their able-bodied contact. Ignorance and fear of disability will prejudice the initial contact but once made will rarely interfere with its development. On occasions, pity or sympathy or a genuine wish to help the disabled person will initiate the contact and allow a relationship to develop. The same ignorance and incompetence in understanding the complexities of a relationship may also account for some of the stresses placed on a previously mature relationship after the onset of disability. Time, care, patience, and the development of an understanding of each other's needs hopefully will lead to a successful and long-lasting relationship.

Thus, a husband who asks for assistance to obtain an erection the first time he and his partner are alone after an SCI is probably going to put their marriage under strain, whereas those who enjoy their privacy and relearn intimacy will be in a better position to overcome the new physical problems. It is probably through a process of exploration, experimentation, and discovery that a new relationship develops or an old relationship thrives. A relationship based on pity or guilt is probably doomed.

In the past, there has been much discussion in the spinal injury literature and patient care manual of sexual pleasure being derived from the stimulation of erogenous zones in the sensory areas above the level of injury, not just from stimulating the breast or nipples, if spared, but from exploring all parts of the body where sensation is present. Then, penetrative sex is supposed not to be necessary to provide adequate fulfillment. This may have been overplayed by medical staff caring for the spinally injured person. However if stimulation to sexual gratification and even orgasm can be relearned by a combination of central imagery and peripheral stimulation in the context of a mutually rewarding relationship, then that it is obviously to be supported and encouraged. We in the medical field have much to learn from the originality of our patients in this.

Thus far we have discussed sexual intercourse from either the male or female perspective. Of course such orientation-fixated viewpoints are themselves vastly oversimplified. A full and mature relationship goes way beyond that to a mutual giving and receiving of pleasure. In a normal relationship, each partner gains pleasure from and is excited by the other being turned on—it becomes a mutual interdependence. After SCI the same hopefully also develops, although with differing components. Thus a man with SCI may find ways of stimulating his partner that lead to the gratification of both. This pleasure, when sensation is absent from his lower body, not only allows gratification for both parties but helps him to maintain an ego with a sexual component. In this respect there seems to be no intrinsic difference between men and women.

It would be unfair to romanticize the development and maintenance of sexual relationships after SCI: many people fail to develop or sustain them. We have heard of people after SCI having to endure their partners going elsewhere for sexual pleasure, which must be very difficult to adjust to, or to fully condemn, forcing the patient to face and explore his or her inadequacy and invalidity as a person each time it happens.

The inadequacy in performance that men may feel after their SCI finds its parallels in women in slightly different ways. Asentient women engaging in sex may feel used "as a vessel," and it is important in such cases for men to realize the importance of making their partners aware of their femininity.

IV. CONCLUSIONS

With the general evolution of medical management of spinally injured patients during the last 50 years, recognition of their sexual needs has lagged behind other considerations. It is time that we, in the United Kingdom at least, included this aspect along with all the others. This may lead us to listen to our patients more and learn from them. It may lead to the establishment of named specialist practitioners in spinal units, for the relationship between patient and doctor may not be ideal for discussing such matters. Almost certainly it will mean more openness and willingness to talk.

Having said that, it would be unfair not to mention the difficulties encountered with reduced sexual self-esteem, and support must be with both physical advice and psychological support. We cannot ignore the differences between men and women in this respect. Although gender roles have been much discussed during the last 20–30 years as being genetic or social, there is no doubting that such differences reach to our very cores. In the spinal cord-injured population, it does seem that women may fare worse.

The female spinally injured population is smaller (less than 20% of the total injured population), and they are often older than male patients. If not already in a stable relationship at the time of their injury, they may find new relationships difficult to initiate and sustain. Completely dependent males may marry, but we have only experienced one female patient, a C6 tetraplegic, marrying and this was when both partners held strong religious beliefs.

It does not seem entirely dismissable that men initially are attracted to women physically and are deterred by disability. They also may find it more onerous to embark on a longer-term relationship with a disabled person. Without seeking to underestimate the power of physical sexual attraction for women, they may also have wider, more humane, criteria when reaching out to men and so find it easier to enter into a relationship that may develop further. This is a cross women have always had to bear, but it may be made heavier when disability is considered.

As in the general public, strains may be put on a relationship by problems other than sexual after an injury. There can be financial strain resulting from the loss of employment, and anger and guilt as a result of the accident. The alteration of the daily routine, partners having to spend time together after the loss of employment, and the dependency of the disabled partner on the spouse with its attendant guilt all contribute. The posttraumatic strains on the relationship are complicated, and the sexual ones are but one facet. Greater recognition of sexual problems, hopefully, will lead to greater understanding and exploration of ways of reducing this most private and yet important aspect of what it is to be human.

On the positive side, several studies have shown that life satisfaction, quality-of-life ratings, and other indicators of well being are either unrelated or minimally related to SCI and to its level (5,6). The adaptability and resourcefulness of the human spirit is a source of continuing wonder.

ACKNOWLEDGMENTS

We are grateful to an anonymous female SCI patient and to our wives for discussions about this subject.

REFERENCES

1. Whipple B, Komisaruk BR. Sexuality and women with complete spinal cord injury. Spinal Cord 1997;35:136–138.
2. Gautier-Smith PC. Sexual dysfunction and the nervous system. In Aminoff MJ, ed. Neurology and General Medicine. New York and Edinburgh: Churchill-Livingstone, 1989;471–487.

3. Whipple B, Gerdes CA, and Komisurak BR. Sexual response to self-stimulation in women with complete spinal cord injury. J Sex Res 1996;33:231–240.
4. Dijkers MP, Abela MB, Gans BM, Gordon WA. The aftermath of spinal cord injury.
5. Cushman LA, Hassett J. Spinal cord injury: 10 and 15 years after. Paraplegia 1992;30:690–696.
6. Lundqvist C, Siosteen A, Blomstrand C. Spinal cord injuries: Clinical, functional and emotional status. Spine 1991;16:78–83.

29

The Palliative and Terminal Care of Patients with Spinal Cord Disease

Tony O'Brien

St. Patrick's Hospital and Cork University Hospital, Wilton, Cork, Ireland

I. INTRODUCTION

Palliative care focuses on the management of patients with advanced, progressive, and potentially fatal disease. At the outset, the specialty developed in response to the needs of patients with advanced cancer, and for many years concerned itself almost exclusively with the care of such patients. In later years, it became evident that the skills and philosophies that had been developed in hospices were equally applicable to a much broader cohort of patients and in a greater variety of settings.

The application of "hospice care" or "palliative care" is not confined to freestanding hospice units or to dedicated beds within a general hospital. Rather, hospice and palliative care denotes a concept of care that is applicable in all settings, both inpatient and community based. As such, the provision of good palliative care becomes the responsibility of every health care professional.

In a world where medical developments are frequently dependent upon further technological advances, patients and their families can often feel dehumanized and deskilled by the investigative and management process. Of course, the technologies are both necessary and welcome, but we should not sacrifice the art of medicine for the science. Both are necessary, working together in close harmony, if we are to offer patients and families an optimal level of care.

In the minds of the general public, and indeed in the minds of many health care professionals, palliative care equates exclusively with the care of dying patients. This betrays a fundamental attitudinal problem and misconception. Primarily, palliative care is concerned with enabling patients and their families to live full, rewarding, enriching, and meaningful lives within the obvious limitations of their illness. The emphasis is very much placed on life and living. If we can harness all that scientific medicine has to offer and combine that with a dedicated compassion for individuals and their families, we can create the scope and opportunity for people to live their lives to their own maximum potential.

Kearney (1) highlighted the need for a basic attitudinal change when he wrote:

> Patients with incurable illness must no longer be viewed as medical failures for whom nothing more can be done. They need palliative care, which does not mean a hand-holding second rate soft option, but treatment, which most people will need at some point in their lives, and many from the time of diagnosis, demanding as much skill and commitment as is normally brought into preventing, investigating and curing illness.

II. PALLIATIVE CARE: A DEFINITION

Palliative care is the continuing, active, total care of patients and families by a multiprofessional team at a time when the medical expectation is not to cure and the primary aim of treatment is no longer to prolong life. The goal of palliative care is the highest possible quality of life for both patient and family. Palliative care responds to physical, psychological, social and spiritual needs. If necessary, it extends to support in bereavement (European Community, Europe Against Cancer Committee).

By definition, therefore, palliative care is concerned with the management of patients whose disease is not responsive to curative treatments. For many patients, it will be evident from the moment of first diagnosis that they will not ultimately be cured of their disease. Ideally, there will be a period of overlap during which the referring service and the palliative care service will both be involved in management. As the disease progresses, it may well be appropriate for the palliative care service to steadily increase its involvement coinciding with a gradual reduction in the involvement of the referring service.

III. TERMINAL CARE: A DEFINITION

Terminal care is the final phase of palliative care and defines that period in which it is clear that death is imminent. The chances of a patient achieving a good and peaceful death will be greatly enhanced if he or she has received an optimal level of palliative care from the outset. Similarly, the provision of an effective palliative care service and support structure for families will help to reduce the incidence of bereavement morbidity.

IV. PRINCIPLES OF PALLIATIVE CARE

The essential principles of palliative care may be considered as follows.

A. Symptom Control

All patients must be offered an optimal level of pain and symptom control. Even if the underlying cause of the symptom cannot be corrected or reversed, there is still much to be done to achieve and maintain a good level of pain and symptom control.

B. Total Patient Care

We cannot and should not reduce the human condition to a series of mechanical and biochemical processes. We must consider each person as a unique individual, encompassing a complex interaction of physical, psychological, social, and spiritual dimensions. If we focus all of our efforts on the physical aspects of care and selectively ignore these other dimensions, our care will inevitably be fragmented and will fall far short of the ideal.

C. The Family Is the Unit of Care

Care must not simply be confined to the patient but must be extended to include the needs of the family. The family may well need help and support in coming to terms with their new situation. In addition, the family will be a most valuable resource to the professional caring team.

D. Good Communication

The development of any disease of the spinal cord is a frightening and confusing experience. As health care professionals, we have a responsibility to ensure that patients and their families are given adequate and appropriate information, in a manner and at a pace appropriate to their individual needs. It will require a number of meetings to enable patients to seek clarification and explanation and to encourage discussion of the real implications of the diagnosis. By avoiding such discussion, we leave patients confused, bewildered, and totally unprotected from their fears and their fantasies.

This approach is important in all situations, but particularly so in the case of spinal cord disease. Many diseases of the spinal cord are comparatively rare, and for most patients and families it will be the first time that they are made aware that such a condition exists. Careful explanation, perhaps supplemented by a simple explanatory leaflet, is vital.

E.   Interdisciplinary Teamwork

Palliative care requires input from a variety of professional disciplines. Each individual will bring to the situation not just their specific professional skills and expertise, but also something of their personal selves. In order to function well as part of an interdisciplinary team, it is essential that individuals are both competent and confident in their own area of practice. They must also have a healthy appreciation of the role that others have to play and a willingness to involve them appropriately.

V.   SYMPTOM CONTROL

In the early stages of disease, symptoms serve a useful function by alerting the patient that something is wrong and thereby prompting him to seek medical attention. To mask symptoms at this early stage, without a comprehensive assessment to determine the cause of the symptoms, would be harmful. Such an action may delay or prevent the introduction of curative treatments.

In established disease states, when it has been demonstrated that the disease process cannot be cured or reversed, it is imperative that we use every means at our disposal to achieve and maintain an optimal level of pain and symptom control. Indeed, it is precisely because the disease cannot be cured that all efforts must focus on good symptom control.

We all must take great care not to communicate directly or indirectly with patients and families that appalling declaration that "there is nothing more to be done." There is always more to be done.

A.   Pain Control

In advanced disease, pain is the symptom that is most expected and most feared by patients. In the past, chronic pain was not well understood and in many instances was inadequately treated. Indeed, for many patients the fear of uncontrolled pain is a greater source of anguish than the reality of their impending death.

Pain is a uniquely individual experience and as such has virtually defied definition. Perhaps the most widely accepted definition is that proposed by the International Association for the Study of Pain (IASP) (2):

> Pain is an unpleasant sensory and emotional experience associated with actual or potential tissue damage, or described in terms of such damage. Pain is always subjective. Each individual learns the application of the word through experiences related to injury in early life. It is unquestionably a sensation in a part or parts of the body but it is also always unpleasant and therefore an emotional experience.

Melzack and Wall commend this definition for highlighting the association between tissue damage and pain, although it is by no means consistent, and also for identifying the emotional dimension of the pain experience. However, they are concerned that the word "unpleasant" is wholly inadequate to describe the "misery, anguish, desperation and urgency that are part of the pain experience" (3).

In the clinical setting, the IASP definition of pain has two vital elements. First, it clearly emphasizes the simple but often ignored fact that pain is always subjective. As clinicians, we must actively resist the temptation to question the validity or reliability of a patient's history when we fail to understand his or her pain in terms of its pathophysiology or, more particularly, when our best therapeutic efforts are consistently ineffective. As a starting point, we must begin by learning to believe patients when they complain of pain.

Second, the IASP definition emphasizes the importance of emotional factors in the appreciation and interpretation of pain. Twycross (4) has described pain in terms of a "dual phenomenon." One part of this phenomenon is the perception of the stimulus and the other is the patients emotional response to the stimulus. Consequently, the potential of any given stimulus to cause distress and suffering will be influenced by the emotional state of the patient at that time. For example, a patient who is feeling frightened, angry, sad, or isolated will experience a greater degree of suffering than one who is feeling supported, understood, and loved.

Although the pain perception threshold (the least experience of pain that an individual can recognize) may be relatively constant for all individuals, the pain tolerance threshold (the greatest level of pain that an individual is willing to tolerate) is subject to considerable variation. The capacity of emotional and spiritual factors to influence the pain tolerance threshold must be fully recognized and appreciated.

B. Evaluation of Pain

When a diagnosis of spinal cord disease is made, whether it be of malignant or nonmalignant origin, there is sometimes the assumption that all pains are therefore caused directly by that disease process. This is not the case. Patients may experience a number of distinct and etiologically separate pains and each will require separate evaluation and management.

In general, pain may be caused by one or a combination of the following factors:

1. Pain may be caused directly and exclusively by the underlying disease process.
2. Pain may be caused by the treatment, e.g., surgery, chemotherapy, other drug treatments, and radiotherapy.
3. Pain may be caused by general weakness, debility, or immobility.
4. Pain may be totally unrelated to the underlying disease process or its treatment.

The evaluation process will therefore involve taking a careful history, particularly a pain-related history. The site(s), severity, quality, intensity, exacerbating and relieving factors, and temporal relationships of the pain must all be recorded. When interpreting this information, it will be necessary to take full cognizance of concurrent medical conditions and the influence of psychological or emotional factors and spiritual concerns.

After taking a detailed history, the clinician should elicit any physical signs that might be relevant to the pathogenesis of the pain. It may also be necessary in selected circumstances to undertake laboratory, electrophysiological, and/or radiological investigations to define the precise cause(s) of the pain(s). An integral part of the overall assessment will include an assessment of the extent to which the patient is distressed or inconvenienced by these various pains; i.e., does the pain limit mobility, interfere with sleep and concentration, and so on.

A number of clinical and research tools are commonly used to measure pain. The verbal rating score (none, mild, moderate, severe) and the visual analog scale are both designed to measure pain in a single dimension—intensity. The McGill pain questionnaire is designed to identify and measure three major categories of pain experience—sensory, affective, and evaluative.

C. Approach to Physical Pain

Approaches to physical pain must include an assessment of the cause(s) of the pain(s). Based on this assessment, appropriate treatment choices are selected. Once any treatment is initiated, it is vital that we systematically and regularly assess the outcome of this treatment in terms of its benefits and adverse effects.

1. Opioid-Sensitive Pains

Analgesic drugs form the mainstay of our management approach. They are divided into one of three categories based on their relative potencies: nonopioids, weak opioids, and strong opioids. If, for example, a patient is on an adequate dose of a weak opioid, yet continues to experience uncontrolled pain, there is no merit in choosing another drug of similar potency. In this instance, a move to a more potent strong opioid is indicated.

There is now general acceptance of the value of opioid drugs in the management of patients with malignant disease. However, many doctors are reluctant to use opioids in nonmalignant conditions, fearing the prospect of addiction. There is no convincing evidence to support the view that opioids, when used appropriately in the clinical setting, cause addiction in patients with pain of nonmalignant origin. Physical dependence will develop after a time, but this can be easily managed by gradually reducing the dose. Portenoy (5) and Melzack (6) both believe that opioids should not be withheld from such patients, provided that their use is necessary to relieve the pain.

The timing of the introduction of a strong opioid must be based on an accurate assessment of the nature and severity of the pain and the extent to which the pain is responsive to opioids. Their introduction should not be influenced by the histology of the lesion or any crude assessment of the likely prognosis.

A number of myths and misunderstandings can delay the appropriate introduction of opioids to patients who are experiencing severe pain. In particular, fears of addiction, tolerance, and respiratory depression are grossly exaggerated and essentially without foundation when opioids are used appropriately in the clinical setting in the management of severe pain.

Analgesic drugs should be given orally whenever possible. Severe pain per se is not an indication for parenteral therapy. On occasion, it will be necessary to use the parenteral route for those patients who cannot tolerate oral medication because of severe weakness, nausea/vomiting, or dysphagia. The frequency with which all analgesic drugs are given will be based on the duration of their clinical effect. It is essential that we give drugs regularly and in anticipation of pain. Patients whose pain is reasonably well controlled with regular analgesia should also have rescue or breakthrough analgesia available.

Morphine

Morphine is the strong oral opioid of choice. The dose required for individual patients may vary from 10 mg per day to several hundred milligrams per day or more.

After oral administration, morphine is well absorbed, predominantly in the duodenum and upper small bowel. There is extensive first-pass metabolism. The liver is the main site of morphine metabolism and the principal metabolites found in the plasma are morphine 6 glucoronide and morphine 3 glucoronide. Morphine 6 glucoronide accounts for much of the analgesic activity of morphine. The major metabolites of morphine are excreted through the kidney, and particular care must therefore be exercised in patients with impaired renal function.

The correct dose of oral morphine for an individual patient is the lowest dose that effectively controls the pain. A starting dose of 2.5–5 mg every 4 hours (standard release) or 5–10 mg every 12 hours (modified release) is recommended. The dose of morphine is then gradually titrated against the clinical response. The following are common side effects associated with the use of morphine.

Nausea/Vomiting.   About 30% of patients will experience nausea/vomiting when morphine is first introduced. The prophylactic use of an antiemetic is recommended at the commencement of morphine therapy.

Constipation.   All patients on regular morphine will require a laxative.

Dry Mouth.   There is a clear association between the use of morphine and the development of a dry mouth. This occurs independently of the multiplicity of other factors that predispose patients to a dry mouth. Strict attention to oral hygiene is essential.

Myoclonus.   Myoclonus is a descriptive term applied to shock-like involuntary muscular contractions due to a variety of causes. It is a useful and early sign of opioid neurotoxicity, thought to be mediated through the metabolite normorphine.

Subjective Voice Changes.   Some patients complain of a change in the quality of their voice. They may describe a weakening of their voice or may complain that their ears are blocked. A modest reduction in the dose of morphine will usually solve the problem.

Drowsiness/Confusion.   Patients may experience a transient sense of drowsiness when morphine is first introduced. If it persists beyond a few days, it should prompt either a reduction in the dose or a search for some other cause. Patients receiving a stable dose of morphine show no evidence of cognitive impairment. The dose of morphine is titrated to one of two clear end points:

1. Relief of pain. Once the pain is controlled, the dose of morphine is continued in whatever form is most convenient and acceptable to the patient. It is necessary to monitor and to treat any side effects and to continue to review the dose regularly.
2. Pain continues with unacceptable side effects. Some pains are less responsive to morphine. As the dose of morphine increases, the patient will develop evidence of morphine toxicity without any further improvement in pain control. In these circumstances, it is necessary to explore alternative treatment options.

2. Pains Less Sensitive to Morphine: Alternative Opioids

It is now widely recognized that patients can exhibit very variable responses to different opioid drugs. This phenomenon is recognised in both malignant and nonmalignant pain (7). When using pure agonist opioids, the upper limit of dosage is defined by toxicity. In practice, when a patient continues to experience pain despite rapidly escalating doses of morphine, and exhibits features of dose limiting toxicity (confusion, drowsiness, hallucinations, myoclonus, nausea/vomiting, etc.), it is necessary to consider the role of an alternative opioid.

Hydromorphone is a semisynthetic congener of morphine, and like morphine, is a μ-selective full opioid agonist. Both drugs share similar pharmacological actions. Following administration of hydromorphone, it is extensively metabolized to hydromorphone 3 glucuronide. Oral hydromorphone is approximately 7.5 times stronger than oral morphine. However, as there is considerable interpatient variability in the response to different opioids, the dose for each patient should be titrated carefully.

Other opioids including oxycodone, fentanyl (transdermal preparation), and methadone may all have a useful role in the management of severe pain. deStoutz et al. have concluded that the symptoms of opioid toxicity can be relieved by opioid rotation, and that a choice of two or three different opioids is necessary to obtain satisfactory long-term pain control (8).

3. Pains Less Responsive to Opioids: Alternative Approaches

Neuropathic Pain

Neuropathic pain describes those pains that are induced by mechanisms that cause injury or damage to the nervous system, resulting in a functional abnormality of the nerves. Clinically, patients will complain of an atypical but very unpleasant pain. Indeed, many are reluctant to describe it as pain, yet it is distinctly unpleasant. It may occur in association with a number of sensory abnormalities including causalgia (a syndrome of sustained burning pain) and allodynia (pain due to a stimulus that does not normally provoke pain). Neurological examination may reveal motor or reflex abnormalities in addition to the sensory changes already described.

Opioids, are typically less effective in the management of neuropathic pain. Sutherland has proposed the theory of "spinal turbulence" to explain this phenomenon (9). In spinally mediated neuropathic pain, there is spontaneous hyperactivity of the spinal pain transmission neurones, with impulses conducted in an erratic, turbulent fashion. Opioids work better in nociceptive pain, where the impulse is transmitted in a smooth laminar fashion. The origin of the impulse and the manner of its transmission accounts for the relative lack of efficacy of opioids in this condition.

Tricyclic antidepressants have a useful action in neuropathic pain that is independent of their effects on mood. There are of particular benefit in "burning" pain. A starting dose of amitriptyline 25 mg daily, increasing in increments to 100 mg daily, is usually adequate. The onset of relief may be less than 1 week, but Glynn recommends that treatment should be given a trial of 6 weeks before it is considered to be a failure (8).

Anticonvulsant drugs have also been used with benefit in neuropathic pain. They are particularly indicated in "shooting" or "stabbing" pains. The NMDA receptor channel blocker, ketamine, is of benefit in the management of neuropathic pains that are unresponsive to tricyclic antidepressants and/or anticonvulsants.

A variety of other drug therapies have also been tried in the management of neuropathic pains with varying degrees of success. These drugs include dexamethasone, clonidine, flecainide, mexilitine, naloxone, and baclofen. Nondrug measures may also be of benefit, e.g., transcutaneous nerve stimulation. Patients with more difficult neuropathic pain that fails to respond to standard measures may benefit from anaesthetic intervention.

Musculoskeletal Pain

Musculoskeletal pain and pain associated with prolonged immobility will often respond to a nonsteroidal anti-inflammatory agent. There are a wide range of such agents available and the clinician is advised to become familiar with perhaps three or four from different classes. Many of these drugs are now marketed in a modified-release format, which reduces the frequency of doses. Also, many are available in liquid or suppository form if required.

Dyspnea

Dyspnea is a subjective sensation of an increased awareness of or increased difficulty with breathing. As with pain, there are two components to the symptom. The first is the perception of the symptom, i.e., the increased work associated with breathing; the second is the patient's reaction to that sensation, i.e., the subjective distress associated with the symptom.

The cause of dyspnea is usually multifactorial and the initial assessment will therefore include an assessment of the various contributing factors. Reversible factors such as cardiac failure, infection, and pleural effusion, must be identified and specific therapies started.

In many instances, it will not be possible to reverse all of the underlying causes, and symptomatic measures must then be employed. The purpose of symptomatic treatments is to reduce the subjective sensation of dyspnea, even though these treatments will not affect the underlying pathology. The efficacy of these various interventions can only be measured by the patients own assessment and not by objective measurements such as spirometry.

Opioids can offer useful palliation of dyspnoea. By reducing the sensitivity of the respiratory center and peripheral chemoreceptors to various stimuli, opioids will lead to a reduced rate and depth of ventilation resulting in greatly enhanced patient comfort. Fears of respiratory depression and concern that the use of opioids will somehow hasten death are ill founded. The principles governing the use of opioids in pain apply equally in the management of dyspnea, although the doses employed are typically lower.

The use of benzodiazepines will also benefit patients with dyspnea. This effect is thought to be mediated by the potentiation of gamma-aminobutyric

(GABA) neural inhibition in the brain and spinal cord, thus reducing muscle spindle mismatch. Nondrug therapies include physiotherapy, behavioral therapies, counseling, and simple supportive aids such as a bed-side fan.

Dysphagia

In a study of 124 patients with motor neurone disease, 79% experienced some degree of dysphagia at the time of referral to a palliative care program (9). The management of neurological dysphagia will require input from a range of professional disciplines. Early assessment should be undertaken by a multidisciplinary team.

Video fluoroscopy may be of benefit in defining the level and the extent of the problem. Decisions regarding the use of percutaneous gastrostomy feeding systems must involve the patient, the family, and professional caregivers. If a percutaneous gatrostomy feeding system is started, the patient and family will need a lot of ongoing support and advice.

VI. TOTAL PATIENT CARE

In the high-technology world of hospital medicine, many patients feel that they are somehow reduced to a complex series of biochemical and mechanical processes that they are ill equipped to understand. The very essence of the person, of the human condition, is secondary to or is made to feel secondary to the technologies.

As clinicians, we must ensure that each person is recognized to be a unique individual, encompassing physical, psychological, social, and spiritual dimensions. The care that we offer cannot be fragmented and confined to a single dimension of the individual.

In trying to understand some of the complexities of the human condition, it is helpful to use the model of "total pain" described by Dame Cicely Saunders. In this model, the pain that a patient describes may be seen as the tip of an iceberg. Underlying this pain are a whole range of factors—physical, emotional, social, and spiritual—each contributing to the total pain experience and each inextricably entwined.

It follows, therefore, that if we focus all of our efforts on achieving control of the physical symptoms without regard to these other factors, it is highly unlikely that we will achieve an optimal level of success.

Case history: J.K. was a 37-year-old man who was admitted to the hospice with an established paraplegia associated with metastatic carcinoma of kidney. He had many physical symptoms and required total nursing care. He was a married man with four children, ranging in age from 3 to 11 years. Much of his pain and anguish stemmed from his loss of role as parent, partner, and provider; he found his enforced dependency and reliance on others very difficult to accept. He resented his body and felt humiliated by his condition.

He frequently stated that he had never smoked and never took alcohol in excess. This latter comment was a profound spiritual statement as he struggled in vain to find some meaning or purpose in his life, in his suffering and in his dying. "Why is this happening to me? What did I ever do to deserve this?" As clinicians, we must recognize that there are pains that do not carry opioid receptors and that are beyond the scope of even the most carefully placed anesthetist's needle. There are questions for which we can provide no answers; but we can at least undertake to be with people and to accompany them on their own unique and individual journey.

"There is always more to analgesia than analgesics" (10).

VII. FAMILY IS THE UNIT OF CARE

The impact of serious illness is not confined to the patient but will reverberate throughout the entire family structure. In this context, the family will include both blood relatives and also a number of other significant people. As professional caregivers, we must consider people in the context of their families and not as isolated entities.

Within families, serious illness can rapidly lead to a devastating breakdown in communication. Individuals may feel that they must not show their feelings as this may upset others and there may be a strong statement in the group of the need to protect one another. They will have to cope with a variety of stresses, including uncertainty about the future and taking on new and unfamiliar roles, such as managing the home and domestic chores, conducting business affairs, and dealing with banks and insurance companies. The physical burden of caring is yet another facet of the problem and people often find it difficult to ask for help: "If the positions were reversed, he would do it for me." "I always promised him that I would look after him at home."

Individuals within the family will all be at different stages in their lives and each will have a separate and unique relationship with the ill person. A spouse will be losing a partner; daughters and sons will be losing a parent; parents will be losing a child; brothers and sisters will be losing a sibling; and friends and colleagues will be losing a much loved companion and confidante.

It is vitally important to recognize and address the specific needs of children. They are part of the family and must not be made to feel excluded at a point when they will be feeling particularly confused and vulnerable. Adults will often seek to exclude children in a well-intentioned but misguided attempt to protect them. Thus, children are left isolated, confused, and unprotected from their fears and their fantasies.

Children know when something is wrong within the family structure, but they are ill equipped to understand why. It is precisely because they do not understand what is happening that they will need opportunity to talk about it and to have their questions answered in a factually clear, sensitive, and understandable way. This can sometimes feel like a dangerous thing to do. Children who are facing the death of a parent have the capacity to arouse strong feelings in all of us. Their vulnerability and innocence reminds us of our own vulnerabilities, regardless of how sophisticated we like to believe that we are.

Children have the capacity to ask the most pertinent questions. When meeting recently with a family who were facing the death of their father, Emma, age 8, asked if Dad would be alive on January 26th. When asked why January 26, she said, "It's my birthday. I'd like to have Dad home for my birthday." We explained gently that Dad would not be home for her birthday. After a few moments silence, Billy, age 6, announced that he had a question. "Will my Dad be able to come home on January 7? That's my birthday." Again, we replied in the negative. Dad died in the hospice on Christmas Day with his wife and children present.

In addressing the needs of children, we must take care to reinforce the role of the parents in caring for their children. Professionals should not take over this role, but rather work in a supportive and advisory capacity to the parents. Consideration must also be given to the fact that in addition to the immediate impact of the illness, families may also have to cope with a range of concurrent stresses and anxieties, such as financial and business worries, fears of redundancy and unemployment, and strained relationships and family feuds.

In recognizing the above, it is important that professional caregivers resist the temptation to seek to rectify all of these problems. We must have clearly defined and well-recognized goals and objectives. We can help to support families by at least meeting with them and trying to harness their skills and resources. We can provide a conduit for people to channel their fears and anxieties and thus we try to prevent the angry explosions that will occur if people hold on to painful and agonizing emotional burdens for too long.

VIII. GOOD COMMUNICATION

Good communication is fundamental to good clinical practice. The importance of good communication is increasingly being recognized and specific training on the subject is now an integral part of undergraduate training in most medical schools.

A comprehensive program of care for any patient will inevitably involve a range of disciplines, both medical and nonmedical, and probably in a variety of settings—home, hospital, and hospice.

It is vital for all those involved in providing care to have rapid access to accurate and relevant information. It is extremely frustrating for patients and professionals alike when management decisions have to be deferred because one professional caregiver has not received a communication from another. This sense of frustration and anger at the apparent fragmentation of care often prompts patients to seek redress in the courts. In addition to providing information regarding the presentation, investigation, and management of each patient, we must also take care to document exactly what information has been given to the patient and family regarding the disease process and its likely progression. Again, it is extremely frustrating and confusing for patients when they receive conflicting signals and messages from different care providers.

One aspect of communication that falls to the doctor is the communication of bad news. Sadly, this important task is often delegated to a relatively junior and inexperienced colleague who is ill equipped to perform the task and is often unable to deal with the issues that will inevitably arise. Buckman and Maguire have described five stages in breaking bad news (11).

A. Planning the Meeting

A diagnosis of serious illness brings particular pressures to bear on patients and their families. The manner in which bad news is given, and the extent to which patients and families feel supported with this news, will have a major influence on their capacity to cope. It is important to recognize that breaking bad news is not a one-shot affair, and patients will need a number of opportunities to seek clarification, explanation, and reassurance. Forward planning is essential; who should be there, where should the meeting take place, when should the meeting be held, and how should we proceed. In general, it is desirable to see people together and in a private and comfortable location. The practice of breaking bad news to a patient who is alone in the middle of an open ward or in a busy hospital corridor is to be deplored.

B. Assessing the Situation

Before giving the information, take the time to establish just what exactly the patient understands about his or her condition. As doctors, we sometimes assume that patients will know only what we have told them. This is invariably wrong. Patients pick up cues from a variety of sources and in a range of different ways. Much of what is communicated is done so by nonverbal means. Questions such as, "You have been unwell for some time now. What do you make of it all?" or, "What do you think is causing all of these problems?" will be of enormous value in making this assessment.

Having established what the patient knows, the next step is to establish what exactly the patient wishes to know. Remember that the agenda belongs to the patient and family and not to the professionals. We can help by trying to establish key concerns, such as what is most worrisome right now. Does the patient have particular concerns about the future for self or family? The patient may well want some more information regarding condition and prognosis but may not wish to have all the facts confirmed at this meeting. In this regard, the importance of sensitivity and pacing cannot be over emphasized. This process will require the doctor to be capable of picking up nonverbal factors and to really listen to and recognize the signals that the patient is sending.

C. Giving the Information

No doctor will enjoy giving bad news. We may seek to minimize the personal impact on ourselves in a number of ways. We may be less than honest with the patient, we may choose to use technical and ambiguous language, or we may talk too quickly, thereby not allowing the patient the opportunity to express his or her feelings. Remember that pacing is vitally important. Be sensitive to the patient's need to have time to absorb the reality of this new situation. Patients may not hear much of what you say at this first meeting. Breaking bad news is a gradual process during which patients slowly come to a fuller understanding of their position.

D. Handling the Reactions

Breaking bad news is never easy and often feels particularly risky. We sometimes feel a sense of helplessness and we fear that the patient and family may blame us for perceived delays in diagnosis. We may wish to avoid a prolonged tearful and angry outburst, and may feel anxious about our ability to cope with these reactions.

Personal fears of illness and discomfort regarding our own mortality will serve to compound the problem. All of these factors may cause the doctor to behave in a way that is perceived as being unhelpful, dismissive, uncaring, or defensive. There is no format of words that we can use to make patients feel good about hearing that their life span is short or that they will now be confined to a wheelchair. Regardless of how skillfully and sensitively one breaks bad news, the net effect is to radically alter that person's reality.

If patients choose to cry out in anger and despair or if they become sullen and withdrawn on hearing bad news, that is their own way of dealing with the news they have just received. The patient's reactions are not the fault of the doctor and we should not blame ourselves for these reactions.

Among the common reactions that one will see are shock, numbness, sadness, anxiety, fear, and anger. Patients may enter a phase of complete denial: "It can't be true, they must have got my tests mixed up" or they may bargain, "Well, I know that it's serious, but I don't mind once I'll be well enough to see my daughter get married in 2 years." Patients use denial and bargaining when the truth is simply too painful to bear. We need to tread gently in these instances and take care not to destroy all of their defenses. It is always possible to communicate a gentle truth and we can at least undertake to be with patients and to offer them ongoing support.

E. Ending

When ending the meeting, it is useful to summarize what has been said to ensure that the messages are clear and unambiguous. Typically, a first meeting will raise more questions than provide answers. Patients and families need time to reflect on their situation and to consider privately the implications of their new reality. Make a firm commitment to meet again to provide an opportunity for these other issues and questions to surface. A summary of the meeting should be recorded as an integral part of the patient's case notes.

IX. INTERDISCIPLINARY TEAMWORK

No one individual person or discipline will possess the range of skills necessary to provide a comprehensive program of care for patients and their families. We therefore rely on the timely and appropriate intervention of an array of professional disciplines. It is vital that all concerned are both competent and confident in their own professional skills. Each should have a healthy appreciation of personal limitations, combined with an appreciation of the unique contribution of other disciplines and a willingness to involve them appropriately.

X. TERMINAL CARE

When it is evident that death is fast approaching, it is essential that medical and nursing staff reorientate themselves to the new reality. Prescribing priorities must change and all but essential medication should be withdrawn. The precise benefit of all interventions, e.g., intravenous fluids/therapies, must be reevaluated in the light of the changed circumstances. The objective at this stage is to ensure that the patient can die peacefully and with dignity.

Patients must continue to receive adequate analgesic medication. At the point when they are no longer able to tolerate oral medication, administration is most conveniently achieved by using a portable syringe pump. The medication required over a 24-hour period can thus be infused subcutaneously without the need for frequent injections. Other medications, including hyoscine hydrobromide, and midazolam, can also be administered in this way. Family members should be encouraged to participate in the care of their loved one and must not be made to feel excluded by our apparent professionalism. It is important to explain to the family precisely what is happening and to give them the opportunity to ask questions and to seek explanation and reassurance. Remember, many people have never witnessed a death and will appreciate information on what to expect.

Individual family members may have something important to say to the patient and it is always wise to facilitate this even if the patient is barely responsive. At the time of death, families will experience profound shock and sadness, however much the death has been expected. They need time to absorb what has happened and staff must be careful not to intrude. Families need space and privacy at this stage and may wish to be left alone with the body. A little later, it may be appropriate to help to contain the shock and panic by uniting the group in a common activity, such as saying some prayers or even serving tea or coffee. Family members may wish to help wash and dress the body, and again this should be facilitated. Nursing staff should take care to inform other patients on the ward that a patient has died and the primary care physician will certainly welcome telephone notification of the death.

Ideally, families should be seen together at some convenient time after the death. This is an opportunity to say goodbye and to encourage acceptance of the reality of the death. We can alert them to the fact that they are likely to experience a complex array of powerful and sometimes conflicting emotions in the period ahead. They will have a multitude of "if onlys" and will need reassurance that they did all that could be reasonably expected of any family.

The process of grieving is generally not well understood and certainly takes considerably longer than many people seem to realize. However, "grief is a normal and inevitable human journey, not an illness. Most people will successfully accomplish the task of grief with the help of their family, friends, and local community" (12).

Staff members who were involved in caring for the patient and the family must be sensitive and attentive to their own needs. It is useful and constructive for multidisciplinary teams to formally review their performance and to audit and monitor consistency in the quality of the service that they provide.

XI. MOTOR NEURON DISEASE/AMYOTROPHIC LATERAL SCLEROSIS

Motor neuron disease/amytrophic lateral sclerosis (MND/ALS) is the neurological disorder that has attracted most attention from hospice and palliative care services over the years. It is a condition ideally suited to palliative care because it is a progressive and potentially fatal disorder of unknown etiology associated with a multiplicity of symptoms. The problems and difficulties facing a family caring for a patient with MND/ALS are profound, and a comprehensive management program will require input from a range of professional disciplines, both hospital and community based. The importance of clear, accurate, and unambiguous communication at each stage of the disease is paramount.

MND/ALS is virtually unique among incurable diseases in it's capacity to evoke a sense of therapeutic impotence and despondency in physicians. This excessively negative and despairing attitude is reflected in many standard textbooks of medicine. Sadly, in descriptions of MND/ALS in such textbooks, the reader will find little information on the practical and symptomatic management of the disease.

In a review of 124 patients with MND/ALS who were referred for palliative care, the control of symptoms was stated as a reason for referral in only 15% of cases. Yet these patients had a variety of symptoms as summarized in Table 1. Although MND/ALS is a relatively rare disorder, many of the symptoms and problems associated with the disease are extraordinarily common. Symptoms such as constipation, pain, cough, dyspnea, and insomnia respond to the application of standard treatment regimens, which do not require any detailed knowledge of MND/ALS per se, and which should fall easily within the realm of all hospital- and community-based doctors.

Bulbar problems are more difficult to manage and will require input from a multidisciplinary team. The role of nutritional support in the form of perecutaneous gastrostomy feeding or ventilatory support will require skilled specialist assessment and follow-up. A detailed account of the management of bulbar symptoms in MND/ALS may be found in Hillel and Miller (15).

One of the fears shared by many patients with MND/ALS is the mode and

Table 1 Symptoms of Patients with MND/ALS on Admission to Hospice Care

Symptom	n = 124
Constipation	81 (65)
Pain	71 (57)
Cough	66 (53)
Insomnia	59 (48)
Dyspnea	58 (47)
Dribbling saliva	47 (38)

Source: Ref. 11.
Figures are numbers (percentages).

manner of death, and in particular the fear of choking. Data from O'Brien's study indicate that of 113 patients who died in the hospice, 58% deteriorated rapidly and died within 24 hours of this deterioration. This rapid deterioration was attributed to a sudden decompensation in respiratory function resulting in acute or acute on chronic respiratory failure. No patient choked to death. The airways were entirely free of foreign matter in each of the 19 patients who had a postmortem examination performed.

The term *choking* is highly emotively charged and is both inaccurate and inappropriate in describing the cause of death in MND/ALS. It's use must be abandoned. The distress associated with a sudden collapse in respiratory function is relieved by an injection of a low dose of opioid in combination with hyoscine hydrobromide. Rectal diazepam may be administered with good effect in the home setting by family caregivers while awaiting the arrival of a physician or nurse.

XII. CONCLUSION

Inspired by the pioneering work of Dame Cicely Saunders at St. Christopher's Hospice, London, and earlier at St. Joseph's Hospice, London, palliative medicine has evolved as a specialist area of care. In the foreword to her biography, Bishop John Taylor describes Dame Cicely as the person who has tackled and overcome one of the greatest unspoken fears that haunts human beings today, the fear of a painful and humiliating death from an incurable disease.

It was while working as a medical social worker that Dame Cicely met David Tasma, a young Polish man who was dying in a London hospital from an inoperable cancer. David was acutely aware of the need to improve the care being offered to patients who were dying. He summarized precisely what he required from his professional carers in the immortal phrase: "I only want what is in your mind and in your heart."

The challenge facing all of us involved in palliative care, and this includes all health care professionals regardless of their training or specialty interest, is to offer all that is in our minds and in our hearts. That we should appropriately apply all of the technical skills at our disposal to alleviate suffering and to relieve distress is essential, but it is not enough. Equally, we must concern ourselves with the psychological, social, and spiritual well-being of all those patients and families who come under our care.

This statement, that patients only want what is in your mind and in your heart, encapsulates the very essence of hospice and palliative care—the union of scientific medicine with a compassionate and dedicated concern for the individual and family.

REFERENCES

1. Kearney M. Palliative care in Ireland. Irish Coll Phys Surg 1991; 20(3):170.
2. IASP. Pain. J Int Assoc Study of Pain. Supplement 3, 1986; S 217.
3. Melzack R., Wall P. The Challenge of Pain. London: Pelican Books, 1988; 45.
4. Twycross RG, Lack SA. Pain—a broader concept. In: Symptom Control in Far Advanced Disease—Pain Relief. London: Pitman, 1983.
5. Portenoy RK. Chronic opioid therapy in non-malignant pain. Pain Sympt Management 1990; 5:S46–62.
6. Melzack R. The tragedy of needless pain. Sci Am 1990; 162:19–25.
7. Galer BS, et al. Individual variability in the response to different opioids: report of five cases. Pain 1992; 49:87–91.
8. deStoutz et al. Opioid rotation for toxicity reduction in terminal cancer patients. J Pain Sympt Management. 1995; 10(5):378–384.
9. Sutherland S. Nerve and nerve injuries. Edinburgh: Churchill Livingstone, 1978; 399–400.
10. Glynn C. An approach to the management of the patient with deafferentation pain. Pall Med 1989; 1:13–21.
11. O'Brien T, Kelly M, Saunders CM. Motor neurone disease: a hospice perspective. Br Med J 1992; 304:471–473.
12. Twycross RG. Cancer Pain—A Global Perspective. In: The Edinburgh Symposium on Pain Control and Medical Education, 1989, 6.
13. Buckman R, Maguire P. Why won't they talk to me? Video Series Sponsored by Norwich Eaton, Newcastle upon Tyne, England.
14. O'Brien T, Monroe B. Twenty four hours before and after death. In: Saunders CM (ed.), Hospice and Palliative Care—An Interdisciplinary Approach. London: Edward Arnold, 1990, 53.
15. Hillel AD, Miller RM. Management of bulbar symptoms in amyotrophic lateral sclerosis. Adv Exp Biol 1987; 209:255–263.

Index

Abscess, spinal, 223
Acquired immune deficiency syndrome,
    221, 259, 270
  demyelinating neuropathy, 262
  tumors, 267
  vacuolar myelopathy, 267–268, 404
Acute demyelinating polyradiculopathy,
    242
Acute disseminated encephalomyelitis,
    403
Acute hemorrhagic viral conjunctivitis,
    215
Acute inflammatory demyelinating poly-
    neuropathy neurophysiology, 571
Acute inflammatory polyradiculopathies,
    235
Acute intermittent porphyria, 235
Acute motor axonal neuropathy, 242
Acute motor and sensory axonal neurop-
    athy, 242
Acute necrotizing myelitis, 221
Acute sensory neuropathy, 253
Acute pandysautonomia, 254

Alar ligament, 137
Allodynia, 616
Alternative opioids, 652–653
Amyotonia congenita, 176, 189
Amyotrophic lateral sclerosis (ALS),
    413–442
  neurophysiology, 570
  terminal care, 661–663
Aneurysmal bone cyst, 293
Ankylosing spondylitis, 444–453
  clinical features, 446
  differential diagnosis, 444, 451
  epidemiology, 445
  extraskeletal features, 448
  HLA typing, 450
  management, 451
Anterior cord syndrome, 125
Apgar, 181
Arachnoid cysts, 303
Arachnoiditis, 212
Arterial supply of cord, 463–464
Arteriovenous malformations, 404, 467–
    468

Arthropathy, neuropathic, 170 (*see also* Charcot joints)
Astrocytoma, 315
Ataxia telangiectasia, 115
Atrophy, spinal muscular, 176
Autonomic dysreflexia(e), 9, 157, 586
  radiology, 554–556

Bacterial infections, 223–237
Bad news, communication of, 657–660
Batson's plexus, 339
Benign intracranial hypertension, 244
Beta-interferon, 408
Birth injuries of cord, 175–197
  diagnosis, 181–190
  pathophysiology, 176–181
  treatment, 190–191
Bladder
  clinical effects of spinal injury, 584–586
  management of problems, 589–595
  neurological control, 579–581
  physiological changes after spinal cord injury, 561–584
  surgery, 594–595
  voiding, 581
Bone cyst, 293
Botulism, 235, 244
Brachial plexus, 180
Brain-derived neurotrophic factor, in MND, 435
Breech, 177, 179
Brown-Séquard syndrome, 12, 131, 159, 290, 499
Brucellosis, spinal, 454
Bubbles, in decompression illness, 475–477
Bulbar involvement in MND, 417
Bulbar palsy, 108–112
Bulbar symptoms, management of in MND, 662
Bulbocavernous reflex, 125
Bunina bodies, in MND, 416

Campylobacter infection and GBS, 243, 248

Capsaicin, 593
Carcinoma, renal, 386
Caudal regression syndrome, 56
Cavitron, 306, 321
Central cord syndrome, 125, 148
Cerebral palsy, 176
Cerebrospinal fluid, 3–4
  in GBS, 244
  in MS, 405
  in syphilis, 233
  in TB, 230
Cervical disc disease, radiology, 548
Cervical laminectomy, 506–510
Cervical myelopathy
  MRI features, 501–504
  natural history, 500–501
  neurophysiology, 504–505
  pathophysiology, 496–498
  surgical treatment, 506–510
  symptoms, 498–500
Cervical spine
  anatomy, 495–496
  cervical spondylosis, 495–515
Cervical spine injury
  C1-C2 vertebrae, 136–140
  epidemiology, 121
  low cervical vertebral, 140–148
  management, 134
  pathophysiology, 122
  occiput-C1, 135
Cervical subluxation, rheumatoid, 456
Cesarean section, 193
Charcot joints, 170, 200
Chemotherapy, 309
Chiari malformations
  classification, 67–72
  clinical presentation, 83–85
  diagnosis, 87
  epidemiology, 72
  etiology, 73–80
  treatment, 89
  pathology, 80–83
Chinese paralytic syndrome, 246
Chordoma, 295
Chronic inflammatory demyelinating polyradiculopathy, 236, 251–252

Chronic neuropathic pain, 617–618
Ciliary neurotrophic factor, in MND, 434–435
Clinical neurophysiology of
  acute inflammatory demyelinating polyneuropathy, 571
  amyotrophic lateral sclerosis, 570
  multifocal motor neuropathy, 570
  multiple sclerosis, 572
  polio and postpolio, 570
  radicular disease, 568–569
  root disease, 569–570
  spinal muscular atrophy, 572
  syrinx, 571–572
Cloward's procedure, 507–508
Cockayne's syndrome, 116
Communication of bad news, 657–660
Computed tomography, 537
Contraception, 637–638
Conus Medullaris syndrome, 160
Cord syndromes, 159
Corpectomy, 368
Costotransversectomy, 307
Cotrel-Dubousset instrumentation, 168
Crutchfield tongs, 134
Cu/Zn SOD gene mutations, in MND, 413, 436
Cyst(s)
  arachnoid, 303
  epidermoid and dermoid, 282
  neurenteric, 302
Cystic degeneration, 199
Cystometrogram, 189
Cytomegalovirus, in AIDS, 264

Deafferentation pain, 617
Decompression illness, 471–494
  classification, 472
  neurological pathogenesis, 474
  treatment, 476–480
Deformity, postoperative, 329
Degenerative disc disease, radiology, 544–548
Dementia, in MND, 420–421
Dermoid, 301
Dermoid cyst, 53

Desmopressin, 593
Detrusor hyperreflexia, treatment of, 591
Detrusor sphincter dyssynergia, 584
Devic's disease, 404
Diastematomyelia, 45–48
Diastrophic dwarfism, 190
Diethylcarbimazine myelitis, 237
Diffuse idiopathic skeletal hyperostosis, 459
Diplegia, 101
Discography, 540
  bilateral facet, 146
  unilateral facet, 146
Diving, long-term neurological consequences, 481–485
Divorce after spinal injury, 640–641
Dominantly inherited ataxias, 116
DREZ lesions for pain, 621
Dural hemorrhage, 177
Dural laceration, 177
Dura mater, 3
Dysarthria, 112
Dysphagia, 112, 655
Dyspnea, 654

Ejaculation, 635
Electromyography, 562–563
Embryology of the cord, 16–25
  theories of development, 27–28
Endarteritis, spinal, 233
Endoscopy, 207
Enteroviral infections, 214
Ependymomas, 315, 322
Epidermoid, 300
Evaluation of pain, 649–650
Evoked potentials, 125
  motor, 567
  somatosensory, 565–567 (see also Somatosensory evoked potentials)
Ewings sarcoma, 352
Experimental allergic neuritis, 247

Familial MND, 423
Family unit, in terminal care, 656–657

Fertility, 637
Filum terminale, thickened, 48
Forrestier's disease, 459
Fracture
  burst, 163
  compression, 162
  hangman's, 138
  Jefferson, 136
  thoracolumbar, 162–164
Friedrich's ataxia, 115
Fungal disease of the cord, 237

Gadolinium, 319
Ganglioneuroma, 296
Gangliosides, 167
Gardner-Wells tongs, 134
Glascow Coma Score, 124
Glioma, 315
Guam Disease 421
Guillain-Barré syndrome, 214, 227,
    241–251
  diagnostic criteria, 243
  neurophysiology, 571
  treatment, 248–250

Halo ring, 134
Halo-vest, 134
Hartnup disease, 114
Hemangioma, 293
Hematomyelia, 134, 186
Hemorrhage
  epidural, 177
  subarachnoid, 177
Hereditary motor and sensory neuropa-
    thy, 106
Hereditary motor neuropathy, neuro-
    physiology, 572
Hereditary spastic paraparesis (paraple-
    gia), 104, 404
Herniation, disc, 148
Herpes zoster radiculopathy, 222
Hexosaminadase deficiency, 426
HTLV-1 associated myelopathy, 219,
    404
Hyaline membrane, 181

Hydrocephalus, 65, 330
Hyperammonemia, 114
Hypokalemia, 135
Hypotonia, 176

Infarction, 182
Infections, 211
  bacterial types, 212
  viral, 212–223
  viral types, 212
Infectious spondylitis, 454
Injuries
  birth, 175–194
  brain, 181
Insulin-like growth factor, in MND, 435
Intermittent catheterization (of urinary
    bladder), 590–591
Intracavernosal injection, 633
Intramedullary tumors, 315–334
  incidence, 316
  management, 320
  presentation, 316
Intrauterine, 181

Juvenile-onset MND, 424

Kennedy's syndrome, 419, 423–424
Konzo, 424

Laminectomy, 191
Larsen's syndrome, 190
Laser evoked potentials, 568
Leptomeninges, 3
Lesions, meningeal, 177
L'Hermitte's phenomenon, 103
Libido, 638
Lipid peroxidation, 123
Lipomas, 281–282
Lipomyelomeningocele, 49–52
Lumbosacral disease, radiology, 544–
    548
Lyme disease, 234–235, 252–253

Magnetic resonance imaging, 539
Management of bladder problems, 589

Mannitol, 135
Marriage after spinal injury, 640–641
Meningiomas, 280, 299
　radiology, 551
Meningocele, 25
　anterior sacral, 57–59
Meningotheliomatous, 299
Metastases to spine
　diagnosis, 343
　neurological classification, 346
　stages, 341
　treatment, 362–386
Metabolic disorders with ataxia, 114–115
Metastatic bone disease of the spine, 462
Methylmethacrylate, 368
Methylprednisolone, 123, 135, 166
Miller Fisher syndrome, 252
Monitoring, 308 (see also Somatosensory evoked potentials and Motor evoked potentials)
Morphine, 651–652
　side effects, 652
Morquios disease, 190
Motor evoked potentials (MEPs), 306, 327, 567
　in cervical myelopathy, 505
Motor neuron disease, 413–442
　clinical features, 417–419
　dementia, 420–421
　El Escorial criteria, 415, 428
　familial, 423
　investigations, 428–430
　lymphoma and, 425
　pathogenesis, 427
　pathology, 4157
　terminal care, 661–663
　treatment, 431–436
Motor neuropathy, 419
Multifocal motor neuropathy, 422–423
Multiple sclerosis, 399–412
　clinical features in cord, 401–403
　differential diagnosis, 404
　management, 406

[Multiple sclerosis]
　neurophysiology, 572
　pathophysiology, 399–401
Muscle cramps, in MND, 417
Myelography, 534–537
　complications, 537
Myelomalacia, 184, 186
Myelomeningiocele, 25
Myelopathy, 212
　ischemic, 464–465
Myeloschisis, 25
Myelotomy, 207, 323

N-Acetylcysteine, in MND, 435
Naloxone, 135, 167
Nerve conduction studies, 560–561
Neurenteric cyst, 52–53, 302–303
Neurofibroma, 297
Neurogenic pain, 614–615, 616
Neurogenic shock, 124, 157
Neurolathyrism, 425
Neuromatrix model for pain, 622
Neuronophagia, 122
Neuropathic pain, 612–614, 617–618, 653–654
Neurophysiology of closed spinal malformations, 44
Neurostimulation for pain, 620
Neurosyphilis, 232–234

Obstetrical, 178
Occipitocervical fusion, 136
Omental transposition, 602–607
　results, 604–607
　technique, 603–604
Opioid sensitive pain, 650–652
Oppenheim's disease, 176, 189
Ossification of the posterior longitudinal ligament, 519
　presentation and management, 526
　prognosis, 528
　subtypes, 522
Osteoblastoma, 288, 292
Osteoid osteoma, 288, 292
Osteomalacia, 462

Osteoporosis, 460–461
Onuf, Nucleus of, 13
  in MND, 418

Paget's disease, 461–462
Pain, 12, 611–625
  with benign spinal tumor, 289
  control in palliative care, 648–654
  evaluation, 649
  incidence in spinal disease, 611–613
  with metastatic spinal disease, 344
  neuromatrix model, 622
  pathophysiology, 616–618
  treatment, 618–623
Palliative care, 645–664
  definition, 646
  principals, 647
Palsy
  Erb's, 177
  Klumpke's, 177
Paraplegia, 101
  hereditary spastic, 104
Parasitic disease of the cord, 237
Parkinson's disease, 13
Penile erection, 631–632
  enhancement of, 632–634
  implants, 633
  intracavernosal injection, 633
Penile sensation, 631
Plexopathy, 182
Poliomyelitis, 213–215
  neurophysiology, 570
Porphyria, intermittent, 214, 235, 244
Posterior longitudinal ligament, 517–
  518
Postherpetic neuralgia, pain in, 615
Postinfectious/postvaccinial myelitis,
  223
Postpolio syndrome, 214
Pott's paraplegia, 227
Pregnancy, 637
Priapism, 182
Primary lateral sclerosis, 420
Progressive multifocal leukoencepha-
  lopathy, in AIDS, 264
Progressive muscular atrophy, 414

Pseudobulbar palsy, 108
Pseudosubluxation, 176

Rabies, 215
Radiculitis, syphilitic, 233
Radiculopathy, 212
Radiography of
  cervical disc disease, 548
  degenerative lumbosacral disease,
    544–548
  extradural pyogenic infection, 551
  spinal cord compression, 549–554
  trauma, 540–544
  vascular malformations, 554
Radiotherapy, 309
Reiter's disease, 453
Renal carcinoma, metastases to spine,
  386
Renal disease after spinal cord injury,
  588
Respiratory failure in MND, 432
Rheumatoid disease of spine, 455–457
Riluzole, in MND, 433
Root avulsion, pain in, 615

Sacral root stimulation, 634
Sacral sparing, 159
Sacrococcygeal teratoma, 56
Sarcoidosis, 231–232
Schistosomiasis, 237
Schwannoma, 297
Scintigraphy, 540
Scoliosis, 288
Secondary hyperalgesia, 616
Sexual intercourse, 634
Sexuality after spinal cord injury, 638–
  640
Sexual problems, 629–643
Shunt
  syringoperitoneal, 205
  syringopleural, 205
  syringosubarachnoid, 205
  syrinx-cisternal, 207
Somatosensory evoked potentials
  (SSEP), 125, 158, 186, 306, 326,
  565–567

Spasticity, 169
  in MND, 432
  prevention and treatment, 107–108
Spastic paraplegia, 101, 498
  acquired, 102
  inherited, 104
  symptoms and signs, 103
Spinal angiography, 539
Spinal arteries, 463–464
Spinal cord
  anatomy, 6
  physiology, 6–11
Spinal cord compression, radiology,
  549–554
Spinal cord injury, 9
  bladder control, 10, 581–586
  blood pressure, 10
  epidemiology, 156
  marriage and divorce after, 640–641
  pathophysiology, 165, 600
  management, 166–169
  radiography, 540–544
  rehabilitation, 169–170
  sexual problems after, 628–643
  visceral effects, 10–11
Spinal cord malformations, open, 28–40
  clinical features, 29–33
  epidemiology, 28
  long-term outcome, 37–40
  management, 34–37
  prenatal diagnosis, 29
Spinal cord malformations, closed, 40–
  58
  clinical features, 40–43
  management, 44–45
Spinal cord monitoring, 572–574
Spinal ischemia, 465
Spinal muscular atrophy, 418, 425–427
  neurophysiology, 572
Spinal shock, 58, 125
Spinal stenosis, 459
Spine
  cervical, 121–148
  thoracolumbar, 155–170
Spinocerebellar degeneration, 112
Spondylolisthesis, 458

Spondylolysis, 458
Spondylopathies, 444–453
Spondylosis, 457
Spondyloepiphyseal dysplasia, 190
Stenosis, of spine, 459
Syphilis, 232–234
  in AIDS, 267
Syrinx, neurophysiology, 571–572
Systemic lupus erythematosus, 467
Steele-Richardson-Olzewski syndrome,
  13
Strumpell-Lorrain syndrome, 104
Subarachnoid space, 3
Syringomyelia, 170
  clinical presentation, 85–87
  diagnosis, 88
  etiology, 76–80
  pathology, 82–83
  posttraumatic,199–208
  treatment, 91
Syringostomy, 204, 205
Syrinx, 184
  late consequence of spinal cord in-
  jury, 170, 199–209

Tay-Sachs disease 426
TENS, 620
Teratoma, 301
Terminal care, 660–661
  definition, 646
Total patient care, 655
Toxoplasmosis, in AIDS, 262
Transverse myelitis, 104, 403
Tricyclic antidepressants, in pain, 653
Tropical spastic paraparesis, 219
Tuberculoma of the cord, 229
Tuberculosis, spinal, 225–231, 454
  in AIDS, 266
  radiology, 551
Tumors, 275–286
  benign, 287–309
  classification, 277
  clinical effects, 283–284
  intradural-extramedullary, 296–303
  intramedullary, 283
  malignant, 330

[Tumors]
  metastatic, 282–283, 335–391
    biology, 338
    biopsy, 359
    in children, 387
    classification, 346
    complications, 388–390
    diagnosis, 343
    prevalence, 336
    surgery, 365–385
      anterior, 370
      cervical, 378–385
      posterior, 375–378
    treatment, 362–365
  primary intramedullary, 315–332
    surgical complications, 328
    surgery, 320

Ultrasonography, 185
Urodynamics, 589

Vertebral column, 1
Vitamin E deficiency, 116
von Recklinghausen's neurofibromatosis, 280–281

Wernig-Hoffman disease, 176,189,
  426
Winking owl, 291
Wohlfart-Kugelberg-Welander disease,
  426

Xanthochromia,189
Xeroderma pigmentosa, 116

About the Editors

GORDON L. ENGLER is Professor of Clinical Orthopaedics and Neurological Surgery and the Director of Scoliosis and Spinal Surgery at Los Angeles County Hospital/University of Southern California Medical Center, Los Angeles, California. The author of over 35 articles, Dr. Engler is a past President of the Scoliosis Research Society. He received the B.S. degree (1958) from the University of Michigan, Ann Arbor, and the M.D. degree (1963) from the Chicago Medical School, Illinois.

JONATHAN COLE is Honorary Senior Lecturer in Clinical Neurological Sciences at the University of Southampton and Southampton University Hospital, England. Additionally, he is a Consultant in Clinical Neurophysiology at Poole Hospital, England, and Salisbury Hospital, England. He is the author or coauthor of numerous articles as well as two books. Dr. Cole is a Fellow of the Royal College of Physicians and a member of The Physiological Society. He received the B.A. (1974), M.Sc. (1977), and D.M. (1984) degrees from Oxford University, England, and the M.B./B.S. degree (1978) from the Middlesex Hospital, London, England.

W. LOUIS MERTON is Consultant in Clinical Neurophysiology at St. Mary's Hospital and Director of Clinical Support Services, Portsmouth Hospitals NHS Trust, Portsmouth, England. Dr. Merton is a Fellow of the Royal College of

Physicians and the Royal Society of Medicine, and a member of the British Society for Clinical Neurophysiology and the Association of British Clinical Neurophysiologists. He received the B.Sc. degree (1977) with Honors in physiology and the M.B./B.S. degree (1982) in medicine from University College, London, England.